HANDLING BIRTH TRAUMA CASES

HANDLING BIRTH TRAUMA CASES

VOLUME 1

STANLEY S. SCHWARTZ

**Member of the Bar
of the State of Michigan**

NORMAN D. TUCKER

**Member of the Bar
of the State of Michigan**

WILEY

Wiley Law Publications

JOHN WILEY & SONS

New York · Chichester · Brisbane · Toronto · Singapore

Library of Congress Cataloging in Publication Data

Handling Birth Trauma Cases
Schwartz, Stanley S.
  (Wiley law publications)
  Includes index.
  1. Obstetricians—Malpractice—United States.
2. Tort Liability of hospitals—United States.
3. Childbirth—United States.   I. Tucker, Norman D.
II. Title.   III. Series.
KF2910.G943S39   1985   346.7303'32   85-12076
ISBN 0-471-83024-0 (V.1)   347.306332
ISBN 0-471-50846-2 (Set)

Printed in the United States of America

10 9 8 7 6 5 4

ACKNOWLEDGMENTS

We wish to express our gratitude and appreciation to Richard Toth and Wendy I. Fields for their helpful suggestions and research.

Southfield, Michigan   STANLEY S. SCHWARTZ
June, 1985   NORMAN D. TUCKER

SUMMARY CONTENTS

DETAILED CONTENTS

PART I

LEGAL PRINCIPLES APPLICABLE TO BIRTH TRAUMA CLAIMS

CHAPTER 1

INTRODUCTION

§ 1.1 Birth Trauma and Medical Malpractice

Birth trauma claims arise in the context of the medical care and treatment preceding, during, and immediately following the delivery of a child. In the cases which will be examined throughout this work, we will look at the potential liability of doctors, residents and interns, nurses, and hospitals for negligent acts contributing to the birth of a physically or mentally defective infant. Such liability is usually brought to the attention of our judicial system through the institution and litigation of a claim for medical malpractice.

Medical malpractice is a subspeciality of tort law which often intimidates novice attorneys by its nuances and subtleties. We shall make no attempt here to cover the subject in all of its depth—there are many fine works already extant which perform this task quite admirably—but we will present a general overview of the basic principles of medical malpractice law in order to assist attorneys contemplating a potential birth trauma claim in identifying the more significant legal issues which such a venture entails. Generally, this book serves as a forewarning of the many traps and snares placed along the path of medical malpractice litigation which the wary attorney must be prepared to recognize and sidestep in pursuing her client's claim. The advocate of an injured child bears a heavy responsibility to her client, one which should encourage the attorney to use utmost diligence throughout the course of litigation. The attorney cannot afford to compromise either issues of fact or of law.

Medical malpractice law is among the most customized in terms of jurisdictional eccentricities. Consequently, any broad statements regarding malpractice law must be read with a caveat allowing for deviations among the several states. For example, it may be stated broadly that the distinguishing feature of a medical malpractice case is that the liability of a defendant is governed by the standard of care; however, this standard itself may mean one thing in Michigan yet quite something else again in Indiana. In reviewing the law of medical malpractice, as discussed in this book, each reader must make allowance for the special rules which may be applicable in her own jurisdiction. Also, since the law is never static, no statement made here should be taken as forever fixed in stone. Each new birth is an introduction to new life; each new birth trauma case lays a foundation of new precedent.

§ 1.2   Overview of the Book

This book is divided into three parts. In the first eight chapters, we present a general overview of the substantive law of medical malpractice. These chapters are designed to acquaint the reader with some of the peculiarities and unique problems associated with malpractice law. Where possible, we have tried to tie these malpractice principles directly to birth trauma litigation, but in aiming to be comprehensive, the scope of these chapters is not focused solely on birth trauma cases, and may be helpful to attorneys comtemplating any type of medical malpractice claim.

The second part of this work shifts to the medical aspects of birth trauma litigation, examining in some detail the processes of birth and the art and skill required of physicians, nurses, and hospitals in assisting in that process. The purpose of these chapters is to establish the criteria expected of medical professionals and to identify the problems which arise when appropriate professional standards are not followed. The final chapters of this book offer a review of some of the pragmatic issues involved in actually litigating a birth trauma case. Here we present examples of litigation techniques which counsel may follow in pursuing a birth trauma claim.

In preparing this book, our goal was to provide a practical guide to the practicing lawyer, one offering assistance in handling these unique, often dramatic, and occasionally heart-rending birth trauma claims. We hope that those who turn to this book in pursuing a birth trauma claim will find it both informative and helpful.

CHAPTER 2

IDENTIFYING THE DEFENDANTS

INTRODUCTION

§ 2.1 The Complexity of Modern Medical Practice

Today, the practice of medicine is not confined to the family physician or the town doctor. With increased medical knowledge has come increased specialization. With improved medical technology has come the multifaceted medical institution. Only by specializing can a physician become fully conversant with all the advances and new techniques of a particular subject. Only by sophisticated methods of capitalization and organization can a hospital keep pace with the rapid developments and costs of modern medical equipment. Paralleling these trends is the increasingly complex legal forms and relationships under which the medical care of patients is undertaken.

The modern hospital, where the vast majority of babies now are born, provides a setting in which numerous actors function and interact with one another in a bewildering matrix of legal relationships. Within the few days stay that accompanies a normal birth, a mother may, quite unknowingly, encounter half dozen distinct and separate legal entities at the hospital. She may, for example, have her own obstetrician visit her. This specialist, she might be surprised to learn, is an *independent staff physician*, a confusing phrase that fails to honestly convey its actual meaning. Normally, the word staff connotes someone who is an employee of a corporation, such as a staff of design engineers working for an auto company. Here, however, the emphasis must be on the word independent, for one who is an independent staff physician is, in essence, an independent contractor. Being on staff merely means that the doctor has staff privileges at the hospital: the right, that is, to utilize the hospital facilities and its auxiliary personnel for the treatment of one's own private patients. Of course, those staff privileges may carry with them some active obligation towards the hospital itself. Often, teaching hospitals will require, as a condition for the granting of staff privileges, that the private physician spend some part of the year giving instruction to the hospital's residents, interns, or other employees. Governmental or charitable hospitals might demand that the doctor spend a portion of his time attending to clinic patients having no regular private physician of their own. Thus, a doctor may find himself slipping in and out of various roles even as he walks down the hospital corridor— here for his own patient as an independent contractor, there for the clinic patient in the next room as an ostensible agent of the hospital, and next for the instruction of the residents, reviewing their treatment of a third patient, as an actual agent of the hospital.

Our hypothetical independent staff doctor, on the advice of his attorney, may also have incorporated himself as a professional corporation (P.C.). Or

he, like many other physicians are now doing, may have become but one partner or shareholder in a medical clinic or professional corporation associating
several physicians. So, when this doctor does look upon a patient in the hospital, he may be representing only himself, or his own corporation, or a corporation of which he is only one of several shareholders, or a partnership, or the
hospital. It's all a matter of perspective and the underlying facts.

It is not unusual today to find that an emergency room P.C. is running a
hospital's emergency room facilities, that an obstetrics P.C. is directing the
hospital's obstetrical program, or that an outpatient P.C. is in charge of the
hospital's outpatient clinic. Like tectonic plates, the modern hospital is becoming fractured by the devolution of its functions upon P.C. subcontractors,
each group crunching and sliding against each other within the hospital's
walls.

The expectant mother, when not being visited by her obstetrician, is likely
to come under the observation of a hospital resident, intern, or nurse. A *resident*, for general discussion, is usually a full-fledged general physician who has
continued his stay at the hospital in order to take advanced training in a particular field. This may lead, ultimately, to his *board certification* by the
American Medical Association, a kind of honorarium which identifies the
physician as a specialist in some subcategory of medical knowledge. In contrast, an *intern* (not to be confused with an internist, a specialist in internal
medicine), is usually a medical school graduate undergoing the practical experience of patient care preparatory to qualifying for a state endorsed license to
practice medicine.

The nursing staff represents a wholly separate and distinctly complex hierarchy of talents, ranging from specialists (certified Registered Nurse Anesthe-
tists, for example) through varying degrees of more general service provided
by registered nurses, licensed practical nurses, and nurse's aides. To this professional world must be added a polyglot mixture of ward clerks, lab technicians, maintenance workers, administrators, food preparers, dieticians,
volunteers, and other auxiliary personnel which complete the picture of a
modern hospital in operation.

§ 2.2   —Significance to the Plaintiff's Attorney

An understanding of this array of medical and hospital personnel is crucial to
the practicing attorney pursuing a medical malpractice claim. Negligence
may be simply an individual act, but given the multiple participants involved

in patient care, an act of negligence may be compounded by the failure to the hospital's internal system of checks and balances to contain and neutralize an individual's mistake. A doctor may wrongly prescribe an intravenous injection for a patient, but his neglect may cause no harm if the nurse to whom the actual administration of the drug is delegated is cognizant of the error and has the courage to point out the mistake before proceeding. A resident may apply too much force upon forceps being used to deliver a baby, but his personal error may be directly the result of the obstetrician's failure to supervise the resident, or of his initial decision to allow the use of forceps when such a method of delivery is not necessary. With proper cooperation and true professionalism, most of the human errors which lead to tragedy can be avoided. Sadly, in our experience, we have all too often seen egocentrism, jealousy, pride, prejudice, and all the spectrum of human folly sowing discord and dissension within a hospital's walls, causing a breakdown of communication, disruption of harmonious teamwork, and contributing, at least in part, to the injury of a patient.

Consequently, today's malpractice case rarely focuses on the neglect of a single individual. This is especially true of birth trauma cases arising out of events taking placed within a hospital's obstetrics ward. When everything works right, when everyone does his job and acts in accord with his fellow professionals, then rarely will a tragedy occur giving rise to a suit. However, in the complicated division of labor current in modern medicine, a simple error of judgment, a minor breakdown in technique, a failure of a diagnosis, anywhere along the line, may multiply up and down the rank and file of functionaries, becoming progressively worse until snowballing into a catastrophe. A lapse in charting, confusion over who should make a phone call, inadequate communication with the patient, a momentary distraction from observance of a monitor, these are the seeds of a malpractice suit. Yet, individual errors of this kind usually only grow into significant mistakes when others involved in the treatment of the patient neglect their own duties and fail to discover and countercheck these errors before they cause harm. More often than not, we find that the birth of a defective child results from an almost surreal compounding of errors by a number of different personnel, each of whom, at one point, was in a position to dam the flow of neglect that precipitated the tragedy, but each of whom failed in his duty towards the patient.

Additionally, each of these medical professionals and auxiliary personnel bears a certain legal relationship to one another which can have major significance in determining the potential liability of each person. Not every physician liable for an errant cut is the one who held the knife. Not every nurse liable for the injection of the wrong drug is the one who held the needle. The complex warp and weave among medical practitioners has its parallel in the complex intertwining of legal responsibility for the wrongful acts of individuals. The lawyer's job is not over when he finds the actual culprit who committed the crucial error injuring his client. That individual may be the most culpable, but might not be the most collectable, nor the sole defendant legally responsible for his wrongful act. A lawyer must be fully aware of all the nuances of vicarious liability and must search down all the paths that might connect one defendant to another.

There are many advantages to be gained by increasing the number of potential defendants. The first and most obvious is that there is likely to be more insurance coverage available for the plaintiff. If a million dollar injury was caused by the mistake of a resident personally carrying only a hundred thousand dollar policy, it is readily apparent that bringing the hospital into the case as the employer of the resident, with its own million dollar policy, is a necessary strategy to maximize the potential of the case. For this same reason, multiple defendants are more willing to negotiate an acceptable settlement. Each defendant having something to contribute to a claim sees the benefit of encouraging other defendants to do the same to resolve the case. Lurking in the shadows of each adjuster's nightmares is the horrible possibility that a jury might find his insured to be the only culpable party, leaving his company responsible for the full amount of plaintiff's damages. Thus, self-interest spurs multiple defendants, if separately insured, to actively seek an equitable settlement. An interest in self-preservation also causes each of the defendants to point a finger at each other at trial should the attempts at settlement fail. Often a plaintiff can benefit as the defendants prove each other's liability for him. The hospital marshals its witnesses to prove that the independent staff doctor committed the critical mistakes, while the doctor parades in his experts to show how the hospital's employee independently made the error that caused the injury. Rarely do multiple defendants bend over backwards to try to exonerate each other.

Identifying the actual breach of the standard of care is the first step toward filing a malpractice suit, but an equally important second step is identifying the culpable defendants who may be held *legally* responsible for that act of professional negligence. Understanding the complexity of modern medical procedures should sharpen the lawyer's ability to pick out multiple breaches of the standard of care by one or a number of actors involved in the treatment of the patient. Understanding the legal relationships between these actors will assist in determining exactly which individuals or entities should be brought into the suit. Obviously, the person or persons who have actually and personally committed the breach of the standard of care are the most logical candidates to stand before the bar to answer for their mistakes. Occasionally this proves to be impossible (because of some legal impediment such as immunity or the expiration of a limitations statute), impracticable (no insurance), or insufficient (little insurance). Then, the plaintiff's attorney has an obligation toward his client to diligently seek out alternative or additional defendants answerable for the injuries to the plaintiff. In doing so, some of the legal concepts discussed in the remaining subsections of this chapter may prove helpful.

PHYSICIAN'S LIABILITY

§ 2.3   The Physician's Liability Generally

The central character in the practice of medicine is the physician. He may be a specialist. He may be an M.D. or a D.O. (osteopath). He may be a podiatrist, a psychiatrist, a chiropractor, dentist, or any of a dozen licensed subspecialists. Whatever he is, he takes pride in his professionalism and his independence. Indeed, these are the earmarks of a workable definition of a physician. He is a person holding a license from the state allowing him to make an independent professional judgment regarding the condition and treatment of his patient. The verbs that describe his function derive from diagnosis and prescription—he is the one who diagnoses, he is the one who prescribes.

He is also the one on whom liability will fall if the diagnosis is faulty or if the prescribed treatment fails in its purpose. This is *direct liability*, liability which arises out of his own personal breach of professional standards. This is the model malpractice case, a suit against a physician whose own breach of the standard of care proximately results in the plaintiff's injury.

Today's physician, however, does not operate in a vacuum. He works with a multitude of fellow professionals and interacts with them in a dozen different ways. Thus, he may, under appropriate circumstances, become responsible not just for his own acts, but for the acts of others with whom he is associated in some legally significant way. Through such interactions, a physician may find himself liable for the negligent acts committed by another. Let us look at some of these situations in §§ 2.4 through 2.8.

§ 2.4   Liability of a Physician for the Acts of an Agent, Employee, or Assistant

A physician who employs an assistant or agent to help him care for a patient may be held liable, under principles of *vicarious liability*, for the negligent acts of such assistant or agent. This is an obvious rule of respondeat superior, but often it is not clear who may be properly identified as an assistant or agent of the defendant physician. Naturally, the rule may extend to nurses, apprentices, and any other professional or lay persons actually employed by the physician to serve him in an ongoing master-servant or principal-agent relationship.[1] Under certain circumstances, however, another person may become the physician's assistant in an ad hoc basis, triggering vicarious liability absent a formal or continuing employment of agency. A physician, for example, may become liable for the acts of a fellow physician, intern, or nurse who assists the first in an operation. This situation arises so frequently that in many jurisdictions it has come to be known as the *captain of the ship* doctrine.

One of the earliest and leading cases endorsing this captain of the ship doctrine is a birth trauma case, *McConnell v. Williams*.[2] Defendant Dr. Williams had been engaged by plaintiffs to attend to the pregnancy and delivery of their expected child. Defendant requested that an intern from the hospital where this delivery was to take place assist him in the delivery. When the child was born, he was turned over to the intern for application of a solution of silver nitrate to the child's eyes. Plaintiffs claimed that the intern applied more than the required drops of silver nitrate and failed to properly irrigate the eyes afterwards, causing the loss of sight in the child's right eye. The real question confronted by the court was whether the defendant, as attending physician at the delivery, should be held vicariously liable for these alleged negligent acts of the intern. Noting that the determination of whether one is the servant of another or not depends essentially on whether or not he is subject to the latter's control or right to control, the court went on to state:

> And indeed it can readily be understood that in the course of an operation, (the "operation" in the present case including the tying of the cord and the insertion of the silver nitrate solution in the infant's eyes) he is in the same complete charge of those who are present and assisting him as is the captain of a ship over all on board, and that such supreme control is indeed essential in view of the high degree of protection to which an anaesthetized, unconscious patient is entitled,—a protection which Mrs. McConnell could justify claim in this case by reason of her trust and confidence in, and necessary reliance upon, the surgeon she employed to take care of her and her child when born.[3]

This doctrine has been adopted in most jurisdictions, even if the phrase captain of the ship is not employed.[4] Normally, this doctrine is only employed

---

[1] Thompson v. Brent, 245 So. 2d 751 (La. Ct. App. 1971); Barnes v. Mitchell, 341 Mich. 7, 67 N.W.2d 208 (1954). Both cases holding a doctor liable for the negligent acts of nurses directly employed by the doctor.

[2] 361 Pa. 355, 65 A.2d 243 (1949).

[3] *Id.* at 246.

[4] *See, e.g.,* Johnson v. Ely, 30 Tenn. App. 294, 205 S.W.2d 759 (1947) ("The rule is that a surgeon is liable for the negligence of nurses and operating assistants while under his special

where the physician is actually present at an operation, and the doctrine requires some evidence of the physician's actual supervision or control (or right of supervision and control) over the attendant personnel.[5] In most cases, the issue of supervision or control becomes a question of fact to be resolved by the trier of fact.[6] Where these conditions are met, the physician in charge will be held vicariously liable for the negligent acts of others over whom he has the right to exercise supervision or control.

The captain of the ship doctrine is closely related to, but not exactly identifiable with, the *borrowed servant* doctrine. This latter phrase is specifically associated with the negligent acts of hospital employees during their attendance upon the patient. While the borrowed servant rule frequently arises in situations involving operations, this potential for vicarious liability need not be limited to such instances. Likewise, there may be occasions where a surgeon under the captain of the ship doctrine is liable for the acts of others in attendance at the operation who are borrowed from the hospital; as for example, where the operating surgeon has asked another independent staff physician to assist him, the operating surgeon may be liable under the captain of the ship doctrine.[7] Consequently, these legal precepts are distinct.

---

supervision and control during the operation"); Orozco v. Henry Ford Hosp., 408 Mich. 248, 290 N.W.2d 363 (1980) ("He [the doctor in charge of the operation] had a non-delegable duty to see that the operation was performed with due care"). Some recent examples of the application of the captain of the ship doctrine, whether so named or not, are Kitto v. Gilbert, 39 Colo. App. 374, 570 P.2d 544 (1977); Miller v. Atkins, 142 Ga. App. 618, 236 S.E.2d 838 (1977); McCullough v. Bethany Medical Center, 235 Kan. 732, 683 P.2d 1258 (1984).

[5] *Compare,* for example, Parker v. St. Paul Fire & Marine Ins. Co., 335 So. 2d 725 (La. Ct. App. 1976) (operating surgeon not liable for acts of assisting nurses who, out of his direct supervision and control, mismatched blood used in transfusion during operation), and Sparger v. Worley Hosp., Inc., 547 S.W.2d 582 (Tex. 1977) (emphasizes that caption of ship doctrine is merely an extension of the borrowed servant rule of agency and merely raises a factual issue dependent upon the physician's right of control; the case specifically disapproves of the captain of the ship doctrine, at least insofar as it falsely suggests that the mere presence of the surgeon in the operating room makes him liable as a matter of law for the negligence of other persons).

[6] Kitto v. Gilbert, 39 Colo. App. 374, 570 P.2d 544 (1977); Sparger v. Worley Hosp., Inc., 547 S.W.2d 582 (Tex. 1977).

[7] Where a surgeon specifically selects another doctor to assist him in an operation, he may be held liable for the negligence of that doctor. This may be either through application of the captain of the ship doctrine or by simply applying the legal principle that the respective doctors are acting jointly to care for the patient and hence are jointly and severally liable for each others acts. See Ales v. Ryan, 8 Cal. 2d 82, 64 P.2d 409 (1936); Kitto v. Gilbert, 39 Colo. App. 374, 570 P.2d 544 (1977); Voss v. Bridwell, 188 Kan. 643, 364 P.2d 955 (1961); Orozco v. Henry Ford Hosp., 408 Mich. 248, 290 N.W.2d 363 (1980); Frazier v. Hurd, 6 Mich. App. 317, 149 N.W.2d 226 (1967), aff'd, 380 Mich. 291, 157 N.W.2d 249 (1968). Of

Essentially, the broad rule capable of supporting both doctrines is that a physician will be held liable for those who assist him in the care and treatment of a patient if their negligent acts fall within activities over which the physician either has the right and duty to supervise or control, or over which he has as immediate opportunity to exercise supervision or control. In a surgical procedure (including the delivery of a newborn), this means that the physician in charge, for example, generally will be found liable for negligent acts committed by his assistants since it can usually be shown that the assistants are acting under his direct supervision and control. Whether the physician will be also held liable for their negligent acts before or after the operation depends upon the degree of control he exercises within the framework of the borrowed servant principle.

§ 2.5   Liability of Physician for Acts of Employees of a Hospital

As a general rule, a private physician will not be held liable for the negligent acts of a hospital employee not acting under his direct supervision and control nor pursuant to his direct orders.[8] Hospital employees are deemed to have an independent responsibility for the care of patients admitted to the hospital, and private physicians have the right to rely upon such employees to perform their duties competently and without negligence.[9]

However, modern medical practice does not draw a sharp dividing line between the acts of the independent staff physician and those of hospital employees. Often in the treatment of a patient, hospital employees are called upon to exercise independent judgment regarding the welfare of the patient. For example, when a mother begins labor, with contractions far apart, the obstetrician may leave the hospital with an order to be called if anything abnormal develops. He is trusting the hospital employees to use their own judgment to determine when a condition may be sufficiently abnormal to warrant a call to

---

course the fact that one physician is in charge of an operation and thus may be vicariously liable for the negligence of another physician attending to give assistance, does not relieve the negligent physician from his own personal liability towards the patient. *See* Conrad v. Lakewood Gen. Hosp., 67 Wash. 2d 934, 410 P.2d 785 (1966).

[8] Bernardi v. Community Hosp. Ass'n, 166 Colo. 280, 443 P.2d 708 (1968); Hospital Auth. v. Smith, 142 Ga. App. 284, 235 S.E.2d 562 (1977); Striano v. Deepdale Gen. Hosp., 54 A.D.2d 730, 387 N.Y.S.2d 678 (1976); Burke v. Pearson, 259 S.C. 288, 191 S.E.2d 721 (1972).

[9] Adams v. Leidholt, 38 Colo. App. 463, 563 P.2d 15 (1976), *aff'd*, 195 Colo. 450, 579 P.2d 618 (1978).

the doctor. At other times the physician and hospital employees share a mutual responsibility to the patient such as when the doctor orders medicine to be administered, but leaves the actual administration of the medicine to the skill of the hospital nurse. Other occasions may make the physician primarily responsible to the patient, leaving little or no decisions to the hospital employees acting on his orders, e.g., an obstetrician ordering an assistant resident to use forceps to complete delivery of a child.

Consequently, there are many factual circumstances in the course of treating a patient where the clear distinction between the acts of the physician and those of the hospital employee becomes blurred. Sometimes the actual direct control which the physician exercises over the hospital employee may be sufficient to support the conclusion that the hospital employee has become the agent or employee of the physician. Under these circumstances, it may then be appropriate to hold the physician vicariously liable for the employee's negligent acts. Such liability is often discussed in the context of the borrowed servant doctrine.

The *borrowed servant* doctrine arises directly out of the law of agency.[10] An agent or servant of one master may be directed or permitted by his principal to become a servant or agent performing services for another. This accurately describes what frequently occurs in hospitals, where nurses, residents, and interns perform ancillary services for the physician which are only available through the hospital. Hospital personnel often serve as the conduits through which the physician provides care and treatment to his patient. Nurses administer the drugs that the physician prescribes; interns or residents perform the treatment he recommends; radiologists take the x-rays that he requests; and other hospital technicians perform the tests which the physician decides are needed. A physician's own direct contact with the patient, or with the hospital personnel involved with the patient, represents only a small percentage of the actual care or treatment rendered to the patient. For example, during a long and difficult labor, hospital nurses, interns, and residents are likely to have more frequent contact with the expectant mother, monitoring her condition and making important decisions about her comfort and care, than the obstetrician-gynecologist (OB-GYN) physician who is called in only at the time of actual delivery.

At what point do such hospital employees become temporary employees or borrowed servants of the attending physician so as to render that physician liable for their wrongful acts? Are they servants of the physician when they are left broad discretion to exercise their own judgment regarding patient care? Probably not. Are they servants of the physician when they are acting directly in response to his orders under his immediate supervision and con-

---

[10] *See, e.g.,* Restatement (Second) Agency, § 227 (1957).

trol? In most cases the borrowed servant rule will impose vicarious liability under these circumstances. What remains is the difficult area where the physician, by note or by phone, gives orders or directions to hospital personnel but leaves the execution of such matters to their own discretion. In these cases, there are no concrete rules to determine if the physician is vicariously liable.

Consider two examples. In many operations a physician is assisted by a nurse anesthetist. The physician may direct the nurse anesthetist to anesthetize his patient, but leaves the means and method to the nurse's discretion. If the patient is injured due to the negligence of the nurse anesthetist, should the physician be held liable? According to at least one case, the mere fact that the nurse received instructions from the physician as to the work to be performed was held insufficient to render the nurse the legal servant or agent of the physician.[11] Yet several cases have held that where the physician has selected the kind of anesthetic to be administered and told the nurse when to begin and when to stop the anesthesia, the physician could be held vicariously liable because of his right and exercise of control over the nurse anesthetist.[12] Nurses are also left with the responsibility of making the sponge count following surgery before closing the wound. According to some cases, the operating physician is not liable for a sponge left in the operating site due to a negligent sponge count.[13] Yet other cases have found the physician liable, either on the basis of his own neglect in leaving a sponge in the wound, or on the basis that as the surgeon in charge he was responsible for the sponge count performed by his borrowed servant.[14]

Contradictory precedents such as these demonstrate that it is not possible to propose any fixed criteria for establishing when a hospital employee is, or is not, a borrowed servant of the private physician. Some cases have attempted to draw a finer definition of the borrowed servant rule by distinguishing the performance of administrative or clerical acts on behalf of the physician, for which there is no vicarious liability running to the physician, from medical or ministerial acts for which the physician may be held vicariously liable.[15] However, such an approach merely adds confusion to what might be best left

---

[11] Sesselman v. Muhlenberg Hosp., 124 N.J. Super. 285, 306 A.2d 474 (1973).

[12] Foster v. Englewood Hosp. Ass'n, 19 Ill. App. 3d 1055, 313 N.E.2d 255 (1974); Voss v. Bridwell, 188 Kan. 643, 364 P.2d 955 (1961); Jackson v. Joyner, 236 N.C. 259, 72 S.E.2d 589 (1952); Whitfield v. Whittaker Memorial Hosp., 210 Va. 176, 169 S.E.2d 563 (1969).

[13] E.g., Worley Hosp., Inc. v. Caldwell, 552 S.W.2d 534 (Tex. Civ. App. 1977).

[14] Burke v. Washington Hosp. Center, 475 F.2d 364 (D.C. Cir. 1973); Martin v. Perth Amboy Gen. Hosp., 104 N.J. Super. 335, 250 A.2d 40 (1969).

[15] Buzan v. Mercy Hosp., 203 So. 2d 11 (Fla. Dist. Ct. App. 1967); Porter v. Patterson, 107 Ga. App. 64, 129 S.E.2d 70 (1962). See the valid criticism of this dichotomy in Bing v. Thunig, 2 N.Y.2d 656, 143 N.E.2d 3, 163 N.Y.S.2d 3 (1957).

to the singular determination of whether the physician has exercised sufficient supervision or control over a hospital employee to justify imposing liability upon him for that employee's negligent act, regardless of the nature or character of the act itself.

Focus on the borrowed servant doctrine, however, should not blind counsel to other factual situations in which a private physician may be held liable for the acts of a hospital employee. It has been held that the chief anesthesiologist of a hospital, nominally a private physician, having the responsibility to assure that safe and adequate practices are performed by the anesthesiology staff may be held liable on an agency theory for the negligent acts of anesthesiology residents of the hospital.[16] Likewise, specialists on staff of a hospital who have undertaken the responsibility to teach, advise, and supervise the advanced training of residents may be liable if they fail to use reasonable care to ascertain that surgery performed by a resident is properly and competently done.[17] The question cousel should ask in each case should not be limited to some facile formula. Rather, the question to be asked is whether under the facts of the case, a physician's interaction with a hospital employee creates circumstances where a court may find it appropriate to hold the physician liable for the acts of that employee.

§ 2.6   Partnership Liability

Folklore depicts the physician at the turn of the century as a universal healer who carried all his medical instruments in a little black bag. Until recent decades, it was certainly true that the majority of doctors were general practitioners, and the state of the art produced only a handful of reliable and proven devices to aid in healing the sick. Under such conditions, and before the imposition of high rates of income taxation, a good living could be made by a general physician with a modest investment of capital.

Medical science, in recent years, has radically altered this prosaic picture. Not only is there much more to be known about the human body and mind, which was not known even 50 years ago, but science has also provided medicine with remarkable tools to assist in the diagnosis and treatment of disease. The stethoscope is not replaced, but is supplemented, by the electrocardiogram, which far more accurately hears and depicts the beat of the heart. X-rays, CAT-scans, and many similar instruments probe the very rhythms

---

[16] Schneider v. Albert Einstein Medical Center, 257 Pa. Super. 348, 390 A.2d 1271 (1978); see also Grubb v. Albert Einstein Medical Center, 255 Pa. Super. 381, 387 A.2d 480 (1978) (applying similar rule to orthopedic staff member).

[17] McCullough v. Hutzel Hosp., 88 Mich. App. 235, 276 N.W.2d 569 (1979).

and structures of life. However, the equipment needed to display these images no longer fits into the traditional black bag, and, more significantly, few single practitioners can afford to purchase all the sophisticated devices which complete medical care requires.

A doctor, as we have seen, can have access to such equipment by obtaining staff privileges at a hospital. However, having all of one's patients routinely admitted to a hospital in order to properly treat them can be terribly inconvenient, and expensive. Consequently, two alternatives, not mutually exclusive, help to preserve the direct relationship between patient and physician outside of the hospital setting.

First, a physician can help limit the expense of equipment for his private practice by specializing. A specialist needs only to invest in the equipment needed to practice his specialty. A podiatrist need not purchase a fetal heart monitor and an obstetrician rarely needs a gripometer. But specializing means that a physician only sees his patient for a particular problem. When the patient has different requirements for treatment, he must look elsewhere.

So, the second alternative is for physicians to form linkages with other physicians—partnerships or the popular professional corporation (P.C.). Partnerships or corporations among physicians practicing the same specialty provide a means for such specialists to share in the expense of buying expensive diagnostic and remedial equipment. Partnerships and corporations among physicians having different specialities have a similar benefit of capital investment, but also have the benefit of providing at one clinic, complete health care for the patient. If partner A, a family physician, finds that one of his patients has a skin problem, he can refer the patient to partner B, a dermatologist. When Dr. B is asked by one of his own patients to recommend a physician to treat chicken pox in the family, Dr. B merely points down the hall to the office of Dr. A.

This book is concerned with liability for malpractice, not with the principles of partnership law corporate law with all of its financial shadings. What is important here is that the physician who is a member of a partnership or a P.C. no longer acts solely for himself. He is a representative of the partnership or corporation to which he belongs. Legally, he is an agent and under the law of respondeat superior, and his partnership or corporation may be liable for his acts.

When physicians combine to form a partnership they may each be assuming vicarious responsibility for the acts of one another. If one partner commits malpractice, then each other partner may find himself vicariously liable for the offending partner's act. Each member of a partnership is liable for a tort committed by a co-partner acting within the scope of partnership business.[18]

---

[18] Grubb v. Albert Einstein Medical Center, 255 Pa. Super. 381, 387 A.2d 480 (1978); *see also* Flynn v. Reaves, 135 Ga. App. 651, 218 S.E.2d 661 (1975); Martin v. Barbour, 558 S.W.2d 200 (Mo. Ct. App. 1977).

For such a rule to apply, there must, in fact, be a formal partnership and the mere sharing of office space will be insufficient to impose vicarious liability.[19]

If the plaintiff decides to sue only the offending physician and not the remaining partners, the culpable physician may not himself bring an action against his co-partners in the hope of compelling them to contribute their share to plaintiff's damages. As in any other vicarious liability situations, if the partners are held liable for the acts of a co-partner, they would have right of indemnity against the partner who was actively negligent.[20]

§ 2.7   Professional Corporations

Unlike a partnership, the association of physicians into a professional corporation provides the members insulation from the negligent acts of a co-employee of the corporation. As stated in one Illinois case:

> A physician-shareholder has the same privileges and liabilities as a shareholder in any other Illinois corporation. In this state a shareholder, officer, director, agent or employee of a corporation is insulated from personal liability for the tortious acts of the corporation and its officers, agents, employees and shareholders in which he does not participate and resultant injuries to which he does not contribute. . . . Thus, under basic corporate law doctrine, Dr. Feldman, like any other shareholder of an Illinois corporation, is not vicariously liable for the alleged malpractice of a fellow physician-shareholder who rendered services for the corporation.[21]

Consequently, absent some direct involvement with the patient, one physician member of a professional corporation will not be held personally liable for the negligent acts of a fellow physician member of the corporation.

However, a physician member may be held personally liable for the negligent acts of the corporation's nonmedical clerical staff. In *Boyd v.*

---

[19] Feigelson v. Ryan, 108 Misc. 2d 192, 437 N.Y.S.2d 229 (1981); *see also* Impastato v. DeGirolamo, 117 Misc. 2d 786, 459 N.Y.S.2d 512 (1983).

[20] Flynn v. Reaves, 135 Ga. App. 651, 218 S.E.2d 661 (1975).

[21] Fure v. Sherman Hosp., 55 Ill. App. 3d 572, 371 N.E.2d 143, 144 (1977); *see also* Birt v. St. Mary Mercy Hosp., 175 Ind. App. 32, 370 N.E.2d 379 (1978); Ballard v. Jayakrishnan, 427 So. 2d 665 (La. Ct. App. 1983).

Badenhausen,[22] a Kentucky case, the plaintiff sought medical treatment from Dr. Badenhausen, a member of a P.C. She claimed negligence in that he delayed treatment of her condition. This delay, the evidence suggested, resulted from the misfiling of plaintiff's medical records by the corporation's clerical staff. The defendant contended that as he was not personally responsible for this error, he could not be held personally liable. The Kentucky corporation laws,[23] however, provide in substance that the corporate form shall not affect the physician-patient relationship, and the court held that just as a physician is responsible for the negligence of nurses or hospital attendants employed to assist him, so is he responsible for the derelictions of persons employed by a corporation to carry out the clerical details that are necessary to the successful performance of his duty to render skillful care and attention to whomever he accepts as a patient. "Placing a layer of other people, by whomsoever they may be employed, between the physician and his patient does not alter the situation," the court said, "because the physician's professional duties are not susceptible of being delegated or diffuse."[24]

Of course, where negligence or malpractice is committed by a physician himself who is a member or employee of a professional corporation, the corporation itself will be liable under respondeat superior principles.[25]

§ 2.8   Physician's Direct Liability for Negligent Referral or Consultation

In the practice of modern medicine, so fragmented into fields of special competence, the *referral* has become a commonplace activity. A physician may refer his patient to another physician, or recommend another physician to his patient, for any number of reasons. The original physician may be going out of town for a few weeks vacation, yet anticipates that his patient might need medical services while he is away. He might then conscientiously suggest to his patient the name of a fellow physician within his own area of expertise. Or

---

22 556 S.W.2d 896 (Ky. 1977).

23 Ky. Rev. Stat. § 274.055 (1981).

24 556 S.W.2d at 899.

25 Peters v. Golds, 366 F. Supp. 150 (E.D. Mich. 1973); McGuire v. Sifers, 235 Kan. 368, 681 P.2d 1025 (1984); Lenhart v. Toledo Urology Assocs., Inc., 48 Ohio App. 2d 249, 356 N.E.2d 749 (1975); *see also* Jines v. Abarbanel, 77 Cal. App. 3d 702, 143 Cal. Rptr. 818 (1978) (emphasizes that such corporations are not mere alter egos of the physicians and must be separately sued). *Cf.* Connell v. Hayden, 83 A.D.2d 30, 443 N.Y.S.2d 383 (1981) (recognizing that the P.C. must be separately sued, but holding that service on physician could toll running of statute of limitations against P.C. because of unity of interest).

the patient may have received a disquieting diagnosis, and the physician may suggest another name so that his patient can receive a second opinion. The most typical case of referral arises when the original physician recognizes that his patient's problem falls outside his own area of competence, and thus requires the expertise of another to treat. For whatever reason, occasions do occur quite often in which a patient submits himself to one physician's care and treatment because another physician has made a referral or a recommendation encouraging the patient to seek out the professional services of the recommended physician.

When the recommended physician's negligence causes injury to the patient, does any liability lie against the orginal physician who made the referral? This question is best answered in a Montana case, *Llera v. Wisner*: "We find no case law cited by plaintiff or by our research of the question, that holds a recommendation of a physician to another will subject the latter to liability for the recommendation, absent a showing of partnership or employment or agency. . . ."[26]

Since physicians are nominally independent contractors, once a second physician takes charge of the patient, his acts cannot be attributed to the physician who referred the patient to him. We should note that although there appear to be no precedents holding a referring physician liable for the negligent acts of the recommended physician, the cases which have considered this issue have emphasized that such nonliability is proper when the referring physician uses due care in selecting the recommended physician, and the recommended physician is competent.[27] The inference which may be drawn from such language is that if it can be shown that a physician referred his patient to another who was not competent, and who was known to the referring physician to be not competent, then the referring physician might be held liable for his own negligence in making the referral. Whether, in a proper case, liability for a bad referral will be upheld is presently purely conjectural.

Public policy is probably best served by this rule of law preventing one physician from being held liable for the negligent acts of another to whom he has referred his patient, for in many cases the best interests of the patient require that he be referred to a specialist capable of properly treating his health problem. The first physician, in recognizing the need for a referral to a specialist, should not be restrained by any fear that he is in some way vouching for the competency of the recommended physician and might himself be held liable if the recommended specialist commits malpractice.

---

[26] 171 Mont. 254, 557 P.2d 805, 809 (1976); *see also* Nelson v. Sandell, 202 Iowa 109, 209 N.W. 440 (1926); Stovall v. Harms, 214 Kan. 835, 522 P.2d 353 (1974).

[27] Stovall v. Harms, 214 Kan. 835, 522 P.2d 353 (1974).

In fact, public policy leans to the opposite side, for cases have held that a physician who recognizes that his patient's problem requires the application of skills beyond his own competence may be liable if he fails to refer the patient to a competent specialist. Where a plaintiff can establish that the appropriate standard of care would require a referral to a specialist, the physician's failure to direct, or delay in directing, his patient to the proper medical specialist may render him liable for any injuries or damages which results from that failure or delay.[28]

As a corollary to this doctrine, a physician who proceeds to treat a condition which he knows should be treated by a specialist when the standard of care requires a referral of the patient to a specialist, will be held liable for any injuries resulting from his failure to treat the condition with the same skill and care of a specialist.[29]

Consultation between physicians also raises some interesting problems of liability. A *consultation* is a request by one physician to another for advice or assistance in the treatment of the former's own patient. As a general rule, each physician remains an independent contractor liable to the patient for his own individual acts of negligence, but not liable for the negligent acts of the other.[30] One case has held that one physician may be held liable for the negligent acts of another which he personally observed, or in the exercise of reasonable care, should have observed.[31] Of course, the situation may develop where the one physician allows himself to come under the actual supervision or control of the other in the treatment of the patient, creating an agency relationship (see § 2.4) rendering the physician in charge liable for the negligent acts of one he has asked to assist him.[32]

---

[28] Erickson v. Waller, 116 Ariz. 476, 569 P.2d 1374 (1977); Valentine v. Kaiser Found. Hosps., 194 Cal. App. 2d 282, 15 Cal. Rptr. 26 (1961); Morgan v. Engles, 372 Mich. 514, 127 N.W.2d 382 (1964); Lowery v. Newton, 52 N.C. App. 234, 278 S.E.2d 566 (1981); Osborne v. Frazor, 58 Tenn. App. 15, 425 S.W.2d 768 (1968).

[29] Larson v. Yelle, 310 Minn. 521, 246 N.W.2d 841 (1976).

[30] Brooker v. Hunter, 22 Ariz. App. 510, 528 P.2d 1269 (1974); Scruggs v. Otteman, 640 P.2d 259 (Colo. App. 1981); Josselyn v. Dearborn, 143 Me. 328, 62 A.2d 174 (1948).

[31] Rodgers v. Canfield, 272 Mich. 562, 262 N.W. 409 (1935).

[32] *See, e.g.,* Frazier v. Hurd, 6 Mich. App. 317, 149 N.W.2d 226 (1967), *aff'd,* 380 Mich. 291, 157 N.W.2d 249 (1968).

HOSPITAL LIABILITY

§ 2.9   Traditional Limitations of Hospital Liability

Not all that long ago hospitals were rarely named as defendants in medical malpractice suits. Early attempts to hold hospitals liable in malpractice met with serious objections of a technical nature. Hospitals were, after all, corporations, not individuals, and as such were not licensed by the state to practice medicine. Thus, the argument went, hospitals, not being licensed to practice medicine, could not themselves be guilty of malpractice which related only to the negligence of a licensed professional.[33]

This archaic view of hospitals stems from an era when hospitals were looked upon as being merely extensions of the little black bag of private physicians. Hospitals were considered somewhat as specialized hotels, a place in which sick people were housed at the request of their private physicians. They offered a bed for the patient to lie down in, the maid and cook service one might expect in a public accommodation, and a few specialized pieces of equipment which the physician might employ to treat his patient. For the purposes of this present work, it may be added that until the mid-twentieth century few babies were ever born in hospitals. Today, of course, few babies are born anywhere else.

Under this image of the hospital, its liability to patients would only arise under those circumstances where a hotel might be held liable to one of its guests. A patient might sue in general negligence if injured by a slippery floor or by a dark and dangerous stairway, but not if he received substandard medical care or attention. Hospitals might be held liable in the general negligence of its employees, but usually not for their malpractice. Up until the late 1940s many states continued to draw a distinction between the administrative acts of a hospital, for which it might be held liable, from its medical acts, to which no liability could attach.[34]

---

[33] *See, e.g.*, Rosane v. Senger, 112 Colo. 363, 149 P.2d 372 (1944); Smith v. Duke Univ., 219 N.C. 628, 14 S.E.2d 643 (1941).

[34] Some examples of hospitals being liable for burns, cuts, bruises, and so forth, resulting from the negligence of a nurse or other hospital attendant are: Norwood Clinic v. Spann, 240 Ala. 427, 199 So. 840 (1941) (fall on slick entrance-way sidewalks); Corey v. Beck, 58 Idaho 281, 72 P.2d 856 (1937) (79 year old patient fell while being assisted to lavatory); Petry v. Nassau Hosp., 267 A.D. 996, 48 N.Y.S.2d 227 (1944) (unattended patient fell from examination table).

§ 2.10   Charitable and Sovereign Immunity

In addition to the historical restraint upon malpractice claims against hospitals (see § **2.9**), in many jurisdictions private charitable hospitals were considered immune from tort suit under the doctrine of charitable immunity. Many fine hospitals were founded at the bequest or gift of a benefactor and were (and still are) maintained as charitable institutions. Case law 50 years ago held that imposing tort liability upon such charitable institutions would intrude upon the trust of funds established to maintain the hospital, and would diminish or destroy the benevolent purposes for which the trust was created. Since the founder of the trust had not intended the funds to be used to compensate the victims of the hospital's neglect, any judgment against the hospital to compensate a tort victim would be contrary to the purposes of the trust. From such reasoning, now largely discredited, the principle of charitable immunity evolved which kept many of these hospitals out of court for years.[35]

Similarly, public hospitals have frequently been held to enjoy the protection of sovereign or governmental immunity. Like charitable immunity, this defense often prevented patients in such hospitals from seeking damages for injuries arising from negligent care or treatment rendered by employees of such public institutions. In several jurisdictions vestiges of this sovereign immunity remain.[36]

§ 2.11   Modern View of Hospital Liability

The modern hospital is not merely a place where a private physician, in solitude, medically serves his patient while hospital employees look passively on, awaiting the doctor's instructions. The modern hospital takes an active, participating role in patient health care, sharing responsibility with the physician for the course and method of treatment employed to cure those received within its walls. This change in the role of hospitals is reflected in this oft-quoted passage from *Bing v. Thunig*,[37] a New York case which abolished hospital charitable immunity in that state:

---

[35] The seminal charitable immunity case in this country appears to be McDonald v. Massachusetts Gen. Hosp., 120 Mass. 432, 21 Am. Rep. 529 (1876). The development of this doctrine is discussed in Parker v. Port Huron Hosp., 361 Mich. 1, 105 N.W.2d 1 (1960).

[36] *See, e.g.,* Perry v. Kalamazoo State Hosp., 404 Mich. 205, 273 N.W.2d 421 (1978); Papenhausen v. Schoen, 268 N.W.2d 565 (Minn. 1978).

[37] 2 N.Y.2d 656, 143 N.E.2d 3, 163 N.Y.S.2d 3 (1957).

The conception that the hospital does not undertake to treat the patient, does not undertake to act through its doctors and nurses, but undertakes instead simply to procure them to act upon their own responsibility, no longer reflects the fact. Present-day hospitals, as their manner of operation plainly demonstrates, do far more than furnish facilities for treatment. They regularly employ on a salary basis a large staff of physicians, nurses, interns, as well as administrative and manual workers, and they charge patients for medical care and treatment, collecting for such services, if necessary, by legal action. Certainly, the person who avails himself of "hospital facilities" expects that the hospital will attempt to cure him, not that its nurses or other employees will act on their own responsibility.[38]

Charitable immunity, as mentioned in § 2.10, has been abandoned as a valid defense in the jurisdictions which had adopted it. Governmental immunity in most jursidictions, as it applies to public hospitals, is on the retreat. The archaic concept that hospitals, as corporate entities, could not themselves be held liable for malpractice (or, more precisely, held liable upon respondeat superior principles in the professional negligence of its own employees) has been discredited. The courts have recognized that hospitals are major institutions actively involved in the health care of their patients, and as such should be held responsible for the negligent delivery of such care.

Modern hospitals, whether publicly, privately, or charitably operated, provide indispensible health care services to the general public. The health needs of the public cannot be fully attended to without the ancillary services of a well-equipped hospital. Properly, the broadening of liability insures that these hospitals will exercise great care in serving the medical needs of the community, for just as immunity can be rightly criticized as fostering neglect, the imposition of liability encourages those responsible for operating hospitals to maintain high standards of professional competence with regard to its agents and employees. We will now look in §§ 2.12 through § 2.17 to some of the ways in which a hospital may incur liability to its patients.

§ 2.12   Vicarious Liability: Actual Agency

Obviously, a hospital, being either a corporate or quasi-corporate body, acts primarily through its servants, employees, and agents. The well-established principles of respondeat superior serve to impose liability on the hospital for the neglect of the nurses, residents, and interns, and auxiliary personnel actually employed by the hospital to perform the hospital's multifunctional tasks.

---

[38] 143 N.E.2d at 8.

As indicated in § 2.9, hospitals have long been held liable for the administrative acts of these salaried employees. Today, they may also be held liable
for negligent medical treatment which is rendered by a nurse,[39] resident,[40]
intern,[41] or other professional[42] employed by the hospital to care for patients.

The doctrine of respondeat superior embraces such professional and
pseudoprofessional employees in their professional negligence as well as the
general negligence of ward clerks, orderlies, security guards, cooks, and other
nonprofessionals who service the daily routine of the hospital.

In § 2.4, we discussed the borrowed servant rule under which hospital employees may temporarily come under the supervision and control of a private
physican so as to render the latter vicariously liable for their acts of negligence. In some jurisdictions such exercise of control makes the liability of the
physician and of the hospital mutually exclusive—-that is, while a hospital employee is being supervised or controlled by the doctor, only the doctor is vicariously liable for the borrowed servant's negligence and the hospital is relieved
of its respondeat superior liability.[43] In at least one jurisdiction, an attempt is
made to distinguish between the ministerial acts of hospital employees and
their medical acts, with the hospital being vicariously liable for the former
acts, and the physician liable for the latter.[44] The more enlightened and reasonable rule, however, holds that such a borrowed servant remains a servant
of both the physician and the hospital, so that both may be held vicariously
liable for the borrowed servant's negligence.[45] Such a rule has the advantage
of avoiding fine distinctions between medical and ministerial acts while at the

---

[39] Beardsley v. Wyoming County Community Hosp., 79 A.D.2d 1110, 435 N.Y.S.2d 862
(1981) (hospital liable for brain damage of six year old child negligently administered excessive amount of salt-free fluid by a nurse, apparently contrary to treating physicians' orders);
see discussion in Fraijo v. Hartland Hosp., 99 Cal. App. 3d 331, 160 Cal. Rptr. 246 (1979);
see also Hiatt v. Groce, 215 Kan. 14, 523 P.2d 320 (1974) (hospital liable for failure of nurse
to inform doctor of maternity patient's labor); Ramsey v. Physicians Memorial Hosp., 36
Md. App. 42, 373 A.2d 26 (1977).

[40] Register v. Wilmington Medical Center, Inc., 377 A.2d 8 (Del. 1977) (hospital's liability for
negligence of obstetrical resident recognized).

[41] City of Miami v. Oates, 152 Fla. 21, 10 So. 2d 721 (1942); Emory Univ. v. Lee, 97 Ga. App.
680, 104 S.E.2d 234 (1958); Stuart Circle Hosp. Corp. v. Curry, 173 Va. 136, 3 S.E.2d 153
(1939).

[42] South Miami Hosp. v. Sanchez, 386 So. 2d 39 (Fla. Dist. Ct. App. 1980) (physiotherapist).

[43] Moore v. Carrington, 155 Ga. App. 12, 270 S.E.2d 222 (1980); St. Paul-Mecury Indem. Co.
v. St. Joseph Hosp., 212 Minn. 558, 4 N.W.2d 637 (1942); Hull v. Enid Gen. Hosp. Found.,
194 Okla. 446, 152 P.2d 693 (1944).

[44] Beaches Hosp. v. Lee, 384 So. 2d 234 (Fla. Dist. Ct. App. 1980).

[45] City of Somerset v. Hart, 549 S.W.2d 814 (Ky. 1977); Simpson v. Sisters of Charity, 284 Or.
547, 588 P.2d 4 (1978); Tonsic v. Wagner, 458 Pa. 246, 329 A.2d 497 (1974).

same time recognizing the mutual responsibility of the private physician and the hospital in providing skilled and competent care to the patient.

Where vicarious hospital liability is recognized, a subsidiary issue arises concerning the standard of care to be applied. This is discussed in greater detail in § **4.9**.

A hospital clearly plays a dual role in caring for a patient through its personnel. Some of these employees—nurses, residents, radiologists, interns, and the like—are employed to render professional services to patients, and the hospital may be liable for their acts only if it can be established that the employee breached his or her professional standard of care, i.e., that malpractice was committed. Other employees serve the patient in a more custodial fashion, providing food service, housekeeping, or similar assistance to provide for the patient's safety and comfort. Here the simple negligence of the employee may render the hospital vicariously liable. Sometimes these functions overlap. Consider, for example, a registered nurse who drops a newborn baby. Is it malpractice or is it negligence? The hospital may be liable in either case, but coping with procedural and evidentiary rules of law (statutes of limitations and the need for expert testimony, for example) may require a determination of which theory of liability applies.

§ 2.13   Vicarious Liability: Ostensible Agency

Traditionally, the law looks upon the private physician who treats his own patient at the hospital as having a relationship to the hospital as that of an independent contractor. This is not, of course, a wholly accurate depiction of the realities. A hospital does not really contract with private physicians to perform services for the hospital in the same way that a homeowner, for example, contracts with a painting firm to paint his house. The hospital is more analogous to a private club which owns certain equipment which it allows only its members the privilege of using. Hospitals grant staff privileges to private physicians in the community served by the hospital, which in turn, enable the physician to utilize the hospital's facilities in the treatment of his own patients. But the physicians remain autonomous and independent of the hospital. No formal agency or employment relationship is created by this symbiotic association, even when staff privileges are maintained only by a commitment by the physician to perform detailed obligations on the hospital's behalf, such as teaching residents or administrating its departments.

The *independent contractor* concept more accurately describes the physician-patient relationship which arises outside and independent of the hospital setting. When, in fact, a private physician has had his own patient admitted to a hospital, the hospital will not be held vicariously liable for the physician's own negligent acts which injure that patient. The hospital may be vicariously liable for the negligent acts of its own agents or employees in carrying out the staff physician's orders or directly liable for its own separate negligence as described later in this section, but a firm wall is erected by the nature of the physician-patient relationship which insulates and protects the hospital from being held answerable for the physician's mistreatment of his own patient.

However, not all physician-patient relationships arise outside of the hospital setting. Not every patient who enters a hospital does so through his own doctor's admission procedures. Not every independent staff physician who looks in on him at the hospital is a doctor with whom the patient had prior contact before entering the hospital. In fact, it is becoming increasingly common for persons to look to the hospital itself for health care, and not to some specific family doctor. In emergency situations, especially, the hospital is viewed as the primary health care provider, its own reputation as a place of healing overriding any considerations of the quality of care rendered by an individual physician.

Several jurisdictions have found it appropriate to hold hospitals liable for the acts of those independent staff physicians which it places in the position of treating patients who have initially looked to the hospital for medical care. Realistically, when a mother comes to term and goes into sudden labor and is rushed to the hospital for delivery, she doesn't ask and isn't concerned with whether the men and women wearing white frocks and stethoscopes are employees of the hospital or independent staff physicians. To her the terms would be meaningless in any event. What she does know, and all that she cares about, is that the hospital to which she has been precipitously taken, by gesture, by suggestion, by the mere circumstances of the case, has represented, or held out, these persons as being qualified to assist her and to serve her medical needs. Her own doctor, should he arrive in time, does not fall into this category, for she herself selected him and she has independently weighed and judged his competency to help her. His acts of negligence are chargeable only to himself. But anyone which the hospital has placed in a position of treating her acts not just for himself, but for the hospital as well.

This doctrine, referred to in the cases as the doctrine of *ostensible agency*, apparent agency, agency by estoppel, or inaccurately, implied agency, is essentially founded upon two propositions—that the patient has had no prior relationship with the alleged culpable physician and that the hospital has represented the physician as qualified to render professional care and treatment to the patient. We might call these two elements the *look to* and the *holds out* rules. If the patient has looked to the hospital for treatment, and the hospital has held out the culpable physician as capable of providing such treatment, then the doctrine will apply and the hospital will be held vicariously liable for the culpable physician's acts. The hospital will simply be estopped from denying that the physician was its employee or agent.[46]

These elements should not be taken literally. A patient need not be considered looking to the hospital for treatment. In fact, in many emergency room situations the patient is brought in unconscious; however, certainly the friends and relatives or stranger who brought the patient to the hospital did so because they looked to the hospital as a place of healing. Alternatively, the patient may have been admitted by her own private physician; nevertheless, except for her private physician, she looks to the hospital to provide her with the proper monitoring, supervision, and medical care rendered between her own physician's visits. With respect to the other leg of liability, the hospital need not do anything dramatic to hold independent staff physicians out as persons qualified to treat the plaintiff. Simply the setting itself, and the traditional attitude that the patient need not be told anything of what is going on round her, suffices to create the proper impression. When a physician, not her own private physician, pops in and begins feeling her pulse or checking her chart, or chatting about her complaints, he rarely wears a badge that announces to the patient that he is an independent staff physician acting solely on his own judgment and discretion, and that the hospital is not his principal and should not be held liable for his mistakes. Simply placing a physician in the position of treating the patient is usually sufficient evidence that the hospital has held that physician out to be its agent.

This doctrine certainly represents a hybrid between traditional vicarious liability (see § 2.12) and direct corporate liability (see § 2.14). It is *vicarious* in the sense that the theory of recovery is the principal-agent relationship between the hospital and the physician. It is *direct* in that the hospital itself, by placing that physician in a position to treat a patient who has looked to the hospital for medical care, has by its own action created the circumstances engendering the liability. However characterized, this doctrine represents a significant departure from the traditional view that hospitals are absolved from responsibility for the acts of the independent staff physicians who commit negligence within its walls.

Before leaving this discussion, a nod must be given to a modern trend by many hospitals to erect a three tiered hierarchy over the treatment of a pa-

---

[46] Brown v. Moore, 247 F.2d 711 (3d Cir. 1957); Seneris v. Haas, 45 Cal. 2d 811, 291 P.2d 915 (1955); Stanhope v. Los Angeles College of Chiropractic, 54 Cal. App. 2d 141, 128 P.2d 705 (1942); Irving v. Doctors Hosp., 415 So. 2d 55 (Fla. Dist. Ct. App. 1982); Mehlman v. Powell, 281 Md. 269, 378 A.2d 1121 (1977); Grewe v. Mt. Clemens Gen. Hosp., 404 Mich. 240, 273 N.W.2d 429 (1978); Mduba v. Benedictine Hosp., 52 A.D.2d 450, 384 N.Y.S.2d 527 (1976); Rural Educ. Ass'n v. Tacoma Gen. Hosp., 20 Wash. App. 98, 579 P.2d 970 (1978). *Contra*, Smith v. Duke Univ., 219 N.C. 628, 14 S.E.2d 643 (1941).

tient. Hospitals today operate primarily through specialized departments— the emergency room, OB-GYN, occupational health, cardiac care, and so forth. There is a growing trend among hospitals to contract with professional corporations to service one or more of their departments to, in effect take over for the hospital the functional operation of a department. For example, an OB-GYN P.C. might enter into a contract with a hospital to service the hospital's OB-GYN ward. The contract might encompass the responsibility of staffing the ward with proper assistants including providing its own members to staff the ward, to teach residents, and to otherwise handle the administrative chores of the ward. Under such a system, a maternity patient may be treated by an OB-GYN physician who is an employee or shareholder of an OB-GYN P.C. which has a contract with the hospital.

This farming out of hospital functions to specialized P.C.'s does not add any insulation between the patient and the liability of the hospital. It may be legitimately argued that the P.C. is the actual agent of the hospital, particularly as hospitals in such arrangements usually reserve significant contractual control over the P.C. inconsistent with any independent contractor claim. Also, we might suggest that the duty of the hospital to provide certain services to the public is nondelegable, so any acts of the P.C. are legally the acts of the hospital itself. However, most often a patient may simply rely upon the doctrine of ostensible agency to reach the P.C.[47] People do not go to the hospitals because of the independent reputation of the P.C. staffing the hospital's department. Departmental P.C.'s do not put up large signs or make public address announcements disclosing their involvement in the hospital. The vast majority of patients have absolutely no idea when, or if, they are being treated by agents of the hospital or of some P.C. which the hospital has engaged to service one of its departments. Nor do they care; nor does it make any difference with respect to the hospital's liability. By hiring a P.C. to service a hospital department, the hospital has made an obvious declaration holding out the P.C. to be the hospital's agent for this purpose.

Thus, the inclusion of service contract P.C.'s does not seriously alter the hospital's vulnerability to suit. Such arrangements only serve to provide yet another defendant to be added to the list of defendants. It is becoming increasingly common to find one incident of malpractice blossoming into a claim naming a private physician, his own P.C. or partnership, a hospital, a

---

[47] *See, e.g.,* Schagrin v. Wilmington Medical Center Inc., 304 A.2d 61 (Del. Super. Ct. 1973); Baloney v. Carter, 387 So. 2d 54 (La. Ct. App. 1980); Hannola v. City of Lakewood, 68 Ohio App. 2d 61, 426 N.E.2d 1187 (1980); Rural Educ. Ass'n v. Bush, 42 Tenn. App. 34, 298 S.W.2d 761 (1957); Jenkins v. Charleston Gen. Hosp. & Training School, 90 W. Va. 230, 110 S.E. 560 (1922). *Contra,* Pogue v. Hospital Auth., 120 Ga. App. 230, 170 S.E.2d 53 (1969).

hospital's employee, and a servicing P.C. as a community of defendants answerable for the resultant injuries.

§ 2.14 Corporate Liability of the Hospital

A hospital may be held liable for the negligent acts of its actual or ostensible agents (see §§ 2.12 and 2.13). Such vicarious liability focuses upon a specific actor; a plaintiff, in order to recover, must establish that some breach of due care by an employee or agent of the hospital was a proximate cause of plaintiff's injuries.

Direct or corporate liability, on the other hand, exposes a hospital to liability upon broader principles.[48] Here the negligence is the negligence of the hospital staff, performing its functions through its administrative committees and rules of operation. The hospital is liable as an entity, not because of its own legal duties toward the patient. Basically, this is the duty to provide the patient with quality health care while the patient is in the hospital.

Not so long ago there existed no well-formed concept of direct liability applicable to a hospital. But medical science has changed, and the law, more slowly, has also evolved theories of liability appropriate to modern circumstances. At this time, the corporate liability of a modern hospital is premised essentially upon the public policy which recognizes that hospitals are no longer the passive stages upon which physicians perform, are no longer merely extensions of the physician's black bag, but have become active and independent participants in providing full health care and treatment to the patient. The modern hospital, in this view, shares with the physician the responsibility of medical care and treatment. The patient who enters the hospital expects the hospital, as much as the physician, to provide skilled and professional services

---

[48] The term corporate liability is probably more accurate, for even under this species of liability the hospital is still acting through its employees and agents, i.e., through nurses who fail to report bad medical practices, through paid administrators, or through independent staff physicians acting on behalf of the hospital, credentials or review committees. Basically, the liability stressed here is that growing out of the hospital's corporate responsibility to the patient. In other words, it is direct liability only in that this liability grows out of the direct responsibilities which the hospital owes to its patient to provide for the patient's well being. Consequently, although the application of this doctrine under the circumstances described in this section are new, this liability grows out of older traditions which recognize that a hospital owes to its patients a duty of protection and must exercise reasonable care to a patient as his known condition may require. See, e.g., Rice v. California Lutheran Hosp., 27 Cal. 2d 296, 163 P.2d 860 (1945); Stansfield v. Gardner, 56 Ga. App. 634, 193 S.E. 375 (1937); Paulen v. Shinnick, 291 Mich. 288, 289 N.W. 162 (1940); Flower Hosp. v. Hart, 178 Okla. 447, 62 P.2d 1248 (1937).

for the patient's benefit, and to protect the patient from avoidable injury and harm.

What this means, in practical terms, is that theories of liability are evolving which hold a hospital liable for its own failure to supervise and monitor the health care provided within its walls, even when such health care is rendered by one of the independent staff physicians privileged to use its facilities. Basically, the concept of direct or corporate liability is another assault upon the traditional view that independent staff physicians are independent contractors for whose negligence the hospital itself bears no responsibility. This doctrine proposes that under some circumstances the hospital is responsible for the negligence of a staff physician through its own negligence in allowing that physician to proceed in a way causing harm to his, and the hospital's patient.

§ 2.15   Corporate Liability: Staff Privileges

In granting staff privileges to a private physician, the hospital, acting through its credentials committee, is making a positive statement about the ability of the physician receiving those privileges. This grant of privileges and the periodic continuation or renewal of such privileges, represents a kind of endorsement by the hospital that the doctor possesses sufficient training and skill to be awarded the privilege of utilizing the valuable equipment and services which only the hospital can economically provide. Suppose, however, that the credentials committee fails to make a proper investigation of a physician's background before granting these privileges, and that such an investigation would have turned up a dire history of mistreatment and patient mismanagement by the physician raising serious doubts as to his professional skill. Or, suppose that the hospital continues to renew a physican's staff privileges each year, even though the physician has become unstable, alcoholic, senile, as all his colleagues whisper about with knowing nods and misplaced sympathy. Then, imagine that the physician in question mistreats one of his own patients at the hospital, a patient who would not have been under that physician's care at the hospital if his privileges had been denied or revoked, or whose care by the physician might have been monitored by another physician if the hospital had placed the errant physician on a probationary status. Should the patient be entitled to sue the hospital for having given the physician the privileges which placed him in a position to harm the patient? The answer increasingly being given by our courts, as shown in the cases discussed below, is yes.

The granting and perpetuation of staff privileges to a known incompetent physician (or one whose incompetency should have been known to the hospital had it exercised due care) might be seen as analogous to the theory of negligent entrustment. If an automobile owner allows a person who he knows to have a bad driving record to drive his car, he is liable to someone injured by the driver because of his negligence of entrusting this instrumentality to someone lacking the competency to properly use it. Certainly, the instruments and services provided by a hospital have all the sophistication of an automobile, if not more so, and should not be placed into the hands of someone who, through lack of experience, skill or physical, or emotional stability, is wholly unfit to be trusted with them.

The duty of the hospital respecting staff privileges has been stated to be a duty to exercise reasonable care to permit only competent medical doctors the privilege of using the hospital facilities. The screening of the qualifications of its staff physicians is one of the primary functions of a hospital. In *Johnson v. Misericordia Community Hospital,*[49] the Wisconsin Supreme Court summarizes comprehensively both the legal duty and the practical standards required to discharge the hospital's duty respecting the granting of staff privileges:

> In summary, we hold that a hospital owes a duty to its patients to exercise reasonable care in the selection of its medical staff and in granting specialized privileges. The final appointing authority resides in the hospital's governing body, although it must rely on the medical staff and in particular the credentials committee (or committee of the whole) to investigate and evaluate an applicant's qualifications for the requested privileges. However, this delegation of the responsibility to investigate and evaluate the professional competence of applicants for clinical privileges does not relieve the governing body of its duty to appoint only qualified physicians and surgeons to its medical staff and periodically monitor and review their competency. The credentials committee (or committee of the whole) must investigate the qualifications of applicants. The facts of this case demonstrate that a hospital should, at a minimum, require completion of the application and verify accuracy of the applicant's statements, especially in regard to his medical education, training and experience. Additionally, it should: (1) solicit information from the applicant's peers including those not referenced in his application, who are knowledgeable about his education, training, experience, health, competence and ethical character; (2) determine if the applicant is currently licensed to practice in this state and if his licensure or registration has been or is currently being challenged; and (3) inquire whether the applicant has been involved in any adverse malpractice action and whether he has experienced a loss of medical organization membership or medical privileges or membership at any other hospital. The investigating committee must also evaluate the information gained through its inquiries and make a reasonable judgment as to the approval or denial of each application for staff privileges. The hospital will be charged with gaining and evaluating the knowledge that would have been acquired had it exercised ordinary care in investigating its med-

---

49 99 Wis. 2d 708, 301 N.W.2d 156 (1981).

ical staff applicants and the hospital's failure to exercise that degree of care, skill and judgment that is exercised by the average hospital in approving an applicant's request for privileges is negligence. This is not to say that hospitals are insurers of the competence of their medical staff, for a hospital will not be negligent if it exercises the noted standard of care in selecting its staff.[50]

Although *Johnson* describes this corporate liability in the context of initially granting staff privileges, it should not be thought that the duty of the hospital to monitor a physician's competency ends once the doors of the hospital are opened to him.[51] It is increasingly apparent that this duty does not merely arise when staff privileges are granted or renewed; instead, this duty is a continuous one.

§ 2.16   Corporate Liability: Monitoring Health Care

The landmark case both for the hospital's duty to monitor the quality of care rendered by physicians in the hospital and for the hospital's duty to enforce its own rules is *Darling v. Charleston Community Memorial Hospital*.[52] In this Illinois case, the nurses and employees of the defendant hospital stood by and were silent while a patient undergoing treatment for a broken leg was improperly casted and then negligently cut during uncasting by an emergency room staff physician. The court held that the hospital was negligent both for failing to require consultation and for failing to review the work of the doctor. *Darling* suggests that a hospital's duty to its patients includes the duty to supervise the health care provided to the patient by its own independent staff physician. In this, *Darling* ventures significantly beyond the view that hospitals are mere facilities for the treatment of patients absolved from any responsibility to oversee the activities of the staff physicians who employ those facilities.[53]

---

50 *Id.* at 174 (footnotes omitted).

51 Additional cases discussing hospital liability in respect to staff privileges are: Tucson Medical Center Inc. v. Misevch, 113 Ariz. 34, 545 P.2d 958 (1976); Purcell v. Zimbelman, 18 Ariz. App. 75, 500 P.2d 335 (1972); Elam v. College Park Hosp., 132 Cal. App. 3d 332, 183 Cal. Rptr. 156 (1982); Mitchell County Hosp. Auth. v. Joiner, 229 Ga. 140, 189 S.E.2d 412 (1972); Ferguson v. Gonyaw, 64 Mich. App. 685, 236 N.W.2d 543 (1976); Corleto v. Shore Memorial Hosp., 138 N.J. Super. 302, 350 A.2d 534 (1975); Hannola v. City of Lakewood, 68 Ohio App. 2d 61, 426 N.E.2d 1187 (1980).

52 33 Ill. 2d 326, 211 N.E.2d 253 (1965).

53 For a contrast to Darling, *see* Fiorentino v. Wenger, 19 N.Y.2d 407, 227 N.E.2d 296, 280 N.Y.S.2d 373 (1967), which finds that a hospital has no duty to determine if a private physician has obtained the informed consent of his patient to a high risk operation since the hospital only serves a function as a specialized facility and not as a direct healing institution

A most curious case which ties together these principles comes from the Supreme Court of Arizona in *Fridena v. Evans*.[54] Following a motorcycle accident, the plaintiff was seen by Dr. Fridena who placed a pin in plaintiff's leg and hip. Later, at the defendant hospital, Dr. Fridena attempted a leg lengthening operation which was unsuccessful due to Dr. Fridena's alleged negligence. Dr. Fridena was an independent staff doctor of the hospital but he was also chief surgeon, chairman of the board of trustees, medical director, and controlling stockholder of the hospital. The court noted that except when acting as shareholder or while operating on his patients, Dr. Fridena was an agent of the hospital in these other roles. The court latched upon this point to supply what defendant hospital claimed was a missing element of plantiff's corporate liability claim—that the hospital had notice of the incompetency of Dr. Fridena. Because the law conclusively presumes that an agent will give notice to his principals of knowledge acquired by them in the scope of their authority, the court concluded that Dr. Fridena, in his role as agent, had knowledge imputable to the hospital regarding the competency of Dr. Fridena in his role of private surgeon. Finding that the hospital has a duty to supervise the quality of care rendered by independent staff physicians in the hospital, the court apparently held the hospital liable for Dr. Fridena's failure to supervise himself.[55]

Not every jurisdiction may recognize the liability of a hospital for negligence in monitoring the competency of its staff physicians, and those that do recognize such liability draw differing perimeters around its scope. Even in Illinois, where the *Darling*[56] case was decided nearly two decades ago, the courts have not expanded this rule to abnormal lengths. The hospital is not held to the standard of an insurer of the competency of its staff physicians; it does not warrant that they will do no harm. In *Pickle v. Curns*,[57] an Illinois Appellate Court refused to hold a hospital liable for the negligent administration of a electroconvulsive therapy by one of its staff physicians whom the plaintiff had independently employed. Other cases have likewise been reluctant to find any duty imposed upon the hospital from the failure to supervise

---

and should not intrude upon the decisions of a privately retained physician; *see also* Cooper v. Curry, 92 N.M. 417, 589 P.2d 201 (1979). *But see* Magana v. Elie, 108 Ill. App. 3d 1028, 439 N.E.2d 1319 (1982) (duty to require staff physician to give advice on risks of operation recognized).

[54] 127 Ariz. 516, 622 P.2d 463 (1981).

[55] *Id.* at 466-67.

[56] *Darling*, 211 N.E.2d 253 (1965).

[57] 106 Ill. App. 3d 734, 435 N.E.2d 877 (1982).

the acts of an independent staff physician personally engaged by the plaintiff.[58] Obviously, to state a viable cause of action against the hospital, something beyond the physician's negligence and a general allegation of the hospital's failure to supervise is required.

What is usually required to charge a violation of the hospital's duty to supervise an independent staff physician is evidence of awareness by hospital employees that the physician is mistreating his patient. When such facts can be alleged, the hospital cannot escape liability for resulting injuries on the ground that it had no obligation to interfere or to criticize the treatment rendered by an independent contractor. For example, in *Utter v. United Hospital Center, Inc.*,[59] the hospital was held liable for the negligence of the nurses who fail to observe or call attention to the worsening condition of plaintiff's limbs two days after casting by his doctor. The court noted that a nurse has a duty to seek consultation with the doctor if harboring any doubts about the care being provided to the patient. Similarly, in *Poor Sisters of St. Francis Seraph of Perpetual Adoration, Inc. v. Catron*,[60] nurses remained silent despite observing an endotracheal tube being left in a doctor's patient beyond the normal three days they knew to be proper. The court said:

> Thus, if a nurse or other hospital employee fails to report changes in a patient's condition and/or to question a doctor's orders when they are not in accord with standard medical practice and the omission results in injury to the patient, the hospital will be liable for its employee's negligence.[61]

§ 2.17   Corporate Liability: Enforcement of Rules and Regulations

Negligent supervision of patient care is only one theme which may be drawn from *Darling*.[62] *Darling* held the hospital liable not only because it failed to monitor the competency of the physician, but also because it failed to require consultation. To reach these conclusions the court looked to state regulations, the accreditation standards of the American Hospital Association, and the

---

[58] Jeffcoat v. Phillips, 534 S.W.2d 168 (Tex. Civ. App. 1976); Pedroza v. Bryant, 101 Wash. 2d 226, 677 P.2d 166 (1984).

[59] 236 S.E.2d 213 (W. Va. 1977).

[60] 435 N.E.2d 305 (Ind. Ct. App. 1982).

[61] *Id.* at 308.

[62] Darling v. Charleston Community Memorial Hosp., 33 Ill. 2d 326, 211 N.E.2d 253 (1965); see § **2.16.**

hospital's own by-laws to determine the nature of the duties owed by the hospital to its patient.

The granting of staff privileges, as has been noted, is similar to awarding someone membership to a private club. While the honor extends to the recipient certain benefits, it is also usual to require the member to follow certain established rules and regulations of the club.

The hospital, of course, is an institution, a corporation. As such it physically acts through its agents and employees, while its thoughts are expressed by its rules and regulations. These can cover a broad range of subjects, both administrative and operational, and a significant fraction deals directly with the quality of health care being rendered to its patients.

The hospital itself is not necessarily the author of all these rules and regulations. Some are mandated by agencies of the government, often establishing the minimum requirements for health care to which a hospital must affirm its compliance in order to be licensed by the state. A large number of these rules and regulations will be adapted from the standards promulgated by national organizations such as the Joint Commission for Hospital Accreditation. Finally, the hospital itself will promulgate by-laws governing its daily operations. Yet, regardless of the source, each rule or regulation attempts to fix a procedural protocol of tested efficacy and proven success.

There is some controversy respecting the role of rules and regulations as measures of the standard of care. This issue shall be discussed more fully in § 4.20. Here, the issue is not whether a particular rule should be followed, but whether a hospital may be liable for failing to enforce its rules and regulations. This issue will come up, of course, in those cases where a physician has failed to follow an established hospital policy and injury has resulted. If the hospital could have taken steps to assure that its policy would be followed by a staff physician, and the hospital failed to take those steps, then liability might be against the hospital.

Several cases demonstrate the potential liability of a hospital for its failure to promulgate proper rules or its failure to enforce its rules and regulations. *Magana v. Elie*,[63] may be viewed as a failure to promulgate rules case in that the Illinois Court of Appeals sustained a complaint charging the hospital with negligence in failing to require staff physicians to advise patients of the risks of and alternatives to surgery. *Utter v. United Hospital Center, Inc.*,[64] looked to the rules of the hospital's advisory department to find that hospital nurses had a duty to take action when observing improper medical treatment by a staff

---

[63] 108 Ill. App. 3d 1028, 439 N.E.2d 1319 (1982).

[64] 236 S.E.2d 213 (W. Va. 1977).

physician. In *Johnson v. St. Bernard Hospital*,[65] the hospital was found liable for failure to use reasonable efforts to assist an emergency room to obtain a consultation as required by its by-laws. Finally, in *Duckett v. North Detroit General Hospital*,[66] where the evidence showed that a 16 year old hospital patient had not been seen by a doctor for two days, the Michigan Court of Appeals found that the hospital had violated the state's administrative code which required hospital patients to be seen by a physician daily.

What these cases establish is that the modern hospital owes a duty of care to a patient which often transcends the physician-patient relationship between the patient and his own private doctor. The hospital must take steps to assure that in granting and continuing staff privileges to private physicians that they have the qualifications and skills to perform medical treatment within these privileges competently. When the hospital, through its employees, sees that a patient is not being rendered proper treatment by his physician, then it must take appropriate action to correct the situation. The hospital must follow regulations and promulgate proper rules for the well being of its patients, and it must also see to the enforcement of those rules or be held liable for injuries caused by the breach.[67] In sum, as we have repeatedly emphasized, the hospital must play an active role in responding to the health care needs of its patients, and may be held accountable when it fails to take action to protect patients from violations of the standard of care by independent staff physicians under the special circumstances described here.

---

[65] 79 Ill. App. 3d 709, 399 N.E.2d 198 (1979); *see also* Kakligian v. Henry Ford Hosp., 48 Mich. App. 325, 210 N.W.2d 463 (1973).

[66] 84 Mich. App. 426, 269 N.W.2d 626 (1978).

[67] Of course, in order to be liable in damages to the injured patient, the breach of duty by the hospital must be a proximate cause of the injury. Thus in Ferguson v. Gonyaw, 64 Mich. App. 685, 236 N.W.2d 543 (1976), the court agreed that a hospital has a duty to assure that physicians granted staff privileges are competent, but found that the evidence failed to disclose that had a proper investigation of the physician's credentials been undertaken that the decision to grant staff privileges would have differed. In Bost v. Riley, 44 N.C. App. 638, 262 S.E.2d 391 (1980), the court recognized that the hospital was negligent in not enforcing its bylaw requiring the keeping of progress notes, but found the injuries not to have been proximately caused by their neglect.

HOSPITAL EMPLOYEES

§ 2.18   Liability and Settlement

In addition to physicians and hospitals, the individual employees of the hospital—interns, nurses, residents, technicians, and so forth—are personally liable for their own acts of malpractice or negligence which cause injury to a patient. Although in most malpractice cases arising from the negligent act of a hospital's (physician's) employee, the preferred or target defendant will be the hospital itself (or the physician), in many cases counsel must seriously weigh the merits of also naming the actual errant employee as a defendant. The decision to name the employee should not be automatic. If the employee makes a sympathetic defendant or there are indications that the employee may be more cooperative if left out of the suit, then the wiser course may be to reach some accommodation with the employee before trial to gain a tactical advantage in the case.

That an agent or employee remains personally liable for his torts despite acting on behalf of a corporation is an axiom of tort law requiring no further elaboration. Counsel should be conscious, however, of the relationship between the tortfeasor and the vicarious liability of the principal or employer. This becomes particularly important when a settlement with one of the tortfeasors is contemplated. At common law, in many jurisdictions, the *release* of the agent or employee was deemed the release of the vicariously liable principal or employer, and vice versa.[68] Consequently, caution should be exercised in reaching a settlement with a nurse, intern, resident, or other employee to avoid entering into any agreement which might be construed to release the hospital from liability. In some jurisdictions the common law snare can be avoided by entering into *covenant not to sue* rather than a release.[69] The agent or employee seeking to avoid further litigation by settlement should have no objection to accepting a covenant not to sue in lieu of a formal release, thereby avoiding any unintentional compromise of claims against nonsettling defendants.

---

[68] Charouleau v. Charity Hosp., 319 So. 2d 464 (La. Ct. App. 1974); Smith v. Flint School Dist., 80 Mich. App. 630, 264 N.W.2d 368 (1978); Ericksen v. Pearson, 211 Neb. 466, 319 N.W.2d 76 (1982).

[69] Thomas v. Checker Cab Co., 66 Mich. App. 152, 238 N.W.2d 558 (1975). *But see* Holcomb v. Flavin, 34 Ill. 2d 558, 216 N.E.2d 811 (1967).

CHAPTER 3

PARTIES PLAINTIFF

§ 3.1   Birth Trauma Plaintiffs

§ 3.2   Fetal Injuries

§ 3.3   Injuries at or after Birth

§ 3.1   Birth Trauma Plaintiffs

Having looked at the potential defendants in a medical malpractice suit in **Chapter 2**, some brief consideration of the plaintiffs is in order. In most medical malpractice cases the identities of the parties plaintiff are not hard to discern. The principal plaintiff is the party injured, physically or mentally, by the alleged negligent acts of the physician and/or hospital. Should the injury be fatal, his estate shall be the plaintiff under an appropriate wrongful death act. A spouse of the injured plaintiff may join the suit to pursue a loss of consortium claim. Birth trauma cases, however, often present an unusual set of circumstances because the individual most likely harmed by malpractice is either an unborn or a newborn child. Such harm to the child may accompany harm to the mother or to both parents of the child. Special problems may arise with divorced or putative fathers, stepfathers, and perhaps someday, with surrogate mothers. Under some circumstances only the child might have a cause of action, whereas other circumstances would permit only the parent to state a claim.

For example, in wrongful birth or wrongful life actions (these are discussed in detail in **Chapter 8**), only the parents will have a cause of action. The gravamen of a *wrongful birth claim* is that the parents have become financially burdened with a normal, but unplanned child.[1] In *wrongful life claims* the child is victimized by birth defects which are not directly attributable to the defendants, and the law of most jurisdictions recognizing a claim for

---

[1] Of course, the mother may also recover damages for any personal pain or suffering resulting from the pregnancy and delivery. *See* Troppi v. Scarf, 31 Mich. App. 240, 187 N.W.2d 511 (1971).

wrongful life permits the parents, but not the child, to recover damages resulting from these birth defects.[2]

Wrongful birth and wrongful life claims involved unique problems not typical of most birth trauma or infant injury cases. Usually, these cases focus on a direct injury to the child by the negligence of the defendant. Such an injury can occur before, during, or after the birth of the child.

§ 3.2 Fetal Injuries

When a fetus is injured through the negligence of a third party, provided the injury is not fatal, according to the modern weight of authority, a cause of action may be brought on the child's behalf to recover damages for any birth defects attributable to that injury.[3] If the injuries are fatal, however, causing the death of the fetus, either in the womb or shortly after birth, then case law is divided as to whether a separate wrongful death claim can be brought on behalf of the child's estate. In some cases an attempt has been made to distinguish between a viable (capable of sustaining life outside the womb) and a nonviable fetus. Courts have held that there is no action for wrongful death which may be maintained on behalf of a fatally injured nonviable fetus.[4] Other cases have ignored the issue of viability, indicating that if the fetus does not survive birth it does not become a person for whom a wrongful death action may be brought.[5] In either situation, only the parents may have any cause of action for their personal injuries or loss. Where wrongful death actions are allowed for a fatally injured fetus,[6] appropriate pleadings on behalf of the unborn's estate should be filed.

---

[2] Becker v. Schwartz, 46 N.Y.2d 401, 386 N.E.2d 807, 413 N.Y.S.2d 895 (1978); *see also* Eisbrenner v. Stanley, 106 Mich. App. 351, 308 N.W.2d 209 (1981); Jacobs v. Theimer, 519 S.W.2d 846 (Tex. 1975); Dumer v. St. Michael's Hosp., 69 Wis. 2d 766, 233 N.W.2d 372 (1975). *But see* Procanik v. Cillo, 97 N.J. 339, 478 A.2d 755 (1984).

[3] Womack v. Buckhorn, 384 Mich. 718, 187 N.W.2d 218 (1971).

[4] Rapp v. Hiemenz, 107 Ill. App. 2d 382, 246 N.E.2d 77 (1969); Toth v. Goree, 65 Mich. App. 296, 237 N.W.2d 297 (1975); Poliquin v. MacDonald, 101 N.H. 104, 135 A.2d 249 (1957).

[5] McKillip v. Zimmerman, 191 N.W.2d 706 (Iowa 1971); Leccese v. McDonough, 361 Mass. 64, 279 N.E.2d 339 (1972).

[6] O'Neill v. Morse, 385 Mich. 130, 188 N.W.2d 785 (1971) (death of eight month old viable fetus *en ventre sa mere*).

§ 3.3 Injuries at or after Birth

When the child is injured during or after birth, then no difficulty arises in recognizing the child's own cause of action. However, the child is under a legal disability because of her minority and will have to sue through a guardian, next friend, personal representative, or whatever appropriate designee is required under the laws of the jurisdiction where suit is pursued.

The separate claims of the parents cannot be ignored. In **Chapter 6**, the distinct damages recoverable by parents, and by injured minors, are discussed in detail. What is important is the recognition that when a child is injured, her parents also have their own separate claim for damages resulting because of the child's injuries (loss of support, loss of society and companionship, medical expenses). Also, in many birth trauma cases it is not unusual to find that the mother has herself sustained some personal injury for which a claim should be asserted.

A principle concern in birth trauma cases is to bring suit within the limitations period. While the infancy of the injured child usually tolls the statute of limitations, the statute will run against the claims of her parents. Because these separate parental claims may be substantial, counsel should make every effort to preserve these claims against the bar of the limitations statute.

CHAPTER 4

STANDARD OF CARE

§ 4.1   Standard of Care in Malpractice Cases

The cause of action which is most likely to arise from injuries sustained as a result of a traumatic birth is one for medical malpractice. The word, malpractice, unfortunately, all too often conjures up an image of some specialized species of the law that lies beyond the understanding of the average legal practitioner and which strikes fear into the heart of a medical professional. Let us take a moment, at the outset, to demystify this concept.

Malpractice is the liability which the law imposes on the professional acts of a person licensed to practice a specialized calling. Traditionally, it was a term applied only to physicians and attorneys, although in some jurisdictions this term has been extended to other licensed professionals.[1] What is important to keep in mind, however, is that regardless of who may be sued in malpractice, the essential nature of the suit is one of professional negligence—the failure of the defendant to exercise the reasonable care required by professional standards. When we remember that malpractice is merely a form of negligence—a professional's negligence—and thus subject to the same four elements applied in all negligence cases—duty, breach, proximate cause, and damages—then the concept becomes one which can be more readily analyzed and understood.

While malpractice law in a particular jurisdiction may be surrounded by certain procedural idiosyncracies that give it an identity separate from that of the general negligence cases in the jurisdiction (such as a shorter statute of limitations and peculiar restrictions on evidence), the only essential feature that distinguishes a malpractice case from other torts is the applicable standard of care. In general, our common law imposes upon all persons (including legal persons, such as corporations) an obligation to exercise reasonable care under the circumstances. The standard against which human actions are measured is, of course, the standard of what a hypothetical reasonable person of ordinary care and prudence would do under the circumstances. Even doctors and lawyers who are acting outside of their professional capacities are subject to this same standard, for obviously their professional standing does not entitle them to special treatment when they engage in nonprofessional activities.

However, the law presumes that persons whose profession calls upon them to exercise professional judgment, a judgment based upon precepts lying outside the common knowledge of an average lay person, must exercise a degree of care which is measured against the standards of their profession. Malpractice, quite simply, is a breach of this standard—the failure to exercise the care which a similar professional of ordinary prudence and care would exercise under the same or similar circumstances.

Of necessity, this measure of negligence, this standard of care, is not a fixed or predetermined pattern of behavior which can be categorized for each and every circumstance which arises in a professional activity. The medical professional, in applying special skills to the treatment of a patient, does not always follow a fixed set of commonly known guidelines like a car following traffic signs along the road. The signs (symptoms) that guide his response to the patient require special knowledge to interpret; often the appropriate re-

---

[1] See Sam v. Balardo, 411 Mich. 405, 308 N.W.2d 142 (1981).

sponse to a medical problem requires the professional to use his best judgment in the selection of one course of treatment over several alternatives. Consider, for example, the decision to induce labor through chemical means. At what stage of labor is such action justified? At what stage of labor will its application be truly beneficial to the mother and child? What are the risks involved and how should these be balanced against the benefits? Most importantly, from a legal standpoint, when can it be said that in balancing the risks against the benefits, the doctor made a mistake in either failing to induce labor, waiting too long to induce labor, or acting too precipitously to induce labor? The average layperson, which is to say, the average juror, is simply without sufficient training, knowledge or experience to properly evaluate these issues. To simply present the bare facts to a jury ("defendant induced labor at 10:30, three hours after the mother's membrane ruptured") and to ask the jury of untrained laypersons to reach a decision regarding the reasonableness and prudence of the physician's actions is, of course, absurd and illogical. The jury needs the additional guidance of being informed what the standard of care requires.

This chapter discusses the concept of standard of care from several points of view. Who creates this standard? What is the standard of care under particular circumstances? Under what circumstances will proof of the standard of care be rendered unnecessary? And, most importantly, how is the standard of care to be proven—which is really an evidentiary issue, but one so crucial to the litigation of a malpractice case and so intimately tied to these other issues, that it needs to be presented as part of this general discussion.

§ 4.2   The Measure of Duty—Generally

In the ordinary negligence case, the acts of the defendant are measured against the standard of a reasonable person of ordinary prudence. This character of legal fabrication has, of course, no real point of reference. The law has no particular individual in mind. This reasonably prudent person is a hypothetical creation, nonexistent except in the common sense and experience of each juror which contributes ultimately to a collective judgment of what behavior is safe, proper, reasonable, and prudent, and what behavior, failing those tests, constitutes negligence. In the broadest, most philosophical perspective, society as a whole creates this standard of care. More pragmatically, we might simply say that this reasonably prudent person is a tool created by the courts to fix some parameters upon a negligence action.

In a case of professional negligence, this general measure of the standard of care breaks down and fails to provide an appropriate legal measure for a professional's performance of his services. Clearly, a physician's actions, in most cases, which are determined by his special skill, education and training, are not comparable to the actions of the ordinary layperson of reasonable prudence. It follows that a different or amended standard is required, and by a simple process of logic it is apparent that a physician's conduct should be measured against the acts of a reasonable physician of ordinary prudence acting in the same or similar circumstances.

Unfortunately, this logical solution is incomplete. The reasonable person of ordinary prudence, as we have seen, is a purely hypothetical being, created out of the common sense of the community. However, the hypothetical, reasonable physician of ordinary prudence does not exist in the average layperson's experience. To find this person, the jury must receive guidance. The *standard of care* in a medical malpractice case is ultimately based not on the actions of an imaginary prudent physician, but upon the actual behavior of fellow physicians from which a jury can construct or comprehend the conduct against which the acts of defendant are to be measured. In a very real sense, as some courts have observed, the medical profession itself sets the standard of care.

The real dilemma of establishing this standard of professional medical care lies in determining the breadth of the control group to be surveyed to establish the requisite standard. The practice of medicine is compartmentalized and specialized; there are different schools of practice and different specialities within each school. While each individual doctor adds his contribution to the medical community, at the same time each individual practitioner learns from, and has his conduct governed by the precepts established by either the medical community as a whole or by a particular group of physicians pursuing specialized skills. Consequently, at one extreme the standard of care could be measured against the conduct of all other medical professionals in all the disciplines of all the schools of practice. At the other extreme, recognizing that no two doctors ever treat their respective patients exactly the same, the standard of care might be measured simply against the acts of an individual practitioner. Both extremes, of course, are unworkable, so the courts have devised rules which find a standard of care, depending upon the circumstances, pulsating somewhere in between.

In so doing the courts have attempted to give recognition to the various disciplines through which medicine is provided to patients in this country so that the standard of care is customized according to the school of practice of the defendant. The courts also acknowledge the different degree of skill separating specialists from general practitioners, which also modifies the standard of care. In addition, factors such as the state of scientific knowledge, the availability of medical facilities and auxiliary personnel, and, in some states, social or political demographics, have also influenced the standard of care.

§ 4.3   —Standard of Care Related to Disciplines

The practice of medicine is fragmented for historical reasons beyond the scope of this work. There are obvious distinctions between dentists and medical doctors (M.D.s, also called allopaths), for example, and less obvious ones between M.D.s and osteopaths (D.O.s). The licensing laws of most states reflect this fragmented nature of medical practice by providing for the separate licensure of medical doctors, osteopaths, chiropractors, dentists, optometrists, podiatrists, registered nurses, licensed practical nurses, dermatologists, and psychiatrists—to name some of the usual professions regulated by legislation.

Similarly, the case law of malpractice acknowledges this array of professions by restricting the standard of care applicable to a particular defendant to that discipline the defendant professes to practice. The law presumes that one who seeks out an osteopath or chiropractor for treatment, expects to receive the type of treatment practiced by that school of medicine, and the obligation of the doctor is only to render the care mandated by his own discipline.[2] Consequently, it is uniformly recognized that a professional defendant shall only be liable to a plaintiff if the defendant breached the standard of care followed within his own school.[3]

An exception to this, which applies not only here, but generally, is that regardless of the school, discipline, or speciality of the practitioner, when he proceeds to render treatment which lies beyond the scope of his licensed profession, then he will be held to the standard of care of the discipline into which he is intruding.[4]

Most birth trauma cases will involve claims against medical doctors or osteopaths and the applicable standard of care, depending on which discipline is involved, shall be either the standard of care for medical doctors or that of osteopathic doctors. This is the first criteria which must be met, and in preparing any suit against a doctor, the attorney for the plaintiff must keep in mind that he will be required to prove the standard of care as it exists for the discipline practiced by the particular defendant being sued.

---

[2] State v. Smith, 25 Idaho 541, 138 P. 1107 (1914); Van Sickle v. Doolittle, 173 Iowa 727, 155 N.W. 1007 (1918); Janssen v. Mulder, 232 Mich. 183, 205 N.W. 159 (1925). Some of these early cases also express the fear that an expert from one discipline may be biased against the practices of a competing discipline. *See, e.g.,* Force v. Gregory, 63 Conn. 167, 27 A.1116 (1893).

[3] Bryant v. Biggs, 331 Mich. 64, 49 N.W.2d 63 (1951); Bush v. Cress, 181 Minn. 590, 233 N.W. 317 (1930); Forthofer v. Arnold, 60 Ohio App. 430, 21 N.W.2d 869 (1938); Floyd v. Michie, 71 S.W.2d 657 (Tex. Civ. App. 1928); Ennis v. Banks, 95 Wash. 513, 164 P. 58 (1917).

[4] Kelly v. Carroll, 36 Wash. 2d 482, 219 P.2d 79 (1950) (holding chiropractor subject to standard of care of medical doctor).

§ 4.4 — Standard of Care Related to Specialty

Just as case law has uniformly recognized that each medical practitioner should be held to the standard of his or her own school of discipline, so also have the cases uniformly stated that a specialist, within any school or discipline, is held to the standard of care of similar specialists and not to the standard of care of the average general practitioner.[5]

Yet, while the various jurisdictions are in complete agreement with this distinction drawn between specialists and general practitioners, there is less agreement with what this means in terms of actual legal practice. First of all, when is a practioner a specialist? Several cases apply the specialist standard of care to one who simply holds himself out to be a specialist.[6] While such a rule is workable, it may create problems if the defendant should deny that he ever held himself out as a specialist, even though he has limited his practice to one area. An alternative approach may be to hold a physician to the standards of a specialist if he acts as a specialist.[7] An even more practical test is whether or not the physician has been board certified, which is usually the requirement which must be met in order to represent oneself as a specialist.[8]

Having determined that the physician is a specialist, what practical effect does this have on the standard of care? As will be discussed in §§ **4.5** and **4.6**, one of the critical restrictions on establishing standard of care is the *locality* or *similar community rule* which requires proof of what the standard of care is in a particular area. In some states this locality rule is not altered by a finding that the defendant is a specialist, for his actions will still be judged by the standard of care of specialists practicing in the same or in similar communities.[9] In other jurisdictions, where the locality rule is still applied to general

---

[5] Barnes v. Bovenmyer, 255 Iowa 220, 122 N.W.2d 312 (1963); Naccarato v. Grob, 384 Mich. 248, 180 N.W.2d 788 (1970); Park v. Chessin, 88 Misc. 2d 222, 387 N.Y.S.2d 204 (1976); Belk v. Schweizer, 268 N.C. 50, 149 S.E.2d 565 (1966).

[6] Valentine v. Kaiser Found. Hosps., 194 Cal. App. 2d 282, 15 Cal. Rptr. 26 (1961); McClarin v. Grenzfelder, 147 Mo. App. 478, 126 S.W. 817 (1910); Belk v. Schweizer, 268 N.C. 50, 149 S.E.2d 565 (1966).

[7] *See* Pratt v. Stein, 298 Pa. Super. 92, 444 A.2d 674 (1982) (hospital resident held to standard of a specialist when the resident is acting within his field of specialty); *see also* McCullough v. Hutzel Hosp., 88 Mich. App. 235, 276 N.W.2d 569 (1979); Larson v. Yelle, 310 Minn. 521, 246 N.W.2d 841 (1976); *cf.* Callaghan v. William Beaumont Hosp., 67 Mich. App. 306, 240 N.W.2d 781 (1976) (specialist doing rotation in emergency room held to general standard of care when acting outside his specialty).

[8] *See* Roberts v. Tardif, 417 A.2d 444 (Me. 1980); Francisco v. Parchment Medical Clinic, P.C., 407 Mich. 325, 285 N.W.2d 39 (1979).

[9] Poulin v. Zartman, 542 P.2d 251 (Alaska 1975); Carmichael v. Reitz, 17 Cal. App. 3d 958, 95 Cal. Rptr. 381 (1971); Halligan v. Cotton, 193 Neb. 331, 227 N.W.2d 10 (1975); Belk v.

practitioners, a finding that the defendant is a specialist will subject him to a general *nationwide* or *universal standard*.[10] See § **4.7** for a discussion of the universal standard.

Whether judged by a locality or nationwide standard, the specialist will be expected to bring to his care of his patients the special degree of skill normally possessed by other specialists who have devoted special study to the disease or injury involved, having regard to the state of scientific knowledge.[11] An unusual case which emphasizes this last point is *Toth v. Community Hosp. at Glen Cove*.[12] In this New York case a pediatrician had authorized the administration of oxygen to twins incubated shortly after birth. As a result of such treatment the children suffered blindness. Although the case involved many issues, including the physician's liability for the failure of the hospital nurses to carry out his orders (the court found that he could be held liable for his own failure to check on whether his orders were being properly carried out), the discussion of the standard of care is especially worth noting. Conceding that the law "generally permits the medical profession to establish its own standard of care," the court nevertheless rejected the pediatrician's argument that he should not be held liable for the administration of oxygen to the infants since at the time his treatment fell within the acceptable practice of the community. As the evidence showed that defendant was himself knowledgeable of the risks of such treatment and was acquainted with scientific evidence critical of this medical practice, the court found that his mere adherence to what the standard of care of his fellow practitioners would allow was insufficient.

> Evidence that the defendant followed customary practice is not the sole test of professional malpractice, the court said. If a physician fails to employ his expertise or best judgment, and that omission causes injury, he should not automatically be freed from liability because in fact he adhered to acceptable practice. There is no policy reason why a physician, who knows or believes there are unnecessary dangers in the community practice, should not be required to take whatever precautionary measures are deemed appropriate.[13]

Schweizer, 268 N.C. 50, 149 S.E.2d 565 (1966). Some of these decisions are influenced by statutes specifically enforcing a locality rule.

[10] Shilkret v. Annapolis Emergency Hosp. Ass'n, 276 Md. 187, 349 A.2d 245 (1975); Naccarato v. Grob, 384 Mich. 248, 180 N.W.2d 788 (1970); Freed v. Priore, 247 Pa. Super. 418, 372 A.2d 895 (1977); Shier v. Freedman, 58 Wis. 2d 269, 206 N.W.2d 166 (1973).

[11] Grosjean v. Spencer, 258 Iowa 685, 140 N.W.2d 139 (1966); Wood v. Vroman, 215 Mich. 449, 184 N.W. 520 (1921); McClarin v. Grenzfelder, 147 Mo. App. 478, 126 S.W. 817 (1910); Lewis v. Read, 80 N.J. Super. 148, 193 A.2d 255 (1963).

[12] 22 N.Y.2d 255, 239 N.E.2d 368, 292 N.Y.S.2d 440 (1968).

[13] 239 N.E.2d at 373.

The specialist, therefore, will be expected to exercise sound judgment, and that judgment will be measured against the light of scientific knowledge. This may be viewed as a higher standard of care. In fact, it is merely a more exacting standard of care which does not allow the specialist to avoid liability if all he has done for the patient is to provide the average care of a general practitioner.

In birth trauma or infant injury cases, especial attention should be given to the standard of care applicable to specialists in the jurisdiction, for in most instances the physician subject to a birth trauma or an infant injury claim will fall into one of two categories widely recognized as specialties of medical practice—obstetrics-gynecology (OB-GYN), or pediatrics. Many cases have recognized that obstetrician-gynecologists and pediatricians are specialists and are held to the standard of care of specialists.[14]

§ 4.5 —Standard of Care and the Locality Rule

When suing a physician, the standard of care should reasonably be that followed by all similar physicians in the same discipline under the same or similar circumstances. Such a rule would be a simple adaptation from the broader negligence standard of care which required individuals to act as a reasonably prudent person would act in the same or similar circumstances. In general negligence cases, there is no locality rule. One would not expect that to prove negligence it would be necessary to show what reasonable and prudent behavior in a particular community would be, for it is inconceivable that standards of reasonable care would vary from place to place. However, in medical malpractice cases, tradition and precedent have saddled litigants with a curious quirk in the law known as the locality rule.

The rule appears to have originated in American jurisprudence in the 1870s.[15] At the time it was supported by the rationale that a small town or

---

[14] Pediatricians: Poulin v. Zartman, 542 P.2d 251 (Alaska 1975); Shilkret v. Annapolis Emergency Hosp. Ass'n, 276 Md. 187, 349 A.2d 245 (1975); Naccarato v. Grob, 384 Mich. 248, 180 N.W.2d 788 (1970); Koury v. Follo, 272 N.C. 366, 158 S.E.2d 548 (1968). Obstetricians/gynecologists: Robbins v. Footer, 553 F.2d 123 (D.C. Cir. 1977); Harris v. Campbell, 2 Ariz. App. 351, 409 P.2d 67 (1965); Carmichael v. Reitz, 17 Cal. App. 3d 958, 95 Cal. Rptr. 381 (1971); Fitzmaurice v. Flynn, 167 Conn. 609, 356 A.2d 887 (1975); Steele v. St. Paul Fire & Marine Ins. Co., 371 So. 2d 843 (La. Ct. App. 1979); Roberts v. Tardif, 417 A.2d 444 (Me. 1980); Shilkret v. Annapolis Emergency Hosp. Ass'n, 276 Md. 187, 349 A.2d 245 (1975); Halligan v. Cotton, 193 Neb. 331, 227 N.W.2d 10 (1975); Lewis v. Read, 80 N.J. Super. 148, 193 A.2d 255 (1963); Belk v. Schweizer, 268 N.C. 50, 149 S.E.2d 565 (1966); Bly v. Rhoads, 216 Va. 645, 222 S.E.2d 783 (1976).

[15] The roots of the locality rule have been traced to Tefft v. Wilcox, 6 Kan. 46 (1870); Smothers v. Hanks, 34 Iowa 286 (1872); and Hathorn v. Richmond, 48 Vt. 557 (1876),

rural medical practitioner should not be held to the same sophisticated standard of care which might be found in metropolitan areas. Thus, in a sense, the rule was a response to the urbanization of society when medical advances taking place in larger communities might not reach, or be available to, the general practitioner residing in the smaller towns or rural areas of the country. At a time when communication was still by telegraph and mail, and transportation by railroad or horse and buggy, this locality restriction on the standard of care seemed both sensible and necessary to protect small town and rural doctors from being held liable for failing to treat their patients in accordance with improved techniques which might not be known or available to them.

Unfortunately, the rule has outlasted its rationale, lingering into this century of electronic communications and rapid transportation. The minority of physicians who continue to serve the needs of our residual rural and small town citizens have continual access to medical information that keeps them abreast of the present state of medical and scientific knowledge. In fact, it could be argued that any physician who fails to keep current with such knowledge is guilty of inexcusable neglect towards his professional responsibilities.

The original locality rule has come under increasing attack, and it has been significantly modified over the years in many jurisdictions in response to valid criticisms of its harshness and unfairness. Before briefly reviewing these trends, the scope of the rule and the nature of the criticisms should be noted.

The original locality rule, as expressed in some of the earliest cases, suggested (it is not absolutely clear that they mandated) that a physician's standard of care should be measured by the standard of care of doctors in the same "neighborhood" or "locality."[16] This *strict locality rule*, rejected in the majority of jurisdictions, essentially says that in determining the standard of care applicable to a physician—or, more importantly, in determining whether or not he breached that standard of care—the courts would not look beyond the practices of the physicians professionally servicing the same locality. This strict rule allowed the medical community of which the defendant was a member to establish, in effect, its own standard of care, one which outsiders could not criticize.

The two most obvious defects of this rule were, first, that this often allowed a small medical community to establish whatever standard of care it wished, to the detriment of the public being served, and, second, that in a close-knit medical community it became virtually impossible for a plaintiff to find a witness in the locality who was familiar with the local standard of care and willing to testify against a fellow physician. It was this draconian doctrine of law

---

although possibly the most influential early decision was Small v. Howard, 128 Mass. 131, 35 Am. Rep. 363 (1880).

[16] Tefft v. Wilcox, 6 Kan. 46 (1870); Small v. Howard, 128 Mass. 131, 35 Am. Rep. 363 (1880).

which gave life to the popular conception that there was a conspiracy of silence among medical professionals which obstructed plaintiffs seeking to recover damages from a doctor. It was believed, rightly or wrongly, that when a doctor in a community was sued, the other doctors, out of professional pride, friendship, and self-preservation, closed ranks behind the sued doctor and mutely protected him from accusations of having breached their local standard of care.[17]

§ 4.6 —Modifications of the Locality Rule

Recognizing the injustice of permitting a lone practitioner in a community, or a small close-knit group of practitioners, to set the standard of care for themselves, thereby precluding any injured patient from ever obtaining redress no matter how gross defendant's medical mistreatment might be, most jurisdictions adopting the locality rule also adopted some modification of this rule. A few jurisdictions have expanded the locality to include the entire state, so that the standard of care is that established by the practice of physicians with the same state as the defendant.[18] However, by far the most common rule now prevailing in this country is the *same or similar communities rule* whereby a physician's actions are measured against the standard of care operative in his own locality or in any community which is *similar* to the one in which he practices.

This same or similar localities rule is an improvement over the strict locality rule for it opens the door to a plaintiff to secure expert testimony from outside the defendant's own community. If an expert can establish that he practices in, or is familiar with, the practices of a community similar to defendant's, then he may be able to provide evidence of the standard of care and how it was breached by the defendant.

However, this modified locality is not without flaws, as will be noted later in this section. Hence, a few courageous courts have taken the bold steps of abolishing the locality rule, either generally, or at least as it applies to specialists.[19] In so doing, these courts have recognized that radical changes in medi-

---

[17] *See* Shilkret v. Annapolis Emergency Hosp. Ass'n, 276 Md. 187, 349 A.2d 245 (1975) for a summary of criticisms of the locality rule.

[18] *See, e.g.*, Fitzmaurice v. Flynn, 167 Conn. 609, 356 A.2d 887 (1975); King v. Murphy, 424 So. 2d 547 (Miss. 1982). Such a standard has also been adopted by statute in Virginia, Va. Code § 8.01-581.20 (1984), and Washington, Wash. Rev. Code Ann. § 7.70.040 (Supp. 1985).

[19] *E.g.*, Blair v. Eblen, 461 S.W.2d 370 (Ky. 1970); Shilkret v. Annapolis Emergency Hosp. Ass'n, 276 Md. 187, 349 A.2d 245 (1975); Pederson v. Dumouchel, 72 Wash. 2d 73, 431

cal practice since the 1870s have abolished the need to rely upon geographical factors in determining the standard of care. In *Shilkret v. Annapolis Emergency Hospital Association*,[20] the Maryland Court of Appeals stated:

> We agree with these courts that justification for the locality rules no longer exists. The modern physician bears little resemblance to his predecessors. As we have indicated at length, the medical schools of yesterday could not possibly compare with the accredited institutions of today, many of which are associated with teaching hospitals. But the contrast merely begins at that point in the medical career: vastly superior postgraduate training, the dynamic impact of modern communications and transportation, the proliferation of medical literature, frequent seminars and conferences on a variety of professional subjects, and the growing availability of modern clinical facilities are but some of the developments in the medical profession which combine to produce contemporary standards that are not only much higher than they were just a few short years ago, but also are national in scope.
>
> In sum, the traditional locality rules no longer fit the present-day medical malpractice case.[21]

The locality rule can be abolished without doing violence to the original factual premises on which it was based. Through modern communications, the standardization of most medical training and continuation of education through national organizations have virtually eliminated the importance of most local factors which may have once had an influence on the quality of medical services in a particular community; however, abandonment of the locality rule does not mean that such local factors need to be ignored where they still may have an impact upon the standard of care. Certainly, a doctor in a small rural town should not be criticized for failing to employ some medical treatment regularly employed by fellow professionals in a major city when that technique requires the utilization of medical facilities which are not available to him. These are factual differences which can be developed in litigation without resort to any artificial limitation based upon geography alone.

Unfortunately, despite the obvious erosion of the rationale supporting the continued application of the locality rule to standard of care, in the majority of jurisdictions this demographic requirement remains viable. As discussed in § 7.6, the legislatures in some states where the locality rule was in jeopardy have passed statutes preserving some form of locality rule. In other states the courts have simply rejected invitations to abolish the rule. Consequently, for

---

P.2d 973 (1967). *But see* Wash. Rev. Code Ann. § 7.70.040 (Supp. 1985); Shier v. Freedman, 58 Wis. 2d 269, 206 N.W.2d 166 (1973).

[20] 276 Md. 187, 349 A.2d 245 (1975).

[21] *Id.*

most attorneys pursuing a birth trauma claim, the locality rule, either in its strict, statewide, or similar communities form must be directly confronted.

In adopting the similar communities modification, many jurisdictions have eliminated the worst features of the strict locality rule which contributed to the conspiracy of silence and the difficulty of finding cooperative expert witnesses. However, the principal failing of the similar communities rule is that no fixed criteria exists for determining when communities are sufficiently similar to allow a physician from one community to testify against a physician in a different community. Courts have not clearly articulated the demographic criteria which must be met to qualify the proposed expert from a different community. Some factors have been noted, such as the size of the communities, respective populations, geographical proximity to one another or to a common metropolitan area, and the availability of similar hospital facilities,[22] however, there are no hard or fixed rules for determining when communities are sufficiently similar so that an expert familiar with the standards of a community like that of defendant's can describe the standard of care. Consequently, the similar communities rule still leaves an attorney fairly much at the mercy of the trial judge who, having been presented with such evidence, might nevertheless conclude that a proper foundation for the expert's testimony has not been laid.

§ 4.7 —Towards a "Universal" Standard of Care

As noted in § 4.6, in many cases specialists have been held to be subject to a nationwide standard of care. Some cases have recognized that despite the continued application of a locality rule, certain medical practices have become so standard that no variation exists from one community to the next. Hence, while still adhering to the basic premise of a locality rule, an expert from outside of defendant's community may often be qualified to testify to the standard of care applicable to the defendant simply by demonstrating that the medical issues relate to a practice or procedure which is *universally* recognized, and thus, by logical progression, is a practice or procedure necessarily followed in defendant's locality.

In *Webb v. Jorns*,[23] for example, plaintiff's expert testified respecting the administration of anesthesia that "there are certain minimum safe and ac-

---

[22] *See, e.g.*, Slayton v. Brunner, 276 Ark. 143, 633 S.W.2d 29 (1982) (similar hospital facilities); Sinz v. Owens, 33 Cal. 2d 749, 205 P.2d 3 (1949) (defendant's and expert's communities both satellites of the same metropolitan area); Kirchuer v. Dorsey & Dorsey, 226 Iowa 283, 284 N.W. 171 (1939) (expert familiar with standards in towns the same size as defendant's).

[23] 488 S.W.2d 407 (Tex. 1973).

cepted practices and procedures that cannot vary in any locality or between nurses and anesthesiologists, since the human tolerance to certain conditions is uniform and apply to all persons wherever they may be." The Texas Supreme Court, while nodding to the community standards rule, acknowledged that the trial court had discretion in applying the rule since any other treatment of the rule "would mean that some communities would be measured by standards which fall below those universally regarded as ordinary medical standards."[24] Similarly, in *Clapham v. Yanga*,[25] a wrongful birth case from Michigan, where the locality rule still prevails as to general practitioners, the court of appeals rejected the claim of defendant, a general practitioner, that the trial court had erred in failing to instruct the jury in accordance with the same or similar communities standard. Noting that the case involved defendant's failure to conduct a pregnancy test when his patient displayed symptoms of pregnancy, the court said:

> In *LeBlanc v. Lentini*, 82 Mich. App. 5, 17-19, 266 N.W.2d 643 (1978), lv den 403 Mich. 807 (1978), this Court recognized that in some cases local standards might be uniform throughout the United States. After reaching this conclusion, the Court upheld a decision to allow a medical expert to testify on the standard of care in the local area, even though he was unfamiliar with the locale. The record in this case suggests that such a nationwide locality standard exists in respect to the tests and treatment to be performed on one who has missed menstrual periods and complains of dizzy spells and fainting. This being the case, it would make no difference if the standard of care instruction was tied to a specific locality or explicitly posited as having nationwide applicability. While the latter instruction would be technically defective, since the substantive standard is the same, it would be unnecessary and inappropriate to reverse the case for a new trial.[26]

A few other cases have acknowledged that local standards may be universal or uniform throughout the country,[27] and that an expert familiar with the nationwide standard may testify to that standard of care. Such cases may encourage a more liberal approach in applying the locality rule so as to temper some of the pragmatic problems which result from its persistance in malpractice law. In birth trauma cases today, it is truly absurd to believe that geographical

---

[24] *Id.* at 411.

[25] 102 Mich. App. 47, 300 N.W.2d 727 (1980).

[26] *Id.* at 731.

[27] DeWitt v. Brown, 669 F.2d 516 (8th Cir. 1982) (applying Arkansas law); Martin v. Bralliar, 36 Colo. App. 254, 540 P.2d 1118 (1975) Faulkner v. Pezeshki, 44 Ohio App. 2d 186, 337 N.E.2d 158 (1975); Swan v. Lamb, 584 P.2d 814 (Utah 1978); Hundley v. Martinez, 151 W. Va. 977, 158 S.E.2d 159 (1967).

differences play any major role in qualifying the standard of care. Natural processes do not display local variations or idiosyncracies. Women giving birth to babies in Detroit go through the same physiological and chemical changes as women giving birth in Dallas. Physicians who preside over the natural processes leading to birth are thus limited in their reactions to the activity—certain things must be done at certain times, the signs and symptoms of distress calling for a response are universally recognized, and the appropriate way of dealing with a crisis usually provides only extremely narrow margins for variation. Consequently, in birth trauma cases, the courts are becoming more and more inclined to accept the proposition that the standard of care is not one which is tied to any locality, but is one which requires the medical personnel in attendance upon the mother and child to employ the same skills and techniques in their care and treatment which are employed by fellow practitioners throughout the nation.

Thus, today, while nodding acquiesence is still given to the same and similar localities rule, in actual practice the standard of care to which medical personnel involved in the care and treatment of pregnancy, birth and prenatal care are subject is the standard of care promulgated by a nationwide fraternity of physicians, hospitals, and nurses who have established the working guidelines for what should or should not be done. Most professional individuals involved in this area of medical practice are, in name or in fact, specialists in their fields. In most instances they will follow procedures and engage in treatment which leaves little room for local variations or personal or professional eccentricities. Courts, the medical profession, and the public should be intolerant of any suggestion that the standard of professional care in the care and treatment of pregnancy and birth should be anything less than that which obtains generally among all similar professionals involved in this universal process.

§ 4.8 Standard of Care and the Need for Expert Testimony

The discussion of standard of care in §§4.1 through 4.7 is mere academic interest to the legal profession. The primary importance of identifying the standard of care lies in determining the means of proving that a physician, nurse, or hospital has breached its duty to the plaintiff by performing some act or omission which falls below the appropriate standard. This proof, in most malpractice cases, requires the testimony of expert witnesses.[28]

---

[28] Clary Ins. Agency v. Doyle, 620 P.2d 194 (Alaska 1980); O'Connor v. Bloomer, 116 Cal. App. 3d 385, 172 Cal. Rptr. 128 (1981); Grody v. Tulin, 170 Conn. 443, 365 A.2d 1076

Because malpractice requires a showing that defendants have breached a standard of care which is created and maintained by members of defendant's own profession, courts, rightly, are reluctant to allow untutored lay jurors to assess what that standard of care is or how it was breached.[29] Although there are rare cases where the wrongful act is so gross and apparent that a breach of standard of care is indicated even without expert testimony (see § **4.16**), for the most part a malpractice case demands the introduction of testimony to educate lay jurors as to the standard of professional practice against which defendants' acts are to be judged. Thus, malpractice litigation does usually reduce itself to a battle of the experts.

The ideal expert, from a strictly legal standpoint, would be a fellow practitioner of the defendant, someone belonging to the same discipline, a board certified specialist in the same field if defendant is a specialist, and someone residing and practicing in the same locality during the same time period as the defendant. This ideal is often impossible to coax out of reality. Doctors practicing in the same community will be reluctant to testify against a fellow practitioner, someone they are likely to know personally, someone who may even be a friend. One's fellow physicians may look upon a doctor willing to testify against another as a traitor to his peers, and this attitude, whether open or implied, would make it extremely difficult for any qualified local witness to come forward to speak against a local physician. Indeed, this legally ideal witness is more often found on defendant's side of the bench.

Even if this legally ideal witness did step forward, this would not necessarily make him the best witness from a practical viewpoint. The legal system is an adversarial one, and the obligation of counsel to his client is not just to present the truth to the jury, but to present it in a way which the jury will understand and react to. An expert witness must be more than simply academically knowledgeable. He must also be articulate and persuasive. An untainted reputation and a willingness to testify for the sake of the truth, and not just for the payment of a fee, are also prerequisites to effective expert testimony. These qualities are not that easy to find in one individual expert, and these prerequisites narrow the harvest of experts significantly. In a particular case, the best expert might practice on the opposite coast,[30] he might be a specialist

---

(1976); Walski v. Tiesenga, 72 Ill. 2d 249, 381 N.E.2d 279 (1978); Starr v. Providence Hosp., 109 Mich. App. 762, 312 N.W.2d 152 (1981); Folger v. Corbett, 118 N.H. 737, 394 A.2d 63 (1978); Hale v. State, 53 A.D.2d 1025, 386 N.Y.S.2d 151 (1976); Harris v. Grizzle, 625 P.2d 747 (Wyo. 1981).

[29] Walski v. Tiesenga, 72 Ill. 2d 249, 381 N.E.2d 279 (1978).

[30] Katsetos v. Nolan, 170 Conn. 637, 368 A.2d 172 (1976) (one of plaintiff's four experts in suit against Connecticut physicians and hospital lived and practiced in California); Naccarato v. Grob, 384 Mich. 248, 180 N.W.2d 788 (1970) (Los Angeles pediatrician qualified to testify as to standard of care applicable to Detroit area pediatrician).

where defendant is a general practitioner,[31] or an M.D. where defendant is a D.O.[32] He might have been a resident when defendant committed the alleged malpractice.[33] In other words, he may not fit defendant's mold, but a mold of his own which causes the judge's eyebrows to be raised and a puzzled look to enter his eyes when the expert is called to the stand to testify against the defendant. In every trial the first hurdle to overcome is the inevitable objection from the opposite number, "Your Honor, Dr. Johnson is not qualified to testify against my client respecting the standard of care."

The riskiest part of any malpractice case is qualifying one's expert witness to testify to the standard of care. An important, well-prepared malpractice case can fall apart if the key expert witness fails to satisfy the minimal conditions to permit the introduction of his testimony respecting the standard of care. Often, the success or failure of qualifying one's expert depends on the judicial philosophy of the jurisdiction in which the case is tried. Some courts, quite simply, are conservative and strict in evaluating the credentials of a witness, and will insist that the expert share significant characteristics with the medical profile of defendant to convincingly demonstrate his ability to render an opinion regarding the standard of care.[34] More liberal courts, inspired in part by the modern rules of evidence respecting expert witnesses, follow the axiom that so long as the witness testifies that he is familiar with the standard of care applicable to a practitioner such as defendant, and can support this assertion with facts, then his testimony may be received and the appropriate weight to be given to his testimony will be left for the jury to decide.[35]

---

[31] Berwald v. Kasal, 102 Mich. App. 269, 301 N.W.2d 499 (1980).

[32] Fridena v. Evans, 127 Ariz. 516, 622 P.2d 463 (1981); Musachia v. Terry, 140 So. 2d 605 (Fla. Dist. Ct. App. 1962).

[33] See, e.g., Dickens v. Everhart, 284 N.C. 95, 199 S.E.2d 440 (1973) (where court found that expert pathologist who was a medical student in Ohio at time alleged malpractice was committed by North Carolina physician was qualified to give expert testimony); see also Harvey v. Silber, 300 Mich. 510, 2 N.W.2d 483 (1942) (holding that expert who was a medical student at time defendant negligently treated gunshot wound was qualified to testify where it was admitted that proper treatment of gunshot wounds had not changed). But see Swanek v. Hutzel Hosp., 115 Mich. App. 254, 320 N.W.2d 234 (1982) (witness who had not completed his residency in 1972 held not qualified to testify to standard of OB-GYN care at that time.)

[34] E.g., Koch v. Gorilla, 552 F.2d 1170 (6th Cir. 1977); Smith v. Hospital Authority, 161 Ga. Ct. App. 657, 288 S.E.2d 715 (1982).

[35] White v. Mitchell, 263 Ark. 787, 568 S.W.2d 216 (1978); Francisco v. Parchment Medical Clinic, P.C., 407 Mich. 325, 285 N.W.2d 39 (1979); Ives v. Redford, 219 Va. 838, 252 S.E.2d 315 (1979).

§ 4.9   Standard of Care Experts—The School of Practice

Defendants often urge that the expert witness must belong to the same school as the defendant—that M.D.s should not be allowed to testify against D.O.s, for example. However, where the test is one of familiarity with the appropriate standard of practice, this criteria is artificial and unsupportable. Despite the categorization and specialization of medical practice, there are still many areas of medicine where the various disciplines overlap. The scientific principles of anesthetics, for example, are the same regardless of whether anesthetics are administered by an M.D. anesthesiologist, a D.O. anesthesiologist, or a certified registered nurse anesthetist. The same is true of many other medical procedures. Consequently, the courts often allow experts from one discipline to testify against another, so long as some evidence is presented to show as a foundation for his testimony that he is familiar with the standard of care of defendant's discipline.[36]

Thus, in a birth trauma case a plaintiff may be successful in utilizing M.D.s to testify as to the standard of care of D.O.s, or D.O.s to testify as to the standard of care of M.D.s. The reason for this is simple and can usually be factually supported at trial through the witness testimony. Osteopaths and medical doctors study the same basic textbooks covering obstetrics and gynecology, and recognize the same books as authoritative. They often attend the same lectures, learn from the same teachers. During intern and residence periods, osteopaths and medical doctors may find themselves working side by side. They will subscribe to the same medical journals. In treating pregnancy and birth, they will be limited by the same physiological and chemical processes; they will be expected to recognize and interpret diagnostic signs in the same way and to apply the same skills and techniques which are universally recognized regardless of one's discipline. Thus, there are significant parallels between the standard of care of medical doctors and osteopaths in overseeing pregnancy and birth so as to create a basis for allowing members of one school to testify as to the standard of care of the other.

---

36 Fridena v. Evans, 127 Ariz. 516, 622 P.2d 463 (1980); Hundley v. St. Francis Hosp., 161 Cal. App. 2d 800, 327 P.2d 131 (1958); Foster v. Thornton, 125 Fla. 699, 170 So. 459 (1936); Harris v. Bales, 459 S.W.2d 742 (Mo. Ct. App. 1970); James v. Falk, 226 Or. 535, 360 P.2d 546 (1961).

§ 4.10 —Specialists and General Practitioners

While courts are usually willing to allow a practitioner of one school to testify against a practitioner of another school where there is a basis for finding that the expert is actually familiar with the standard of care of defendant's school, there appears to be a greater reluctance to accept the testimony of a specialist against a general practitioner (G.P.) and vice versa. Courts adopting and abiding by the *familiarity rule* will be consistent in expressing the principle that so long as the expert is familiar with the standard of care applicable to defendant the witness may testify. However, it is often more difficult, as a practical matter, to qualify a specialist or a general practitioner against his opposite. A specialist, of course, is likely to be familiar with the standard of care of a general practitioner since he was probably a general practitioner before becoming a specialist. However, when a specialist testifies against a general practitioner, the court will be concerned with the possibility that the general practitioner will be held liable, not for violating his own standard of care, but for violating the more exacting standards of a specialist in the field.[37] This, of course, would be improper, and counsel who seeks to present a specialist against a G.P. should be careful to emphasize that the specialist is familiar with, and only testifying to, the standard of care of general practitioners and not as to the standard of his own specialized practice.

For different reasons, counsel may find it extremely difficult to qualify a G.P.'s testimony against a defendant specialist. Since being a specialist connotes a degree of education, skill, training, and experience beyond that of a general practitioner, a court may well doubt that a general practitioner has sufficient background to be familiar with the specialist's standard of care. Of course, if counsel can show that the alleged negligent act of defendant breached a standard which even general practitioners uniformly adhere to, and one which a specialist, being even better trained, certainly should have followed, then the general practitioner's testimony might be admitted because of the universality of the standard of care.[38]

---

[37] *See, e.g.*, Smith v. Guthrie, 557 S.W.2d 163 (Tex. Civ. App. 1977).

[38] Fitzmaurice v. Flynn, 167 Conn. 609, 356 A.2d 887 (1975); Carbone v. Warburton, 11 N.J. 418, 94 A.2d 680 (1953); Lewis v. Read, 80 N.J. Super. 148, 193 A.2d 255 (1963). *Contra* Harris v. Campbell, 2 Ariz. App. 351, 409 P.2d 67 (1965).

§ 4.11   —The "Universality" Rule

The uniform, universal, or nationally recognized medical practice rule deserves a separate discussion. As indicated in § 4.9, certain medical techniques and applications are so basic to the treatment of patients or are so subject to unvarying scientific law that they apply across the whole spectrum of medical disciplines. Frequently, in birth trauma cases, for example, the issues of malpractice will center around some medical diagnosis, treatment, or lapse of treatment which is related to a universal standard of medical practice subject to no significant geographical, interdisciplinary, or temporal variation. The issue may still be very complex and esoteric and may still require an expert to illuminate the medical principles involved. However, the expert can be from any school of practice, can be from any locality, can be a specialist or a general practitioner, and still be qualified to testify as to what the basic standard of care requires in dealing with the issue.[39]

An attorney should never go to trial, however, hoping to qualify his expert on the sole basis of the universality rule, for what the attorney may see as being universal, the court may find subject to the locality rule. The better approach is to view the universality rule as a cushion to fall back on when all else fails to qualify the proposed expert. Expert testimony is crucial to a malpractice case. No matter how severely injured the plaintiff might be, or unsympathetic the defendant, no matter what the skills of counsel or the depth of preparation, the role of the expert witness remains the focus of the suit. Whenever possible, the expert should be capable of demonstrating his familiarity with the standard of care in the same locality of the defendant or of a similar community, identified by evidence such as population, the availability of medical facilities, the nature of surrounding communities (next to an urban center, for example, or near a major university hospital), the number of hospital beds, the number of physicians, and any other factors which counsel can employ to establish a firm conviction that the expert knows the standard of care applicable to defendant. When a defendant is a specialist, then the expert should also, whenever possible, be a specialist in the same field, familiar with the national standard of care prevailing in the speciality. It is less important that the expert be in the same discipline as defendant, though certainly such compatability will make it easier to qualify the expert.

As a supplement to these criteria for qualifying an expert, or as a substitute argument when all else fails, counsel should establish that the issues involved in the suit concern matters of such universal medical concepts and that the standard of care pertinent to the response to such issues is not affected by

---

[39] *See, e.g.,* Katsetos v. Nolan, 170 Conn. 637, 368 A.2d 172 (1976).

factors of locality, professional standing, or schools of practice. Then the expert, based upon his own training, experience, education and skills, may validly testify to such standard of care regardless of the fact that the patterns on his coat do not perfectly match those on defendant's.

§ 4.12   —Time of Practice

One final problem of qualification needs to be discussed which may arise in birth trauma cases more often than in any other type of malpractice cases. A birth trauma case concerns an injury to a child at or near the time of birth. Most states provide a tolling provision which preserves a child's cause of action against the running of the statute of limitations until the child reaches majority. Consequently, it is not impossible for such suits to be filed against defendants several years after the event of birth. Occasionally, this may lead to a question of what the standard of care *was*, rather than what the standard of care *is*, for medical practice is not stagnant and unchanging—indeed, it is often very dynamic and improving. Under circumstances where there has been a significant gap in time between the alleged act of malpractice and the suit, should counsel be concerned to find an expert who actually was engaged in practice at the time of the alleged wrong doing and who returns a memory of the standard of care? Certainly such a witness, if otherwise qualified, would be the witness of choice, yet it might be difficult to find such a witness if 10 or 20 years have intervened. When such a witness is not available, then counsel's next step is to find an expert who was at least in training to become a physician at the time and thus exposed to the prevailing standard of care through his studies. When this, too, proves impossible, the final resort is to find an expert who, aside from his professional training, also has the skill to research and comprehend the historical evolution of patient care and who, based on his present study of prior practices, can illuminate the standards of the dim past.[40]

---

[40] A useful precedent, although not a birth trauma case, is Harvey v. Silber, 300 Mich. 510, 2 N.W.2d 483 (1942). In holding that an expert who was a medical student at the time defendant allegedly committed malpractice in treating a gun shot wound was qualified to testify as an expert, the Michigan Supreme Court noted, first, that the practice of treating gun shot wounds had not changed, and second, that an opinion could be formed from study of the subject. *See, e.g.,* Dickens v. Everhart, 284 N.C. 95, 199 S.E.2d 440 (1973) (where court found that expert pathologist who was a medical student in Ohio at time alleged malpractice was committed by North Carolina physician was qualified to give expert testimony); *see also* Harvey v. Silber, 300 Mich. 510, 2 N.W.2d 483 (1942) (holding that expert who was a medical student at time defendant negligently treated gunshot wound was qualified to testify where it was admitted that proper treatment of gunshot wounds had not changed). *But see* Swanek v. Hutzel Hosp., 115 Mich. App. 254, 320 N.W.2d 230 (1982) (witness who had not

§ 4.13   —Basis for Opinion

Another significant issue in qualifying expert witnesses, is determining when is an expert truly an expert. Laying aside all other considerations about disciplines, locality, professional status, and so forth, the question still remains as to whether a proposed witness does have sufficient experience, training, or background to be deemed an expert. This, of course, is a problem which is not unique to malpractice cases, but is a general issue in any litigation where expert testimony is proposed. Thus, it has been treated in depth in many publications. Perhaps the best, most cogent response to the question of when and how an expert becomes an expert is found in the Federal Rules of Evidence, which, by court rule or case law, finds parallels in most jurisdictions on this issue. Quite simply, an expert becomes such "by knowledge, skill, experience, training, or education,"[41] and may express an opinion based upon facts or data "perceived by or made known to him" at or before the trial.[42] No more firm or fixed rule is needed nor would serve the purposes of litigation. But counsel must always be prepared to meet any challenge to his expert by laying an evidentiary foundation, establishing that the witness has the requisite knowledge, skill, experience, training, or education to testify as to his opinion.

§ 4.14   —The Defendant and His Agents

All states contain some type of adverse witness statute, court rule, or rule of evidence which permits a party in civil litigation to call the opposite party to the stand to face cross-examination. Most statutes contain the modifier that the adverse party can be cross-examined "as to facts." This has led to some real controversy over whether a defendant, who is a professional and an expert in his own right, can also be cross-examined as to his expert opinion. Standard of care is not strictly a factual issue; it is established by witnesses qualified to give their opinion as to what the appropriate standard of care is. It has been argued, therefore, that as an adverse witness can only be cross-examined as to facts, he cannot be asked to render his own private and personal opinion as to what the standard of care is.[43] It has also been argued with occasional success that opinions are a property right to those qualified by training and

---

completed his residency in 1972 held not qualified to testify to standard of OB-GYN care at that time.)

[41] Fed. R. Evid. 702.

[42] Fed. R. Evid. 703.

[43] *E.g.*, Osborn v. Carey, 24 Idaho 158, 132 P. 967 (1913).

experience to hold them, and that the courts cannot compel a defendant doctor to relinquish his property right to his opinion regarding the standard of care.[44]

These arguments are rightly discredited in most jurisdictions,[45] for they conflict with modern principles of litigation. The opinion of standard of care is only technically an opinion—it is a real fact in a malpractice case which the plaintiff has the obligation to prove, along with such other facts as who did what, when, and to whom. The standard of care is no one's private secret or special property; a defendant becomes subject to this standard by virtue of his professional activities, and it is the profession as a whole which develops this standard of care. In asking the appropriate question, counsel is not so much eliciting defendant's opinion as probing defendant's knowledge. There is really no distinction here between asking, "Did you know the light was red when you ran it?" and "Did you know what the standard of care required you to do when you did what you did?"

Thus, in most jurisdictions today, a plaintiff can, if necessary, prove a medical malpractice case out of defendant's own mouth.[46] Whether plaintiff should want to, or attempt to do so, is another matter. The defendant's own testimony is likely to be self-serving, and his own view of the standard of care will normally be one which justifies his actions. While a vigorous cross-examination of defendant should play a vital part in the presentation of plaintiff's case, evidence of the standard of care should be established through one's own expert witnesses whenever possible.

A corollary to this issue is whether a plaintiff can use the expert testimony of an agent of the defendant physician or of an agent or employee of a defendant hospital as evidence against the defendant physician or hospital. This contemplates a much more controversial use of the adverse witness principle, and the answer will depend upon the language of the statute or rule which permits cross-examination of an opponent. Where such language embraces within the definition of "adverse party" the agents and employees of an adverse party, no logical reason exists to preclude nurses, residents, interns, or physicians who

---

[44] Hull v. Plume, 131 N.J. L. 511, 37 A.2d 53 (1944).

[45] *See, e.g.,* McDermott v. Manhatten Eye, Ear & Throat Hosp., 15 N.Y.2d 20, 203 N.E.2d 469 255 N.Y.S.2d 65, (1964).

[46] Lawless v. Calaway, 24 Cal. 2d 81, 147 P.2d 604 (1944); State v. Brainin, 224 Md. 156, 167 A.2d 117 (1961); Giocabazzi v. Fetzer, 6 Mich. App. 308, 149 N.W.2d 222 (1967); Anderson v. Florence, 288 Minn. 412, 181 N.W.2d 873 (1970); Rogotzki v. Schept, 91 N.J. Super. 135, 219 A.2d 426 (1966); McDermott v. Manhattan Eye, Ear & Throat Hosp., 15 N.Y.2d 20, 203 N.E.2d 469, 255 N.Y.S.2d 65 (1964); Iverson v. Lancaster, 158 N.W.2d 507 (N.D. 1968); Oleksiw v. Weidener, 2 Ohio St. 2d 147, 207 N.E.2d 375 (1965).

are agents or employees of the named defendant from being called upon to render expert opinion evidence concerning the issues in the case.[47]

§ 4.15   Standard of Care—Special Circumstances

Several extraordinary issues relating to the standard of care remain to be discussed. In an occasional case, specific proof of the professional standard of care is made unnecessary by the fact that defendant's acts are so clearly negligent that lay jurors need no expert to tell them that defendant failed to exercise due care (see § **4.16**). Likewise, some jurisdictions recognize the doctrine of res ipsa loquitur which effectively shifts to the defendant the burden of establishing the propriety of his acts (see § **4.17**). Lastly, the liability which the law imposes upon hospitals, requires a slightly different focus on the hospital's standard of care (see §§ **4.18** through **4.20**).

§ 4.16   —Obvious Acts of Negligence

Malpractice is the name the law gives to the failure of a professional to exercise due care, and usually the measure of due care is the standard of care of his or her own profession. Yet, instances do arise where, in treating or caring for a patient, a professional person commits an act or omission which is clearly a failure to exercise due care without any reference to professional standards. A gross example might be a nurse who drops a newborn infant in the delivery room. No one needs to be told that the professional standards for nurses require the nurse to hold onto a neonate with caution and care, and it does not take a parade of experts to explain that dropping an infant is a breach of professional responsibilities. In cases of this nature, expert testimony is not required since the failure of the professional defendant to act with due care is a matter within the common knowledge of laypersons.[48]

---

[47] *See, e.g.,* Frazier v. Hurd, 6 Mich. App. 317, 149 N.W.2d 226 (1967), *aff'd*, 380 Mich. 291, 157 N.W.2d 249 (1968) (holding that physician who assisted defendant in performing an operation became defendant's agent who could be called upon to give testimony under the adverse witness statute); *cf.* Mayers v. Litow, 154 Cal. App. 2d 413, 316 P.2d 351 (1957) (physician called in by defendant for consultation held an independent contractor who could not be called for cross-examination by plaintiff as an adverse witness).

[48] Revels v. Pohle, 101 Ariz. 208, 418 P.2d 364 (1966) (steel suture material left in operating site); McKnight v. St. Francis Hosp. & School of Nursing Inc., 224 Kan. 632, 585 P.2d 984 (1978) (leaving ill 75 year old patient standing unattended); Clapham v. Yanga, 102 Mich. App. 47, 300 N.W.2d 727 (1980) (failing to perform pregnancy test on nonmenstruating teenager); Turney v. Onspaugh, 581 P.2d 1301 (Okla. 1978) (sponge left in operating site);

This legal principle, that certain acts of negligence are obvious even when committed by a professional person and waive any need to establish the standard of care and its breach through expert testimony, does not require a lengthy dissertation. This is a firmly established principle which is well known to the legal profession. Rather, what is important is to caution attorneys against placing too much reliance on this doctrine.

Knowledgeable attorneys may find it easy to succumb to the temptation of treating a malpractice case as an ordinary negligence case whenever defendant's actions may seem obviously improper. Malpractice cases, which require expert testimony, a careful review of medical records, long, unending hours of preparation, and the physical and mental strain of litigation, are not the most economical cases which a busy, cost-conscious attorney can pursue, and any short-cut that might lessen the expense and burden is eagerly embraced. Attorneys are themselves professional people, and personal injury attorneys became particularly knowledgeable regarding physical injuries and medical procedures. Consequently, what may seem to an attorney to be a clear case of ordinary negligence may, in fact, be seen by a court or a jury in an entirely different light. Not every case involves a dropped baby or a needle left inside a wound. More often, cases which appear to involve simple negligence in fact hover in a vague middle ground where there is room for a difference of opinion.[49]

To avoid any unpleasant surprises, every case naming a nurse, physician, or hospital as a defendant should be treated as a malpractice case rather than as an ordinary negligence case. Cases involving injuries to infants are too important to risk being dismissed for failure to have an expert witness available to testify to the standard of care, even when, in the attorney's judgment, such testimony is unnecessary.

§ 4.17   —Res Ipsa Loquitur

In several jurisdictions, the courts recognize the doctrine of res ipsa loquitur ("the thing speaks for itself"). Basically, this is a case law created of evidence

---

Runnels v. Rogers, 596 S.W.2d 87 (Tenn. 1980) (failure to remove wire from oozing and running foot wound).

[49] *E.g.*, Crowley v. O'Neil, 4 Kan. App. 2d 491, 609 P.2d 198 (1980) (surgeon cut healthy portion of patient's body in performing surgery, held incident not within "common knowledge" exception); Cox v. Dela Cruz, 406 A.2d 620 (Me. 1979) (risk of injury to fetus from x-rays held not to be obvious); Waatti v. Marquette Gen. Hosp. Inc., 122 Mich. App. 44, 329 N.W.2d 526 (1982) (not common knowledge that leaving seizure patient in bed with guard rails down constitutes negligence).

which is designed to assist a plaintiff in meeting his burden of proving negligence by creating a rebuttable presumption or inference that negligence has occurred, thereby shifting to defendant the burden of presenting evidence to contradict this presumption. Perhaps the best example of res ipsa loquitur applied to a malpractice situation is the landmark case of *Ybarra v. Spangard*.[50] Plaintiff submitted himself to surgery by the defendant physicians, nurses, and hospital. This surgery did not involve his upper arms and shoulders which, until after the operation, were essentially normal and healthy. However, after the surgery, which plaintiff endured under a general anesthetic, he discovered severe pain and soreness in his shoulders, which progressed and caused plaintiff unexpected discomfort and annoyance. Unable to ascertain, and failing to plead, the specific act of negligence that caused this condition, plaintiff's suit was dismissed by the lower court. The California Supreme Court reinstated the case, applying the principle of res ipsa loquitur to salvage plaintiff's claim. The court explained:

> Without the aid of the doctrine, a patient who received permanent injuries of a serious character, obviously the result of someone's negligence, would be entirely unable to recover unless the doctors and nurses in attendance voluntarily chose to disclose the identity of the negligent person and the facts establishing liability. . . .[51]
>
> [W]here a plaintiff receives unusual injuries while unconscious and in the course of medical treatment, all those defendants who had any control over his body or the instrumentalities which might have caused the injuries may properly be called upon to meet the inference of negligence by giving an explanation of their conduct.[52]

The traditional doctrine of res ipsa loquitur, which is seen in play here, depends upon a showing (1) that the injury which occurred was of a type which ordinarily does not occur unless caused by someone's negligence, (2) that at the time of the injury the instrumentality responsible for the injury was actually or inferentially in the exclusive control of the defendant, and (3) that the plaintiff did not himself contribute to his injuries. The rule is also surrounded by a halo of idiosyncrasies and local variations far too complex and esoteric to be treated at any length here.

As can be seen from *Ybarra*, the application of res ipsa loquitur is seen by some courts to be a necessary aid to a plaintiff confronted by bewildering silence or insufficient revelations in seeking an explanation for his injury. Sym-

---

[50] 25 Cal. 2d 486, 154 P.2d 687 (1944).

[51] *Id.* at 689.

[52] *Id.* at 691.

pathy is especially merited to the unconscious patient who has no opportunity to even see or sense the source of his injury, although it might also be argued that most lay persons are so perplexed by the administration of medical treatment even when conscious of their surroundings, that unconsciousness alone is not the touchstone of the application of this rule. What does seem to be crucial is that the patient suffers an injury which is of a kind which would only be suffered because of someone's negligence, for the doctrine will not apply simply because the care or treatment rendered by the defendants was unsuccessful or led to a bad result.[53]

Res ipsa loquitur, where it is recognized, is a potent addition to a plaintiff's trial arsenal. The rule, however, can be abused, for an attorney can often be misled into placing too much reliance on the rule, inducing sluggishness in the preparation of the case. Wherever possible, using the tools of modern discovery practice, an attorney should try to determine exactly how and why an injury occurred and who was responsible, and should rely upon specific expert testimony to prove the negligence of defendants. Only when this becomes impossible should the attorney in a medical malpractice case look to this doctrine for assistance in proving the plaintiff's case.[54]

§ 4.18   Standard of Care of Hospitals—Generally

In discussing the standard of care in medical malpractice cases, special attention must be given to the standard of care applicable to hospitals. Hospitals, as discussed in §§ 2.9 through 2.17, stand in a unique relationship to the patient, and may be held liable under a variety of legal theories. As a corporate entity, it may be held vicariously liable for the wrongful acts of its own employees and agents. Some of these employees or agents may be engaged in providing nonmedical services to the patient, services of an administrative or custodial nature. Other employees, such as nurses, residents, and interns, are licensed professionals who may provide medical care and treatment to patient, sometimes exercising their own independent medical judgment while at other

---

[53] Borghese v. Bartley, 402 So. 2d 475 (Fla. Dist. Ct. App. 1981); Van Zee v. Sioux Valley Hosp., 315 N.W.2d 489 (S.D. 1982). In many cases the res ipsa loquitur rule merges with the common knowledge rule. *See, e.g.*, Nixdorf v. Hicken, 612 P.2d 348 (Utah 1980).

[54] The res ipsa loquitur doctrine may still require that expert testimony be presented to show that the injurious result is one which would not have occurred but for someone's negligence. *See, e.g.*, Fox v. Cohen, 160 Ga. App. 270, 287 S.E.2d 272 (1981), where burns on the back of a child following electrosurgery did not trigger application of res ipsa loquitur doctrine in absence of expert testimony rebutting defendant's testimony that such burns were rare, but not unheard of, complication of such surgery.

times acting under the direct supervision and control of the patient's private physician. The hospital's vicarious liability can arise through such acts as the negligence of a ward clerk who fails to clean up a spill in a hallway, or the improper suturing of a wound by a resident operating under a physician's directions. Each particular circumstance may call into play a different standard of care.

We have also noted in §§ 2.14 and 2.15 that hospitals may be held liable for failure to oversee the competency of the independent physicians to whom staff privileges have been granted. This direct, corporate liability, likewise, raises an issue concerning the standard of care applicable to the hospital's performance of its corporate obligations to the patient. All of these considerations are intertwined with the usual standard of care issues such as the viability of the locality rule and the need for expert testimony.

In an earlier era, before hospitals were recognized as subject to liability for malpractice, but were only liable for the negligence arising from its administrative, ministerial, or custodial responsibilities to the patient, the hospital's standard of care was most often expressed as the exercise of such reasonable care as required for the comfort and safety of the patient commensurate with the known, or should have known, physical or an mental condition of the patient. This is a general negligence standard of care which is still frequently echoed in the case law, especially in cases involving injuries to a patient not arising from medical care and treatment.[55]

Injuries which do arise from the medical care and treatment of the patient by hospital personnel have generated litigation against hospitals which have inspired a variety of statements concerning the standard of care. As a general statement, this standard of care for hospitals parallels the standard of care applicable to physicians in the jurisdiction. If the jurisdiction applies a form of the locality rule, or requires expert testimony, in establishing a physician's standard of care, such requirement is likely to color the standard of care of hospitals in the jurisdiction. Consequently, in some states, where a strict locality rule applies, courts have indicated that a defendant hospital has the duty to provide the degree of skill and diligence expected of a reasonably competent hospital in the same community, area, or locality.[56]

---

[55] *E.g.,* Bivens v. Detroit Osteopathic Hosp., 77 Mich. App. 478, 258 N.W.2d 527 (1977), *rev'd on other grounds,* 403 Mich. 820, 282 N.W.2d 926 (1978); Sylvester v. Northwestern Hosp., 236 Minn. 384, 53 N.W.2d 17 (1952); Miller v. Trinity Medical Center, 260 N.W.2d 4 (N.D. 1977); Utter v. United Hosp. Center, Inc., 236 S.E.2d 213 (W. Va. 1977).

[56] Emory Univ. v. Porter, 103 Ga. App. 752, 120 S.E.2d 668 (1961). *But see* Smith v. Hospital Auth., 761 Ga. App. 637, 288 S.E.2d 715 (1982); Roark v. St. Paul Fire & Marine Ins. Co., 415 So. 2d 295 (La. Ct. App. 1982); Charouleau v. Charity Hosp., 319 So. 2d 464 (La. Ct. App. 1975); Gridley v. Johnson, 476 S.W.2d 475 (Mo. 1972); Nelson v. Peterson, 542 P.2d

Just as a plurality of states have adopted a same or similar communities standard for physicians, it is not surprising to find a plurality of jurisdictions expressing the standard of care of hospitals as being that degree of skill and diligence used by hospitals in the same or in similar communities.[57] And, of course, a few states have abandoned the locality rule altogether.[58]

Most of these cases state the standard of care as being the standard of care applicable to the hospital itself. A few cases, however, have recognized that this approach may not be technically correct in those cases where the hospital is being held vicariously liable for the acts of its employees. Sensibly, these cases have recognized that the hospital's standard of care is really a matter of standard of care applicable to the employee or agent whose acts render the hospital liable.[59] In *Garfield Memorial Hospital v. Marshall*,[60] the federal court of appeals made an interesting comment linking the hospital's standard of care to that of private physicians:

> If a hospital undertakes to render services customarily performed by physicians, it must perform such services with the same degree of care to which a private physician is held; that is to say, the physician employed by the hospital must exercise the ordinary skill and care which is exercised generally by members of his profession in the community, giving consideration to medical learning.[61]

The conclusion which is readily apparent from these cases is that where a hospital is being sued because of the negligent medical treatment provided by one of its professional employees, then the standard of care for the hospital is going to be the same as that which would be applied to a private physician. This, in most cases (again, except where the act of negligence is gross and within the common knowledge of laypersons), will require the testimony of an

---

1075 (Utah 1975); Leahy v. Kenosha Memorial Hosp., 118 Wis. 2d 441, 348 N.W.2d 607 (1984).

[57] Faris v. Doctors Hosp., Inc., 78 Ariz. App. 264, 501 P.2d 440 (1972); Hirn v. Edgewater Hosp., 86 Ill. App. 3d 939, 408 N.E.2d 970 (1980); Chandler v. Neosho Memorial Hosp., 223 Kan. 1, 574 P.2d 136 (1977), Foley v. Bishop Clarkson Memorial Hosp., 185 Neb. 89, 173 N.W.2d 881 (1970); Patterson v. Van Wiel, 91 N.M. 100, 570 P.2d 931 (1977); Fjerstad v. Knutson, 271 N.W.2d 8 (S.D. 1978).

[58] Dickinson v. Mailliard, 175 N.W.2d 588 (Iowa 1970); Shilkret v. Annapolis Emergency Hosp. Ass'n, 276 Md. 187, 349 A.2d 245 (1975); Rogers v. Baptist Gen. Convention, 651 P.2d 672 (Okla. 1982).

[59] Wade v. John D. Archibald Memorial Hosp., 252 Ga. 118, 311 S.E.2d 836 (1984); Hirn v. Edgewater Hosp., 86 Ill. App. 3d 939, 408 N.E.2d 970 (1980).

[60] 204 F.2d 721 (D.C. Cir. 1953).

[61] *Id.* at 725.

expert to establish.[62] On the other hand, where the hospital is being sued for a nonmedical act, such an expert may not be required, for in such circumstances the standard of care may simply be one of ordinary negligence. This distinction was noted by the Wisconsin Supreme Court in *Cramer v. Theda Clark Memorial Hosp.*,[63] where it states:

> The general rule is that a hospital must in the care of its patients exercise such ordinary care and attention for their safety as their mental and physical condition, known or should have been known, may require. . . . If the patient requires professional nursing or professional hospital care, then expert testimony as to the standard of care is necessary. The standard of nonmedical administrative, ministerial or routine care in a hospital need not be established by expert testimony because a jury is competent from its own experience to determine and apply such a reasonable care standard.[64]

§ 4.19   —Medical and Nonmedical Acts

Of course, broad statements of principle do not diminish the confusion as to when an act is medical—and requires expert testimony—or nonmedical. Expert testimony, for example, has been held not to be required where plaintiffs have alleged that the hospital was negligent in the way it permitted vaginal examinations with unsterilized hands,[65] in applying a post-partum douche which burned the patient,[66] and in failing to call a doctor when the birth of a baby was imminent.[67] Yet, in each of these cases the courts could have as

---

[62] Charouleau v. Charity Hosp., 319 So. 2d 464 (La. Ct. App. 1975); Chandler v. Neosho Memorial Hosp., 223 Kan. 1, 574 P.2d 136 (1977).

[63] 45 Wis. 2d 147, 172 N.W.2d 427 (1969).

[64] *Id.* at 428. Other cases have distinguished between medical and nonmedical care, though not with consistent results. For example, in the following cases the professional care rendered by a hospital was noted to be subject to the same or similar communities rule, while the administrative or ministerial care standard was held to be merely such reasonable care as the patient's condition required. Kastler v. Iowa Methodist Hosp., 193 N.W.2d 98 (Iowa 1971); M.W. v. Jewish Hosp. Ass'n, 637 S.W.2d 74 (Mo. Ct. App. 1982). *But* in Wade v. John D. Archibald Memorial Hosp., 252 Ga. 118, 311 S.E.2d 836 (1984), the court recognized the distinction between professional and ministerial care, yet seems to apply a "same or similar communities" standard to the latter.

[65] Inderbitzen v. Lane Hosp., 124 Cal. App. 462, 12 P.2d 744 (1932).

[66] Mills v. Richardson, 126 Me. 244, 137 A. 689 (1927).

[67] Hiatt v. Groce, 215 Kan. 14, 523 P.2d 320 (1974).

readily found that the actions complained of were matters of professional judgment requiring expert testimony to prove a breach of the standard of care.

The hospital's direct or corporate liability, growing out of the hospital's negligent selection of a private physician on staff to treat a hospital patient, its negligence in determining the competency of a physician to be granted staff privileges, or its failure to supervise the care and treatment rendered to a patient by an independent staff physician where it knows, or in the exercise of reasonable care should know, that improper care is being provided to its patient, involve a more serious problem with respect to standard of care. These supervisory acts are nonmedical, and thus might arguably call for the application of an ordinary negligence standard of care. Yet, at the same time, each of these acts calls for the exercise of judgment which may be beyond the common experience of laypersons. Consequently, there is confusion as to what standard of care is applicable.

In *Johnson v. Misericordia Community Hospital*,[68] for example, a leading staff privileges case, the Wisconsin Supreme Court specifically held that the procedures ordinarily employed by hospitals in evaluating applications for staff privileges are not within the ordinary experience of mankind, and thus expert testimony was required (and was here presented) to prove that defendant hospital had been negligent in reviewing the credentials of the offending staff physician. However, in *Darling v. Charleston Community Memorial Hospital*,[69] the landmark negligent supervision case, it does not appear that plaintiff presented any expert testimony to prove that the hospital had failed to act in accordance with the standards of similar hospitals when defendants medical staff failed to take appropriate action in response to the obviously questionable treatment by the attending physician. The Illinois Supreme Court was satisfied that plaintiff had shown the hospital's breach of its duties of care to the patient, which duty was established, in part at least, by the "regulations, standards and bylaws which plaintiff introduced into evidence" and which "performed much the same function as did evidence of custom."

§ 4.20   —Rules and Regulations

Darling v. Charleston Community Memorial Hospital[70] may be read as adhering to the requirement that a hospital be held to the standard of care customarily followed by hospitals in the same or similar community if it is

---

[68] 99 Wis. 2d 708, 301 N.W.2d 156 (1981).

[69] 33 Ill. 2d 326, 211 N.E.2d 253 (1965).

[70] 33 Ill. 2d 326, 211 N.E.2d 253 (1965).

understood that the regulations, standards, and by-laws take the place of expert testimony to prove that standard. Other cases have noted that the hospital's failure to follow its own bylaws may be sufficient to show a breach of the standard of care, or at least is evidence of negligence.[71] Similarly, a hospital breach of a state regulation may be evidence of negligence.[72] Several cases have held that such regulations, standards, and bylaws establish the hospital's standard of care,[73] or at least are admissible as evidence of the standard of care.[74] Also, it has been stated that a hospital has the duty to promulgate and follow reasonable rules and regulations for the care of its patients.[75]

The corporate liability of hospitals may be subject to the same standard of care applicable when the hospital is vicariously liable for the acts of its employees, if that standard is taken in the broadest sense as requiring the exercise of reasonable skill and diligence as the condition of the patient requires. However, when a hospital is subject to suit on its corporate liability, that standard may be proven by its own rules and regulations, by those of national hospital organizations which give accreditation to hospitals, as well as by state statutes and regulations. Of course, such liability might also still be proven by appropriate expert testimony, which can identify the applicable standard of care either through such rules and regulations or independently, and which can demonstrate in what manner that standard of care has been breached. Then, the task which remains is to prove that the breach was a proximate cause of the plaintiff's injuries.

---

[71] Van Steensburg v. Lawrence & Memorial Hosps., 194 Conn. 500, 481 A.2d 750 (1984), Fjerstad v. Knutson, 271 N.W.2d 8 (S.D. 1978).

[72] Kakligan v. Henry Ford Hosp., 48 Mich. App. 325, 210 N.W.2d 463 (1973); Distad v. Cubin, 633 P.2d 167 (Wyo. 1981).

[73] Pedroza v. Bryant, 101 Wash. 2d 226, 677 P.2d 166 (1984).

[74] Purcell v. Zimbelman, 18 Ariz. App. 75, 500 P.2d 335 (1972); Boland v. Garber, 257 N.W.2d 384 (Minn. 1977); Foley v. Bishop Clarkson Memorial Hosp., 185 Neb. 89, 173 N.W.2d 881 (1970).

[75] Williams v. St. Claire Medical Center, 657 S.W.2d 590 (Ky. Ct. App. 1983); Burks v. Christ Hosp., 19 Ohio St. 2d 128, 249 N.E.2d 829 (1969).

CHAPTER 5

PROXIMATE CAUSE IN MALPRACTICE

§ 5.1   The Need for an Expert Witness

Proximate cause is that indefinable path of reason and logic that connects the wrongful act of a defendant to the damages suffered by the plaintiff. It is a difficult enough concept to deal with a case of ordinary negligence. In malpractice cases, and especially birth trauma cases, it is a monster waiting in the woods to snare the unwary just before reaching the goal of a verdict.

This colorful analogy is made for emphasis, for all too often the mistake is made of overlooking the need to establish that defendant's breach of the standard of care proximately caused plaintiff's injuries.[1] In ordinary negligence cases, where the test of proximate cause is simply one of reasonable foreseeability, the relationship between the tort and the injury is usually open and apparent to anyone having the powers of reason. It is reasonably foreseeable that in running a red light, an automobile accident may result. It is reasonably foreseeable that a banana peel left on the floor may result in someone's fall. It is reasonably foreseeable that a defectively designed stamping machine may amputate a worker's hand. The common experiences of life equip most nor-

---

[1] *See, e.g.,* Lindsey v. Clinic for Women P.A., 40 N.C. App. 456, 253 S.E.2d 304 (1979), where evidence was presented showing that the defendant obstetricians were negligent in their treatment of plaintiff mother, but were discharged from liability due to the absence of expert testimony showing that their negligence proximately caused a stillborn birth; *see also,* Caldwell v. Parker, 340 So. 2d 695 (La. Ct. App. 1976); Parker v. St. Paul Fire & Marine Ins. Co., 335 So. 2d 725, (La. Ct. App. 1976); Carman v. Dippold, 63 Ill. App. 3d 419, 379 N.E.2d 1365 (1978).

mal sentient adults with the mental tools necessary to relate cause to effect. Only lawyers have made this relationship complicated in their attempt to clothe it with the raiments of the law.

In malpractice cases, the law requires clearer proof of this cause and effect relationship, generally for the same reason that the law creates a special standard of care to measure a medical practitioner's breach of the duty of due care. The law correctly presumes that laypeople are not sufficiently knowledgeable in the art and science of medicine to determine, without being educated by an expert, that the medical practitioner has failed in her professional duties. Likewise, the law considers the relationship between the failure of a medical practitioner to perform medical services properly and the resulting injury to be outside of most laypeople's experiences and also will require proof through expert testimony.[2] Birth trauma cases provide some of the best examples of this. If a newborn child exhibits the signs and symptoms of brain damage, for instance, it is impossible to determine, without expert testimony, whether this results from some natural process—a genetic malfunction, a prenatal disease, an aberrant development of the fetus in the womb—or from some human error committed by a physician, resident, intern, or nurse in attendance at the pregnancy or delivery. Even when human error is suspected, liability depends upon showing which human error contributed to the problem, how that error could cause the problem, and elimination of the role of natural factors as the possible cause of the problem independent of the human error.

Malpractice law recognizes that in the usual case, a person seeks out medical care because of some ailment already existing. The law holds that physicians, hospitals, and nurses are not guarantors of the results of their ministrations. A bad result, a negative response to treatment, does not necessarily mean that some neglect of the doctor proximately caused subsequent deterioration of the condition. Someone stricken with cancer, for example, might still die from the disease despite the best, even heroic, efforts of medical practitioners to effect a remission or cure of the disease. Even if it can be shown that in treating the patient the doctor committed the gross errors of diagnosis or treatment, the errors may well have had absolutely no effect upon the progress of the disease, nor have altered one iota the unfortunate conclusion of the case. Consequently, in a medical malpractice case the plaintiff will

---

[2] "Moreover, when the medical causal relations issue is not one within the common knowledge of laymen, proximate cause cannot be determined without expert testimony." Ellis v. United States, 484 F. Supp. 4 (D.S.C. 1978); *see also* Grody v. Tulin, 170 Conn. 443, 365 A.2d 1076 (1976); Gerety v. Demers, 92 N.M. 396, 589 P.2d 180 (1978); Martinez v. Meek, 540 S.W.2d 774 (Tex. Civ. App. 1976); Harris v. Grizzle, 625 P.2d 747 (Wyo. 1981).

have the burden of proving, by the preponderance of the evidence, that a causal relationship exists between the alleged act of negligence and the injury.[3]

A plaintiff need not prove his relationship as a certainty, but must at least prove that the relationship is probable.[4] The standard found stated in the case law is often one of a "reasonable degree of medical certainty."[5] Plaintiff must present facts from which a causal relationship may be reasonably inferred,[6] and this usually means presenting an expert who can testify to a definite probability that the injury would not have occurred but for the negligence of defendant.[7] Any less testimony, any weak testimony to the effect that such a relationship is merely possible, can be fatal to the case for failing to lift the issue of proximate causation above the level of mere speculation and conjecture.[8]

Birth trauma cases differ from the usual negligence case only in that here medical attention is sought to prevent an adverse situation from developing. However, this very fact only increases the confusion between cause and effect. Pregnancy and child birth are fraught with perils which medical attendance and care can only assist in reducing. Human history provides the common knowledge that without medical attention and care, pregnancy and birth exposes mother and child to unacceptably high risks of injury and death. For a pregnant woman, the doctor's office and modern hospital is not a place of cure, but a place of refuge, a place of security. The quest is for a normal, healthy baby. The fear is that the fates will be unkind. Medical care and attention are sought to increase the odds against birth defects, yet a pregnant woman is painfully aware that no one can insure that the fetus' journey of nine months within her womb will conclude with the delivery of a perfectly formed and mentally sound child.

Thus, in a birth trauma case, as in any malpractice case, there may be negligence and there may be injury, but there might not be any relationship be-

---

[3] Wise v. St. Mary's Hosp., 64 Ill. App. 3d 587, 381 N.E.2d 809 (1978).

[4] Abille v. United States, 482 F. Supp. 703 (N.D. Cal. 1980).

[5] Hamil v. Bashline, 481 Pa. 256, 392 A.2d 1280 (1978); Martinez v. Meek, 540 S.W.2d 774 (Tex. Civ. App. 1976). A workable definition of this term is found in Boose v. Digate, 107 Ill. App. 2d 418, 246 N.E.2d 50 (1969):

> When a doctor is asked to base his opinion on a reasonable degree of medical certainty, the certainty referred to is not that some condition in the future is certain to exist or not to exist. Rather, the reasonable certainty refers to the general consensus of recognized medical thought and opinion concerning the probabilities of conditions in the future based on the present conditions.

[6] Harvey v. Kellin, 115 Ariz. 496, 566 P.2d 297 (1977).

[7] Van Vleet v. Pfeifle, 289 N.W.2d 781 (N.D. 1980).

[8] Grody v. Tulin, 170 Conn. 443, 365 A.2d 1076 (1976); Shapiro v. Burkons, 62 Ohio App. 2d 73, 404 N.E.2d 778 (1978); Martinez v. Meek, 540 S.W.2d 774 (Tex. Civ. App. 1976).

tween the negligence and the injury. Such a relationship may be suspected, but mere suspicion is insufficient to support a claim. To overcome the fatal criticism that this causal relationship is based only in speculation or conjecture, convincing evidence must be introduced to prove that the defendant's professional negligence contributed to the injury. The same expert who gives an opinion as to standard of care and its breach, might not be the same expert who can give testimony relating the breach to the plaintiff's injuries or vice versa. To successfully prove a malpractice case there usually must be some expert testimony proving each of these separate elements. Ideally, the expert witnesses called by counsel will be able to testify both to standard of care and causal relationship, and the attorney examining the expert should make sure that her expert does not leave the stand until both elements have been treated.

§ 5.2   Proximate Cause and Statistical Evidence

To prove the causal relationship, the expert may have to resort to statistical evidence and scientific studies. How detailed her explanation must be, how technical her testimony should become, what kind of evidence should be presented primarily depends upon the circumstances of the particular case. Consider, for example, claims involving birth control pills. There is an ample body of medical literature which demonstrates a statistical relationship between an increased level of estrogen and blood clotting in women on the pill. Yet, the actual chemical processes which cause an increased coagulability of blood is only obscurely understood. A plaintiff claiming to have suffered an injury caused by clotting and by the renewal of her prescription by a defendant who knew or should have suspected clotting, would have a difficult time proving proximate causation is required to prove exactly how the pill causes an increase in coagulability. In such cases, it will be sufficient merely to show the statistical evidence which unquestionably shows a causal relationship even though the scientific mechanism inducing this relationship is unknown.[9] On the other hand, the deprivation of oxygen to the brain has adverse results which are more clearly understood. While statistical evidence should not be discarded, in a case claiming brain damage to a newborn due to insufficient oxygenation, a detailed explanation of the relationship between brain cells, blood cells, and the role oxygen plays in the chemistry of the body is a far more efficient and dramatic means of establishing the proximate cause between the negligent act contributing to the diminished supply of oxygen and the resulting brain damage.

---

[9] See, e.g., Klink v. G.D. Searle & Co., 26 Wash. App. 951, 614 P.2d 701 (1980).

These examples bring to notice another aspect of expert testimony which might cause some concern to counsel when attempting to enter proof of causation. Rarely will a medical expert, a person involved with the actual practice of medicine, have the qualifications of a research scientist. Ideally, the persons most competent to testify to cause and effect are those who make a career of studying and conducting experiments to establish such relationships. In the above example, for instance, the most qualified witness to testify to the effect of estrogen on coagulability would probably be a biochemist who has spent considerable years studying this phenomenon, and the same would be true regarding the effect of oxygen deprivation on brain cells. However, if parties to litigation are required to produce experts at each level of causation to establish proximate cause, trials would become woefully unwieldly and the fact finders wearily confused. Courts usually have permitted, and in most cases should permit, such evidence of causation to come in through the medical witnesses normally presented to testify to malpractice. Although these witnesses may not have been personally involved in the research studies which probe the effects of chemistry and disease upon humans, they are certainly qualified, in most instances, by virtue of their own special education and training, to appreciate the significance of such studies which often lay the foundation for the actual care and treatment of patients. A witness who obtains knowledge of a scientific topic through reading the authoritative reports and by keeping abreast of current developments is as well qualified to illuminate these issues for a jury as a person actually involved with the procedures generating the underlying data. So long as the expert witness is conversant with the terminology, has the background, education, and experience to comprehend and interpret the reported studies, and can affirm upon her own knowledge the reliability of the studies or the reputation of the authors, then the expert's testimony should be admitted.[10]

§ 5.3 Proximate Cause—Loss of a Chance and Increased Risk

In birth trauma cases, as in many other types of malpractice cases, statistical evidence is often crucial in establishing certain types of damages which, without such testimony, might be objected to as speculative. There are two special

---

[10] *See, e.g.,* Gaston v. Hunter, 121 Ariz. 33, 588 P.2d 326 (1978); Brown v. Colm, 11 Cal. 3d 639, 522 P.2d 688, 114 Cal. Rptr. 128 (1974); Hawkins v. Schofman, 204 So. 2d 336 (Fla. Dist. Ct. App. 1967); Harvey v. Silber, 300 Mich. 510, 2 N.W.2d 483 (1942); Ragan v. Steen, 229 Pa. Super. 515, 331 A.2d 724 (1974); Quinley v. Cocke, 183 Tenn. 428, 192 S.W.2d 992 (1946).

categories of causation which frequently arise in these cases, although pragmatically they are but two facets of the same problem. These are identified as the loss of a chance and the increased risk issues of liability. An act of malpractice may cause a plaintiff to lose the chance of mitigating her injury or it may cause a plaintiff to face an increased risk of suffering additional deleterious effects in the future.

Consider the situation of a neonate who suffers a skull fracture due to negligence attributable to the defendant. Although the skull fracture may heal and, by the time of trial, no further problems in the child's development have been manifested, it is a scientific fact that because of such skull fracture, the injured child faces a statistically signficant *increased risk* of suffering diseases such as epilepsy and meningitis over that of a child who has not been subject to such trauma. Meningitis, for example, is an infection of the meninges, the area coating the skull, and a skull fracture may leave miscroscopic areas of damage in the meninges which can become more readily infected than would otherwise be the case if the meninges had not been traumatized. This creates a legal question of whether damages may be properly awarded for a tort which has caused merely an increased risk of meningitis, rather than the actual presence of the disease by the time of trial.[11]

The *loss of chance* problem of proximate causation may be illustrated using this same disease. Here we deal with a child, a neonate, in whom the infection of the meninges has already developed and its signs and symptoms are already displayed. Meningitis is a good example to use because the precursor signs are relatively patent—a loss of appetite, a pale appearance, the presence of sputum mucus—and there is a diagnostic test (examination of spinal fluids) which gives certainty to a diagnosis of the disease. Also, meningitis is progressive, and it is treatable. Left untreated, the infection progresses and will eventually cause severe brain damage or death. Diagnosed and treated promptly, the adverse effects of the disease can be minimized or even eliminated. Suppose, then, that due to the neglect of physicians or nurses overseeing the care of a neonate, there is a delay in the diagnosis and treatment of the disease, perhaps resulting in treatment being started twelve hours after its onset instead of seven hours. The child, after the disease is subdued, displays the horrible signs of brain damage. Brain damage may have occurred even if treatment had been started earlier, when the disease first manifested itself. Here the best that expert testimony can prove is not that the brain damage would have been

---

[11] Examples of increased risk cases are: Southwest Freight Lines v. Floyd, 58 Ariz. 249, 119 P.2d 120 (1941); Boose v. Digate, 107 Ill. App. 2d 418, 246 N.E.2d 50 (1969); Dunshee v. Douglas, 255 N.W.2d 42 (Minn. 1977); Feist v. Sears Roebuck & Co., 267 Or. 402, 517 P.2d 675 (1973); Schwegel v. Goldberg, 209 Pa. Super. 280, 228 A.2d 405 (1967); Bell Helicopter Co. v. Bradshaw, 594 S.W.2d 519 (Tex. Civ App. 1979).

avoided had treatment been started earlier, but only that by delaying treatment the child has lost a certain percentage of chance for complete recovery or for sustaining a lesser degree of brain damage. Once again, a legal question is posed as to whether the child should be allowed to recover damages for the loss of this chance.[12]

In both situations, the law does recognize the validity of the claim. A wrongful act which increases a risk of future injury to a person, or which causes a person to lose a chance of diminishing the effects of an injury, entitles the victim of the tort to recover damages for such increased risk and lost chances. This is not an entirely novel or modern concept, for it has its roots in a number of earlier cases, but in recent times this doctrine has been given a more definite structure. The supporting judicial policy is one which casts the risk of damages on the tortfeasor. As a number of cases state, echoing a 1905 Missouri case, *Granger v. Still*,[13] "it does not lie in the defendant's mouth" to say that the same results would have ensued even without her negligence, or that her negligence has not increased a risk of injury. It is necessary, of course, that the plaintiff establish the probability, or at least possibility, that defendant's act has increased a risk of harm or has caused a diminution of a chance, and most cases require that such be proven with "reasonable medical certainty." However, this term should not be construed to require certainty in the particular case, that, for example, the skull injury is certain to cause the plaintiff meningitis in the future or that the delay in treatment had certainly caused the child to lose a chance of improvement. Rather, it need only be shown, within reasonable medical certainty, that there is a significant probability of future problems, or that there was a significant probability that had prompt action been taken the degree of injury would have been minimized.[14]

The precise degree of proof required in such cases is a subject of some controversy. In *Hamil v. Bashline*,[15] the Pennsylvania Supreme Court appears to waive the medical certainty test with respect to proving that harm would not have resulted even in the absence of defendant's negligence. The court indi-

---

[12] Examples of loss of chance cases are: Hicks v. United States, 368 F.2d 626 (4th Cir. 1966); Jeanes v. Milner, 428 F.2d 598 (8th Cir. 1970); James v. United States, 483 F. Supp. 581 (N.D. Cal. 1980); Kallenberg v. Beth Israel Hosp., 45 A.D.2d 177, 357 N.Y.S.2d 508 (1975); Hamil v. Bashline, 481 Pa. 256, 392 A.2d 1280 (1978); Martinez v. Meek, 570 S.W.2d 774 (Tex. Civ. App. 1976); Whitfield v. Whittaker Memorial Hosp., 210 Va. 176, 169 S.E.2d 563 (1969).

[13] 187 Mo. 197, 85 S.E. 1114 (1905).

[14] James v. United States, 483 F. Supp. 581 (N.D. Cal. 1980); Boose v. Digate, 107 Ill. App. 2d 418, 246 N.E.2d 50 (1969); Feist v. Sears Roebuck & Co., 267 Or. 402, 517 P.2d 675 (1973); Schwegel v. Goldberg, 209 Pa. Super. 280, 228 A.2d 405 (1967).

[15] 481 Pa. 256, 392 A.2d 1280 (1978).

cates that once the plaintiff introduces evidence that defendant's acts have increased the risk of a harm, the fact finder may find that such an increased risk was a substantial factor in bringing about the resultant harm. In contrast, *Lazenby v. Beisel*,[16] rejects any dilution of the duty to prove proximate causation in cases of this nature and requires the plaintiff to prove more than that defendant's actions destroyed any substantial possibility of recovery. Thus, in Florida, where testimony indicated that had the defendant hospital followed proper procedures the patient still would have had no more than a 50 percent chance of survival, recovery against the hospital was denied in *University Hospital Building Inc. v. Gooding*.[17] Whereas in Pennsylvania, testimony that the patient would have had a 75 percent chance of recovery had defendant administered prompt treatment was held sufficient to allow recovery to the plaintiff.[18]

The measure of damages for such loss of chance or increased risk is, of course, difficult to ascertain, but no more difficult, given proper testimony, than that of measuring the damages of other intangible items such as pain and suffering. A fact finder, hearing that a skull fracture increases the risk of future meningitis, say, 20 to 25 percent over the normal risk to an untraumatized child, can utilize its common sense and experience to place a value upon the concern which this testimony raises for such future medical problems in the same way that it evaluates the future pain and suffering which an injured person may be expected to endure. In loss of chance cases, the measure of damages should be the difference between what condition would have probably obtained but for the negligence of the defendant and the condition that actually occurred. The burden of establishing that the defendant's negligence had a negligable effect on the progress of the condition should be on the defendant, for, as case law has often observed, the risk of any uncertainty as to damages lies with the tortfeasor, not the plaintiff.[19] When there is a probability, however slight or remote, that had the defendant acted properly, the plaintiff would have escaped the injuries for which damages are sought, then holding defendant liable for all the damages is not unfair since defendant's own wrongful act eliminated any possibility of distinguishing between the effects of a natural process and the effects of her tort. This is the same rule which is applied when defendant's negligence combines with a preexisting condition to cause an aggravation or acceleration of the plaintiff's preexisting condition. In such cases, if it is impossible for the trier of facts to separate that part of the harm caused by the negligence of defendant from that caused by

---

[16] 425 So. 2d 84 (Fla. Dist. Ct. App. 1982), *aff'd*, 444 So. 2d 953 (Fla. 1984).

[17] 419 So. 2d 1111 (Fla. Dist. Ct. App. 1982).

[18] 481 Pa. 256, 392 A.2d 1280 (1978).

[19] Routsaw v. McClain, 365 Mich. 167, 112 N.W.2d 123 (1961).

the preexisting disease, the modern view holds that the culpable defendant should be liable for all the damages sustained by plaintiff.[20]

Standard of care, its breach, and proximate causation must all be satisfactorily proven before a plaintiff may recover in a malpractice case—and usually expert testimony is required to provide such proof. Once these elements of the case are established, then plaintiff will be entitled to the damages which can be shown to have flowed out of the defendant's professional negligence.

---

[20] *See, e.g.,* Newbury v. Vogel, 151 Colo. 520, 379 P.2d 811 (1963); McNabb v. Green Real Estate Co., 62 Mich. App. 500, 233 N.W.2d 811 (1975); Fosgate v. Corona, 66 N.H. 268, 336 A.2d 355 (1974).

CHAPTER 6

DAMAGES RECOVERABLE IN BIRTH TRAUMA CASES

§ 6.1   Overview

The focus of this chapter is on the damages recoverable specifically in birth trauma cases. Absent from this discussion are damages for wrongful death, which are subject to the variations found under the wrongful death statutes of every state, and the damages to a mother for a negligently caused abortion. Rather, the assumption is made here that a child has been born alive, but because of someone's negligence, has suffered severe injuries of a lifelong nature. An injury to a child occurring at or immediately after its birth is certainly among the cruelest of injuries to be evaluated under legal principles.

Such an injury is usually permanent and will mark a person for the rest of his life. That life might be unnaturally shortened because of the injury. That life might lack the normal pleasures and enjoyments due to some permanent restrictive damage that can never be repaired. The handicaps imposed by a permanent injury at birth may turn the promise of future success and happiness into a struggle for survival and dignity.

Yet, damages for birth trauma are among the hardest to properly assess. A newborn child is like Locke's *tabula rasa*, an unblemished slate on which nothing is yet written. One of the excitements of birth is knowing that a child comes into the world with unbounded potential, that his story is yet to unfold according to fates and circumstances wholly unforeseen. It is a legitimate argument that damages awarded for an injured child are primarily speculative, a result of conjecture concerning what the child might have been but for his injury. A normal, healthy child might become almost anything—a great statesman, a petty criminal, rich, poor, famous, infamous. How then can we legitimately measure the damages appropriate for a child who has been injured, when the standard is so unfixed? Only by resort to educated guesses based upon experience and averages.

Birth trauma injuries are not solely the burden of the child, but cause hardship and suffering to the parents as well. Thus, these cases also raise a question of damages for the parents of the child, and the need to distinguish these damages. To adequately portray the damages recoverable in a birth trauma case, each element of damage should be separately considered. First, a view of the parents' damages will be undertaken (see §§ **6.2** through **6.7**), followed by a consideration of the child's own separate damages (see §§ **6.8** through **6.11**). At the end, a checklist summarizing these damages is presented (§ **6.15**).

§ 6.2   Damages Recoverable by Parents of an Injured Child

The traditional view indicates that the parents' damages consist of only their pecuniary losses—the loss of the child's possible earnings and services during his minority (more important in the time when children went to work early and were a part of the economic unit of the family), and the medical expenses the parents are obliged to provide for the child, by law, during minority. The mental and emotional anguish suffered by parents of an injured child are generally *not* recoverable (except in rare cases where mental anguish is suffered directly as a result of seeing a negligent injury inflicted on the child). See § **6.7**. Also, the diminution of the child's society and companionship is traditionally not recoverable, although there is some movement towards allowing such additional damages. See § **6.6**.

§ 6.3   —Loss of Earnings and Services

Loss of earnings has long been recognized as an element of damage available to parents of an injured child. At the time when tort law evolved into its modern form, children were frequently additional breadwinners for the family, and any injury that might diminish their earnings would be a significant hardship to the parents who had a common law right to those earnings. Considering that children frequently began working at age 10 or 11, and that their minority lasted until age 21, an injury that affected their earning capacity could cause a substantial loss of income to the parents. Thus, from an early time, it was well established that the parents of an injured child had a right to recover damages for the child's loss of earnings. This right of action (along with that for medical expenditures) is of such a distinct nature that the parent can sue for such damages independent of the child's suit, and the one is not deemed res judicata of the other. As an extension of this, the majority of cases insist that *only* the parent can recover damages for loss of earnings during minority, and these are not usually allowable in an action brought by the injured minor.[1]

Realistically, in our present society, the damages related to a child's loss of earnings during minority are no longer of great economic significance. Most children go to school until reaching the age of 18, which in most jurisdictions is also the age of majority. For all but a few child prodigies and infant entrepreneurs, we are looking at part-time and summer job earnings which contribute only slightly to the finances of the family. In birth trauma cases, where an injury at birth is often of such nature as to destroy the child's potential earning capacity, it is often difficult to evaluate what those lost earnings during minority might have been. (The problem of proving loss of earning capacity in birth trauma cases is discussed further in § **6.9**). Loss of earnings in actual outside employment is, typically, less important in terms of itemizing the damages awardable to the parents than are the other elements of damages to which the parents are entitled.

Loss of services expresses a broader concept which is more considerate of the actual role children play in the modern household. In theory, at least, when a child has been injured the parents should be entitled to recover the

---

[1] *See* Annot., 37 A.L.R. 11 (1925); 32 A.L.R.2d 1060 (1953); 59 Am. Jur. 2d, *Parent and Child*, § 112 (1971); 67A C.J.S., *Parent and Child*, § 137 (1978).

reasonable economic value of those services which, but for the injury, that child may have been expected to provide to the family. Here we are speaking of such domestic chores as doing dishes, shoveling snow, cutting the lawn, helping with the housecleaning, and so forth, as well as any valuable services the child has provided to his parents beyond his minority.[2] As a practical matter, however, proving the actual monetary value of such services, and convincingly demonstrating that these services would have been demanded of the child, without sounding hardbitten, is often difficult.[3] Sadly, when a child is severely and permanently injured the real loss to today's parents is not one which can be measured in economic terms, but consists primarily of the loss of the child's society and companionship. As will be discussed in § **6.6**, a few jurisdictions may allow the parents to recover such damages in a birth trauma or infant injury suit, but most states continue to reject this more humane approach and adhere to the pecuniary loss of earnings and loss of services standards for measuring parental damages.

§ 6.4 —Medical Expenses: Professional Care

The law recognizes that parents of a minor child have a legal obligation to provide for the medical expenses necessary for the health of the child. It follows that when a tortfeasor causes an injury to a minor child which exposes the parents to an increased obligation to provide medical care to treat the injury, the parents have themselves suffered direct loss which they are legally entitled to recover from the tortfeasor. This rule of law is well recognized in every jurisdiction.[4] The only controversy which may arise regarding recovery for medical expenses involves situations where the parents do not actually pay for the medical services made necessary by the injury. Where the minor himself has paid for his own medical care out of his own sources of income or wealth, then the parents may lose the right to recover damages in their action.[5] Where the parents either cannot pay, or, where the medical expenses

---

[2] *See, e.g.*, Gilbert v. Root, 294 N.W.2d 431 (S.D. 1980).

[3] One novel approach taken in Rohm v. Stroud, 386 Mich. 693, 194 N.W.2d 307 (1972), a wrongful death case, is to equate the value of the child's services to the expense of rearing the child, on the theory that a child is "worth his keep" so that a "negligent act which snuffs out their child's life" entitles the parents of lost services at least equal in value "to the amount of their pecuniary outlay." The court also noted that such damages could be required without the parents showing that services were actually rendered or were likely to be demanded in the future.

[4] *See* Annots., 37 A.L.R. 11, (1925); Annot., 29, 32 A.L.R.2d 1060, 1069 (1953); 59 Am. Jur. 2d, *Parent and Child*, § 120 (1971); 67A C.J.S., *Parent and Child*, § 152c (1978).

[5] This rule is stated in dicta in many cases. See, Annot., 32 A.L.R.2d 1060, 1074 (1953).

are paid by a third party (such as by a medical insurer under a parents' employer's health benefits program), a defendant may content that the parents have not actually suffered these damages. Most courts will reject this view, noting that it is the increased obligation of the parents to pay which is the basis of their claim, not the actual expenditure of funds.[6] What is involved here is the *collateral source rule,* which merely recognizes that the expenses caused by a tortfeasor's actions are the responsibility of the tortfeasor to repay as damages, regardless of the fact that plaintiffs were wise enough to provide for, or in a position to obtain, collateral sources of indemnification for personal injuries.[7]

Note that parents are only legally obligated to provide medical care to a child during the child's minority, and this places a temporal limit upon the damages which parents may claim. Parents recover the damages of medical expenses caused by the injury which have been incurred since the time of the injury and which are reasonably likely to be incurred until the date that the child becomes an adult. If any medical expenses are reasonably likely to be incurred because of the injury after reaching majority, then these post-minority expenses are recoverable in the child's own cause of action, and are not recoverable by the parents.[8]

The measure of such expenses is one of reasonableness—the reasonable cost of the medical care and treatment, including nursing care and other assistance, which is reasonably necessary for the health and well-being of the child, and which is reasonably related to the injury caused by the defendant. As seen, such damages are for past, present, and such future medical expenses as may be reasonably expected to be incurred into the future up to the date of the child's majority. Obviously, the award of such damages depend upon the circumstances of the individual case.

§ 6.5   —Medical Expenses: Parental Care

A corollary to the medical expenses recoverable by parents of an injured child are damages to the parents for the extraordinary services and nursing care which the parents themselves may be obligated to perform for the child as a result of the child's injury. If a child's injury is of such severity that he re-

---

6 Degen v. Bayman, 241 N.W.2d 703 (S.D. 1976).

7 In some states this collateral source rule has been modified by statutes, particularly in medical malpractice cases. These statutes are discussed further in § 7.9.

8 Apodaca v. Haworth, 206 Cal. App. 2d 209, 23 Cal. Rptr. 461 (1962); Beyer v. Murray, 33 A.D.2d 246, 306 N.Y.S.2d 619 (1970). *But see* Peer v. Newark, 71 N.J. Super. 12, 176 A.2d 249 (1961).

quires more than just the usual parental attention, there exists no reason for depriving parents of damages for the time and sacrifice required to provide additional services to the child as a result of the child's injuries. Such services are not "voluntarily" undertaken, even though the parent may willingly, out of affection and love, provide the necessary attention and care, for the injury is the unsolicited and unwelcomed cause of such services. Of course, this element of damages does not incorporate the usual household tasks which would be provided even in the absence of injury—cooking, housekeeping, mending clothes, and normal instruction and guidance. Rather, it encompasses such special obligations as bathing a child who, because of his injuries, cannot bathe himself as children of his age might normally do, cutting up his food if his hands are crippled, dressing him if he is paralyzed, carrying him from place to place because he cannot walk, cleaning and changing bandages, massaging or manipulating his limbs, changing and cleaning a catheter, administering medicines, supplementing special education because of reduced mental capacities, driving him to hospitals, clinics, doctors' offices, rehabilitation centers, and other similar activities which call for close attendance and care paralleling that which a professional nurse or paid attendant would otherwise provide.

Wherever this element of damages has been considered, the courts have acknowledged that damages for such extraordinary services and nursing care are recoverable by the parents (unless these have been recovered in the child's claim).[9] The courts have recognized that if the parents had not themselves provided such services, then they would have had to have hired third persons to perform these tasks, and this cost would be taxable against defendant's liability as a medical expense. Defendant should gain no advantage because the parents themselves have shouldered the responsibility for such care. To deny such damages, in fact, would only endorse a policy of hiring a stranger to serve the child's needs, which might be of less benefit to the child and to the family as a whole.

The only real controversy regarding this element of damages is in the proper measure of damages. The rule usually followed is to award the parents damages which reflect the reasonable cost of what it would take to employ a nurse or attendant to perform the same tasks.[10] Often, however, the child's injuries have compelled a parent to make an even greater sacrifice by forcing the parent to take time off from, or even quit, lucrative employment, but few

---

[9] Smith v. Richardson, 277 Ala. 389, 171 So. 2d 96 (1965); Mancino v. Webb, 274 A.2d 711 (Del. Super. 1971); Armstrong v. Onufrock, 75 Nev. 342, 341 P.2d 105 (1959); Woodman v. Peck, 90 N.H. 292, 7 A.2d 251 (1939).

[10] Smith v. Richardson, 277 Ala. 389, 171 So. 2d 96 (1965); Armstrong v. Onufrock, 75 Nev. 342, 341 P.2d 105 (1959).

cases have measured these damages by what the parent has financially lost because of caring for the child.[11]

There is no sound reason, with a catastrophically injured child whose damages are permanent, why these damages to the parents should be cut-off when the child reaches majority. If he continues to require extraordinary care and services after majority, and the parents continue to provide these services and care, a legitimate argument can be made for awarding damages past minority. However, as a practical matter, damages for these services should be part of the child's action, where the temporal yardstick would be the child's life expectancy rather than that of the parents who provide such care.

§ 6.6   —Loss of Society and Companionship

As seen in the discussion in § 6.3 concerning loss of services, traditionally parents were restricted to recovering damages only for their pecuniary, out of pocket, losses caused by the child's injury.[12] Today, we recognize that a child contributes more to the family than his occasional earnings. In fact, in most households, a child's earnings are unimportant to his role in the family. Children today are not valued for their breadwinning abilities, but for the pleasure (and occasional pain) they give in simply being children.

Many wrongful death acts allow recovery for the loss of the society and companionship of the decedent. Increasingly, courts are recognizing that even injuries which do not result in death can nevertheless seriously impair or diminish the society and companionship provided by a loved one. Between married couples the law has recognized this fact by permitting recovery for loss of consortium when a spouse is injured, a concept which has long ago expanded beyond the sexual connotation this concept once had. Some courts have now accepted that an injury to a child likewise damages the society and companionship which a child normally shares with his parents, and have allowed parents to recover for his injury.[13] Given the changed role of a child in the family

---

[11] In Nichols v. Hodges, 385 So. 2d 298 (La. Ct. App. 1980), the court allowed to stand an award of damages to a mother which was based on the present value of her lost wages for the job she quit in order to provide nursing services to her injured daughter. However, this was probably allowed only because such dangers were actually less than the salary which would be paid to a licensed practical nurse to perform the same nursing services.

[12] Smith v. Richardson, 277 Ala. 389, 171 So. 2d 96 (1965); Baxter v. Superior Court, 19 Cal. 3d 461, 563 P.2d 871, 138 Cal. Rptr. 315 (1977); Beyer v. Murray, 33 A.D. 2d 246, 306 N.Y.S.2d 619 (1970).

[13] Hayward v. Yost, 72 Idaho 415, 242 P.2d 971 (1952); School City of Gary v. Claudio, 413 N.E.2d 628 (Ind. Ct. App. 1980); Shockley v. Prier, 66 Wis. 2d 394, 225 N.W.2d 495 (1975). *Contra*, Wilson v. Galt, 100 N.M. 227, 668 P.2d 1104 (1983) (holding parent has no action

unit, damages for loss of society and companionship are frankly more realistic elements of recovery in the parents' action than the loss of the child's earnings and pecuniary services. Eventually, more jurisdictions will acknowledge this fact and will allow parents of injured children to recover damages for the loss of the child's society and companionship in lieu of, or as supplement to, the pecuniary damages now permitted to be recovered in the parents' suit.

§ 6.7 —Mental Anguish

Although an injury to a child, particularly a devastating injury to a newborn child, is certain to cause severe emotional and mental distress to the parents of the child, our present case law rigidly refrains from allowing parents to recover damages for such mental anguish except under very limited circumstances that will rarely arise in birth trauma cases.

Only recently has tort law recognized the right of a person to recover damages for mental distress, absent any physical injury to that person, where that distress arises only from witnessing the infliction of injury upon another. Indeed, the few cases which have permitted such recovery have shackled such causes of action within a narrow framework. Generally, the injured person must be a close relative of the plaintiff, the plaintiff must have actually observed the infliction of the injury upon the injured person, and, usually, the mental anguish must have manifested itself in some physical or physiological way to negate, oddly, any risk of feigning mental distress.[14]

Human beings, we hope, are not so cold as to be unmoved or undisturbed by seeing a stranger injured, but the law necessarily restricts recovery to loved ones of the injured party simply to keep the number of potential plaintiffs within reasonable limits. Thus, this first limitation is based on pragmatics and a logic that a tortfeasor owes no duty to an unforeseen stranger of tender sensibilities.

The requirement that the plaintiff observe the infliction of the injury also has its pragmatic purposes, again to arbitrarily limit the potential claims. The likelihood of mental distress occurring whenever a person hears of an injury to a loved one is a well known fact of life, and if the rule of contemporaneous observation of the tort were waived, the law would have to recognize this element of damage in a cause of action on behalf of parents, children, or spouses in nearly every personal injury case.

---

for loss of filial consortium). In Iowa such damages are allowed by court rule, Iowa R. Civ. P. § 8.

[14] Dillin v. Legg, 68 Cal.2d 728, 441 P.2d 912, 69 Cal. Rptr. 72 (1968); Portee v. Jaffee, 84 N.J. 88, 417 A.2d 521 (1980).

This restriction requiring the plaintiff to have actually observed the wrongful act causing the injury has, we must add, been the barrier preventing recovery of damages for mental anguish in malpractice cases, especially in birth trauma cases.[15] A mother might watch her child being stillborn, might witness a child born to her defective of limb, might watch, helplessly, the steady decline, deterioration, and death of her child due to the neglect of a doctor, yet be barred from all recovery for her emotional distress on the rather dubious proposition that, being unversed in medical knowledge, she could not have known that what was done by the defendants to bring about the injury or death to her child was wrong.

This concept is truly unsupportable. In the same state which might bar a mother who sees her child go through an agonizing fatal illness made unnecessary by a defendant's misdiagnosis and mistreatment, the mother might recover mental distress had she instead seen her child struck by a negligent motorist. The argument made to prohibit mental distress damages in the first instance, that the mother lacked sophisticated medical knowledge and thus could not comprehend that a wrong was being done to her child, is a woefully lame defense when viewed against the second instance where recovery is allowed. The mother who can claim mental distress damages for seeing a car hit her child, receives such damages because of witnessing the injury, not the wrong. She may have absolutely no idea of what the wrong is at the time of her observation—maybe the driver ran a stop sign, maybe he was speeding, or drunk, or failed to make a proper observation—these things, however, are not the thoughts that cause the mental distress. The distress is caused by the injury, and if, subsequently, it can be established that the injury was caused by defendant's negligence, then recovery should be allowed.

The third limitation, that mental distress manifest itself through some physical change (vomiting, loss of weight, nervousness) is designed to weed out cases where a plaintiff may feign such damages. This requirement of physical

---

15 Justus v. Atchison, 19 Cal. 3d 564, 565 P.2d 122, 139 Cal. Rptr. 97 (1977); Hair v. County of Monterey, 45 Cal. App. 3d 538, 119 Cal. Rptr. 639 (1977); Jansen v. Children's Hosp. Medical Center, 31 Cal. App. 3d 22, 106 Cal. Rptr. 883 (1973); Aquilo v. Nelson, 78 A.D.2d 195, 434 N.Y.S.2d 520 (1981). *But see* Mobaldi v. Regents of Univ. of Cal., 55 Cal. App. 3d 573, 127 Cal. Rptr. 720 (1976), where a foster mother who watched an overly strong solution of glucose administered to her foster child, who went into convulsions, became comatose and died; the foster mother was allowed to recover damages for emotional distress manifested by her weight loss, insomnia, and depression. *See also* Vaccaro v. Squibb Corp., 97 Misc. 2d 907, 412 N.Y.S.2d 722 (1978) (parents recovered damages for emotional distress of child born with drug related birth defects); Vaillancourt v. Medical Center Hosp. of Vermont, Inc., 139 Vt. 738, 425 A.2d 92 (1980) (mother, but not father who was not present, entitled to damages for emotional distress in witnessing birth of a still-born child); Friel v. Vineland Obstetrical & Gynecological Professional Ass'n, 160 N.J. Super. 579, 400 A.2d 147 (1979) (mother entitled to damages for emotional distress of an unattended birth).

manifestation is also unsupportable. Fact finders are all capable of under-standing the mental anguish which a parent may feel in seeing a child stricken with a horrible, permanent, life-threatening injury; their intelligence should not be insulted by parading before them the mandated details, "Yes, I was sick to my stomach. Yes, I've lost twenty pounds, and I can't sleep at night." Common sense suggests, without such proofs, that watching a loved one, espe-cially one's child, tormented by some pain or hurt, is a source of emotional disturbance.

Yet, these restrictions remain, not so much out of stubborn adherence to precedent as out of the fear of the consequences if such restrictions were not imposed to restrain these claims. The emotional distress of giving birth to a defective child is one of the most "real" elements of damage a parent can suffer, certainly of greater significance to modern families than any potential loss of earning. The child himself may recover damages for his emotional distress supplementary to his other damages, which is often cruelly ironic, as in severe brain damage cases, where the child may not be capable of appreciat-ing the emotional distress of his own injury. Yet this restriction on the par-ents' right to recover mental distress remains in force throughout the states, probably for no better reason than to restrain fact finders from giving consid-eration to the one element of damage having an indefinite, immeasurable, and perhaps unbridled value. Awarding damages for the mental distress of parents of an injured child comes too close to being a gesture of sympathy, and this is the real justification for locking the door. Until the courts become willing to allow parents to recover all the damages they suffer as a result of a traumatic birth, with faith that the fact finders will respond to the claims intelligently and dispassionately, damages for mental anguish rarely will be allowed to the parents of a severely injured child.

A final note: In a birth trauma case, the mother of the child might herself be placed in jeopardy of her life or health by the malpractice of defendant. Clearly such circumstances would give rise to a suit in her own name against the defendant for her own physical *and* mental distress damages. Her hus-band might have a loss of consortium claim derivitive to his wife's claim. These would be in addition to the claims of the parents arising out of the injuries to the child and should be separately pled and proven.

§ 6.8 Damages Recoverable by the Injured Child

In most cases involving nonfatal injury to a child, the principal concern is the damages to which the child himself is entitled. Whereas, the parents' own damages tend to be limited to their economic or pecuniary loss, the child may recover both pecuniary and intangible damages. The *pecuniary element*, however, is only a factor if the injuries are of a permanent nature and will likely cause the child to suffer a lost earning capacity or medical expenses after reaching the age of majority. The *intangible damages*, in contrast, belong to the child from the time of his injury and for the remainder of his life. In a birth trauma case, where the child plaintiff is usually of tender years, the great bulk of these damages lie in the future and the aim of counsel must be to provide a reasonable basis for assessing such future damages to overcome the prohibition against awarding damages which are merely speculative or conjectural.

§ 6.9   —Loss of Earning Capacity

Any permanent injury to a child which partially or totally diminishes the child's potential to earn a wage, including fringe benefits, after reaching majority, entitles the child to recover the difference between what he had the capacity to earn before the injury and his residual capacity to earn wages after the injury.[16] The time period for assessing these damages is from the age of majority through the child's pre-injury work life expectancy. With regard to lost earning capacity, defendant obtains no advantage by virtue of having caused an injury that might shorten the plaintiff's normal life expectancy.[17]

The law has long recognized both the right to such damages and the practical difficulty of establishing such damages when a child is involved. With an adult, or even with an older child, some past work history or measure of performance exists on which to project the probabilities of future earnings. If a rather brilliant high school student having a record of good grades, especially in science classes, has been known to express an interest in becoming a doctor, then a basis exists for awarding to the young person damages for the loss of the earning capacity of a doctor if an injury robs the child of this realistic opportunity. An average student, earning wages as a gas station attendant during the summer months, and showing interest in mechanics, might likewise be entitled to the loss of the earning capacity of an automobile mechanic should an injury cripple his arm or amputate his hand. These cases, involving older children who have established a record of accomplishment in school and who have demonstrated some skills and desires, are relatively easy ones in which to prove the loss of earning capacity.

---

[16] Annot., 32 A.L.R.2d 1060, 1068 (1953); *see* 20 Am. Jur. Trials 513, *Damages for Child Death or Injury*, § 36 (1973).

[17] 22 Am. Jur. 2d, *Damages*, § 92 (1965).

In birth trauma cases, the task is more difficult since the injury occurs before the child has had any opportunity to demonstrate his earning potential. This does not, of course, mean that the child is not entitled to any such damages, but this does require greater creativity to establish a measure of damages for loss of the child's capacity to earn wages. Although courts have observed that, as jurors were all once children, and have seen children develop into adults, they have the general background sufficient to make an educated evaluation of an average child's earning capacity after reaching majority,[18] this item of damages should be proven as specifically as the circumstances allow through appropriate statistical and expert testimony. In these cases, the most important proofs would center on the socio-economic background of the parents, for jurors commonly recognized that children follow in the footsteps of their antecedents. A sad reality still dictates that children born to affluent homes have more educational and social opportunities to succeed to a lucrative employment, while less fortunate youngsters are more likely to stay fettered to a lower productive level of income. Vocational and economic experts should be called upon to describe the projected availability of jobs, the likely income particular types of employment would generate, the effects of economic factors upon the job market and the real value of possible future wages. No one can know for certain what an infant's future earning capacity might have been but for the injury, but family and social factors can be marshalled in most cases to provide a degree of predictability from which some guidance towards these damages may be taken.[19]

§ 6.10 —Medical Expenses

Medical expenses, including rehabilitative training, vocational education, nursing and attendant care, are damages which a permanently injured child is entitled to recover for the period of his life following the age of majority and throughout his remaining post-injury life expectancy. Damages for premajority medical expense, as noted in § 6.4, belong to the parents of an

---

[18] "The jury had all been boys, and were then men. The average juror knows the ability of a man mentally sound to earn wages, and would be just as competent to estimate the loss of earnings due to mental impairment as would any witness who might be called on to express an opinion. . . . The absence of such proof was no bar to the allowance of such sum as the jury might find to be fair and reasonable." Sadlowski v. Meeron, 240 Mich. 306, 215 N.W. 422 (1927).

[19] See Proof of Lost Earning Capacity and of Future Expenses, 16 P.O.F. 701 (1965).

injured person, and only under rare circumstances might these be recovered in the minor's own suit.[20]

A categorization of what falls within this element of damages would certainly include hospital and doctor bills, both for treatment and consultation, the cost of medications, and orthopedic appliances, the cost of physical therapy, occupational therapy, psychiatric or psychological services, home nursing care or attendance, travel to and from doctors' offices and hospitals, and special educational services. The proofs should show the reasonable need for each item claimed relating it to the injury, and the reasonable fee or cost charged for the item. How often the services shall be required, how long, how often an appliance may be needed to be replaced, these are all questions which should be addressed to the medical witnesses, psychologists, social workers, vocational experts, or other witnesses who might be called upon to present the necessary proof of these future damages.

Each case, of course, presents its own unique circumstances and there may be extraordinary types of medical care and treatment or rehabilitative services not falling within any of the above-mentioned categories. Generally, the courts do not draw any hard and fast boundaries between what is and what is not a legitimate medical expense. The usual rule which is followed is that damages may be awarded for any expense which is "reasonable and necessary" to assist the plaintiff to overcome the handicap, disability, or discomfort caused by the injury.[21] This reasonable and necessary test gives the trial court a great deal of discretion respecting those items of damages which might be esoteric, original, or imaginative. Still, such damages cannot be merely speculative, and a firm foundation of proof should be presented to support any claim for a particular medical expense.

§ 6.11   —Intangible Damages

Intangible damages consist of those items incapable of exact monetary determination. They are the damages awarded for the following: pain and suffering, mental anguish, fright, shock, denial of social pleasures and enjoyments, humiliation, embarrassment or mortification, shame, anxiety, nervousness, mental retardation, disability, disfigurement, susceptibility to future injury or disease, loss of sexual potency or drive, diminution of society, companionship, love, and affection, and so forth. All the weighty synonyms can contribute

---

[20] Apodaca v. Haworth, 206 Cal. App. 2d 209, 23 Cal. Rptr. 461 (1962); Beyer v. Murray, 33 A.D.2d 246, 306 N.Y.S.2d 619 (1970). *But see* Peer v. Newark, 71 N.J. Super. 12, 176 A.2d 249 (1961).

[21] *E.g.*, Alt v. Konkle, 237 Mich. 264, 211 N.W. 661 (1927).

pages to this list, but to no real purpose.[22] As a practical matter, neither courts nor juries attempt to unweave the general tapestry of intangible damages to place each skein under a judicial microscope. The law recognizes these words as merely descriptive of an indefinite, imprecise quantum of damages which attaches to all personal injury cases. Just as Laurel is rarely mentioned without Hardy, so pain is rarely distinguished from suffering, or humiliation from embarrassment, or disfigurement from disability. We may find subtle nuances of meanings for each individual item of intangible damages, but in the final account of the fact finders award a lump sum.

In a birth trauma case these damages may constitute a significant part of a child's damages. Unlike medical expenses and lost earning capacity, these damages belong to the child from the instant of injury and are measured against the whole of his life expectancy at the time of trial: past, present, and future.

No fixed figure is possible for such damages; none is expected. The courts will uphold damages which are reasonable, which do not appear to have been influenced by sympathy or prejudice. The amount, within these broad limits, is otherwise left to the sound judgment of the trier of facts. Surprisingly, despite the unbridled range of intangible damages, despite the vague perimeters of instructions and the unlimited discretion placed in their hands, juries almost always come out with a figure which is restrained, sensible, fair, and just.

§ 6.12   Damages Miscellany

Some loose ends about damages need to be separately considered. Punitive, exemplary, or smart damages are recognized in some jurisdictions as an additional element of damages where defendant's wrongdoing has been especially unconscionable, as where his wrongful act was intentional or thoughtlessly and inexcusably reckless. The rules concerning such damages vary from state to state, and the likelihood of recovering those damages in a state allowing their recovery depends entirely upon the peculiar circumstances of an individual case. Each attorney filing a birth trauma case must exercise his own judgment in deciding the merits of pleading and seeking such damages.[23]

---

[22] An intriguing recent development is the argument that one who is seriously injured should be allowed to recover damages for the impairment of his or her capacity to enjoy life. *See* Flannery v. United States, 297 S.E.2d 433 (W. Va. 1982). Whether this adds a new element to the list of intangible damages, or merely provides a catch-phrase embracing all of these other elements, has not yet been satisfactorily resolved.

[23] Punitive damages, if recoverable for an injury to a child, will only be allowed to the child. *See* Annot., 25 A.L.R.3d 1416 (1969).

The various jurisdictions seem to be also divided on the issue of taxes. In evaluating the loss of future earning capacity, the argument has been made that since income taxes are an inescapable part of economics, only the net, after tax, calculations of earning capacity should be used. Most courts still allow the plaintiff to ask for the loss of his gross earning capacity, recognizing that it is not for the defendant to take advantage of speculative tax liabilities.[24]

Regardless of how courts view discounting the future earnings for income tax, almost all jurisdictions continue to require that damages awarded for future losses, including lost future earnings, future medical expenses and future intangibles, be discounted to their present worth.[25] Courts will, unless defendants waive the instruction, charge the jury to calculate the gross future damages and then calculate, according to one formula or another, the present economic value of these damages. That juries actually labor over such calculations is probably wishful thinking on the part of court and litigants, and at least one state has boldly repudiated this present worth concept, recognizing that it is offset by inflation.[26] Perhaps today, in an age of hand calculators and desk top computers, the courts might permit jurors to use electronic aides to make the cumbersome computations, but for the most part, this concern for awarding only the present worth of future damages is an exercise in futility. Jurors usually award to plaintiff what they deem to be a fair verdict, in one lump sum, according to a consensus arrived at through open discussion, negotiation, and compromise, none of which involve the subtleties of account book arithmetic.

Because courts still go through the effort of adjusting future damages to their present worth, other attempts to subject damages to economic rules often show up during the course of a trial. Living, as we are, in an inflationary age, the declining value of the dollar is a real factor to be considered in awarding future damages. A permanently injured child may need round the clock attendant nursing care for the rest of his life. This year, and perhaps the next, he might be able to obtain such professional care for $20,000 a year. But five years ago, this same care might have cost him only $18,000 a year, and five years before that, only $15,000. If a jury determines that $20,000 a year is sufficient compensation to provide such care, what is the effect of their award ten years from now, when this care might cost $40,000 a year. In effect, the

---

24 *See* Flannery v. United States, 297 S.E.2d 433 (W. Va. 1982).

25 Bean v. Norfolk & W. Ry., 84 Ill. App. 3d 395, 405 N.E.2d 418 (1980); Gannaway v. Missouri-Kansas-Texas R.R., 2 Kan. App. 2d 81, 575 P.2d 566 (1978); Abbot v. Northwestern Bell Tel. Co., 197 Neb. 11, 246 N.W.2d 647 (1976); Watkins v. Ebach, 291 N.W.2d 765 (S.D. 1980).

26 Beaulieu v. Elliott, 434 P.2d 665 (Alaska 1967); *see also* Kaczkowski v. Bolubasz, 491 Pa. 561, 421 A.2d 1027 (1980).

verdict is then only sufficient to provide the child with half the nursing care which the jury intended him to receive. Similar considerations involve future wage loss and intangible damages.

Consequently, testimony as to economic trends, particularly inflation, may play a significant role in developing the damages for a personal injury case, especially any case involving permanent injuries over a significant life expectancy, such as a birth trauma case. The jury must be educated that this verdict is one which must sustain the plaintiff throughout the rest of his life and thus should be sufficient to withstand the ravages of future economic uncertainties.[27]

Once again, it is not likely that jurors, upon retiring for their deliberations, will ponderously calculate the effects of inflation any more than they will struggle with formulas of present worth. The object of the economic testimony is to encourage jurors to take a broader, more realistic view towards damages, just as the object of the present worth argument is to induce jurors to adopt a more cautious, deliberative attitude. Perhaps in the long run, instructions for reducing damages to present worth, and testimony regarding the effects of inflation, tend to cancel one another out.[28]

§ 6.13   The Value of Birth Trauma Cases

Here we stretch out upon the precarious limb of our experiences to offer a bold pragmatic market value for the whole of these damages. What is a birth trauma case worth? If the child, as a result of the injury is severely retarded, paralyzed, wholly dependent upon others for survival, blind, seriously deformed, or otherwise so permanently injured as to require constant care and attention throughout a life devoid of most human pleasure, self-reliance, and hope, then at trial the attorney for the plaintiffs should be unafraid to ask for seven to ten million dollars, can hope for a verdict of five to seven million dollars, but should reasonably expect a verdict of one and a half to three million dollars.

These figures can be intimidating, but in todays's economy reflect a realistic appraisal of what it takes to compensate for a shattered, broken life. Medical

---

[27] Rodriguez v. McDonnell Douglas Corp., 87 Cal. App. 3d 626, 151 Cal. Rptr. 339 (1978); Tiffany v. Christman Co., 93 Mich. App. 267, 287 N.W.2d 199 (1979); Bell Helicopter Co. v. Bradshaw, 594 S.W.2d 519 (Tex. Civ. App. 1979); Cords v. Anderson, 80 Wis. 2d 525, 259 N.W.2d 672 (1977).

[28] The U.S. Supreme Court has discussed this issue as it relates to claims brought under the Longshoremans' and Harbor Workers' Compensation Act. *See* Jones & Laughlin Steel Corp. v. Pfeifer, — U.S. —, 76 L.Ed. 2d 768, 103 S. Ct. 2541 (1983).

science, for some, is a two-edged sword. The same miraculous skills and services which today can nourish and maintain a healthy individual throughout
his life, can also salvage and prolong the life of one permanently inflicted with
horrendous injuries. A brain damaged, deformed or paralyzed baby may well
live his allotted three score years and ten, never escaping, through all that
time, from the prison of his injuries.

So, these cases have a value which is greater than most personal injury actions. Still, the ability to collect damages is the practical restraint upon
dreams of unbounded verdicts. Realistically, most birth trauma cases, like
most personal injury cases, settle for somewhat more modest sums. The severity of a child's injury must be balanced against the difficulty of proving malpractice, and together these factors tug both sides towards an accommodation.
More often than not, that accommodation is the negotiation of a structured
settlement which will secure an annuity to the injured child for the rest of his
life.

§ 6.14   Structured Settlements

Because birth trauma cases involve a damaged child, a child who may have to
cope with the effects of an injury for years, perhaps long after his own parents,
the defendant, or even his counsel are gone (or at least retired), these cases are
particularly adaptable to structured settlements. Structured settlements are
advantageous to both plaintiffs and defendants. On the one hand, they provide a virtually guaranteed life time income for the injured child as he grows,
sustaining him and providing for his needs. At the same time, the annuities to
fund a structured settlement may cost defendants dramatically less than any
equivalent lump sum verdict or lump sum settlement.

In negotiating for a structured settlement, an attorney representing an injured child should pay special attention to provisions of guaranteed yearly
payments, periodic increases, lump sum front money, and back-up insurance.
Thus, an ideal structured settlement will guarantee an amount of money to be
paid yearly for X number of years irrespective of any contingency (such as the
child's death); will provide for periodic increases at certain stages of payment
in the future (to adjust for inflation and also the greater expenditures for the
child as he grows older, when it costs more to feed, clothe, and educate the
child, etc.); will pay a certain substantial amount up front in order to immediately assist the child and family and give them funds to help adjust their life-
style to cope with the injury; and will engage a second well-established and
economically sound insurance company to insure the continuance of the pay-

ments should the initial company default for any reason. See **Chapter 28** for a discussion of structured settlement agreements.

Mindful of the utilization of structured settlements in birth trauma cases, the wise attorney who contracts to pursue a birth trauma case will protect his own lien with an appropriate client contract designating how his fee is to be -paid should litigation be terminated in a structured settlement. Without such a contract, an attorney may be restricted to recovering his share of the fee only from the initial lump sum payment, and his fee may be based upon the size of this payment rather than upon the actual value of the settlement. This is a poor reward for the expertise required to negotiate and reach a favorable settlement for one's client.

An attorney who engages to handle a birth trauma or infant injury case should be prepared to cope with financial and economic issues in order to secure the best possible verdict or settlement for his minor client, and for the family of the child, who intimately share the burden of the child's injuries. Damages are usually viewed as compensation for past hurts, but in cases of this nature they are funds which will be used to support and care for a child well into the future, possibly for the remainder of his life. Every legitimate attempt should be made to obtain the maximum benefits for the birth trauma clients so that they can live their future in dignity and in such comfort as their physical or mental condition allows.

§ 6.15   Checklist of Damages

Damages recoverable by parents of an injured minor:

1. Loss of earnings of a child during minority
2. Loss of services of a child during minority
3. Medical expenses, past and future, until the child reaches majority, consisting of, but not limited to, the following:
   a. physicians' charges and fees
   b. hospital charges and fees
   c. cost of medicine and drugs
   d. cost of orthopedic appliances
   e. cost of physical therapy
   f. cost of occupational therapy
   g. ambulance fees
   h. cost of nursing care and attendance
   i. cost of restorative surgery

    j. cost of chiropractic services

    k. cost of psychiatric or psychological services

    l. cost of transportation

    m. extraordinary educational expenses

4. Reimbursement for the extraordinary services, attendance, and nursing care provided by the parents to the child because of the child's injury.

5. Loss of the society and companionship of the child (allowed in some jurisdictions)

6. Mental distress caused by witnessing the negligent injuring of the child (under appropriate circumstances)

Damages recoverable by the minor plaintiff:

1. Loss of future earnings from age of majority to work-life expectancy

2. Medical expenses after majority, consisting of the same and similar charges as those listed above under the parents' medical expenses

3. Intangible charges consisting of damages for:

    a. pain

    b. suffering

    c. mental anguish

    d. fright

    e. shock

    f. denial of social pleasures

    g. embarrassment, humiliation, mortification, shame

    h. reasonably certain future adverse consequences of the injury

    i. disfigurement

    j. deformity

    k. disability

    l. loss of the enjoyment of life

CHAPTER 7

STATUTORY HURDLES

§ 7.1 Special Problems of Malpractice Litigation

Malpractice cases are among the most difficult personal injury cases to litigate. There are several reasons for this. The general public views medical professionals with a high regard, and is skeptical of allegations that a doctor has failed to faithfully perform her professional obligations. At the same time, the public seems more willing to recognize the limits of medical science to effect cures or maintain health, so that adverse results are more often accepted, even by other medically knowledgeable individuals, as the result of natural processes outside of the physician's control instead of being attributable to a professional blunder. The judicial system further handicaps such litigation by adopting restrictive legal doctrines, such as the locality rule which narrows the pool of experts who might be available to willingly testify for a plaintiff in a malpractice case. Even though modern discovery permits attorneys to take a flashlight into the dark forbidding attics of medical records, and to probe the memory of nurses, interns, or others who might supplement with professional observation the vague facts recollected by the untrained lay plaintiff, many of the underlying facts necessary to prove a malpractice case might not be discovered until trial, or never at all. The cost, both in time and money, of pursuing a malpractice claim is a sobering consideration, especially when, as most studies show, the odds of obtaining a successful verdict for the client are less than two in ten.

Despite these difficulties, malpractice cases continue to inspire some of the foremost legal talents to the challenge of pursuing claims of professional negligence. Malpractice suits, encompassing all professions, not just medical practitioners, like product liability suits, have become a highly visible subspecialty of personal injury litigation. This is due, in part, to modern tools of discovery, the willingness of courts to hold medical practitioners subject to a broader, occasionally national, standard of care, members of the medical profession themselves recognizing the need to police the actions of fellow practitioners in order to assure quality care to the public, and, most importantly, an increased public awareness of consumer rights and a growing intolerance towards substandard goods and services in all fields. The increased visibility of malpractice suits has not come about without leaving much anguish and anxiety in its wake, nor without a degree of legitimate criticism and concern for the future relationship between medicine and law. As in any profession, the focus of malpractice litigation upon the horrendous injuries caused by a physician in a moment of professional error, punctuating what might otherwise be a long and successful career, only distorts and unjustly defames the conscientious work of other physicians who pursue their practice with total dedication and faultless care for their patients.

This is not the place to conduct a forum on the serious social, political and jurisprudential issues involved in the dialogue between medicine and the law. Both lawyers and physicians have been known to take unbending defensive postures in the face of criticism, and much unfortunate energy has been lost on the irrational anger which often flares up from time to time as the two professions clash over their respective roles in society. Here our purpose of nodding to these realities is not to advocate a position, but to observe the legislative response which has shaped the new combat zones of medical malpractice suits. Simply stated, the medical profession, concluding that the common law principles which used to protect practitioners from unjust suits have been seriously eroded by the courts, has turned to the legislatures to pass statutes restoring some degree of protection to its embattled profession. Rightly or wrongly, and leaving unanswered here the question of whether there truly is a "medical malpractice crisis," the legislatures in many states have yielded to the concerns of the medical profession by enacting special laws which have a significant impact upon the pursuit of a malpractice claim. The reality which attorneys must cope with today is that in most jurisdictions statutes exist which are applicable solely to malpractice actions and which, for the most part, tend to erect artificial hurdles that must be overcome on the way to a verdict.

Without attempting an exhaustive survey of the legislation of every state, some discussion of these statutes and the judicial reaction to these statutes is warranted so that an attorney pursuing a birth trauma claim may anticipate the difficulties strewn along her path.

§ 7.2   Statutes of Limitations

Statutes of limitations exist in every jurisdiction and are applicable to all types of legal actions. The period of time in which a suit may be maintained against a defendant is viewed as a matter lying exclusively within legislative prerogatives. The law accepts that the limitation periods are entirely arbitrary, and may differ from one cause of action to the next, with no apparent rational basis for the distinction. Statutes of limitation are respected and upheld by the courts whenever applicable, despite the fact that a legitimate and serious claim may be forever barred by the mere passage of a period of time before bringing suit.

In most jurisdictions it is typical to find a distinction drawn between personal injury suits in general and the specific cause of action for malpractice. Usually the malpractice statute of limitations will be shorter.[1] Unless a malpractice suit is timely filed within this specified period, the claim will be lost.

The actual time limit fixed by the legislature for bringing a malpractice suit is often less important than knowing when the period runs. What this involves is the question of when the cause of action accrues so as to start the statute running, and when the statute is tolled or suspended from running due to special circumstances.

Malpractice actions create special problems involving the *accrual of an action*. Most personal injury actions accrue when the wrong to plaintiff causes injury, and this is the date of accrual sometimes found in malpractice limitation statutes.[2] However, by case law interpretation of the statutes, or by statu-

---

[1] *See, e.g.,* Ark. Stat. Ann. § 37-206 (1962) (three years for personal injury actions); Ark. Stat. Ann. § 34.2616 (Supp. 1983) (two years for malpractice claim); Mich. Comp. Laws Ann. § 600.5805(8) (West Supp. 1984) (Mich. Stat. Ann. § 27A.5858(8) (Callaghan Supp. 1984)) (three years for personal injury actions); Mich. Comp. Laws § 600.5805(4) (West Supp. 1984) (Mich. Stat. Ann. § 27A.5805(4) (Callaghan Supp. 1984)) (two years for malpractice claim); N.Y. Civ. Prac. R. 214 (McKinney Supp. 1984) (three years for personal injury actions); N.Y. Civ. Prac. R. 214-a (McKinney Supp. 1984) (two years and six months for malpractice claim).

[2] *E.g.,* Ark. Stat. Ann. § 34.2616 (Supp. 1983); Ga. Code Ann. § 3-1102 (Supp. 1984); Kan. Stat. Ann. § 60-513(7)(c) (1983).

tory enactment, a malpractice cause of action most often will be held to accrue at one of two other possible junctures—either when the patient was last treated by the defendant for the condition giving rise to the suit, or when the patient discovered, or should have discovered, the malpractice.

The *last treatment rule* entered into law as a modification of the date of wrongful act or injury accrual date for medical malpractice action. Several courts have concluded that as long as a physician who had committed a wrongful professional act harming her patient continued to take steps attempting to rectify the error, then the statute of limitations should not begin to run against the claim of a patient willing to submit to such ongoing treatment.[3]

§ 7.3   —The Discovery Rule

Often in medical malpractice cases neither the last treatment accrual date or the date of injury or wrongdoing accrual date seems fair to the injured patient simply because of the patient's failure to recognize or appreciate that she is a victim of a physician or hospital's professional negligence. A patient may suffer the ill effects of malpractice for several years, not realizing that she has been injured by the defendant, attributing such sufferings instead to the normal consequence of either the original disease or to the unavoidable risks of the treatment to which the patient has submitted. A common complaint of concealment arises in the context of surgery where, inadvertently, some foreign object is sewn up inside the operative site. In a sense, the wrongful act of the surgeon is literally buried, out of sight, and it may be several years—and after the statute of limitations would have run under the wrongful act or last treatment rule—before this foreign object may be discovered. In a few states this has led to the adoption of a specific corollary to the malpractice limitations statute, a tolling provision allowing a plaintiff to commence suit within some period of time after the discovery of a "foreign object" left in the body.[4] A different, and a more flexible approach that encompasses not just foreign object claims but all malpractice cases where the patient fails to recognize that his suffering is a result of a physician's wrongful act, is to permit the plaintiff

---

[3] *See* DeHaan v. Winter, 258 Mich. 293, 241 N.W. 923 (1932); Hotelling v. Walther, 169 Or. 559, 130 P.2d 944 (1942); Samuelson v. Freeman, 75 Wash. 2d 894, 454 P.2d 406 (1969); *see also* Strong v. Pontiac Gen. Hosp., 117 Mich. App. 143, 323 N.W.2d 629 (1982), *vacated on other grounds*, 419 Mich. 881, 347 N.W.2d 696 (1984) (held that the course of continuing treatment included treatment by a physician other than the defendant but for whose services defendant had agreed to pay).

[4] *E.g.*, Ark. Stat. Ann. § 34.2616 (Supp. 1983); N.Y. Civ. Proc. R. 214-a (McKinney Supp. 1984).

to bring suit within some time period after the patient discovers, or in the exercise of reasonable care should have discovered, the malpractice of the defendant.

This *discovery rule* is probably prevalent in one guise or another in the majority of jurisdictions. In states adhering by statute to either a wrongful act or last treatment accrual date, the courts have been able to modify these provisions by a liberal interpretation of the "fraudulent concealment" tolling statute found in most jurisdictions. These provide that a statute of limitations is tolled while a potential defendant takes steps to actively conceal from a potential plaintiff the existence of a claim or cause of action. In medical malpractice cases, courts have held that when the defendant physician knows, or in the exercise of reasonable care should know, that she has committed malpractice harmful to her patient, her failure to disclose these facts to the patient may be sufficient to bring into play the fraudulent concealment tolling statute thereby preventing the plaintiff's suit from being barred by the statute of limitations.[5]

Still other courts have simply engrafted onto the limitations statute a discovery rule.[6] Further, in some states the statute of limitations itself has been amended to include a discovery proviso.[7] Where such a rule is operative, a medical malpractice suit may be commenced within some fixed period of time after the plaintiff discovers, or in the exercise of reasonable care or diligence, should have discovered, the malpractice of the defendant.

As a practical point, rarely will parents come into an attorney's office having "discovered" that a defendant's professional negligence has caused an injury to their child. Rarely, in fact, do they even suspect this possibility, for in trying to cope with and endure the tragedy of a severely injured child, parents typically block out of their minds the events of birth and want to believe that the injury was an unavoidable act of fate rather than the result of another's neglect. The physicians involved invariably will leave the parents with the impression that everything that could have been done for the child was done, and will not even hint that someone's malpractice may have caused the child's injury. Until someone plants a seed of suspicion in the parents' minds, they

---

5 Puro v. Henry, 188 Conn. 301, 449 A.2d 176 (1982); Almengor v. Dade County, 359 So. 2d 892 (Fla. Dist. Ct. App. 1978); Weinstock v. Ott, 444 N.E.2d 1227 (Ind. Ct. App. 1983); Brewington v. Raksakulthi, 584 S.W.2d 112 (Mo. Ct. App. 1979); Ray v. Scheibert, 224 Tenn. 99, 450 S.W.2d 578 (1969).

6 *See, e.g.,* Johnson v. Caldwell, 371 Mich. 368, 123 N.W.2d 785 (1963); Teeters v. Currey, 518 S.W.2d 512 (Tenn. 1974).

7 *See, e.g.,* Cal. Civ. Proc. Code. Ann. § 340.5 (West 1982); Fla. Stat. Ann. § 95.11(4)(b) (West Supp. 1984); Mich. Comp. Laws Ann. § 600.5838 (West Supp. 1984); (Mich. Stat. Ann. § 27A.5838 (Callaghan Supp. 1984)). Of course, in some jurisdictions the legislative response to the discovery rule has been to nullify the rule. *See* Littlefield v. Hays, 609 S.W.2d 627 (Tex. Civ. App. 1980); DeBoer v. Brown, 138 Ariz. 178, 673 P.2d 922 (1983).

normally will neither walk nor run to the nearest attorney. Also, being laypersons, even when they do decide to consult an attorney, they usually have no idea whether there is any basis for suspecting malpractice or not. Nor, based upon the initial client interview, does the attorney. Until the medical records are received and reviewed by experts and their reports returned, a malpractice claim is rarely discovered. For the same reason that malpractice defendants insist upon expert testimony to prove their breach of the standard of care at trial, that breach is often not obvious to either the lay plaintiffs nor even to their more experienced counsel.

Consequently, in most cases, to be perfectly candid about the actual events that lead to a suit, the plaintiff really never discovers if there has been a wrong committed by defendant which caused injury until after seeing an attorney and until after the attorney's own experts can report their evaluation of the case. A good malpractice attorney will not risk injuring the reputation of a fine physician by precipitously filing a suit without first obtaining confirmation from experts that a wrong has been committed.

Because of the time constraints imposed by the limitations period, prompt action is required of attorneys in medical malpractice suits to secure all the available information necessary to prepare the detailed pleadings which initiate the cause of action. Although in birth trauma cases it will often be true that the limitations period is tolled with respect to the minor plaintiff, the parents of the child have an independent claim which an attorney must make every effort to preserve. For this purpose she should, during the first client interview, diligently probe into when the parents first suspected wrongdoing on the part of the likely defendants. Using such information, counsel should be able to gauge when the suit must be filed to be timely under the appropriate statute. See **Chapter 30** for further discussion of the initial client interview.

§ 7.4   —Tolling Provisions

The law views an infant as legally disabled from bringing suit, so typically statutes toll the running of the statute of limitations during minority. This, of course, leads to the academically possible situation of a birth trauma suit remaining viable for 18 to 20 years.[8]

---

[8] Legislative attempts to curtail the tolling provision applicable to minors in medical malpractice cases have met with mixed reactions. Both Schwan v. Riverside Methodist Hosp., 6 Ohio St. 3d 300, 452 N.E.2d 1337 (1983) and Sax v. Votteler, 648 S.W.2d 661 (Tex. 1983) have found provisions which would curtail the tolling provision for minors in medical malpractice cases unconstitutional. *But see* Opalko v. Marymount Hosp. Inc., 9 Ohio St. 3d 63,

While it is true that in an unusual case, a birth trauma claim might not be filed until nearly two decades after the events giving rise to the suit, such a delay in filing a birth trauma claim is rarely justified. Plaintiffs, and their counsel, obtain no benefit from delaying the pursuit of legitimate malpractice claims. Injuries to a child impose an economic and psychological burden on a family which, if anything, merely makes plaintiffs in a birth trauma suit even more impatient to have their day in court in the hope of obtaining a favorable verdict. A significant portion of damages recoverable in such suits is for the parents (medical expenses and loss of earnings to majority, for example; see §§ 6.2 through 6.7), and unless the parents themselves are under the age of majority at the time of the child's birth, no tolling provision will protect their claim from the statute of limitations. Consequently, every incentive exists to place a birth trauma case into court as swiftly as possible. The tolling provisions are there to assist the unusual case, to protect minors whose parents or guardians are less efficient or enthusiastic in pursuing or protecting their rights.[9] They are not there to excuse or permit sloth on the part of counsel undertaking to investigate and pursue a birth trauma claim. In a birth trauma case, tolling provisions on behalf of the injured minor, together with the discovery rule on behalf of the parents, usually suffice to postpone the running statute beyond the actual time period prescribed by legislation. This does not mean that an attorney should slacken her efforts to file suit as soon as possible, or should ignore the running of the statute. Eventually suits will be time-barred unless the appropriate steps to bring the case to court are taken.

§ 7.5   Good Samaritan Statutes

In the 1960s a popular movement occurred to protect physicians performing medical services in an emergency from being subsequently sued for any malpractice committed under such circumstances. Legislatures in most states passed *good samaritan statutes* to accomplish this purpose, limiting the types of claims which may be asserted against medical personnel who respond to an emergency, usually providing that a potential defendant can only be sued for her gross negligence.

Little actual litigation has developed under these statutes and their effect has been sharply curtailed by the case law construing their application.

---

458 N.E.2d 847 (1984), finding that under amended malpractice statute of limitations all claims, including those of minors, are barred four years after the wrongful act occurred.

[9] The appointment of a guardian is held not to affect the tolling provision on behalf of a minor. Mason v. Sorrell, 260 Ark. 27, 551 S.W.2d 184 (1976); Kolsky v. Dick, 359 Mich. 615, 103 N.W.2d 618 (1960). *See*, Annot., 86 A.L.R.2d 965 (1962).

Courts have narrowly interpreted what constitutes an emergency triggering the operation of such statutes, and, looking at the intent of the legislatures in passing these laws, have restricted their application to pure volunteers who do not have any prior commitment to render care or treatment to the plaintiff or hold themselves out to the public as ready to render emergency medical assistance.[10]

As a practical matter, good samaritan statutes will rarely be involved in a birth trauma case. Despite human interest stories of births occurring under unusual circumstances, the reality is that labor is usually a lengthy process which permits a woman enough time to reach her preselected physician and be admitted to her preselected hospital or clinic before actually giving birth. The processes of birth are not such that can be usually categorized as an emergency, and absent an extremely rare case of an unexpected birth occurring in a nonmedical setting and attended to, purely coincidentally, by a doctor who volunteers her assistance, these special protective good samaritan statutes will not have any impact on most birth trauma medical malpractice suits.

§ 7.6　Statutes Fixing the Standard of Care

As discussed in the **Chapter 4** reviewing the development of standard of care, many courts are adopting an increasingly flexible attitude toward the parameters of this standard and towards the nature of expert testimony needed to prove the standard. As a direct reaction to this trend, several legislatures have been persuaded to pass statutes which attempt to codify the standard of care. In Michigan, for example, the supreme court issued a decision previewing a possible abandonment of the locality rule,[11] and the legislature was quick to respond with a statute which specifies that in a malpractice case brought against a general practitioner, the plaintiff must present expert evidence that the defendant failed to follow the standard of care as practiced in the same or similar communities.[12] Examples of even more restrictive statutes are found in Arizona, which applies a state-wide standard,[13] and Delaware, where the statute goes so far as to restore a strict locality rule.[14]

---

[10] *See* Annot., 39 A.L.R.3d 222 (1971).

[11] Siirila v. Barrios, 398 Mich. 576, 248 N.W.2d 171 (1977) (Williams, J., concurring).

[12] Mich. Comp. Laws. Ann., § 600.2912a (West Supp. 1984) (Mich. Stat. Ann. § 27A.2912a (Callaghan Supp. 1984)).

[13] Ariz. Rev. Stat. Ann. § 12-563 (1982); *see also* Va. Code, § 8.01-581.20 (1984); Wash. Rev. Code Ann. § 7.70.040(1) (Supp. 1984).

[14] Del. Code Ann. tit. 18, § 6854(a) (Supp. 1984). Under this statute

These statutes portray the currents of the jousting between courts and the legislatures in attempting to define the standard of care applicable to medical malpractice actions. Generally, the courts in recent years have attempted to move away from some of the legal concepts harking back to an earlier era when the practice of medicine was more parochial. As discussed in **Chapter 4**, medical standards of care today are developed on a national scale eliminating local variations. The courts, which gave birth to the locality rule initially, have responded to changing realities by seeking to retreat from the more unreasonable applications of this rule. However, the legislatures in many states,[15] under considerable pressure from the medical profession, have been encouraged to take a reactionary stance either holding the line on the existing locality rule before its further erosion, or in passing acts restoring a more restrictive locality rule than presently found in case precedents. Whether such statutes shall succeed in their purpose remains to be seen, for it must not be forgotten that the courts interpret statutes and through such interpretation some of the intended consequences of these statutes may be avoided.[16] Where such statutes are a factor, counsel should be encouraged to use imaginative arguments to nullify their restrictive intent.

§ 7.7   Mediation and Arbitration

Several states have responded to the phantom medical malpractice crisis of the past few years by adopting mediation or arbitration statutes. There is some confusion in the nomenclature employed in such legislation, and here we will try to distinguish the two procedures by restricting the term *mediation* to

---

> No person shall be competent to give expert medical testimony as to the applicable standards of skill and care unless such person is familiar with the degree of skill ordinarily employed in the community or locality where the alleged malpractice occurred, under similar circumstances, by members of the profession practiced by the health care provider; provided, however, that any such expert witness need to be licensed in the state.

See Loftus v. Hayden, 391 A.2d 749 (Del. 1980); *see also* Idaho Code § 6-1012 (1979).

[15] In one state the legislature has gone along with the liberalizing trend, passing a statute codifying a national standard of care. *See* Okla. Stat. Ann. tit. 76, § 20.1 (West 1983); *see also* N.H. Rev. Stat. Ann. § 508.13 (19—); Vt. Stat. Ann. tit. 12, § 1908.(1) (Supp. 1984).

[16] *See, e.g.,* Butler v. Alatur, 419 A.2d 938 (Del. 1980); and Thomas v. St. Francis Hosp., Inc., 447 A.2d 435 (Del. 1982), both pointing to a judicial modification of Delaware's statutory strict locality rule. In Butler, the Delaware Supreme Court says, "Nor do we find that the statute or the *Loftus* case require the words 'community or locality', terms which together appear deliberately flexible, to be construed in every instance as limited to the bounds of Delaware."

those statutes providing for a nonbinding review of malpractice claims as a condition precedent to a jury trial, in contrast to *arbitration* statutes which endorse a binding nonjudicial resolution of malpractice claims as a substitute for jury trial.

Under these definitions, most states which have adopted such statutes have opted for the procedure here referred to as mediation. While the details may differ from state to state, essentially mediation statutes create a nonjudicial panel, usually a tribunal consisting of at least one medical practitioner, which is designated to review and pass on the merits of a plaintiff's malpractice claim before plaintiff may proceed to trial.[17]

To give some muscle to these nonbinding decisions, the statutes provide for a variety of sanctions to impose on a plaintiff who persists on going to trial after receiving an unfavorable mediation verdict. The plaintiff may be required to pay actual litigation costs should she be unable to secure a jury verdict significantly in excess of the mediation award. In some jurisdictions, the report of the mediation panel may be later introduced as evidence at trial, coated with varying degrees of evidentiary weight which must be nullified or overcome by plaintiff's proofs.[18] Receipt of an unfavorable mediation decision may subject a plaintiff to a requirement to post a bond in order to preserve her right to proceed to trial.[19]

These mediation procedures have been principally criticized, sometimes successfully, as imposing an unnecessary and unconstitutional delay in the litigation of legitimate malpractice claims.[20] However, in many states, these mediation procedures have overcome constitutional and procedural objections and remain a procedural gatehouse at which all major malpractice cases must

---

[17] Ariz. Rev. Stat. Ann. § 12-567 (1982); Conn. Gen. Stat. Ann. § 38-19b, (West Supp. 1984); Idaho Code § 6-1001 (1979); Ind. Code Ann. § 16-9.5-9-2 (Burns 1983); Kan. Stat. Ann. § 65-4901 (1980); La. Rev. Stat. Ann. § 40:1299.47 (West 1977); Me. Rev. Stat. Ann. tit. 24, § 2803 (Supp. 1984); Md. Cts. & Jud. Proc. Code Ann. § 3-2A-04 (1984); Mass. Gen. Laws Ann. ch. 231, § 60B (Supp. 1984); Mont. Code Ann. § 27-6-101 (1984); N.Y. Jud. Law § 148-a (McKinney 1983); Ohio Rev. Code Ann. § 2711.21 (Page 1981); Tenn. Code Ann. § 29-26-104 (1980); Va. Code § 8.01-581.2 (1984); Wis. Stat. Ann. § 655.04 (West 1980).

[18] *See, e.g.,* La. Rev. Stat. Ann. § 40:1299.47 (West 1977); Md. Cts. & Jud. Proc. Code Ann. § 53-2A-04 (1984) (losing party has burden of proof); N.Y. Jud. Law § 148-a (McKinney 1983); Ohio Rev. Code Ann. § 2711.21 (Page 1981); Tenn. Code Ann. § 29-26-104 (1980); Va. Code § 8.01-5812 (1984); Wis. Stat. Ann. § 655.04 (West 1980). *But see* Mont. Code Ann. § 27-6-101 (Supp. 1984) (decision not admissible).

[19] Mass. Gen. Laws Ann. ch. 231, § 60B (Supp. 1984).

[20] *See, e.g.,* Aldana v. Holub, 381 So. 2d 231 (Fla. 1980); Cardinal Glennon Memorial Hosp. for Children v. Gaertner, 583 S.W.2d 107 (Mo. 1979); Mattos v. Thompson, 491 Pa. 385, 421 A.2d 190 (1980); Boucher v. Sayeed, 459 A.2d 87 (R.I. 1983).

pause and pay a toll.[21] The better malpractice attorneys, of course, will approach mediation with the same enthusiasm and diligence normally employed at trial, for the procedure can provide a real testing ground of the merits of one's case, exposing both strengths and weaknesses. Mediation does have the advantage of a dress rehearsal, and its nonbinding nature still permits a litigant dissatisfied with the outcome to proceed to a jury trial.

The same cannot be said of arbitration, a binding procedure which generally forecloses the opportunity of a jury trial. Most arbitrations arise under private contractual agreements and are limited by their terms to resolving disputes which involve the provisions of the contract. There is a serious question regarding whether a private arbitration agreement, signed by a patient as she contracts to obtain medical services from a physician or hospital, is enforceable, especially when most malpractice claims are not founded upon breach of contract by the physician or hospital, but upon tort law principles which would apply even in the absence of a formal contract. Without legislative endorsement, an arbitration clause contained in a medical contract is likely to be unenforceable or ineffective.[22]

Some states, however, have adopted statutes which permit patients and health care providers to enter into valid arbitration agreements which would permit arbitration panels to enter binding decisions on medical malpractice claims submitted pursuant to such agreements.[23] One of the most comprehensive schemes is that of Michigan, which sets forth detailed procedures for the arbitration of medical malpractice disputes.[24] Although seriously challenged on constitutional grounds because the statutes authorize that at least one member of the three member panel hearing an arbitrated malpractice claim be a physician or a hospital administrator, the Michigan Supreme Court has upheld the validity of the state's medical malpractice arbitration act.[25]

---

[21] Eastin v. Broomfield, 116 Ariz. 576, 570 P.2d 744 (1977); Johnson v. St. Vincent Hosp., 273 Ind. 374, 404 N.E.2d 585 (1980); Vincent v. Romagosa, 425 So. 2d 1237 (La. 1983); Attorney Gen. v. Johnson, 282 Md. 274, 385 A.2d 57 (1978); Paro v. Longwood Hosp., 373 Mass. 645, 369 N.E.2d 985 (1977); Linder v. Smith, 629 P.2d 1187 (Mont. 1981); Beatty v. Akron City Hosp., 67 Ohio St. 2d 483, 424 N.E.2d 586 (1981).

[22] See, e.g., Wheeler v. St. Joseph Hosp., 63 Cal. App. 3d 345, 133 Cal. Rptr. 775 (1976); O'Keefe v. South Shore Internal Medicine Assocs., P.C., 102 Misc. 2d 59, 422 N.Y.S.2d 828 (1979).

[23] Ala. Code § 6-5-485 (1977); Cal. Civ. Pro. Code Ann. § 1295 (West 1982); Ga. Code Ann. § 7-402 (Supp. 1984); Ill. Ann. Stat. tit. 10, 201 (Supp. 1984); Ohio Rev. Code Ann. § 2711.22 (Page 1981); S.D. Codified Laws Ann. § 21-25B-1 (1979); Vt. Stat. Ann. tit. 12, § 7002 (Supp. 1984).

[24] Mich. Comp. Laws Ann. § 600.5040 (West Supp. 1984) (Mich. Stat. Ann. § 27A.5040 (Callaghan Supp. 1984)).

[25] Morris v. Metriyakool, 418 Mich. 423, 344 N.W.2d 736 (1984).

Obviously, these arbitration statutes can be extremely detrimental to patients with serious malpractice claims who, out of ignorance or misinformation, sign away their right to a jury trial. Whatever procedural advantages can be argued on behalf of arbitration, the undeniable fact remains that these advantages are more than offset by the reality that sophisticated arbitrators, especially members of the medical profession, are simply not as generous to personal injury litigants as are lay jurors capable of empathizing with the pain and suffering of a malpractice victim.

Consequently, whenever confronted with an arbitration agreement interposed between a birth trauma claim and the right to a jury trial, counsel are urged to be imaginative and vigorous in their attempts to avoid arbitration.

§ 7.8   Limitations on Damages

Perhaps the most serious threat to malpractice litigation are those statutes which attempt to lessen or limit the potential damages which may be awarded in a medical malpractice case. In several states the legislatures have been induced by the medical profession to pass a variety of acts designed to curb the impact of large medical malpractice awards. Some of these enactments have been found to be constitutional, while others have been struck down.

Essentially, these statutes focus on three approaches to reduce damages. The two least offensive proposals permit a malpractice damage award to be reduced by sums the plaintiff has received from collateral sources of recovery and to be paid through periodic payments. The more draconian legislation seeks to fix a cap or ceiling on malpractice damages, prohibiting any award to exceed an amount arbitrarily decided by the legislature. Although these proposals are usually enacted as a package, we shall briefly discuss them separately in §§ 7.9 through 7.11.

§ 7.9   —Statutes Modifying the Collateral Source
Rule

In the usual personal injury case, a plaintiff who successfully proves the liability of the defendants is permitted to recover damages for medical expenses, lost wages, loss of earning capacity, and such other tangible and intangible damages which she can establish with her proofs. Further, the fact that the plaintiff's medical expenses, lost wages, and so forth, may be paid or reimbursed by disability or health insurance, medicaid, worker's compensation, or other prepaid or state financed programs, will not diminish the defendant's obligation to pay the damages for which plaintiff has recovered such sums. Indeed, the general rule will not even permit defendant to place the fact of such payments into evidence, for the law will not allow a tortfeasor to take advantage of the fact that his innocent victim can obtain financial assistance to alleviate his injuries from third parties. This is known as the *collateral source rule*, and has been adopted uniformly throughout the states, and remains viable in all personal injury actions not subject to special statutes.

However, in several states, legislation has been passed which modifies the general collateral source rule in medical malpractice claims. Basically, these statutes allow a malpractice defendant to reduce her damages by the amount that plaintiff has received from collateral sources as compensation for her injury.[26] (Usually the statutes provide an exception for those amounts paid where a right of subrogation exists.) Although a few cases have found these statutes unconstitutional,[27] others have upheld these malpractice collateral source laws.[28]

§ 7.10   —Periodic Payment Statutes

Periodic payment statutes have been enacted in several states.[29] Basically, these provide that future damages in a medical malpractice case, if in excess of some amount fixed by the statute, may be awarded either as a lump sum to the plaintiff or may be ordered to be paid periodically. The statutes vary in terms the courts' discretion. The Delaware enactment, for example, states that the court *may* order periodic payments of sums exceeding $100,000 if either party requests such payments. The California law more forcefully states that the court *shall* order periodic payments of damages in excess of $50,000 of either party requests. Recently, the California statute was upheld as constitutional.[30]

---

[26] Ariz. Rev. Stat. Ann. § 12-565 (1982); Cal. Civ. Code § 3333.1 (West Supp. 1985); Del. Code Ann. tit. 18, § 6862 (Supp. 1984); Fla. Stat. Ann. § 768.50 (West Supp. 1984); Iowa Code Ann. § 147.136 (West Supp. 1984); N.Y. Civ. Prac. Law, § 4545 (McKinney Supp. 1984); S.D. Codified Laws Ann. § 21-3-12 (1979); Tenn. Code Ann. § 29-26-119 (1981); Wash. Rev. Code Ann. § 7.70.080 (Supp. 1985).

[27] Carson v. Maurer, 120 N.H. 925, 424 A.2d 825 (1980); Arneson v. Olson, 270 N.W.2d 125 (N.D. 1978).

[28] Eastin v. Broomfield, 116 Ariz. 576, 570 P.2d 744 (1977); Pinillos v. Cedars of Lebanon Hosp. Corp., 403 So. 2d 365 (Fla. 1981); Rudolph v. Iowa Methodist Medical Center, 293 N.W.2d 550 (Iowa 1980).

[29] Ark. Stat. Ann. § 34-2619 (Supp. 1983); Cal. Civ. Proc. Code § 667.7 (West 1980); Del. Code Ann. tit. 18, § 6864 (Supp. 1984).

[30] American Bank & Trust Co. v. Community Hosp., 36 Cal. 3d 359, 683 P.2d 670, 204 Cal. Rptr. 671 (1984).

Similar statutes in Florida and in New Hampshire, however, have been found to be unconstitutional.[31]

§ 7.11   —Statutes Fixing a Ceiling on Damages

The most insidious malpractice legislation involves attempts to actually place a limit upon the amount of damages which a plaintiff may recover in a medical malpractice suit. These statutes are now found in several jurisdictions.[32] Where such statutes have faced clear constitutional challenges, the courts have divided on whether such statutes afford due process or equal protection to the victims of medical malpractice. One state, through its courts, has sustained its statutory cap on medical malpractice damages.[33] Other cases have found these provisions to be constitutionally infirm.[34] In these latter cases the courts have criticized such legislation as violating equal protection in treating medical malpractice victims differently from tort victims generally, as violating substantive due process by failing to offer to tort victims a quid pro quo to support the favored treatment afforded to malpractice defendants, and as violating procedural due process in denying the most seriously injured malpractice victims full compensation for their injuries.

Each of these constitutional criticisms of this drastic limitation on damages seem fully justified. These limitations on damages must be of particular concern in pursuing birth trauma claims. The largest statutory limitation is one of one million dollars. The most common statutes limit damages to $500,000. Quite frankly, in light of modern medical costs and economic inflation, these

---

[31] Florida Medical Center Inc. v. Von Stetina, 436 So. 2d 1022 (Fla. Dist. Ct. App. 1983); Carson v. Maurer, 120 N.H. 925, 424 A.2d 825 (1980).

[32] Cal. Civ. Code § 3333.2 (West Supp. 1985) ($250,000 limit on noneconomic damages); Idaho Code § 39-4204 (1977) ($150,000 limit); Ind. Stat. Ann. § 16-9.5-2-2 (Burns 1983) ($500,000 limit); La. Rev. Stat. Ann. § 40.1299.42 (West 1977) ($500,000 limit); N.M. Stat. Ann. § 41-5-6 (1982) ($500,000 limit); S.D. Codified Laws § 21-3-11 (1979) ($500,000 limit); Va. Code § 8.01-581.15 (1984) ($1,000,000 limit); see also the complex malpractice statutes of Wisconsin, Wis. Stat. Ann. § 655.01 et seq. Also see Neb. Rev. Stat. § 44-2801 et seq. (1984) and La. Stat. Ann. § 40.1299.39 (West 1977).

[33] Johnson v. St. Vincent Hosp., 273 Ind. 374, 404 N.E.2d 585 (1980); see also Williams v. Lallie Kemp Charity Hosp., 428 So. 2d 1000 (La. Ct. App. 1983) (upholding limit applied to state health care provider); and Prendergast v. Nelson, 199 Neb. 97, 256 N.W.2d 657 (1977) (upholding elective limitation of damages).

[34] Wright v. Central DuPage Hosp. Ass'n, 63 Ill. 2d 313, 347 N.E.2d 736 (1976); Carson v. Maurer, 120 N.H. 925, 424 A.2d 825 (1980); Arneson v. Olson, 270 N.W.2d 125 (N.D. 1978); Simon v. St. Elizabeth Medical Center, 3 Ohio Op. 3d 164, 355 N.E.2d 903 (1976); Baptist Hosp. v. Baber, 672 S.W.2d 296 (Tex. Civ. App. 1984).

figures are ridiculously low when measured against the lifetime of pain, suffering, and economic hardship which can be predicted to follow brain damage or a crippling disorder at birth. Putting a cap on damages in order to placate the financial concerns of the medical profession and its insurers strikes most persons of reasonable sensitivity as a crude solution to what may not even be a real problem, especially when weighed against the true value of damages sustained by a mother's son who may never walk or a father's daughter who may never cry or laugh. A brain damaged child may require attendance and close care for the rest of her life, and it is easy to demonstrate that the cost of future attendance alone has a present value in excess of the limits imposed by these statutes. Add to this the present value of future lost earnings and pain and suffering over a lifetime, and it is possible to project legitimate, dispassionate, damage figures three or four or five times that of any legislatively imposed ceiling. Singling out victims of medical malpractice to bear for themselves the financial burden of such extensive injuries (while product liability, slip and fall or automobile injury victims do not), in order to appease the medical profession and abate the threat of certain vocal practitioners and insurers to walk away from their professional responsibilities unless given some sort of protection from the consequences of their own errors, must surely be constitutionally wrong. Certainly, such a concept is repugnant to all traditions of tort law, and courts should demand overwhelming proof of the need for such legislation before abdicating to the legislature the judicial power to redress the wrongs done to citizens.

Whether the tide of these protective malpractice statutes shall be stemmed or rolled back depends upon the willingness of the legal profession to vigorously condemn and creatively oppose such legislation both in the judicial and legislative forums. In the meantime, however, attorneys pursuing birth trauma claims must be aware of the statutory hurdles which often intervene in medical malpractice cases and must be prepared to overcome these hurdles as they are encountered.

CHAPTER 8

OTHER ACTIONS

§ 8.1   Breach of Contract

Under some circumstances, it may be possible to bring an action against a physician which sounds in contract as well as, or as an alternate to, an action in tort. Such contract actions are founded upon a specific promise or guarantee made by the physician to effect a specific cure or result, which promise induced the plaintiff to undergo the course of treatment performed by the physician.[1] As with any other contractual warranty, should the promised result not come about, the person who paid consideration on the basis of the promise has a right of action for breach of contract, which allows not just recovery of his consideration, but damages for any consequential injuries which might be reasonably contemplated to result if the agreement is breached.

Birth trauma cases rarely present opportunities for breach of contract claims. Physicians will not usually guarantee that they will deliver a perfectly healthful and normal child, and most parents can hardly make a legitimate

---

[1] *See* Annot., 43 A.L.R.3d 1221 (1972).

claim that they have relied on such guarantees as an inducement to submit to the care of a particular physician. And, of course, the yet to be born child has entered into no contract and would only have standing as a third party beneficiary, if at all.

There are, however, two birth-related areas where a possible breach of contract action may arise from medical treatment that fails to fulfill a contractual promise. Potential parents seeking to avert future pregnancies might engage a physician to perform surgery, usually a vasectomy or tubal ligation, to accomplish this purpose. Most physicians, knowing the risks inherent in any medical procedure, will avoid making any promise that conception will be impossible after surgery. Yet, occasionally, the courts must wrestle with cases of this nature where plaintiffs sincerely affirm that the defendant physician made such an unequivocal promise, thereby creating an express warranty on which to bring a breach of contract action.[2]

The other breach of contract action which infrequently arises involves an obstetrician's promise to deliver a child in a particular manner. For example, a physician might promise a woman undergoing a difficult pregnancy and having a history of past birthing problems that he will perform a cesarean section (C-section) at the appropriate time to protect the health of both mother and child. Should he then fail to keep his promise, and as a result either the mother, the child, or both suffer injury because the promised C-section was not performed, a cause of action for breach of contract as well as for malpractice might be pled and proven against the errant doctor.[3]

As a practical matter, there are few significant advantages to bringing a contract action instead of a tort action. The principal reason for selecting this approach is that contract actions are usually graced with a longer statute of limitations, and thus such an action might be brought to salvage a case barred by the running of the statute against the malpractice claim. In at least one jurisdiction, such promises to cure are caught within the statute of frauds so that no action for a breach of such agreement can be maintained unless the

---

[2] *See, e.g.,* Jackson v. Anderson, 230 So. 2d 503 (Fla. Dist. Ct. App. 1970); Doerr v. Villate, 74 Ill. App. 2d 332, 220 N.E.2d 767 (1966); Mason v. Western Pa. Hosp., 286 Pa. Super. 354, 428 A.2d 1366 (1981). However, in some cases courts have found that the physician's assurances amounted to merely an expression of opinion and not a warranty of successful sterilization. *See* Rogala v. Silva, 16 Ill. App. 3d 63, 305 N.E.2d 571 (1973); Sard v. Hardy, 281 Md. 432, 379 A.2d 1014 (1977) (but court did find evidence sufficient to support a "lack of informed consent" claim).

[3] Stewart v. Rudner, 349 Mich. 459, 84 N.W.2d 816 (1957). *But see* Gilmore v. O'Sullivan, 106 Mich. App. 35, 307 N.W.2d 695 (1981) (insufficient written evidence of contract to take claim out of the statute of frauds).

promise has been reduced to writing.[4] In terms of proof, such contract actions usually resolve themselves into a credibility contest as plaintiff affirms, and defendant denies, that a specific promise to effect a specific result was made. Usually, expert testimony will still be required to prove that defendant had breached the contract and almost always expert testimony is needed to establish that the breach was a proximate cause of plaintiff's damages. Thus, a contract claim is not easier to prove, only different in the focus of its proofs.

§ 8.2   Informed Consent

Informed consent is a distinct species of malpractice suit deriving from common law principles of assault and battery. Today there are two types of informed consent cases. The traditional action is still one based upon assault and battery, and occurs when a physician proceeds to operate on a condition without first obtaining the specific consent of his patient to invade that part of the person's anatomy subject to the physician's ministrations. Because this amounts to an intentional tort, recovery of nominal damages may be allowed, even if the unauthorized procedure is done properly and no serious adverse consequences have resulted. The more common informed consent claim is one based upon negligence principles and arises when the physician fails to inform the patient of the possible adverse consequences of a course of treatment recommended and undertaken by the physician. Because the basic elements and legal rules for each type of action are different, it is important in dealing with informed consent claims to identify which type of claim is being advanced.

In an assault and battery type case, a plaintiff need only show that a physician administered some medical treatment beyond the scope of the consent given by the patient, or, in the case of a minor patient, by the parents of the patient. Where such facts are established, the plaintiff may recover even slight damages for the wrongful invasion of his person, though normally the action will seek actual damages. The typical defenses raised in such cases are, first, that there was consent to the treatment, and, second, that a life threatening emergency situation was present which precluded defendant from having an opportunity to obtain the proper consent before acting to resolve the emergency. The fact that the physician complied with the standard of care in performing the treatment, however, or even that the result was ultimately beneficial to the patient, is no defense to liability if, in fact, the physician ad-

---

[4] Mich. Comp. Laws Ann. § 566.132(g) (West Supp. 1984) (Mich. Stat. Ann. § 26.922(g) (Callaghan 1982)).

ministered medical treatment to a competent patient in a nonemergency setting without first obtaining that patient's consent.[5]

These traditional informed consent cases usually arise out of a surgical procedure where a physician, probing the internal organs of a patient pursuant to an agreement to perform one type of surgery, sees another problem requiring correction and uses the present opportunity to reach beyond the scope of the original surgery to operate on a different organ. While such housecleaning may be medically efficient, it is legally impermissible. If a physician performing a cesarean section (C-section) notices that an ovary is damaged, he will be liable for assault and battery if he goes ahead and decides to remove the ovary without first giving the patient a conscious opportunity to decide for herself that such a course of action should be undertaken. Even if the surgeon is certain that the organ should be removed, that it may cause discomfort to the patient in the future, and that the patient, if apprised of all the facts, will readily agree to the recommended surgery, if no life-threatening emergency exists and if the patient has not agreed to surgery of this type, the surgeon had best sew the patient up and wait for the patient's recovery from surgery in order to discuss the issue with her before proceeding with any additional operation.[6]

Informed consent cases founded upon negligence are more difficult to prove. There are many medical conditions which invite a choice in the patient's selection of a course of action. For example, the delivery of a child may be performed in many different ways, ranging from a wholly natural childbirth, involving minimal medical interference, to the surgical removal of the fetus by a caesarean operation. Sometimes the circumstances preclude a prospective mother from making any choice regarding these matters, but more frequently women are aware of their options and expect to be consulted and to have a say in the method of delivery to be favored. The law recognizes that competent adults have the ultimate right to decide the course of medical treatment to which they are willing to submit themselves, and the role of the physician is to advise and make recommendations, assisting the patient to make the rational decisions necessary for her own well-being. When a patient does consent to a course of treatment, such consent should be an *informed consent*, which means that it should be based upon a proper understanding of the options and of the respective risks inherent in each option. If the physician fails to inform the patient of those options or to adequately discuss the risks of each option with the patient, liability may be found, when adverse consequences occur, because of the lack of such informed consent.[7]

---

[5] *See* 61 Am. Jur. 2d, *Physicians and Surgeons*, § 197 (1981).

[6] *See, e.g.*, Thimatariga v. Chambers, 46 Md. App. 260, 416 A.2d 1326 (1980).

[7] Sard v. Hardy, 281 Md. 432, 379 A.2d 1014 (1977).

Such liability is not, however, premised on assault and battery, because the patient has, in fact, consented to the treatment the physician administered. It is founded instead upon the negligence of the physician, and if it can be shown that the physician, in recommending and administering this particular course of treatment, failed to inform the patient of other options and failed to explain to the patient the actual risks involved in such treatment, then the physician may be liable.

Because this is a negligence cause of action involving professional negligence, these informed consent cases become entangled with all of the problems inherent in medical malpractice cases generally. What the physician should have told the patient, or more usually, how much the patient should have been told, is deemed to depend upon the standard of care for similarly situated physicians. Some risks may be too remote to warrant mentioning, and the physician may consider it important for the well-being of the patient that the patient be put at ease and not unduly worried about unlikely consequences. What other physicians in the community do under these circumstances, the approach taken by similar physicians in discussing options and risks with the patient, determine the standard to be followed and fix the measure of duty against which defendant's actions are judged.[8] In addition, assuming that the physician did breach this duty, plaintiff will still have to make a convincing showing that had he been properly informed of all the options or risks, he would have rejected the treatment administered by the physician.[9] In this type of informed consent case, actual damages must be shown, and plaintiff must prove that any adverse consequences flowing from the treatment administered by the defendant would have been avoided if a different course of action were followed.[10]

§ 8.3   Product Liability—Generally

Occasionally, an injury to a mother or to her newborn child may be caused by the administration of a defective drug or by the use of some defective medical implement. The source of injury may not lie in the decision to use the drug or the instrument, nor in the negligent handling of these products by the physi-

---

[8] Gerety v. Demers, 92 N.M. 396, 589 P.2d 180 (1978).

[9] Dries v. Gregor, 72 A.D.2d 231, 424 N.Y.S.2d 561 (1980). This issue has prompted controversy over whether a subjective or an objective standard should be applied. *See* Dixon v. Peters, 63 N.C. App. 592, 306 S.E.2d 477 (1983).

[10] Some states have adopted informed consent statutes codifying the elements of this cause of action. *See, e.g.,* La. Rev. Stat. § 40:1299.40 (West 1977); N.C. Gen. Stat. § 90-21.13(a)(3) (1981).

cian or nurse, but may be attributable to the dangerous condition of the product itself. In these circumstances, the parents and child may have an action separate from medical malpractice, one which is based on the principles of product liability law as they are applied in the particular jurisdiction.

Through various streams, tributaries, and branches, product liability law has emerged as a significant and far reaching addendum to traditional tort law. Drugs, as a historical note, were among the earliest products to be subject to strict liability concepts, and the proliferation of chemical, mechanical, and electrical devices in the treatment of patients has marched alongside the evolution of theories of product liability law. Medical malpractice cases often grow out of the negligent application of some medical product—administering too much Pitocin, applying too much force to forceps during delivery, causing a needle to break during administration of an anesthetic, for example—or present fact situations where both negligence and a defective product combine to produce injury. Products have become as important to modern medical care as the skill of the physician to diagnose a condition or to surgically repair an organ.

When medical products work, and work precisely as they are supposed to work, they are unabashedly a boon to the care and treatment of patients. However, because of the great dependency modern medical practice places on products, it often sadly follows that when a medical product fails, when it is defective in operation or incorporates some hidden danger which is not adequately described, tragedy results. The human body is a careful balance of physical and chemical forces which nature struggles to maintain adjusted for the well-being of the whole organism. When drugs are administered into that organism to artificially alter that balance, when appliances invade or are connected to that organism to measure, monitor, or correct its behavior, the greatest care must be taken to assure that no serious or permanent harm results. The drugs and instruments of medicine are confined to a narrow tolerance of safety. The most minor defect can cause catastrophic consequences to occur.

§ 8.4   —Basic Elements

Product liability law is the generic term describing the legal principles which apply when a product fails to work in the manner for which it was intended and injury results.[11] The elements of a product liability action are simply stated:

---

[11] While the focus here is upon strict liability in tort, products liability also embraces circumstances where the product associated danger arises from the negligence of the manufacturer

Plaintiff must establish that the product was not reasonably fit for its foreseeable use, i.e., that the product was "defective."

This defect must be shown to have been present in the product at the time the product passed through the hands of the defendant supplier of the product.

Plaintiff's damages must be a proximate result of the defect.[12]

Yet, as simple as these elements may seem, they have been analyzed, discussed, commented upon, and labored over in the courts with the same scrutiny and furor of debate which in an earlier age was reserved for the interpretation of ambiguous passages from the scriptures. There are corollaries and caveats, rules and restrictions, exceptions and encumbrances which have shaped and reshaped these tenets into a myriad of different forms to meet dozens of peculiar circumstances. The ancillary law (statutes of limitations, rules of evidence, viable defenses) of products liability law contributes numerous other complications that vary from state to state. In sum, product liability law can be no more condensed into a universal formula than the law of medical malpractice.

Within the regime of this book, we can only focus on some particular aspects of product liability law which are unique to medical products. Even so limited, we must speak of broad general principles, leaving details to the circumstances of specific cases.

§ 8.5   —Medicines and Medical Equipment

As a general principle, the law will find drug manufacturers liable for failing to adequately test a drug intended for human applications, for marketing a drug which is adulterated or chemically defective, for mislabeling a drug, or, as seen in a majority of products liability cases, for failing to adequately warn the medical profession of the drug's limitations and potential dangers.[13] When the drug passes through the hands of a retailer or pharmacist, they, too,

---

or seller. We make no attempt here to identify the subtle distinctions which define the diverse theories of products liability law. *See, e.g.,* Smith v. E.R. Squibb & Sons, 405 Mich. 79, 273 N.W.2d 476 (1979) (attempting to determine whether a drug manufacturer's inadequate warning is simple negligence or a breach of implied warranty).

12 There are, of course, hundreds of cases identifying these as elements of a product liability action. In Johnson v. Chrysler Corp., 74 Mich. App. 532, 254 N.W.2d 569 (1977), the Michigan Court of Appeals summarizes the whole of product liability law in a single sentence: "It is well settled, and we therefore cite no authority, that a prima facie product liability case consists of proof, 1) that the defendant has supplied a defective product, and 2) that this defect has caused injury to the plaintiff."

13 *See* Annot., 79 A.L.R.2d 301 (1961).

may become liable for acts of negligence endangering the health of the ultimate consumer of the drug.[14] Privity, of course, is no longer a defense, and the plaintiff need not be the one who actually purchased the drug in order to enforce a claim against the manufacturer or seller of the drug.

A more controversial question is a hospital's or physician's liability to a patient for defective products which the hospital or physician utilize to treat the patient. Technically, the physician who prescribes the drug is the supplier of the product to the patient. If the physician orders the hospital staff to give certain drugs to the patient, then the hospital also is the supplier of the product. However, as a general rule, courts will not hold physicians or hospitals liable for the adverse effects of a defective drug or medical device. The most frequently stated reason for insulating hospitals and physicians from such liability is that the hospital and physician are engaged to provide services to the patient and are not sellers or suppliers of products.[15] It seems unlikely that courts shall move from this present position respecting physicians and hospitals in the near future, simply as a matter of public policy.

Hospitals or physicians may be liable, under negligence principles rather than product liability law, if in handling, storing, or using a product they are responsible for contaminating a drug or causing a defect in a product which was not present in the product originally.[16]

Manufacturers of medical devices, as distinguished from drugs, are also subject to product liability law and may be liable for any defects which cause injury when the device is used in a reasonably foreseeable fashion.[17] Electrical devices that cause burns, needles that break, support systems that mechanically fail at crucial times may support a product liability claim. The difficulty with most of these cases from a practical standpoint is that these devices must be operated by human agency, and it is often unclear as to whether the fault lay in the device itself or in the neglect of the person who operates the device. In some cases, the defect may be simply the manufacturer's failure to provide proper instructions on how the device should be used, especially when the device is new and its application to particular circumstances in doubt.

Consequently, failure to warn and failure to instruct defects are the most frequently litigated product liability issues involving drugs and medical appliances.[18] This is to be expected in this field where products are marketed to physicians and hospitals and only actively interact with the public when physicians and hospitals make the decision to employ the products in the treatment

---

[14] *See* Annot., 3 A.L.R.4th 270 (1981).

[15] *See* Annot., 54 A.L.R.3d 258 (1973).

[16] *See* Annot., 9 A.L.R.3d 579 (1966).

[17] *See* Annot., 79 A.L.R.2d 401 (1961).

[18] *See* Annot., 94 A.L.R.3d 748 (1979).

of their patients. Demanding that manufacturers of medical products provide to the medical community detailed and complete information respecting the use of the product, and the risks inherent in such use, is only proper. By recognizing and imposing liability on manufacturers when a failure to communicate vital information regarding their products has caused injury to a patient, the law of product liability will have the salutory effect of making manufacturers more conscious of their responsibility towards the ultimate beneficiary of their commercial efforts.

During pregnancy and birth, a mother and child may be exposed to a myriad of drugs and medical appliances. Consequently, in investigating a possible birth trauma case, counsel should not overlook the possibility that injury may have been caused by a drug or medical implement.[19] Malpractice may have been committed by a defendant who made the decision to use the product, either because the product should not have been employed, or because it was used improperly. Then, again, the product itself may have been defective, in any one of many ways, contributing to the resulting injuries. Whenever the involvement of a product is suspected as possibly causing injuries to the mother or child, a careful effort should be made to identify the manufacturer and to determine whether the product was, in fact, reasonably fit for its intended use.

§ 8.6   Wrongful Birth; Wrongful Life

At the outer boundaries of tort law lie those unique claims which inspire courts to reach back to fundamental principles of law and policy to formulate the elements of new causes of action. Related to birth trauma cases are two such novel actions of relatively recent vintage—actions for wrongful birth and for wrongful life. These are not the same, and although there is some intermixing of the terms, these labels relate to entirely distinct causes of action having different elements and facing different obstacles. Here we shall use the term *wrongful birth* to describe exclusively those actions where parents had sought to avoid the burden of children, but through some act of wrongdoing attributable to a third party suffered the imposition of giving birth to a child

---

[19] Some product related birth defect cases are: Jorgensen v. Meade Johnson Laboratories, Inc., 483 F.2d 237 (10th Cir. 1973); Woodhill v. Parke Davis & Co., 58 Ill. App. 3d 349, 374 N.E.2d 683 (1978); Reeder v. Hammond, 125 Mich. App. 223, 336 N.W.2d 3 (1983); Vaccaro v. Squibb Corp., 52 N.Y.2d 809, 418 N.E.2d 386, 436 N.Y.S.2d 871 (1980); Baker v. St. Agnes Hosp., 70 A.D.2d 400, 421 N.Y.S.2d 81 (1979); Air Shields, Inc. v. Spears, 590 S.W.2d 574 (Tex. Civ. App. 1979); Barson v. E.R. Squibb & Sons, Inc., 682 P.2d 832 (Utah 1984). For cases involving DES, *see* Annot., 2 A.L.R.4th 1091 (1980).

(these are sometimes referred to as wrongful conception cases). *Wrongful life* shall refer to those cases where parents were not informed of the risks of giving birth to a defective child under those circumstances where, had such information been given, the parents would have elected to abort the fetus, and where, as a result of being denied this election, a child is born suffering severe handicaps.

§ 8.7 —Wrongful Birth Causes of Action

Wrongful birth cases, of course, derive from the ability of modern medical science to effect means of contraception so as to avoid unwanted pregnancies and birth. Through birth control pills, mechanical devices, and surgery, doctors can provide to fertile men and women means of avoiding conception. Some of these means are reversible at the option of the party involved—the pill, for example, can be discontinued when the woman decides that she is ready to have children. Other methods are generally irreversible—such as a vasectomy or tubal ligation. However, all chiefly serve to provide to men and women the freedom of choice regarding the responsibility of bearing and raising children, together with the peace of mind of removing from normal sexual relations the fear of an unwanted pregnancy.

Wrongful birth cases can sound in negligence, malpractice, or product liability. A pharmacist who dispenses aspirin in mistake for birth control pills may be liable under negligence principles. A doctor who is shown to have breached the standard of care in performing surgery to tie a woman's ovarian tubes might be liable in a medical malpractice case. A manufacturer of a defective interuterine birth control device may be liable for the failure of the device to prevent a pregnancy under product liability theories. However the action is structured, the essential element of duty and breach is the same—the defendant had the duty to provide to plaintiff the means of avoiding pregnancy and birth, but breached that duty through acts of negligence, malpractice, or product liability.

The traditional objection to wrongful birth actions was that birth itself was of such a benefit to the parent as to overwhelm any objection to any negligence on defendant's part which negated the attempt by the parents to avoid the consequence. No price, after all, can be placed on the value of a normal, healthy child, and public policy, cases have suggested, should not permit parents, giving birth to such a child, to refer to such a blessed benefit as "damages."[20] In many jurisdictions damages for the expense of rearing a healthy

---

[20] Ball v. Mudge, 64 Wash. 2d 247, 391 P.2d 201 (1964); Cockrum v. Baumgartner, 95 Ill. 2d 193, 447 N.E.2d 385 (1983).

child are not recoverable, even though courts will allow parents to recover damages related to the expense and trauma of the pregnancy and birth.[21]

Yet, no matter how art and poetry may portray birth, the reality of modern life is that giving birth is costly and inconvenient, and children impose on parents an awesome responsibility both psychologically and economically. Our society recognizes the right of men and women to determine for themselves when they wish to undertake the obligation of rearing children. The gravamen of the wrongful birth cause of action is that defendant's negligent act has robbed them of this choice by depriving the parents of the means to avoid pregnancy. Wrongful birth actions acknowledge that the birth of a child conveys benefits to the parents, but they also acknowledge the cold reality that children are an expense, and parents who have been negligently placed in the position of being burdened with this expense, an expense they had, in fact, sought to avoid with defendant's help, have, indeed, suffered real and measurable damages. Several courts have now allowed parents of an unplanned child to recover such damages.[22] These damages, in wrongful birth cases, are held to be mitigated by the benefit of the birth of a healthy normal child. This is called the *benefits rule*, and requires juries (in wrongful birth cases) to make the difficult assessment of the dollar value of the child born to the plaintiff parents in order to subtract this figure from the expenses of pregnancy and of rearing the child.[23]

Given this criteria for damages, it is evident that the most successful wrongful birth cases are those in which either a defective, unhealthy child has been born,[24] or those in which the parents are impoverished, already have several

---

[21] Boone v. Mullendore, 416 So. 2d 718 (Ala. 1982); Wilbur v. Kerr, 275 Ark. 239, 628 S.W.2d 568 (1982); Coleman v. Garrison, 349 A.2d 8 (Del. 1975); Schork v. Huber, 648 S.W.2d 861 (Ky. 1983); Mason v. Western Pa. Hosp., 499 Pa. 484, 453 A.2d 974 (1982); Terrell v. Garcia, 496 S.W.2d 124 (Tex. Civ. App. 1973); Beardsley v. Wierdsma, 650 P.2d 288 (Wyo. 1982).

[22] University of Ariz. Health Servs. Center v. Superior Court, 136 Ariz. 579, 667 P.2d 1294 (1983); Custodio v. Bauer, 251 Cal. App. 2d 303, 59 Cal. Rptr. 463 (1967); Anonymous v. Hospital, 33 Conn. Supp. 126, 366 A.2d 204 (1976); Troppi v. Scarf, 31 Mich. App. 240, 187 N.W.2d 511 (1971); Sherlock v. Stillwater Clinic, 260 N.W.2d 169 (Minn. 1977); Betancourt v. Gaylor, 136 N.J. Super. 69, 344 A.2d 336 (1975).

[23] University of Arizona Health Servs. Center v. Superior Court, 136 Ariz. 579, 667 P.2d 1294 (1983); Anonymous v. Hospital, 33 Conn. Supp. 126, 366 A.2d 204 (1976); Troppi v. Scarf, 31 Mich. App. 240, 187 N.W.2d 511 (1971); Sherlock v. Stillwater Clinic, 260 N.W.2d 169 (Minn. 1977); Betancourt v. Gaylor, 136 N.J. Super. 69, 344 A.2d 336 (1975).

[24] Ochs v. Borrelli, 187 Conn. 253, 445 A.2d 883 (1982); Ramey v. Fassoulas, 414 So. 2d 198 (Fla. Dist. Ct. App. 1982); Bowman v. Davis, 48 Ohio St. 2d 41, 356 N.E.2d 496 (1976).

children, and gain little from having another child except the financial burden of having another mouth to feed.[25]

§ 8.8   —Elements of a Wrongful Life Cause of Action

Wrongful life cases are of recent development, having their genesis with *Roe v. Wade*,[26] legalizing the right of a woman to have an abortion. Until this decision, attempts to bring such suits were universally struck down as promoting a cause of action which was contrary to public policy.[27] Today such actions, within restrictive perimeters, are being increasingly recognized as proper and valid.

Exactly what constitutes an action for wrongful life? This action requires an act of negligence by a defendant which prevents a pregnant woman from obtaining information which, had such information been conveyed to her, would have induced her to undergo an abortion rather than bring her child into the world. Modern medicine has now progressed to the point where scientific methods can identify certain risks to fetal development during the early stages of pregnancy. The most well known examples are the risks inherent in rubella and Tay-Sachs syndrome. A woman who, in the course of her pregnancy, is exposed to and contracts rubella has a high risk of giving birth to a defective child. Likewise, certain segments of the population are susceptible to Tay-Sachs syndrome, another cause of defective births. Tests can be conducted on pregnant women during the early stages of pregnancy to ascertain the presence of these diseases, and, when the results are positive, the woman, if informed of the results and the risks involved, can decide to either face the risk and deliver the child after term, or exercise her personal and private option to abort the fetus and avoid the possibility of giving life to a defective child. Wrongful life cases arise when defendants, either knowing of the presence of such diseases, or having the means to ascertain their presence, fail to conduct the proper tests, conduct the tests negligently, or fail to inform the mother of the presence of the disease or of the seriousness of the risks inherent in such disease. In a very real sense, these negligent acts rob the pregnant mother of the opportunity to make her own independent choice regarding the future of her child and of her own well-being.

---

[25] Custodio v. Bauer, 251 Cal. App. 2d 303, 59 Cal. Rptr. 463 (1967); Troppi v. Scarf, 31 Mich. App. 240, 187 N.W.2d 511 (1971).

[26] 410 U.S. 113 (1973).

[27] Gleitman v. Cosgrove, 49 N.J. 22, 227 A.2d 689 (1967).

Unlike a wrongful birth case, in a wrongful life case, the parents have deliberately sought, or at least anticipated, the birth of the child. Consequently, even if the potential defendants have acted negligently in failing to ascertain or inform the mother of known risks, if the child is born normal and healthy, no cause of action arises. These wrongful life cases come about only when the child is, in fact, born burdened with birth defects.

In wrongful life cases, however, these defects are not the result of defendant's negligence. If they were, we would simply be confronted with typical birth trauma medical malpractice cases. The child's defects are caused by a disease over which defendants had no control. Defendants, for example, do not cause the rubella or the Tay-Sachs disease, and the defects which result are caused solely by the operation of these diseases on fetal development. Defendants in these suits are not sued because their negligence caused the birth defects; they are sued because their negligence has taken from the parents, especially the mother, the opportunity of escaping from the consequences of giving life to a defective child through a timely abortion. When abortions were illegal, a pregnant mother who contracted rubella legally had no choice but to give birth to the child, letting nature throw the dice to determine whether the child would be visited with the defects attributable to this disease. But today, the pregnant mother has the option of abortion so that she can either continue with the pregnancy, taking the chance that the child will be normal, or she can remove this risk by having her pregnancy terminated.

Thus, the elements of a wrongful life[28] case are these: the pregnant woman has a disease which creates a high risk of defective birth; the defendants have, in some fashion, negligently withheld from the mother information concerning this risk; the woman can convincingly establish that had she been aware of this risk, she would have elected to have had an abortion; and the woman has given birth to a child having birth defects attributable to the disease. Within this framework, several courts have recognized actions for the benefit of the parents of the defective child.[29]

---

[28] Again, we have used the term wrongful life to distinguish these uniformed risk cases from the unsuccessful sterilization cases discussed above. In many of the cases, this action for the benefit of the parents of the defective child is described as a wrongful birth claim.

[29] Elliott v. Brown, 361 So. 2d 546 (Ala. 1978); Curlender v. Bio-Science Laboratories, 106 Cal. App. 3d 811, 165 Cal. Rptr. 477 (1980); DiNatale v. Lieberman, 409 So. 2d 512 (Fla. Dist. Ct. App. 1982); Eisbrenner v. Stanley, 106 Mich. App. 351, 308 N.W.2d 209 (1981); Berman v. Allen, 80 N.J. 421, 404 A.2d 8 (1979); Becker v. Schwartz, 46 N.Y.2d 401, 386 N.E.2d 807, 413 N.Y.S.2d 895 (1978); Speck v. Finegold, 497 Pa. 77, 439 A.2d 110 (1981); Jacobs v. Theimer, 519 S.W.2d 846 (Tex. 1975); Dumer v. St. Michael's Hosp., 69 Wis. 2d 766, 233 N.W.2d 372 (1975).

§ 8.9 —Wrongful Life: Damages and Claimants

As with wrongful birth cases, however, courts have had little difficulty in accepting or acknowledging these elements of duty, breach or proximate cause. Where the controversy arises in these cases is in the final issue of damages. In wrongful birth cases, as discussed in § **8.7**, the benefits of having a healthy, normal child are highly regarded in the law, and it takes some effort to convincingly show that giving birth to an unplanned child constitutes damage which is actionable. In wrongful life cases, defendants cannot legitimately advance a benefits argument since the child, perforce, is not normal or healthy, but suffers defects which are a burden to the parents. However, defendants in wrongful life cases point out that the only alternative to a child with birth defects (defects, remember, which they did not cause), is an abortion which would have prevented the child's life altogether. Thus, defendants argue in these cases, no measure of damages is possible, for any attempt to measure damages for wrongful life would require juries to weigh the value of a defective life against the value of no life at all, a metaphysical speculation beyond human capacities.

This argument has led most courts which have recognized actions for wrongful life to limit the action to the parents of the defective child, allowing them only to recover the expenses of providing special nursing care or medical care for the child.[30] In this regard, wrongful life cases parallel those for wrongful birth, since both recognize that through someone's negligence parents have been subjected to unexpected or extraordinary financial expenses, expenses which the parents sought, or would have sought, to avoid. In legal terms, the courts have found that as a proximate cause of defendants' breach of their duty to provide parents with the ability to make an intelligent choice regarding the continuation of pregnancy, the parents have been damaged, and the measure of damage is the additional extraordinary expenses made necessary by the defective condition of the child.

In these cases, defendants' negligence has caused the child to become born under circumstances where the only alternative would have been an abortion. Consequently, several courts have held that the child has no cause of action since defendants' negligence has only been a proximate cause of his life, and his damages would be the difference in value between life and nonlife, which

---

[30] Elliott v. Brown, 361 So. 2d 546 (Ala. 1978); Moores v. Lucas, 405 So. 2d 1022 (Fla. Dist. Ct. App. 1981); Strohmaier v. Associates in Obstetrics & Gynecology, 122 Mich. App. 116, 332 N.W.2d 432 (1982); Becker v. Schwartz, 46 N.Y.2d 401, 386 N.E.2d 807, 413 N.Y.S.2d 895 (1978); Nelson v. Krusen, 678 S.W.2d 918 (Tex. 1984); Dumer v. St. Michael's Hosp., 69 Wis. 2d 766, 233 N.W.2d 372 (1975).

cannot be measured, and which, as a matter of public policy, should not be deemed to be damages at all.[31]

This argument, while perhaps technically correct, fails to grasp the reality of defendants' wrongdoing and the policy of tort law to hold persons responsible for the consequences of their wrongful acts. By withholding the pertinent information from the parents, the defendant pulls the lever of the genetic slot machine, wagering that the child, despite the disease, will come into the world healthy and normal. But when the bet is lost, and the disease scars the child with defects, the defendant is allowed to walk away from the consequences, except for the action allowed to the parents. In reality, the measure of damages in cases of this nature should be the same as in any birth trauma case— the difference between the impaired and deformed condition of the child that the defendant's negligence caused to be born, and the normal, healthy condition of the child which would have avoided the cause of action. The fact that some disease was a proximate cause of the defective child, rather than the negligence of defendant, does not lessen the causation factor of the defendant, who was equally responsible for allowing a child to be born handicapped by the inflictions of a disease defendant had diagnosed, or should have diagnosed, and which defendant should have realized might cause the child to suffer a less than normal life.

A few cases, while still recognizing that the comparison between the value of life and the value of nonlife is impossible, have nevertheless extended the cause of action for wrongful life to the defective child. In so doing, they candidly admit that to reach this equitable result some abandonment of traditional tort law concepts must be tolerated. In *Procanik v. Cillo*,[32] the New Jersey Supreme Court observes:

> Law is more than an exercise in logic, and logical analysis, although essential to a system of ordered justice, should not become an instrument of injustice. Whatever logic inheres in permitting parents to recover for the cost of extraordinary medical care incurred by a birth defective child, but in denying the child's own right to recover those expenses, must yield to the injustice of the result.[33]

California,[34] New Jersey,[35] and Washington[36] allow a child born with defects, under the circumstances of a wrongful life claim, to bring a cause of action to

---

[31] "Thus, the cause of action unavoidably involves the relative benefits of an impaired life as opposed to no life at all. All courts, even ones recognizing a cause of action for wrongful life, have admitted that this calculation is impossible." Nelson v. Krusen, 678 S.W.2d 918, 925 (Tex. 1984).

[32] 97 N.J. 339, 478 A.2d 755 (1984).

[33] *Id*. at 762.

[34] Turpin v. Sortini, 31 Cal. 3d 220, 643 P.2d 954, 182 Cal. Rptr. 337 (1982).

[35] Procanik v. Cillo, 97 N.J. 339, 478 A.2d 755 (1984).

[36] Harbeson v. Parke-Davis, Inc., 98 Wash. 2d 460, 656 P.2d 483 (1983).

recover the special damages for medical and other extraordinary expenses. Of course, the parents may also bring an action to recover special damages during the child's minority, and such damages should not be duplicated. The real benefit of recognizing a separate cause of action for the child lies in securing damages for the medical and extraordinary expenses which will likely be incurred after the defective child reaches the age of majority.

§ 8.10   —General Observations

These cases—wrongful birth and wrongful life—demonstrate the need for tort law to keep in touch with scientific and technological advances. Medical science has progressed tremendously over the past half century; it has learned the secrets of genetics; it has evolved methods of diagnosis and treatment which have taken much of the mystery, and most of the risk, out of conception and birth. Indirectly, the law supports and favors such scientific advances and medical improvements, which help to relieve human suffering and improve the quality of life in our society, by imposing a legal duty on those entrusted with diagnosis and treatment to exercise reasonable care in light of present day scientific knowledge. Yet to properly fulfill this role, the law must also remain flexible, and courts must be willing to evolve legal principles which keep pace with science. This often requires the law to rethink old ideas and restructure legal standards to cope with unusual or novel circumstances.

At the core of the law lies a basic premise—that every person has a responsibility for the sufferings which they negligently cause to others. To leave a wrong without a remedy is to leave an inexcusable void in the law which justice cannot tolerate. To mold a proper remedy, the law must sometimes move beyond its technical or traditional rules into areas requiring imagination and insight. Providing such imagination and insight is the responsibility of the legal profession. Wrongful birth and wrongful life cases are examples of suits creatively pursued by lawyers who dared to ask the courts to reach a step beyond prevailing jurisprudence in order to formulate a means of granting relief to clients who had been harmed through another's neglect. These actions are a reminder that the law is neither static nor immovable in the face of technological, scientific or social change, a point to be appreciated by the legal profession in an approaching age of test-tube babies, surrogate parents, genetic engineering, and other wonders affecting the processes of birth and the quality of life.

PART II

MEDICAL ISSUES PERTAINING TO BIRTH TRAUMA CLAIMS

CHAPTER 9

PRENATAL CARE

§ 9.1   Introduction

The goal of prenatal care is to assure that every pregnancy culminates in the birth of a healthy baby to a healthy mother. However, significant improvements in the relatively high perinatal and maternal morbidity and mortality rates can only be made if the attending obstetricians are well-versed in the normal physiological and emotional changes that accompany pregnancy, as well as the signs and symptoms of serious disorders. The importance of strictly adhering to the recommended antepartum and intrapartum protocol, outlined in detail in this chapter and the following one, cannot be emphasized strongly enough. Not only does first-rate prenatal care ensure the mother's good health, but the fetus's health and maturation as well, since its welfare depends almost entirely on its mother's condition during pregnancy. Consequently, by examining each woman as early after conception as possible, and then scheduling a series of frequent examinations throughout her gestation, potentially dangerous abnormalities and warning signs of impending problems can be detected and treated early, *before* they deleteriously influence the outcome of pregnancy.

Throughout the course of the discussion on antepartum and intrapartum care, several sections will be devoted to defining common obstetrical terminology. There is also a glossary included at the end of this book for assistance in defining medical terminology. A familiarity with the professional jargon is vital in order to thoroughly understand what the obstetrician is speaking about, writing down, and referring to in the patient's chart, and reading in medical textbooks and journals. This particular section covers the vocabulary used to describe pregnant women, and the various phases of their gestations.

A *gravida* is a woman who is or has been pregnant. When a prefix is added to the word, it indicates the total number of her pregnancies, regardless of their type, location, duration, method of termination, or outcome. For example, a woman who has had two normal intrauterine pregnancies, one tubal pregnancy, and one abortion is a *multigravida*, or more specifically, a *gravida 4*.

Nulligravida refers to a woman who is not now and has never been pregnant.

Primigravida describes a woman who is pregnant for the first time.

Like the word gravida, the term *para* also reflects the total number of pregnancies, though only those which continue *beyond the 20th week of gestation* (the current definition for the state of fetal viability). It does not indicate the number of babies born. Therefore, a woman who has delivered a set of twins during her first pregnancy (after 40 weeks, for example) is a para 1, not a para 2.

Nullipara refers to a woman who has not yet delivered a viable infant, as would be the case if she had a miscarriage or an abortion before the 20th week.

Primipara describes a woman who has carried one pregnancy beyond the 20th week, regardless of the fetal outcome.

A *parturient* is a woman in labor.

A *puerpera* is a woman after labor, that is, one who has just given birth. The *puerperium* is the period following delivery until the reproductive organs return to their normal prepregnancy size and shape, which usually takes three to six weeks.

The terms *prenatal* and *antenatal* are synonomous, broadly describing the period before birth.

The *perinatal period* begins at 12 weeks of gestation and lasts until 28 days after birth.

The *neonatal period* is from birth to 28 days of age.

The *antepartum period* includes the months before the onset of labor, and the *intrapartum period* is the time during labor.

§ 9.2   Initial Comprehensive Examination

The task of providing complete prenatal services is not only complicated by the diverse prepregnancy medical backgrounds of obstetrical patients, but also by the widely varying degrees of prenatal care these women have received when they first arrive at the obstetrician's office, which is sometimes as late as one-half or three-quarters of the way through their pregnancy. Despite these differences, the patient's first prenatal examination should always consist of a thorough history, initial physical examination, and laboratory studies. The purpose of this detailed examination is to define the health of the mother and the fetus, to determine the gestational age, and to initiate a plan for continuing obstetrical care based on the findings. After such a comprehensive evaluation, the obstetrician will have accumulated the necessary data to determine whether or not any risk factors are present, and if so, she can promptly begin the appropriate treatment to prevent any problems when they may arise. Subsequent prenatal examinations are also mandatory throughout the course of pregnancy in order to quickly detect and treat other later developing high risk complications. At each of these visits, all pertinent data obtained *must* be legibly entered in the patient's prenatal record so that every member of the health care team can understand and interpret it correctly.

§ 9.3   —Initial History

By obtaining a thorough family medical history (the maternal and paternal sides) and inquiring about the outcome of past pregnancies, previous major illnesses (including those from previous gestations because many complications of pregnancy tend to be repetitive), symptoms of any present health problems, and all medication currently being taken, the obstetrician can assess whether the woman is predisposed to hereditary diseases or other disorders during her current gestation. Since her age also significantly influences the outcome of the pregnancy, it must be recorded and taken into account. The period between 20-29 years of age is considered the best time for reproduction due to the relatively lower incidence of complications. Older age groups not only have a greater likelihood of delivery of low birth weight and genetically defective infants, but the women themselves are more liable to suffer from medical disorders that might deleteriously affect the pregnancy. At the other end of the spectrum, teenage pregnancies are also considered high risk gestations because the rates of maternal problems, low birth weight babies, and perinatal mortality, are all increased.

After the history is taken, the physician must then determine the expected date of delivery, an event which typically occurs 280 days (40 weeks) following conception. Using Nagele's rule, the due date can be calculated by adding seven days to the first day of the woman's last menstrual period, subtracting three months from the result, and then adding one year. Whereas about 60 percent of all patients are expected to give birth within one week of the estimated date of delivery, the expected date of confinement (EDC) cannot always be predicted accurately for the remainder because a sizeable percentage of these women did not have regular menstrual cycles when they became pregnant. This makes it almost impossible to pinpoint when fertilization occurred. Errors are most likely to result if the patient has experienced any episodes of vaginal bleeding or has discontinued taking birth control pills just prior to conception. The results may also be unreliable if she becomes pregnant soon after an abortion or a previous pregnancy, since her menstrual periods may not have ample time to reestablish their normal pattern.

Although the Nagele calculation for determining the duration of the pregnancy usually suffices, more *precise* dating (using ultrasound, for example) is sometimes imperative later in the pregnancy in order to optimally treat certain complications which may arise. For instance, if maternal hypertension develops at 38 weeks of gestation (when the fetus is likely to be well-developed and functionally mature), delivery is often beneficial for both the mother and the fetus; but if her high blood pressure begins at 36 weeks of gestation, the same course of action may not be appropriate. As this example is intended to illustrate, a difference of two weeks between the real and the estimated gestational age may cause the obstetrician to induce an early delivery, when it may actually be better to delay delivery of the premature fetus and attempt to correct the maternal disorder instead.

§ 9.4 —Initial Physical Examination

Measuring the mother's blood pressure, pulse rate, and temperature at the first examination provides the physician with a valuable series of baseline measurements with which she can compare the results of her future prenatal visits. After her vital signs have been taken, the mother's height and weight should be recorded. The obstetrician must stress the importance of good nutrition during pregnancy. A weight gain of 24-27 pounds is considered optimal, and great variations in either direction can create a hazardous environment for the mother and/or fetus. The woman's ability to comply with this optimal weight gain directly influences her fetus' health, as reflected by an increased birth weight, and a lower incidence of prematurity and neurologic abnormalities.

Marked deviation from the ideal pregnancy weight, in either direction, also affects the prognosis since various complications are more likely to develop—most notably the frightening correlation between obesity and an increased incidence of preeclampsia. Sudden weight gain in the third trimester usually heralds fluid retention, and can be a warning sign of impending preeclampsia. Also of special concern are patients who lose or fail to gain weight during pregnancy.

A thorough, general physical examination should be performed at the initial visit, and then special attention should be devoted to the areas affected by the pregnancy, namely: the breasts, the abdomen, and the reproductive tract. Manual measurements of the critical pelvic dimensions (the diameters of the pelvic inlet, mid-pelvis, and pelvic outlet) and an evaluation of its general shape are also made at this time.

§ 9.5   —Initial Laboratory Studies

The initial laboratory work-up consists of some basic tests which should be performed as early in the pregnancy as possible. A sample of the mother's blood should be drawn for the following tests: the hematocrit (HCT) and red blood cell (RBC) volume (the two major indices of anemia), a syphilis screen, a rubella screen, a two-hour postprandial blood sugar (to detect diabetes), ABO/Rh (blood group typing), and an identification of any abnormal maternal antibodies. In addition, a specimen of the mother's urine is obtained and tested for the presence of albumin, sugar, blood, and pus. If glucose is present, additional tests are needed to determine if she has diabetes. During the vaginal examination, cervical tissue samples should be obtained for a gonorrhea culture and a Papanicolaou smear (Pap test).

After the history, physical examination, and laboratory studies have been completed, the woman is instructed about general hygiene, clothing, recreation, exercise, rest, medications, smoking, drug and alcohol ingestion, and diet and nutrition. A well-balanced diet is important throughout the prenatal period in order to meet the increased nutritional demands of both the mother and fetus. Whereas most of the essential nutrients can easily be obtained by eating the proper food, diet alone cannot usually supply enough iron, so daily iron supplements are often prescribed during the second and third trimesters to prevent anemia. Finally, the patient is tactfully instructed to *immediately* report the following danger signals to the obstetrician, since they require prompt investigation whenever they occur:

1. Any vaginal bleeding;

2. Swelling of the face, fingers, feet, or ankles;

3. Severe or continous headaches. A headache that does not respond quickly to simple household remedies may be an aura of the first eclamptic convulsion if it occurs without other warnings;

4. Dimness or blurring of vision, dizziness, mental confusion, or spots in front of the eyes are signs of severe preeclampsia;

5. Recurrent pelvic or abdominal cramping. These symptoms may represent the onset of abortion in early pregnancy, or premature or normal term labor in the later months;

6. Spontaneous rupture of the membranes, which is usually signalled by a sudden gush of clear fluid from the vagina;

7. Persistent vomiting;

8. Chills or fever;

9. Any marked reduction in the amount of urine passed. This may be the first sign of fulminant toxemia that the patient can observe.

§ 9.6   Subsequent Prenatal Examinations

In order to carefully observe the course and progress of the gestation, to guard against asymptomatic complications, and to detect the early warning signs of common disorders, subsequent prenatal examinations have traditionally been scheduled at monthly intervals throughout the first seven months, biweekly during the eighth month, and then weekly during the final month of pregnancy. Although some physicians advocate a more flexible appointment schedule to assess the well-being of the mother and the fetus, they all agree that the patient should be instructed to notify her doctor whenever problems arise. If complications are discovered, additional visits may be required, or hospital care may be necessary for further study and treatment.

At each return visit, the obstetrician must inquire about the patient's health since her last appointment, find out whether she has experienced any of the danger signals mentioned above, and measure and record her weight and vital signs. If the expectant mother has high blood pressure, it must be treated immediately, since women with underlying hypertensive disease have a predisposition to develop preeclampsia.

If the patient's initial laboratory results were normal and she does not exhibit any clinical abnormalities, the blood tests do not need to be repeated, except for the hematocrit and red blood cell volume (which should be rechecked at 32 weeks of gestation for evidence of anemia). Some clinicians also remeasure the blood glucose levels in the second half of pregnancy to rule out the possibility of gestational diabetes (diabetes induced by the physiologic changes of pregnancy). Urine specimens should be examined at each visit for the appearance of the previously mentioned abnormal components. Albumin in the urine during the third trimester is a cardinal sign of preeclampsia, and it requires immediate investigation.

A systematic, abdominal examination is also performed at each visit during the last half of pregnancy, since by this time, the intrauterine positioning of the fetus can easily be palpated through the anterior abdominal and uterine walls (using a sequence of four manipulations known as the Leopold maneuvers). After mapping out and recording the fetal position, the height of the uterine fundus (the uppermost region) should be measured to assure that it is progressively enlarging. Since there is a good correlation between the height of the fundus and the age of the fetus between the 18th and 30th weeks of gestation, the duration of pregnancy can be firmly established when this relationship is in agreement.

An internal pelvic examination, done either rectally or vaginally, may also be performed to precisely identify the position and location of the fetus, as well as to evaluate whether characteristic cervical changes have begun. However, this approach for determining the fetal position and location is usually saved for the final month of pregnancy, when it is generally used to confirm the findings of the abdominal examination. If a vaginal examination is needed in the third trimester, it must be done aseptically to prevent introducing pathogenic organisms into the reproductive tract, and it must be conducted carefully, in order to avoid detaching a low-lying placenta from the uterine wall, an accident which could result in severe hemorrhage.

Since the pelvic capacity is one of the major factors responsible for determining whether the baby can be delivered atraumatically through its mother's vagina, or whether a cesarean section must be performed instead to ensure its safe delivery, this parameter must be assessed during one of the subsequent pelvic examinations if it was not done at the first visit. Evaluating the pelvic capacity involves measuring the dimensions of the *true pelvis*, which is comprised of the inlet, the midpelvis, and the outlet. The pelvic inlet is further subdivided into its four characteristic diameters: the anteroposterior diameter, the widest transverse diameter, and the right and left oblique diameters. By making x-ray measurements (called x-ray pelvimetry) of the anterior and posterior sagittal lengths of the anteroposterior diameter, as well as the widest transverse diameter, the obstetrician is provided with instant knowledge of the general shape and capacity of the pelvic inlet, the first region of the birth canal through which the fetus must pass. Despite the fact that the pelvic contours and dimensions can be determined more precisely by x-ray pelvimetry, internal manual measurement of the important pelvic diameters (called clinical or manual pelvimetry) supplies sufficient information in most cases.

Of the four basis types of pelvis—the gynecoid, android, anthropoid, and platypelloid varieties—the gynecoid variety is the type normally present in females. Definitive typing of the maternal pelvis may be necessary in the early months of pregnancy if the pelvis is grossly distorted by rickets or a poorly healed old fracture, or if the baby's size is similar to that of an eight month old fetus, even though the menstrual dates suggest it is younger. However, under normal circumstances, pelvic typing does not provide useful information before eight months of gestation because if delivery occurs prematurely, the baby will be so small that the bony architecture of its mother's pelvis will not affect the course of labor. Besides, clinical evaluation of the pelvis is easier and causes far less discomfort to the patient if it is done about one month before term. The findings are also more meaningful when the examination is performed two to four weeks before term, since the fetus has grown considerably by this time, permitting a more relevant appraisal of the pelvic capacity with respect to the expected fetal size at delivery.

In addition to checking the maternal health, thorough assessment of the fetal condition is also of utmost importance during the prenatal work-up. Proof of a living fetus is provided by hearing the fetal heartbeat, palpating active intrauterine movements, and observing progressive increases in fetal size on successive examinations made several weeks apart. From about the 18th week of gestation, the presence of a healthy fetus can be confirmed by listening to its rapid heart rate (which normally varies between 120-160 beats-per-minute) with a specially designed stethoscope called a *fetoscope*. Another means of monitoring the fetal heart rate is by means of an electronic device known as a *doptone*. Since this instrument is easy to use and provides invaluable information about the fetal status, the fetal heart rate should be auscultated at each prenatal vist.

At some point in her pregnancy, the expectant mother should be thoroughly informed about the beginning signs of labor. Primigravidas should be advised to notify their obstetricians and then report to the hospital when their contractions recur every eight to twelve minutes (every five minutes according to other authorities). However, since labor may ensue very rapidly in multigravidas, these women should be instructed to call their doctors earlier—when they begin feeling unusual pain or discomfort in their lower abdomen or back, near the expected due date. Cramps in this region are the principal signs of imminent labor. Finally, all pregnant women should be requested to eat sparingly as soon as they believe labor is starting because, if anesthesia is required during the delivery, it is safer to administer it when the patient's stomach is empty.

§ 9.7   Terminology: Fetal Orientation in the Womb

The following outline is comprised of important obstetrical terms which describe the orientation of the fetus in the womb. The accompanying percentages are included to give the reader a perspective of the incidence of the various postures at, or near, term.

1. **Attitude**
2. **Lie**
    a. Longitudinal—99%
    b. Transverse—1%
3. **Presenting part (presentation)**
    a. Head
        (i)   Vertex (occiput)—95%
        (ii) Face (chin)—0.3%
        (iii) Brow—0.1%
    b. Buttocks (breech)—5%
        (i)   Frank
        (ii) Complete
        (iii) Incomplete (footling)
    c. Shoulder (transverse)—0.5%
4. Position

The fetal *attitude* describes how the limbs are folded and positioned relative to each other, as well as to the head and spine of the baby. The particular orientation results partly from the way the fetus grows, and partly from how it accommodates to its mother's uterine cavity. In the later months of pregnancy, the characteristic posture is such that the fetal head is completely flexed, with its chin resting on its chest. Below the chin, the arms are typically folded across the chest, the spine is flexed in a smooth curve, and the hips and knees are flexed. Laypersons commonly call this the fetal position.

Depending on the relationship between the long axis of the fetus to the long axis of its mother, the baby can either *lie* longitudinally or transversely. In a longitudinal lie, the fetal and maternal spines are parallel. Whereas the relationship occurs in over 99 percent of term labors, transverse lies are very uncommon and potentially dangerous configurations in which the infant's spine crosses its mother's spine at a right angle. Because of the unfavorable fetal orientation, induction of labor in the presence of a transverse lie is absolutely contraindicated, and this is one of the few instances which unequivocally calls

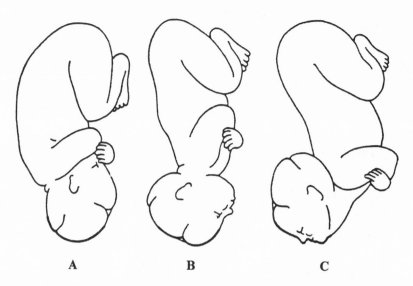

Figure 9-1. Degrees of Deflexion of the Head. The different degrees of deflexion of the head in cephalic presentations. These fetuses are all lying longitudinally, though their spines are each oriented slightly differently. A: Vertex (this baby is in "the fetal position"). B: Brow. C: Face. Reproduced by permission from: Willson, J. Robert, Carrington, Elsie Reid, & Ledger, William J., *Obstetrics and Gynecology*, 7th ed., 372 (St. Louis: The C.V. Mosby Co., 1983).

for a cesarean section. Not only does a transverse lie predispose the mother to uterine rupture, but it also places a tremendous stress upon the fetus, allowing virtually no chance for a living baby to be delivered vaginally.

The *presenting part* is simply the first portion of the fetal body to descend through the birth canal. In a longitudinal lie, the presenting part is either the fetal head or buttocks, giving rise to a cephalic or a breech presentation, respectively. In a transverse lie, the presenting part is usually one of the shoulders. This extremely rare orientation is ominous for the mother and fetus as mentioned above.

Cephalic presentations are classified according to how the head is flexed (see **Figure 9-1**), since this precisely determines which region of the head will emerge first. One of three possible presentations exist: the vertex (also called the occiput or the back of the skull), face (usually referring to the chin), or brow presentations. An attempt should be made to convert a brow presentation to the more favorable vertex presentation, because a baby whose brow is the presenting part cannot advance through the birth canal unless its head is extremely small, or its mother's pelvis is very spacious. If these conditions do

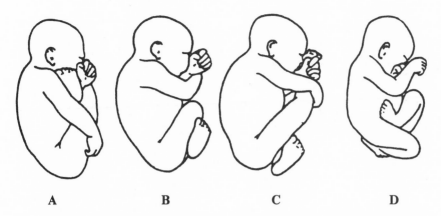

Figure 9-2. Breech Presentations. The different varieties of breech presentations. These fetuses are also lying longitudinally. A: Frank breech. B: Complete breech. C & D: Two types of incomplete breech. Reproduced by permission from: Titus, Paul: *Atlas of Obstetric Technic*, 2d ed., 106 (So. Louis: The C.V. Mosby Co., 1949).

not exist, or if the manipulations are unsuccessful, a cesarean delivery is required.

Like cephalic presentations, *breech presentations* are further categorized according to the relationship of the fetus's legs to its body. See **Figure 9-2**. This potentially hazardous, through relatively infrequent orientation, is discussed in detail in **Chapter 21**, on breech presentations.

Position refers to where the fetus is situated in its mother's pelvis. Using an arbitrarily chosen reference point on the fetus's body based on its presentation (for example, occiput (O) for a vertex presentation and sacrum (S) for a breech presentation), the baby's position is described with respect to the anterior, transverse, or posterior regions of the maternal pelvis. Moving in a clockwise direction around the pelvis, the following eight designations are possible: anterior (the front of the mother's body), left anterior (LA), left transverse (LT), left posterior (LP), posterior (P), right posterior (RP), right transverse (RT), and right anterior (RA). See **Figure 9-3**.

Commonly used abbreviations such as LOA (left occiput anterior, the most frequent fetal position) and RST (right sacrum transverse) are simply formed by combining the pelvic regions with the appropriate fetal reference point. It is worth mentioning that when the word transverse is used in connection with the fetal position, it only refers to an anatomical region of the maternal pelvis, and bears *no* relationship whatsoever to the negative connotation it evokes when describing the fetal lie.

Precise diagnosis of the presentation and position is of little importance before the last eight weeks of gestation for two reasons. First of all, since the

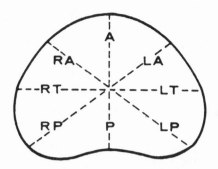

Figure 9-3. Directions of fetal position in maternal pelvis from below. Reproduced by permission from: Willson, J. Robert, Carrington, Elsie Reid, & Ledger, William J., *Obstetrics and Gynecology*, 7th ed., 372 (St. Louis: The C.V. Mosby Co., 1983).

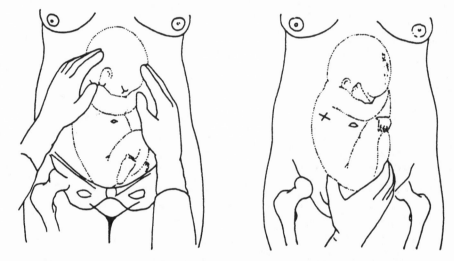

Figure 9-4. Abdominal Palpation. How the abdomen is palpated to determine the position and presentation. This diagram shows the characteristic upper and lower uterine findings in a breech presentation. Reproduced by Permission from: Willson, J. Robert & Carrington, Elsie Reid, *Obstetrics and Gynecology*, 6th ed., 490 (St. Louis: The C.V. Mosby Co., 1979).

fetal position is not yet stable, it frequently changes. Second, abnormal presentations do not threaten to complicate labor during the first six months of pregnancy (should the woman deliver early for some reason) as they do during the last three months of gestation, when the fetus is much larger. At this later stage, assessment of the presentation and position is essential and the physician can usually obtain the necessary information by a clinical examination alone, using abdominal, vaginal, and/or rectal palpation.

A reasonably accurate diagnosis of the fetal presentation and position can be made by abdominal palpation (see **Figure 9-4**) unless certain maternal conditions (such as an unusually resistant abdominal wall, a tender or irritable uterus, or an excessive amount of amniotic fluid) prevent delineation of the fetal landmarks. As long as these factors are not present, the abdominal examination can be performed systematically using the four maneuvers of Leopold. This sequence of manipulations is designed to answer a specific question regarding the orientation of the fetal body to that of its mother's pelvis by pressing down on the appropriate areas of her abdomen.

The first maneuver answers the question: What fetal part occupies the fundus? Palpation of a hard, round structure indicates that the head is located in the fundus, whereas a soft, irregular mass means that the buttocks are there instead. The second maneuver answers the question: On which side is the fetal back? The third maneuver answers the question: What fetal part is situated over the pelvic inlet (for example, the head, shoulder, or buttocks)? The fourth maneuver answers the question: On which side is the cephalic prominence? The cephalic prominence, or the protruding and most readily felt portion of the skull, reveals whether the head is flexed or extended.

§ 9.8   Genetic Counseling

Genetic counseling is a communication process that deals with the human problems associated with the occurrence, or the risk of recurrence, of a genetic disorder in a family. This process involves an attempt by one or more appropriately trained persons to help the individual or family:

1. To comprehend the medical facts, including the diagnosis, probable cause of the disorder, and the available management;

2. To appreciate the way heredity contributes to the disorder and the risk of recurrence in specified relatives;

3. To understand the alternatives for dealing with the risk of recurrence;

4. To choose the course of action that seems appropriate to them in view of their risk, their family goals, and their ethical and religious standards, and to act in accordance with their decision;

5. To make the best possible adjustment to the disorder in an affected family member and/or the risk of recurrence of that disorder.[1]

---

[1] K.F. Swaiman & F.S. Wright, The Practice of Pediatric Neurology (The C.V. Mosby Co., 1982).

The persons choosing to receive testing and counseling include parents of a newborn child with a malformation, syndrome, or disease who are concerned about the possibility of recurrence in a future child. Also included are prospective parents with no family history of genetic defects who want to learn of their risks of having a child with a genetic disorder, and finally, expectant parents who want prenatal testing. Certain categories of people possess a higher risk of having genetically defective children than does the general population. In the general population, approximately a 2 percent incidence of serious birth defects occurs.[2]

These people who have a higher risk of conceiving a genetically defective child, require genetic counseling to guide them through the necessary learning and decision-making processes involved in choosing whether to have a child. The category of patients who most frequently require counseling during the prenatal period are patients conceiving after the age of 35. The risk of having a baby with Down's Syndrome in the population under age 30 is approximately 1 per 2,000 pregnancies. At age 35, the risk increases to 1 per 356 pregnancies, and is increased each year thereafter, reaching 1 in 12 pregnancies at age 49. If a patient has had a previous baby with Down's Syndrome, the risk of this occurring in a subsequent pregnancy is approximately 1 percent regardless of maternal age.[3] Thus, genetic screening and counseling is essential for these women who have a high risk of giving birth to a baby with Down's Syndrome. Screening can determine if the women are carrying a fetus with Down's Syndrome, and thus, they have the option of avoiding the birth of a baby with a genetic disorder.

Another specific category of patients frequently requiring genetic counseling are patients who have given birth to one child with a neural tube defect. These patients have approximately a 5 percent chance of delivering a second child with the problem. The delivery of two such affected children increases the risk of the same occurrence in the third pregnancy to 10 percent.[4]

Even when no family history of genetic disorder exists, couples should choose to receive genetic testing and counseling, if they wish to become informed about the risks of a genetic disorder occurring in their unborn child.

Counselors help the couple make an educated decision, based upon results of genetic testing, on whether to have a child. Therefore, when a couple seeks genetic screening and counseling, they are accepting the responsibility they have to themselves and their unborn child by attempting to avoid the emotionally painful burden of giving birth to a baby with a genetic disorder. The

---

[2] M.E. Rivlin, J.C. Morison & G.W. Bates (eds.), Manual of Clinical Problems in Obstetrics and Gynecology (Little, Brown & Co., 1982).

[3] *Id.*

[4] *Id.*

couple that is negligent by not taking advantage of genetic technology through testing and counseling, probably has not considered the potential social, emotional, and economic consequences of giving birth to a baby with a genetic defect.

Genetic counseling begins with screening procedures which identify those individuals who have a higher risk of producing an offspring with genetic abnormalities than does the population at large. Screening consists of constructing a family pedigree so that all disorders and abnormalities occurring in a family are recorded. Screening also consists of genetic testing such as karyotyping of parents and tests on parents' urine, blood, or cultured skin cells. If the mother is pregnant, test on gene products of the fetus are performed through anmiocentesis, or from cells directly from the fetus. Another procedure is to test the mother's blood for fetal gene products that have leaked into the blood.

Obviously, ideal identification of a high risk couple should occur before, rather than after, the birth of an affected child. However, it is true that a major way of identifying a family at risk for genetic disease is through the birth of a child with an unexpected affliction. When a baby is born with a defect, the parents are shocked, scared, bewildered, and often angered. The job of the counselor at this stage is to explain the nature of the baby's disorder, to explain the short-term prognosis, and to provide as much emotional support as possible. During this initial crisis, many parents worry that they themselves are defective in some way, and they may benefit by having these feelings aired. As the parents become aware of the long-term consequence of their baby's defect, they may become more curious about the cause of the child's disorder, and specifically, whether it may happen again. If genetic counseling is not sought soon after a child's birth, the parents may remain unaware of their high risk and may start another pregnancy, or they may unnecessarily take irreversible measures (i.e. tubal ligation) in an effort to prevent subsequent pregnancies.

It is particularly important for the counselor to inform the parents that there can be no guarantee the couple will have a healthy baby, as there is a risk of recurrence. In order to determine the recurrence risk, the genetic counselor must assign the disorder in question to one of four etiological categories. Those due to:

1. An environmental agent;
2. A chromosomal aberration;
3. A multifactorial interaction;
4. A mutant gene.[5]

---

[5] A.J. Schaffer & M.E. Avery, Diseases of the Newborn (W.B. Saunders Co., 1977).

Defects due to environmental agents will recur only if the environmental agent persists or recurs. When considering defects due to chromosomal aberrations, the counselor should stress that the parents are capable of having normal children, but that when the mother is pregnant, amniocentesis is necessary if the couple wants to be certain that there will be no recurrence.

Recurrence risks of defects caused by a multifactorial interaction have been determined empirically, and can be provided by the counselor for the specific defect and family history. It is essential to inform parents of a child with anencephaly and/or spina bifida of the recurrence risk, since subsequent pregnancies can be monitored by ultrasound and alpha-fetoprotein measurement.[6]

The recurrence risk of defects due to mutant genes depends on both the modes of inheritance of the disorder (for example, autosomal dominant inheritance, autosomal recessive inheritance, x-linked recessive inheritance, and x-linked dominant inheritance), and family history.[7]

When the parents have obtained an understanding of their baby's disorder, the burden that it will impose upon the family, and the risk of recurrence, they will have to decide whether they will have more children, and if not, what options are available. At this time, the counselor may suggest either artificial insemination, if test results indicated the mother's genes as normal, or adoption. The counselor does not tell the parents that they should or should not have children, but the counselor does try to provide helpful support while the parents talk through their problems. Often, counselors will refer the couple to such sources as a priest, social worker, psychiatrist, gynecologist or urologist, whenever they feel it necessary. Thus, the role of a genetic counselor is to act as an information source and as a guide in the couple's critical decision-making processes.

There are many reasons why genetic counseling is important and indispensible to our society. For example, a common misconception is that genetic and chromosomal diseases are so rare they can be dismissed from the minds of prospective parents. A number of human diseases caused by single gene mutations are rare, but in the aggregate, single gene or multi-gene abnormalities account for a significant proportion of human diseases.[8] There is an aggregate

---

[6] Id.

[7] J. Warkany, R.J. Lemire & M.M. Cohen, Mental Retardation and Congenital Malformations of the Central Nervous System 8-11 (Year Book Medical Publishers, 1981).

[8] G.N. Burrow & F.F. Thomas, Medical Complications During Pregnancy (W.B. Saunders Co., 1982).

likelihood of 4 percent to 6 percent for the birth of a child with a specific genetic or chromosomal disease. In any one family, the risk may vary from 1 percent to 50 percent.[9]

Additionally, in the last eight years, the number of women having their first child after the age of 30 has escalated from 58,000 to over 100,000. However, only 10 percent of the 150,000 pregnant women over age 35 in the United States are assessed each year for chromosomal abnormalities.[10]

The escalation in the number of women having their first child after the age of 30, could cause an increase in the possible number of children born with genetic disorders. Since therapy of genetic diseases is as yet very limited, it is of utmost importance to attempt prevention of the genetic diseases. For this pertinent reason, genetic counseling is critical, as these women should be educated about their risks of giving birth to a genetically defected child before conception occurs.

Of the three million babies born each year in the United States, 50,000 to 60,000 have major genetic or congenital diseases.[11] This is another example why genetic counseling is so important. Advanced genetic technology provides the means for a reduction in the number of genetically defective babies born each year through the use of genetic testing and counseling.

Another example of the importance of genetic counseling is that genetic counseling is needed to educate people regarding the cause of genetic defects, and the implications involved in being a carrier of a genetically defective trait. For example, in the 1970s, mass screening for the sickle-cell trait (a single gene for sickle-cell anemia affecting 1 out of 12 American blacks) began. There was no plan at the time to educate the public at large, or the people being screened, regarding what the sickle-cell trait meant. In the words of Dr. Philip Reilly, "Too often the price for this explosion in screening was physiological injury to carriers who had not been adequately counseled."[12] Many people did not realize that people with the trait did not have the disease. As a result, some insurance companies raised their rates for blacks with the trait. In addition, the Job Corps advised blacks with the single gene to choose undemanding work, counseling them to choose electronic assembly, for example, rather than carpentry or automobile body repair.[13] The misimpression that sickle-cell carriers were unhealthy has since been corrected; without genetic

---

[9] *Id.*

[10] M.E. Rivlin, J.C. Morison & G.W. Bates (eds.), Manual of Clinical Problems in Obstetrics and Gynecology (Little, Brown & Co., 1982).

[11] Fraser, *Genetic Counseling*, 26 American Journal of Human Genetics 636-59 (1974).

[12] P. Reilly, Genetics, Law and Social Policy (Harvard University Press 1977).

[13] Andrews, *Genetic Counselors: How They Can Help and How They Can't*, Parent's Magazine, November 1982, at 93.

counseling, the same type of misunderstanding could very easily occur once again. Therefore, where genetic testing informs prospective parents that they are carriers of a disorder, subsequent genetic counseling should be administered. Counseling will eliminate ignorance on the subject of their genetic disorder and the implications involved in being a carrier of a disorder. Knowledge of the risks of occurrence and recurrence of the disorder will help allow prospective parents to make proper decisions concerning reproduction.

For years, there was no way of diagnosing a genetically defective fetus, or of diagnosing that prospective parents were at a high risk of producing a baby with a genetic disorder. However, the present knowledge and skill available to our society enables prospective parents (including parents of a child born with a genetic defect), to accept their responsibility to themselves and their unborn child by taking advantage of genetic counseling. Genetic counseling, by providing the necessary knowledge needed to educate the public on the subject of genetic disorders, guides these people so that they can avoid contributing to the large number of genetically diseased babies born each year. Thus, genetic counseling is a valuable service which is crucial in the prevention of genetic disease.

§ 9.9 Bibliography and Recommended Readings

Allan, Ferguson-Smith, Donald, et al., *Amniotic Alpha-fetoprotein in the Antenatal Diagnosis of Spina Bifida*, 2 Lancet 522 (1977).

Danforth, D.N., Ph.D., M.D., *Obstetrics and Gynecology*, 4th ed. (Harper & Row, Publishers, 1982).

Diagnosis of Genetic Disease by Amniocentesis during the Second Trimester of Pregnancy, Medical Research Council, Report No. 5, Ottawa, Canada (1977).

Hobbins, Grannum, Berkowitz, et al., *Ultrasound in the Diagnosis of Congenital Anomalies*, 135 Am. J. Obstet. Gynecol. 331-46 (1979).

Leonard, Chase, & Childs, *Genetic Counselling: A Consumer's View*, 287 New England J. of Medicine 433 (1972).

Niswander, K.R., M.D., *Obstetrics, Essentials of Clinical Practice* (Little, Brown & Co., Inc., 1981).

Pritchard, J.A., M.D., MacDonald, P.C., M.D., & Gant, N.F., M.D., *Williams Obstetrics* (Appleton-Century-Crofts, 1985).

CHAPTER 10

TECHNIQUES TO EVALUATE FETAL HEALTH

§ 10.1   Introduction

Unlike the normal battery of tests used to appraise every fetus's health during the antepartum and intrapartum periods (see **Chapter 9**), the procedures described in this chapter are primarily geared toward recognizing those fetuses who may be (or already are) endangered by the course of a high risk pregnancy. Early detection of the diagnostic signs of maturity, hereditary disorders, or oxygen deprivation enables the obstetrician to select the appropriate measures needed to treat these babies before permanent injuries or death develop. Although a wide variety of procedures have been developed to identify the ill or distressed fetus, only the most reliable and informative of these (namely, amniocentesis, ultrasound, estriol analysis, fetal heart monitoring, radiography, and amniography and fetography) will be outlined.

§ 10.2   Antepartum Assessment of Fetal Well-Being

Over the past 10 years, several methods of quantifying perinatal risks have been proposed. Taking into account numerous historical, physical, sociologic, and laboratory factors, these methods will identify, prospectively, about one-fourth to one-third of all pregnancies as high risk. From those will arise the majority of the eventual perinatal mortality and morbidity.

In recent years, many surveillance tests have been developed to assess the integrity of the uteroplacental unit. Now, ultrasound assists in identifying intrauterine growth retardation. These tests, combined with an accurate means of assessing fetal pulmonary maturity by the analysis of amniotic fluid, now give the obstetrician the ability to discriminate between the majority of at-risk fetuses (which are doing well and are best left undisturbed) from the few that should be transferred from their hostile intrauterine environment to a neonatal intensive care facility.

Two types of antepartum fetal heart rate testing are currently the most widely known tests of fetal assessment: the contraction stress test (CST), also known as the oxytocin challenge test (OCT); and the nonstress test (NST).

The purpose of both of those tests is to evaluate the fetal heart rate response to induced uterine contractions and spontaneous fetal movement. In pregnancies complicated by uteroplacental insufficiency, these tests will alert the physician as to when, if at all, intervention is necessary. These tests are useful in discriminating between healthy fetuses and those that are destined for stillbirth, intrapartum distress, or related complications.

It can be surmised that given a condition of borderline fetal oxygenation, a test that further stresses the fetus in terms of oxygen deprivation might produce some biophysical sign of such compromise, and that this data might be prognostically important. It can be suggested from animal data that uterine contractions, producing an intra-amniotic pressure in excess of about 30 mm/ Hg (millimeters of mercury) create an intramyometrial pressure that exceeds mean intra-arteriolar pressure. This event thereby temporarily halts the uterine blood flow. A well oxygenated fetus tolerates this limited period of intervillous stasis well. However, hypoxic or "stressed" fetus will manifest abnormal heart rate patterns, which are indicative of decreased placental function.

Those pregnancies considered to be at the highest risk are those complicated by chronic hypertension with preeclampsia and diabetes mellitus.

To perform a contraction stress test, an external monitor is applied to the mother's abdomen. An oxytocin intravenous infusion is then started to stimulate the uterus to contract. When three contractions in a 10 minute period are obtained, the test is completed. The fetal heart rate and contraction pattern is then evaluated for signs of placental insufficiency.

Nonstress testing measures the frequency of fetal movement and the response of the fetal heart rate. To perform the nonstress test, an external monitor is applied to the mother's abdomen and the patient is then instructed to push a button which records each fetal movement the mother perceives. A 20-minute period is then evaluated in terms of the number of fetal movements and the corresponding fetal heart rate pattern. If there are two or more accelerations in 20 minutes, the test is interpreted as reactive (normal) and is concluded. Accelerations are defined as an increase of at least 15 beats-per-minute above the baseline, lasting at least 15 seconds. If there are less than two accelerations in 20 minutes, the test is interpreted as nonreactive (abnormal) and an oxytocin challenge test must be performed.

Thus, one can clearly see that the application of fetal heart rate monitoring to the antepartum period has proven useful as a means of assessing fetal well-being. Observations of the baseline fetal heart rate, and response to uterine contractions, can show signs of fetal compromise from uteroplacental insufficiency. The main value in these tests lies in their ability to assist the obstetrician in analyzing placental function, so as to determine whether or not intervention is necessary.

The volume of amniotic fluid can sometimes assist the obstetrician in determining whether or not there are any complications during gestation. *Polyhydramnios* is a condition where there is a greater than normal amount of amniotic fluid. Polyhydramnios has been associated with an increased number of congenital malformations. *Oligohydramnios* refers to a reduced amount of amniotic fluid. Reduced amniotic fluid is frequently associated with placental insufficiency, severe preeclampsia, essential hypertension, and postmaturity.

Fetal lung fluid flows into the amniotic fluid; analysis of the amniotic fluid will accurately reflect fetal pulmonary maturation and predict the risk of respiratory distress syndrome (RDS). Knowledge that fetal lung maturation has occurred allows the physician to proceed with delivery without fear of subsequent neonatal RDS. Respiratory distress syndrome is also known as hyaline membrane disease and accounts for 50-70 percent of the morbidity associated with premature births.[1] Therefore, one can clearly see the importance in predicting fetal lung maturity.

When a sample of amniotic fluid is required, it is obtained by means of an *amniocentesis*. An amniocentesis is a procedure wherein the physician inserts a needle through the mother's abdomen and withdraws a specimen of amniotic fluid. Amniocentesis generally is an innocuous and simple technique; however, indications and alternatives should be weighed carefully before proceeding. See §§ **10.3** through **10.5** for a further discussion of amniocentesis. Real-time ultrasound is a safe and useful adjunct to locate the placenta, and to determine the fetal position. See §§ **10.6** through **10.8** on the use of ultrasound.

The most popular biochemical method to evaluate fetal lung development is the measurement of the lecithen to sphingomyelin (L/S) ratio. A mature L/S ratio of greater than 2:1 predicts the absence of RDS in newborns with 98 percent accuracy.[2] Other frequently used tests to determine fetal lung maturity are the foam stability test and the optical density measurement.

Intrauterine growth retardation (IUGR) is associated with a significantly increased rate of perinatal mortality and long term morbidity. Improved perinatal outcome is contingent on accurate and early identification. Confirmation of the diagnosis of IUGR by the usual prenatal examinations is inadequate. Therefore, considerable attention has been focused recently on the use of *ultrasonography* in the diagnosis of growth retardation.

Campbell and Dewhurst[3] used serial biparietal diameter (BPD) measurement of the fetal head to predict IUGR. They studied a series of 140 pregnancies complicated by IUGR, and found that in 82 percent the BPD growth was below normal.

Another method used for detection of growth retardation is the head to body ratio. This is of value because in growth retardation, the brain is relatively spared and the body diameter or circumference, will lag behind the head, reflecting reduced growth of the fetal liver. Normally, the average fetal

---

[1] R. Bolognese, M.D., R. Schwartz, M.D., & J. Schneider, M.D., Perinatal Medicine, 2d ed., 196 (Williams & Wilkins, 1982).

[2] *Id.* at 201.

[3] Campbell & Dewhurst, *Diagnosis of Small-for-Date Fetus by Serial Ultrasonic Cephalometry*, 2 Lancet 1002 (1971).

body diameter measured at the level of the umbilical vein should be within 5 mm of the BPD. A body diameter in excess of 5 mm less than the BPD indicates probable growth retardation.

Another means of detecting IUGR is by measurement of the total intrauterine volume. It has been stated that when the volume of amniotic fluid was more than 1.5 standard deviations below the mean for the gestational age, most fetuses are growth retarded.

Abnormalities of the placenta are also frequently associated with IUGR. Although there is no single placental abnormality that is common to IUGR gestations, there are certain lesions of the placenta which are frequently associated with the growth retarded fetus, and these may be identified by ultrasound. These lesions are as follows: (1) placental infarctions, (2) villous vascularity, (3) fibrosis, and (4) nonspecific villous inflammation. Calcification and fibrous maturity rings are found in most placentas near term. However, excessive calcification prior to 36 weeks of gestation indicates possible fetal compromise. Once identification of possible growth retardation has been made, hospitalization is imperative.

The placenta synthesizes or participates in the synthesis of a large number of steroid hormones including progesterone, estrogen, estradiol, and estriol. From a clinical perspective, the most important estrogen is estriol. Estriol production depends on both fetal and placental function; its excretion is related to maternal renal function. Today, it is the most widely used biochemical estimator of fetoplacental function. There are certain conditions of both the mother and fetus which can affect the estriol level, and the physician must be aware of these rare conditions.

The usefulness of estriol as a measure of fetoplacental function arises from the fact that critical enzymatic steps in its synthesis occur in both the fetus and the placenta, with the rate-limiting enzymatic step occurring in the fetal adrenal glands. For normal amounts of estriol to be secreted, there must be a functional fetal hypothalamic-pituitary-adrenal axis, a functioning fetal liver, a functioning fetal placenta, functioning maternal liver, functioning gastrointestinal tract, and kidneys.

Estriol determinations are made from either blood (plasma) or urinary examinations. Clinically, serial estriol determinations are most commonly employed in the management of pregnancy complicated by diabetes, hypertension, suspected IUGR, or postmaturity. Serial determinations are essential; a single value should virtually never be used for assessment or management. In most instances, serial values are compared to a standard curve. Abnormal patterns may be manifest in one of three patterns: (1) progressive downward slope, (2) rapid fall (35-40 percent of baseline established by average values for the preceding three days), and (3) persistent low values.

§ 10.3 Amniocentesis: Procedure

The intrauterine sanctuary of the fetus has always been impenetrable until the recent advent of amniocentesis. By inserting a needle through the mother's abdomen and uterine wall, the physician is now able to enter the amniotic sac and aspirate a sample of amniotic fluid without appreciable risk to either the mother or her baby. The procedure offers tremendous benefits to the unborn child because a large and ever-increasing variety of diagnostic tests can be performed on the amniotic fluid as early as the 14th week of pregnancy to appraise the health of the fetus. As a result, certain problems can be corrected, prevented, or at least anticipated *before* birth, while the fetus is still inside the uterus.

Amniocentesis is performed in the outpatient clinic. To ensure a successful and atraumatic tap, the placenta should be localized, preferably with ultrasound. By clearly displaying the pockets of amniotic fluid on a screen, preamniocentesis ultrasound permits the physician to place the needle exclusively in these areas to obtain blood-free amniotic fluid, without the danger of piercing the placenta or fetus in the process. The site of needle penetration must also be based on the fetal position and a *physical* examination of the placental site. A transabdominal, suprapubic tap is most frequently recommended, especially if amniocentesis is performed without ultrasound, since this area reduces the danger of placental trauma. However, if the suprapubic approach is unsuccessful or contraindicated by the position of the fetus, the needle can alternatively be inserted behind the nape of the fetal neck or in the region of the fetal hands and feet. Regardless of which location is chosen, the procedure should always be done aseptically; the mother's bladder should be emptied and the fetus's heart should be auscultated both before and after the fluid is aspirated. Some clinicians inject a local anesthetic before they begin, yet others oppose this practice on the grounds that it is unnecessary and only compounds the risk by increasing the number of needle insertions needed to withdraw the fluid.

Once the needle is at the proper depth, a small amount of amniotic fluid is aspirated. The exact volume depends on the particular test or tests ordered. The fluid is then usually centrifuged, separating the cellular layer from the cell-free liquid or supernatant. The supernatant, or upper layer, is used for a variety of important biochemical tests; whereas the cellular, or bottom layer, is commonly used for genetic or certain enzymatic studies.

Characteristically, the amniotic fluid has an odor and a slight or moderate degree of turbidity, with varying shades of a faint yellow pigment. However, when contaminants such as blood, meconium, maternal urine, or fetal ascitic fluid enter the amniotic fluid, they are likely to interfere with the analyses and invalidate the results. Similarly, prolonged exposure to light also invalidates certain tests, so the specimen should immediately be covered or placed in a dark container. This is particularly important when bilirubin, the light-sensitive breakdown product of hemoglobin, is being measured. Falsely low bilirubin levels will result if the specimen is unprotected, causing significant cases of hemolytic disease to be overlooked. Anencephaly and certain gastrointestinal obstructions may also result in the misdiagnosis of hemolytic disease, since these disorders elicit pronounced changes in the measurements.

Although meconium also markedly distorts the absorbance of certain substances in the assay, there is some controversy regarding the significance of the meconium itself in the amniotic fluid. Many physicians argue that there is only a limited correlation between meconium-stained amniotic fluid and fetal distress, and they feel its presence is not diagnostic because it is impossible to distinguish an acute or a corrected case of fetal distress from a chronic, ongoing one. Their opponents believe the amniotic fluid should be inspected repeatedly for meconium during the course of labor.[4]

§ 10.4   —Amniocentesis: Uses

Amniocentesis is primarily ordered to diagnose and evaluate the following conditions of the fetus: (1) fetal maturity, (2) genetic aberrations, and (3) hemolytic (RH) disorders. In addition, the procedure is warranted for one maternal reason, namely polyhydramnios.

Fetal Maturity

Information about fetal maturity is mainly needed when either induction of labor or cesarean section is contemplated, but the obstetrician is uncertain whether the fetus is adequately developed to survive outside the womb. Accurate predictions of fetal maturity can now be made, thanks to ongoing medical discoveries. The research has shown that as the levels of several components of the amniotic fluid change during the course of pregnancy, their fluctuations reflect the development and maturity of certain fetal organs.

An evaluation of the fetal pulmonary system is considered one of the most vital indices of maturity, since underdeveloped lungs markedly limit the baby's ability to survive outside of the uterus. Inadequate pulmonary function is one of the major causes of neonatal morbidity and mortality, and can best be

---

[4] R. Bolognese, M.D., R. Schwartz, M.D., & J. Schneider, M.D., Perinatal Medicine, 2d ed., 203 (Williams & Wilkins, 1982).

assessed in utero by measuring lecithin and sphingomyelin (two phospholipids secreted by the lung and found in the amniotic fluid). These substances facilitate and maintain the expansion of the lungs, which is especially critical immediately after birth when the baby must breathe on its own for the first time. Without the essential levels of lecithin and sphingomyelin, the lung collapses each time the infant exhales, and respiratory distress ensues. The syndrome is characterized by tachypnea (more than 70 breaths-per-minute), hypothermia, and cyanosis.

The concentrations of lecithin and sphingomyelin are approximately equal until around the 35th week of gestation, when lecithin suddenly surges and sphingomyelin falls slightly. Because the spurt in lecithin biosynthesis reflects the potential capacity of the lungs to support gas exchange (oxygen and carbon dioxide) outside the womb, the ratio of lecithin to sphingomyelin (L/S ratio) is directly related to the maturity of the fetal lungs. This, in turn, corresponds to the probability that respiratory distress syndrome will occur if the baby is delivered. When the L/S ratio is greater than 2:1, it is extremely unlikely that the newborn will suffer from respiratory distress, unless perhaps, the mother is a diabetic or has received an intrauterine transfusion. However, there may be times when, even though the L/S ratio is less than two, it may be more risky for the fetus to remain inside the uterus than to contend with the possibility of respiratory distress outside the uterus. Despite an immature L/S ratio before birth, approximately 10 percent of term babies still manage to do well postnatally. Because every pregnancy has its own peculiarities, it is the obstetrician's responsibility to carefully evaluate each case rather than rely on generalities. Nonetheless, recognition of pulmonary immaturity and prevention of respiratory distress syndrome is important because it may be fatal. The phrase hyaline membrane disease is often used to describe the lethal sequelae of respiratory distress.

Although the L/S ratio has become the most common determinant of fetal maturity, it is only able to evaluate the pulmonary development. Since other organs may also be underdeveloped when a baby is born prematurely, the measurement of additional constituents or properties of the amniotic fluid have been devised to more thoroughly predict fetal maturity. The most commonly cited indices are the creatinine concentration, the osmolarity, and the presence of specific amounts of lipid-stainable cells. Like the L/S ratio, these properties also change as the fetus develops, but at a rate and degree so slight or so variable that they are generally not considered accurate indices of fetal maturity. The concentration indicative of fetal maturity is usually reached after 37 weeks of gestation and, depending on the particular laboratory technique used, is about 20.0 mg. Errors may occur if the creatinine concentration in the mother's blood (low levels of creatinine are normal in the bloodstream) is increased for any reason. High blood levels cause increases in the creatinine concentration of the amniotic fluid, even though the fetus is not mature. To prevent this error, it is essential to measure the creatinine concentration in the mother's blood to assure it is normal before the results can be valid. In spite of these precautions, the value of the creatinine test remains controversial. Some obstetricians consider it unreliable, whereas others believe it compliments the L/S ratio in assessing the overall fetal maturity.[5]

Genetic Aberrations

Amniocentesis is also indicated when the family history suggests that one parent has, or may be a carrier of, a severe chromosomal or metabolic disorder which the fetus is liable to inherit. However, the procedure should only be ordered when such a genetic or metabolic abnormality can be proven *definitively* by analyzing the fetal cells cultured from the amniotic fluid.

Amniocentesis to detect these disorders, is usually initiated between the 15th and 18th week of gestation. By this time, the amniotic fluid has increased to a volume suitable for safe and easy aspiration, and it is still early enough in the pregnancy for the parents to choose an abortion or to make arrangements for special care if the fetus is found to be abnormal.

Hemolytic (Rh) Disorders

Each person's red blood cells can be typed as Rh-positive or Rh-negative, depending on the presence or absence of a distinguishing chemical structure known as the Rh-factor. Approximately 85 percent of the population is Rh-positive. The other 15 percent are Rh-negative, meaning that they lack the Rh-factor. In the Rh-negative case, if an Rh-factor ever enters their bloodstream, their immune systems react as they would to any other atypical invading foreign substance such as a bacteria or virus, they synthesize antibodies (anti-Rh antibodies in this case) to destroy it.

In the general population, these two blood groups normally never have the opportunity to mix, so no complications arise. This is not true of the pregnant population, since the maternal and fetal circulations generally come into contact with each other in the later months of gestation. Serious problems may develop, but only if the mother is Rh-negative *and* is carrying an Rh-positive fetus *and* has previously been exposed to Rh-positive blood through an unmatched transfusion or past pregnancy. Such a past exposure sensitized or immunized the mother, inducing her to produce anti-Rh antibodies which will now be able to cross the placenta (toward the end of pregnancy), attach to the fetal Rh-positive red blood cells, and then destroy them. This red blood cell

---

[5] *Id.* at 202.

destruction is called hemolysis, and it involves the release of hemoglobin from the cell into the surroundings. As hemolysis continues, the fetal red blood cell supply becomes markedly depleted, leading to jaundice, anemia, and/or death, depending on how much bilirubin (the harmful, though measurable, breakdown product of hemoglobin) is present. This dangerous condition has several names: Rh-disease, hemolytic disease of the newborn, or erythroblastosis fetalis.

Amniocentesis is indispensible because it allows the physician to measure the level of bilirubin present in the amniotic fluid in order to precisely evaluate the fetal condition. Normally, this bilirubin is of fetal origin and it directly reflects the degree of hemolysis, since amniotic fluid typically contains no bilirubin or bilirubin-like pigments toward the end of pregnancy. However, the mother may contribute a significant amount of bilirubin if she has an underlying disease such as sickle cell anemia. *Her* elevated blood levels of bilirubin will cause a rise in the amniotic fluid bilirubin concentration, leading the unobservant obstetrician to mistakenly assume that the fetus is suffering from hemolytic disease.

The timing of the initial amniocentesis depends on the patient's history and anti-Rh antibody titer (that is, a ratio of the level of antibody in her *serum*). An Rh-negative woman who has never been pregnant or has never carried an Rh-positive fetus, will have no anti-Rh antibodies in her bloodstream. However, if she becomes pregnant in the future and then has a high antibody titer, the obstetrician can correctly conclude that the fetus is Rh-positive and some of its red blood cells have crossed the placenta and entered its mother's circulation, inducing her to produce anti-Rh antibodies. Her antibody responses threaten the baby because these newly formed antibodies are capable of crossing the placenta, where they will attach to the baby's blood cells and destroy them. If a critical antibody titer (usually 1:8 or 1:16, depending on the particular laboratory) is reached before it is safe to deliver the baby, the physician must promptly determine how severely the infant is affected. This is accomplished by aspirating some amniotic fluid and measuring the bilirubin concentration.

In sharp contrast to that situation, if a woman has previously delivered an Rh-positive baby, her antibody titers are not entirely diagnostic of the status of her current pregnancy since they also reflect her past Rh-immunization. Therefore, regardless of the antibody titer, an amniocentesis must be performed to measure the concentration of bilirubin. In both of these situations, the initial amniocentesis is generally performed between the 29th and 32d week of gestation, unless very severe hemolytic disease is suspected (in which case amniocentesis may be done earlier). Amniocentesis should then be repeated at 5-21 day intervals to identify a trend in the progress of the disease. When the bilirubin concentration is falling, it is safe to await a natural delivery. On the other hand, a horizontal or rising trend indicates the fetus will die in utero if it is not delivered promptly or given an intrauterine blood transfusion. When the fetus is not mature enough to survive outside the uterus, its life may be saved by an intrauterine transfusion, which involves injecting Rh-negative red blood cells (they blend compatibly with all blood group systems) into the fetal peritoneal cavity, from where they will be absorbed into the fetal bloodstream. These new red blood cells enable the fetus to overcome the severe anemia since the mother's antibodies cannot bind to and destroy them because, unlike the baby's own cells, these lack the Rh-factor.

Polyhydramnios

In addition to the three fetal indications for amniocentesis, the procedure is also warranted for one maternal reason, namely polyhydramnios. However, the underlying causes of the disorder (such as Rh-disease, multiple fetuses, diabetes, and congenital malformations) should be ruled out beforehand. As long as acute polyhydramnios is not associated with these complications, it may be managed therapeutically by repeated amniocentesis to prevent premature labor, and to alleviate the maternal symptoms. Relief occurs almost immediately after the amniotic fluid is withdrawn.

§ 10.5 —Amniocentesis: Safety

Although complications are rarely encountered when amniocentesis is properly performed, the obstetrician should be aware of its potential hazards. The maternal risks are negligible, but they include infection, intraperitoneal hemmorrhage, and amniotic fluid embolism. Only rarely does amniocentesis cause abruptio placenta, or ruptured membranes and the onset of premature labor.

The fetal hazards of amniocentesis are not as negligible as the maternal ones. If the needle pierces the fetus, a vital organ may be punctured, or umbilical cord hematoma or acute blood loss may result. Whenever a bloody specimen of amniotic fluid is aspirated, the source of the bleeding should be determined. If it originates from the fetus, the fetal heart should be monitored continuously, and further tests and evaluation of the fetal condition are mandatory. Immediate delivery may be indicated in some of these cases. Should the physician decide to deliver the baby after performing an amniocentesis, he must closely monitor the newborn's heart rate. Other signs of deteriorating neonatal condition must not be overlooked either, especially if the tap may have been traumatic. Since deaths due to rapidly fatal pneumothorax can be prevented by promptly treating needle wounds in the chest, all infants should be carefully examined immediately following delivery for any evidence of a needle puncture.

Spontaneous abortion may occur if either the fetus or placenta is injured. In fact, if amniocentesis is performed without prior ultrasound placental localization, there is at least a 10 percent risk of placental trauma (however, a transabdominal, supra-pubic tap, when done toward the end of pregnancy, is supposed to reduce the risk), transplacental hemmorrhage and an increased severity of hemolytic disease of the newborn. The latter condition arises following placental perforation since the fetal Rh-positive blood leaks out of its confines and is transferred to the Rh-negative mother, inciting or enhancing maternal Rh-isoimmunization.

Intrauterine fetal injury is also more common when the volume of amniotic fluid is small, relative to the size of the fetus, or when the fluid is thick and does not flow freely through the needle. Because it may be more difficult to withdraw enough amniotic fluid under these circumstances, repeated taps are often necessary, thereby increasing the risks of the procedure. These conditions are encountered more frequently in advanced pregnancies, and especially in post-term pregnancies.

This section has dealt with the immediate complications of amniocentesis. The long-range complications, if they exist, are still unknown.

§ 10.6   Ultrasound: Procedure

The impact of diagnostic ultrasound in perinatal management has been momentous, offering a noninvasive means of visualizing the morphology, physiology, and pathology of the uterus, the placenta, and the fetus throughout the pregnancy. Prior to its introduction, radiographic and radionuclide techniques were the primary imaging techniques used for obstetric evaluation, but they only provided limited information while exposing the mother and fetus to potentially harmful radiation. With ultrasound, in contrast, no deleterious biologic effects have yet been demonstrated in either the maternal or the developing fetal tissues.

Ultrasound is based on the principle that high-frequency sound waves send back (or reflect) echoes whenever they pass through different tissue densities. To initiate this sequence of events, an electric current is applied to a transducer (made of a piezoelectric material) situated on the mother's abdomen. After a coupling agent such as mineral oil is spread on the abdominal skin, the transducer emits a pulse of high-frequency sound waves which pass freely through the soft tissues until they reach an interface between different tissue densities. At this point, some of the energy (proportional to the difference in densities of the adjacent tissues) is reflected, or echoed back to the transducer, stimulating it to generate a small electrical voltage. This voltage is then amplified and displayed on an oscilloscope for easy visualization.

Very slight changes in the nature of a tissue are capable of producing a strong enough echo to be recorded by an ultrasonic scanner. As a result of this sensitivity, the boundaries between the soft tissues of the fetus and the amniotic fluid, between the placenta and the uterine wall, and between the fetal brain and the falx cerebri can all be readily demonstrated. Differences as subtle as these cannot be obtained by the current radiographic techniques, with the possible exception of computerized axial tomography (CAT-scan).

In essence, the pulse-echo technique is able to locate anatomic structures and produce their images by measuring the transition time needed for the ultrasonic waves to reach the structure, to be reflected at the interface, and to return to the transducer. This basic methodology has been applied several ways:

A-mode (amplitude mode): The simplest of the three methods, the A-mode measures the size of structures such as the fetal skull; it is not used too often in obstetrics.

B-mode scan: Using either a conventional black and white picture (a two shade scan) or the recent gray-scale picture (the interfaces of different sound reflectivity are displayed as various shades of gray), the B-mode scan provides a *static* two-dimensional and cross-sectional image; to obtain a composite image, serial scans in the transverse and longitudinal axes are taken. This information allows the size, shape, and location of various anatomic structures to be determined. Static studies such as these are considered better methods of evaluating spatial relationship, and the overall dimensions of the uterus and its contents, than real-time techniques. However, this is not an absolute truth, so each patient's examination must be individualized according to her specific needs.

Real-time ultrasound: Using gray-scale and linear-array imaging, this modality provides *continuous* cross-sectional motion pictures of internal structures; its special transducer is capable of generating multiple pulse-echo systems which can be activated sequentially, enabling the physician to detect fetal activity including breathing, cardiac movement, and blood vessel pulsations. The scan is very versatile and only takes a fraction of the time that a static modality requires. Although the older instruments often had a poorer resolution capability than static scanners, recent innovations have markedly improved the resolution of the newer instrumemts so that they now approach the level of the conventional B-mode scanners.

§ 10.7   —Ultrasound: Uses

Although ultrasound is ordered with increasing frequency for pregnant women, it is not part of the standard antepartum and intrapartum examination,
despite the attempts of some clinicians to make it so. Their efforts may never
be realized since many private practitioners and smaller hospitals will probably be unable to afford the expected price increase of future instruments. Because of the enormous cost it would add to the already high price of giving
birth, *routine* scanning in the United States would have to be thoroughly evaluated, especially in light of the fact that it has not been shown to improve the
outcome of pregnancy. Presently, the most common indications for obstetrical ultrasound are:

1. Determination of the gestational age
2. Localization of the placenta
3. Verification of fetal death
4. Detection of multiple fetuses
5. Detection of congenital malformations
6. Early identification of an intrauterine pregnancy
7. Detection of uterine growths
8. Localization of an intrauterine device
9. Intrauterine Growth Retardation.

Gestational Age

An ultrasonic determination of the gestational age is most commonly indicated when there is an inadequate menstrual history, when pregnancy occurs
following the discontinuation of birth control pills, when there is oligomenorrhea or amenorrhea prior to pregnancy, or when an overlying maternal disorder such as diabetes or hypertension makes it desirable to deliver the fetus
before the onset of labor. In the latter instance, when the physician can accurately estimate the length of the pregnancy, he can schedule a cesarean section
or begin to induce labor without the fear of delivering a premature infant.
    Several fetal structures can be measured by ultrasound to determine the
gestational age. They include the diameter of the gestational sac, the crown-
rump length, and the biparietal diameter (BPD) of the fetal skull. In addition,
as the fetus matures, the placenta develops certain recognizable characteristics
that correspond to the length of the pregnancy.

The diameter of the gestational sac correlates well with the gestational age in the first trimester, particularly between the sixth and eight week. Afterwards, the sac may lose its round and ringlike appearance, so the measurements are no longer valid. The average diameter or the volume of the sac can also be used to reveal early developmental abnormalities.

Another structure which accurately corresponds to the gestational age is the crown-rump length. It is most precise between the 8th and 14th week of pregnancy, after which time, it is difficult to obtain a good measurement on some instruments.

Once the fetal head is well defined, the BPD is the most frequently used index of the gestational age. It is a sensitive measurement, since the fetal head grows at a predictable and decreasing rate from the end of the first trimester to approximately the 34th week of pregnancy. According to most growth curves compiled from ultrasonic data, the BPD correlates most closely to the fetal age between the 15th and 25th week of pregnancy, varying from the true value by only plus or minus 10 days.

Such precision is not possible, however, during the last six weeks of pregnancy because the head grows at a slower and immeasurable rate. If a single measurement of the BPD is taken at this time, it may vary as much as three weeks in either direction. The danger of such misleading information is clearly seen in the following example. If a single measurement indicates that the fetus is 38 weeks old, the infant could potentially only be 35 weeks old because of the three-week range of variability. Assuming that delivery was initiated based on the valid assumption (from erroneous ultrasound conclusions, of course) that a 38 week old fetus should be mature, the obstetrician may inadvertently deliver a premature infant who is unable to survive outside the womb.

As of yet, a universal method for measuring the BPD has not been established since the clinicians cannot concur on the most reliable technique. Reliance upon a single value, particularly one made late in pregnancy, is likely to increase the error.

To avoid any technical errors in the procedure which might misrepresent the gestational age, the pulse-echo must be aimed perpendicularly to the fetal head in order to obtain a horizontal section through the skull. This is not always easy, especially when the fetal head is deeply engaged in the pelvis (since the maternal pelvic bones interfere with the transmission of the sound beam) or in breech presentations (because the relatively free-floating head of the breech baby is not always fixed in one position long enough for the physician to take repetitive readings). Similar problems are encountered in the presence of hydramnios or marked obesity. Consequently, accurate measurements are not possible in about 10 percent of the patients. However, as long as the physician is aware of these limitations, ultrasonic measurement of the BPD is very reliable.

Localization of Placenta

Ultrasound is regarded as the most accurate and noninvasive means of detecting the placental site, particularly during the second trimester. It is also the least painful and least hazardous procedure for the mother and fetus. There are three principal situations when the placental site must be identified: when amniocentesis is ordered, when a cesarean section is planned, and when bleeding occurs in the third trimester.

In order to safely perform an amniocentesis, the placenta must be located so that it will not be punctured when the amniotic fluid is withdrawn. Trauma to the placenta may induce bleeding which may invalidate the current or subsequent test results or, more seriously, it may lead to abortion. Some studies have demonstrated that ultrasound during amniocentesis decreases the number of fetomaternal hemorrhages resulting from pierced placentas. The only time the needle may have to be inserted through the placenta is when the operator is unable to locate a placenta-free area. In these cases, ultrasound is important to locate the site of attachment of the umbilical cord to the chorionic plate, because this area has a large number of blood vessels which must also be avoided.

Advance knowledge of the placental position also enables the surgeon performing a cesarean section to bypass the placenta entirely, or at least warn him of the need to cut through a placenta which cannot be avoided. Probably the most important indication for placental localization is third trimester bleeding. Ultrasound is used to decide if the bleeding is due to placenta previa or some other cause. By depicting the implantation site, the ultrasonogram can implicate previa, though it generally cannot identify the alternate cause of the blood loss if placenta previa is ruled out. In certain situations, however, it may even be difficult to diagnose placenta previa. For example, if the fetus lies deep in the maternal pelvis, it may obscure a low-lying placenta. In addition, whereas a full bladder is essential for accurate placental localization, a markedly distended bladder may alter the ultrasonic appearance of the normal uterine anatomy.

In addition to identifying a placenta previa, ultrasound can also identify the presence of abruptio placenta (an abruption is often identified by the presence of a blood clot behind the placenta). The abruption may also be seen as an area of separation of the placenta from the uterine wall.

Abnormal growth (also referred to as intrauterine growth retardation) is best documented by a combination of ultrasonic measurements, all of which are required since no single parameter is totally reliable. The principal indicators of intrauterine growth retardation are an abnormal head-to-abdomen ratio and decreased measurements of the BPD (taken serially), the head-to-abdomen ratio, the crown-rump length, the fetal thorax and extremities, and the total intrauterine volume. Whenever growth abnormalities are suspected, it is important to notify the physician who performs and interprets the ultrasound so the appropriate measurements will be obtained.

Verification of Fetal Death

Suspected cases of intrauterine fetal death can be confirmed by ultrasound. In the first few hours after death, there is typically an increase in the number of echos coming from within the fetal body and a loss of clarity of the bodily outline. The longer the dead fetus remains inside the uterus, the harder it becomes to identify the head, since it tends to collapse and lose its characteristic echoes and internal structure between five to ten days after death.

However, since it is possible for a dead fetus to appear ultrasonically normal, the most reliable sign of death is a lack of fetal growth. This can be established by serial studies done at intervals far enough apart to ensure that the fetus has stopped growing. Recognizable changes in the BPD usually occur after seven to ten days, so either a reduction in the fetal skull size or no evidence of growth, makes the diagnosis of intrauterine death certain. Even so, an erroneous interpretation could have disastrous consequences, so the ultrasonogram should be repeated seven to ten days later if it suggests fetal death, unless the mother's coagulation tests indicate a coagulopathy.

Detection of Multiple Fetuses

The diagnosis of twins becomes easier after 12 weeks gestation since the heads are readily identifiable then. It is advantageous to show both heads in one picture to avoid confusing twins with a single fetus who changes position during the procedure, and appears like two fetuses.

Detection of Congenital Malformations

By comparing the size of the fetus to the amniotic fluid surrounding it, ultrasound can reveal abnormal amniotic fluid levels, which may be associated with certain congenital deformities. Polyhydramnios, which is characterized by an excessive amount of amniotic fluid, should be suspected when the fetus appears to occupy a relatively small portion of the amniotic cavity. It is often seen in conjunction with neural malformations, anencephaly, and gastro-intestinal disorders.

Ultrasound may also demonstrate hydrocephaly (characterized by a disproportionately large head), large meningoceles, and renal agenesis. Currently, the routine ultrasonic examination of all pregnant women to detect these and other fetal malformations is not considered reasonable.

Intrauterine Pregnancy

Since ultrasound can locate the gestational sac, an intrauterine pregnancy can be diagnosed as early as the eighth week of gestation. In contrast, an ectopic pregnancy, such as one that develops in the Fallopian tubes or the abdomen, is more complicated and cannot be reliably diagnosed with ultrasound.

Detection of Uterine Growths

The presence of solid or cystic characteristics, as well as the extent of many tumors, can be determined by ultrasound. It is important to differentiate an artifact of the scan from a significant anatomic structure, especially since reverberations occur frequently in cyst-like structures. However, they are easily recognized during scanning and should not be mistaken for a solid component, or an otherwise cystic mass.

Localization of Intrauterine Device

Ultrasound has become the examination of choice for detecting an intrauterine device (IUD) within the uterus. Since this contraceptive device is made of a radiopaque material, an IUD shows up entirely differently from the uterine soft tissues on ultrasound.

Intrauterine Growth Retardation

Intrauterine growth retardation (IUGR) is associated with a significantly increased rate of perinatal mortality and long term morbidity. Improved perinatal outcome is contingent on accurate and early identification. Confirmation of the diagnosis of IUGR by the usual prenatal examinations is inadequate. Therefore, considerable attention has been focused recently on the use of ultrasonography in the diagnosis of growth retardation. Once identification of possible growth retardation has been made, hospitalization is imperative.

§ 10.8 —Ultrasound: Safety

Even though there have been no confirmed reports incriminating the diagnostic energy levels used in ultrasound, there have been contentions of possible hazardous biological effects from too frequent or too lengthy examinations. As a precautionary measure, some physicians believe it is wise to limit fetal ultrasonic exposure whenever possible, especially during the first trimester. Others feel that prudent obstetricians ought to explain to their patients that human studies are still crude and difficult to evaluate because environmental factors complicate the issue, so the precise way in which ultrasonic energy interacts with human tissues is still not completely understood.

Despite these potential drawbacks, ultrasound's high degree of resolution offers a reliable and detailed examination of the entire fetal anatomy, allowing more subtle physiologic and pathologic changes to be detected. Until further research proves otherwise, the judicious use of ultrasound is presently regarded as a safe and excellent means of evaluating specific fetal and maternal problems.

§ 10.9 Fetal Heart Rate Monitoring

Fetal heart monitoring is an essential part of intrapartum care, enabling the obstetrician to detect the early warning signs of fetal distress because potentially life-threatening oxygen deficiencies are quickly reflected by alterations in the fetal heart rate (FHR) pattern. Before the introduction of sophisticated electronic detection and recording equipment, periodic auscultation of the fetal heart with a head stethoscope (fetoscope) was the only means of detecting abnormal cardiac patterns. Today, a much wider range of possibilities exist. The new electronic instruments, which continually monitor and record the FHR, can immediately discover deviations in the cardiac rhythm. Besides monitoring the FHR, they also simultaneously measure and record the mother's uterine contractions, since many atypical cardiac patterns arise in response to the pressure changes generated during contractions.

The FHR can be evaluated using one of two vastly different heart monitoring instruments, the traditional fetoscope or the new electronic monitoring and recording equipment. From about the 18th week of pregnancy, the fetal heart sounds can be detected by the fetoscope, a specialized head stethoscope which allows the obstetrician to listen to the fetal heartbeat through the mother's abdomen, and then calculate the number of beats per minute. During labor, this examination is done in the period between uterine contractions, and is usually repeated once every 15 minutes. A major limitation of intermittent auscultation is that a profound alteration in the FHR, which arises in the 14 minute-intervals between auscultations, may easily go unnoticed. In addition, the fetal heartbeat may be obscured by obesity, increased volumes of amniotic fluid, and changes in the maternal and fetal positions. Even though some physicians claim that the fetoscope is unable to discover a significant proportion of FHR abnormalities and reliably detect fetal distress, it is still the most common form of monitoring, especially during labor.

However, a large percentage of physicians now favor *continuous* electronic heart monitors over *intermittent* fetoscopic auscultation, contending that their precision far exceeds that of the human ear.[6] Furthermore, since the factors which interfere with fetoscopic examination do not affect the results of the electronic equipment, virtually 100 percent of the heart rate data can be evaluated by the new heart monitors, which electronically record each beat of the fetus' heart.

A variety of electronic equipment is available, offering two distinct methods of *jointly* monitoring the FHR and mother's uterine contractions: external (indirect) and internal (direct) monitoring. The choice depends on the clinical circumstances during pregnancy and labor. An external monitor can be used for both of the antepartum and intrapartum periods, but it is the technique of choice in the antepartum period because it is noninvasive and can be applied when monitoring is required before the mother's membranes are ruptured and her cervix is dilated. Since the equipment is attached to the outside of the mother's abdomen, the FHR is measured *indirectly*.

Several types of external monitoring are possible, including phonocardiography, fetal electrocardiography, and ultrasonocardiography. Of the three, ultrasonic equipment is used most frequently and is considered more accurate because, unlike phonocardiography and fetal electrocardiography, extraneous environmental noise or electrical signals do not interfere with its measurements. All of the ultrasonic instruments are based on the Doppler phenomenon, whereby high frequency sound waves reflected from a moving structure (in this case, the active fetal heart), return to the transmitter at a different frequency to be converted into the FHR.

Ultrasonocardiography is typically performed by wrapping two belts around the mother's abdomen. The lower belt holds an ultrasonic transducer, which records the FHR, and the upper belt holds a pressure-sensitive tocodynamometer, which simultaneously records the intensity of the uterine contractions. This instrumentation consistently enables the obstetrician to detect the FHR by the 12th week of pregnancy, approximately six weeks earlier than with a fetoscope. Ultrasonocardiography is also valuable to confirm sus-

---

6 Hon, E.H., *Fetal Heart Rate Monitoring*, in Modern Perinatal Medicine, L. Gluck (ed.), (Year Book Publishers, 1974).

pected cases of intrauterine fetal death. If the fetal heartbeat is inaudible by this method, intrauterine death is a virtual certainty.

Whereas external monitoring can be performed any time after the 11th week of gestation, internal monitoring is limited to the final days of pregnancy because it is an invasive procedure which involves passing an electrode through the mother's vagina and attaching it to the baby's presenting part. This can only be done when the mother's membranes are ruptured and her cervix is sufficiently dilated, events which ordinarily do not occur before she is ready to give birth. Changes in the intrauterine pressure resulting from the mother's contractions are measured simultaneously with the FHR, either by a special catheter introduced through the vagina into the uterus (alongside the baby's presenting part) or by the same tocodynamometer used for external monitoring. *Direct* application of the electrode on the fetus's body allows more subtle variations in its heart rate to be detected by the electrocardiogram, making internal monitoring a more accurate technique than external monitoring in the intrapartum period.

During both internal and external monitoring, the mother's blood pressure should be measured periodically. Whenever internal monitoring is chosen, the obstetrician should be prepared to deliver the baby within a reasonable time period following the procedure, because the intravaginal and intrauterine manipulations can introduce micro-organisms into the woman's reproductive tract, which may cause infection if delivery is delayed.

Following its rapid acceptance into the arena of fetal medicine, some physicians began to regard continuous electronic heart monitoring as an intrinsic part of intrapartum fetal care, despite the fact that it is not currently feasible or necessarily justifiable to routinely evaluate the status of every fetus with these new instruments. Although intrapartum hypoxia may occur in any pregnancy, it is much more likely to develop when there are underlying complications. For these reasons, many authorities only recommend continuous monitoring of the FHR in the following high risk situations:

1. If an abnormal FHR is detected by auscultation at a time when immediate delivery is not indicated
2. If meconium-tinged amniotic fluid is discovered when the fetus is in a vertex presentation
3. When there is premature labor
4. When there is poor progress during labor
5. When oxytocin is administered to induce or augment labor
6. When the fetus is compromised or when there are medical complications during the pregnancy associated with insufficient uteroplacental blood exchange, such as preeclampsia, intrauterine growth retarda-

tion, hypertension, bleeding, hemolytic disease, diabetes, and abnormal fetal presentations.

§ 10.10   —Physiology of Electronic Fetal Heart Rate Monitoring

The fetal heart rate (FHR) is believed to be under the direct control of the fetal autonomic nervous system. There are reflex mechanisms involved with hypoxic changes in FHR patterns and variability. With early hypoxia, whether caused by cord compression or uteroplacental insufficiency, the FHR patterns are primarily of neural reflex origin, whereas with *severe* hypoxia and fetal acidosis, the periodic FHR changes are probably primarily due to myocardial depression.

Electronic intrapartum fetal heart monitoring is based on the concept that uterine contractions constitute a repetitive stress that may compromise the fetus, and that the FHR response to this stress may differ greatly from the FHR characteristics between contractions. For descriptive purposes, FHR evaluation is considered to be composed of two categories: (1) the baseline (nonstressed) FHR, and (2) the periodic (contraction-related) FHR. Analysis of a given record requires evaluation of both.

The normal fetal heart rate range is considered to be between the limits of 120-160 beats-per-minute. Fetal heart rate levels less than 120 bpm are classified as bradycardia. Bradycardia is further subdivided into:

1. Moderate (90-120 bpm)
2. Marked (70-89 bpm)
3. Severe (below 70 bpm).

As bradycardia becomes increasingly severe, it is associated with increasing fetal acidosis.

§ 10.11   —Fetal Heart Variability

Variability or reactivity of the baseline is also important in assessing fetal well-being. A reactive baseline is one which fluctuates five beats or more per minute. A nonreactive or silent baseline, often indicates serious compromise and may be associated with placental insufficiency. A favorable fetal heart rate pattern is one which fluctuates five beats or more per minute, but does not fluctuate more than fifteen beats-per-minute with each uterine contraction. *Increased variability has been shown to be the earliest fetal heart rate sign of mild hypoxia.*

§ 10.12   —Fetal Heart Rate Decelerations

A deceleration in the fetal heart pattern is defined as a transient decrease in the fetal heart rate (FHR) below 150 beats-per-minute and is related to a change in intrauterine pressure. In other words, it is not only the decrease in the fetal heart rate that is important, but also the *relation to the contraction* of the decrease in fetal heart rate.

There are three major types of decelerations:

1. Type I or early decelerations
2. Type II or late decelerations
3. Type III or variable decelerations.

§ 10.13   —Early Decelerations

Early deceleration (Type I) refers to a depression of the FHR, usually of the order of 10-20 beats-per-minute, which coincides with a uterine contraction. In early deceleration, the onset occurs with the beginning of a contraction, continues through the height of the contraction, and returns to the baseline as the contraction subsides. This pattern is repetitive with each contraction, is more common during the latter half of the first stage of labor, and is due to vagal stimulation as a result of head compression. Early deceleration has no sinister implications and no therapy is needed. However, it is not a common finding, and its primary importance is that it must not be confused with late deceleration, which may be a most ominous sign.

§ 10.14   —Late Decelerations

Late deceleration (Type II) patterns are thought to be due to acute uteroplacental insufficiency as a result of decreased intervillous blood flow during the contraction. They are of uniform shape and, in the presence of an interuterine pressure gauge, reflect the shape of the associated interuterine pressure curve. If either the amplitude or frequency of this pattern is high, there should be concern that a deteriorating fetal condition exists. In addition to uteroplacental insufficiency, late decelerations may appear when extreme tension is being placed on the cord. Recovery of late decelerations occur more than 15 seconds after the completion of the contractions. The onset and recovery are gradual, and the nadir of the deceleration occurs more than 20 seconds for the peak of the contraction (lag time).

Neonatal depression is found with this pattern, which is likely to be the consequence of hypoxia and associated with metabolic derangements from uteroplacental insufficiency. Late decelerations are frequently associated with high risk pregnancies, uterine hyperactivity, and maternal hypotension.

Attempts to ameliorate the late decelerations may be accomplished by: (1) decreasing uterine activity (or hyperactivity), (2) correcting maternal hypotension, (3) administering oxygen to the mother, and/or (4) changing the maternal position (usually turning the mother on her left side will increase uterine blood flow by removing the weight of the uterus and its contents off the vena cava).

Late decelerations are considered to be an ominous fetal heart rate pattern because of their association with fetal hypoxia and acidosis. Late decelerations are caused by fetal hypoxia usually from inadequate exchange within the placenta which is provoked by the uterine contraction. *Therefore, late decelerations are proportional to the duration and strength of the contractions, and often will be seen with the stronger contractions and be absent with the weaker ones.* Also, the amplitude of the deceleration will usually be proportional to the pressure of the uterine contraction. There is generally a correlation between the magnitude of late decelerations (amount of slowing) and the degree of hypoxia, *but occasionally the most depressed fetuses will have only shallow, late decelerations.*

In addition to the presence of late decelerations, other parameters, such as loss of variability and tachycardia, should be evaluated when the potential of fetal intolerance to hypoxia exists.

According to Dr. Roger Freeman,[7] the most common cause of late decelerations is uterine hyperactivity/hypertonus, usually as a result of excessive oxytocin stimulation.

---

[7] R.K. Freeman, M.D. & T.J. Garite, M.D., Fetal Heart Rate Monitoring, 93 Williams & Wilkins, 1981).

§ 10.15 —Variable Decelerations

Variable decelerations (Type III) are thought to be due to umbilical cord occlusion. They are of variable shape and do *not* reflect the shape of the associated interuterine pressure curve. Their onset occurs at variable times during the contraction phase.

Variable decelerations are related to compression of the umbilical cord. Uterine contractions are the usual cause of intermittent umbilical cord occlusion, especially if the cord is around the fetal neck or fixed in another location, resulting in its impingement during contractions.

Variable decelerations may bear no consistent relationship to the contraction, presumably because the location of the umbilical cord may vary from one contraction to another. The pattern of cord occlusion has therefore been referred to as variable deceleration.

When cord occlusion becomes prolonged, a significant oxygen debt develops, which results in fetal hypoxemia as evidenced by the development of metabolic acidosis reflecting significant anaerobic metabolism. When variable deceleration is severe, the "late component" comes into play. It is believed that this late component is due to myocardial depression, and represents significant hypoxemia and fetal metabolic acidosis.

When intervillous space blood flow is decreased to a point that the fetus becomes hypoxemic, uteroplacental insufficiency (UPI) is said to exist. Clinical UPI may manifest itself in the chronic form with intrauterine growth retardation and/or antepartum fetal death; or in the acute form, the onset of fetal distress during labor, asphyxia neonatorum; and in the extreme, intrapartum fetal death.

Variable decelerations are the most common fetal heart rate patterns associated with clinically diagnosed fetal distress. Variable decelerations are subdivided into four types:

1st degree variable decelerations: Indicate mild cord involvement. They have a precipitous onset and recovery. They are of short duration and have a jagged wave form.

2nd degree variable decelerations: Are indicative of tension being placed on the umbilical cord, and are a prelude to 3rd degree decelerations. These also have a precipitous onset and recovery, however, there is a smoothing of the wave form and loss of the jagged appearance associated with 1st degree variable decelerations. The duration of these decelerations approximates the duration of the contraction. Third degree decelerations again have a precipitous onset, but they have a gradual and late recovery.

3rd degree decelerations: Indicate extreme tension on the umbilical cord. This can occur as the presenting part moves down into the pelvis, and is a sign of progressive fetal compromise.

4th degree variable decelerations: Are indicative of *serious fetal compromise*. They are associated with cord prolapse, tight knots in the cord or any condition that causes complete occlusion of the cord during a contraction. These decelerations are biphasic in nature, and they come back to baseline or near baseline between the biphasic section. They have a precipitous onset and recovery, and the wave form again appears smooth.

Every attempt should be made to ameliorate the stress to the fetus because the longer the decelerations continue, the greater the likelihood of increasing fetal hypoxia and acidosis.

The deceleration is sometimes precipitous, dropping quickly from normal to a rate of 50 beats-per-minute or less, and may be followed by episodes of compensatory tachycardia. Again, varible deceleration is interpreted to mean that the umbilical circulation is impaired (usually by compression of the cord between the fetal head and the maternal pelvis).

Since variable decelerations are sometimes abolished by changing the patient's position (presumably because this alters the baby's position and relieves the pressure on the cord), this simple maneuver should be tried as previously mentioned. There are different degrees of variable deceleration and their interpretation can be difficult. *In general, no major steps need be taken if the fetal heart rate (FHR) remains above 60 beats-per-minute, if the return to average baseline level is prompt and abrupt (not gradual), and if there is no undue tachycardia or smoothness of the baseline FHR.* Preparation for prompt delivery should be made if the baseline FHR is *increasing* and becoming smooth, if the rate consistently drops below 60 beats-per-minute, and if the return to baseline level is gradual rather than abrupt.

In general, fetal heart rate patterns should be observed and assessed to determine which patterns are indicative of potential fetal compromise. Observation of the *baseline* fetal heart rate is important, as well as any observations of tachycardia, bradycardia, and baseline nonreactivity. These abnormal patterns must be identified and documented. Decelerations should be noted, and the frequency of these decelerations recorded. When observing decelerations in the fetal heart rate, the lag time and recover time should also be measured. If either of these increase, insult to the fetus is persistent and progressive.

Every attempt should be made to relieve this stress to the fetus. As the insult to the fetus persists or progresses, fetal compromise becomes more severe.

The previously mentioned palliative measures (such as maternal position changes, nasal oxygen, correcting maternal hypotension and alleviating hypertonic uterine activity if present), do much to reduce the insults. *If, however, the deceleration pattern persists,* fetal compromise should be further investigated by determining fetal scalp pH (if available) and prompt delivery is of utmost importance. See § **10.18** on fetal blood sampling.

§ 10.16   —Beat-to-Beat Variability

The fetal heart rate (FHR) monitor computes, from the interval between every two heartbeats, the projected number of beats that would occur per minute, and this computation provides the fetal heart rate recorded on the paper. Since there is normally some variation in the interval between beats, this is reflected on the strip chart as a normal variability which usually exceeds five beats-per-minute more, or five beats-per-minute less, than the baseline rate. Variability of this kind is a normal, healthy occurrence which can be affected by a number of circumstances. For example, the beat-to-beat variability is normally increased when the baby moves; it is reduced, with consequent flattening or smoothness of the FHR record, by narcotics, atropine, magnesium sulfate, or diazepam (valium) administered to the mother, or by asphyxia. Sometimes, for no apparent reason, episodes of abnormal smoothness are seen; these can be terminated by pressing a finger on the fetal head or by squeezing the buttocks or head through the uterine wall. For lack of a better explanation, these episodes are interpreted as intervals of sleep, which may occur either before or during labor. Smoothness that persists after fetal stimulation may be an ominous sign.

This interval between successive heart beats in the intact fetus is characterized by its nonuniformity. This beat-to-beat variability is known as *short-term variability*. Average interval differences are usually in the magnitude of two to three beats-per-minute, when converted to rate. When variability is diminished, the usual beat-to-beat interval differences average about one beat-per-minute or less.

The *long-term fluctuations* in FHR have a cyclicity of three to five beats-per-minute, and the amplitude is usually from a five to twenty beats-per-minute. A long-term variability of less than five beats-per-minute is considered to be reduced. It has been suggested that short-term variability appears to be reduced early in the course of neonatal hypoxemia with loss of long-term variability being a later change.

The literature indicates that the changes in FHR variability are probably related to changes in the central nervous system (CNS) status. Generally, the intact fetus has good short and long term variability. Drugs that depress the central nervous system, or interfere with autonomic reflexes, will tend to decrease FHR variability.

The major significance of FHR variability is that it may be affected by hypoxemia. Studies have shown that the *earliest effect* of fetal hypoxemia on FHR variability appears to be an *increase in both* long and short term variability. Investigators have shown that *mild* hypoxia resulted in adrenergic discharge and fetal hypertension, causing stimulation of the fetal baroreceptors and a reflex vagal discharge. Thus a general increase in autonomic tone during early fetal hypoxia results in an *increase* in both short and long term variability. It has been well understood, for a long time, that prolonged and severe fetal hypoxia and acidemia, will *reduce* FHR variability, presumably due to the CNS effects of hypoxia and acidosis.

§ 10.17 —Evaluating Electronic Fetal Heart Rate Monitoring

One must always be thinking of fetal heart rate (FHR) patterns in terms of whether they are reassuring of adequate fetal oxygenation, or whether one can no longer be assured of adequate fetal oxygenation.

Reassuring FHR patterns include those with no periodic changes, acceleration, early deceleration, and mild variable deceleration. These patterns have not been associated with an increased risk of fetal acidosis, low Apgar scores, or other parameters of poor outcome due to fetal hypoxia.

Nonreassuring patterns include the more severe forms of variable deceleration. Any degree of late deceleration and various atypical or preterminal patterns. Prolonged decelerations are often a variation of severe variable deceleration, but because they occur under special circumstances and have specific management implications, they should be considered separately from a therapeutic standpoint.

§ 10.18 Fetal Blood Sampling

While continuous monitoring of the fetal heart rate (FHR) and maternal contractions is still the most practical means of identifying the seriously distressed fetus during labor, intrapartum sampling of the fetal scalp blood is a valuable adjunct. It complements electronic monitoring particularly well when the FHR is confusing or difficult to interpret, often enabling the physician to differentiate questionable FHR patterns.

After the mother's membranes are ruptured, an amnioscope is inserted through her vagina in order to obtain a fetal blood specimen from a pin prick made in the baby's scalp. The analysis is based on the principle that whenever the fetus does not receive an adequate amount of oxygen, the acid levels in the blood stream will build up, causing a measurable decrease in its blood pH (the pH measures the acid content of a solution and is inversely proportional to the amount of acid present; therefore, a decreased pH means that the concentration of acid is high).

The degree of the acid derangement in the fetus is proportional to the frequency and severity of umbilical cord compression. Clinically, pH values less than 7.25 are associated with lower neonatal Apgar scores, an increased risk of respiratory distress syndrome and neurologic handicaps. Although the interpretation of fetal blood pH levels has not been uniform, most authors regard values less than 7.20 as critical, values between 7.20-7.24 as suggestive of further evaluation, and values of 7.25 or greater as normal. Sampling of the fetal blood should be repeated immediately, and the maternal acid levels should also be analyzed when low or borderline results are obtained. If fetal acidosis is confirmed, or if the pH continues to fall *and* the mother is not acidotic (in other words, the situation is not elicited by an abnormality in the mother's blood pH), immediate delivery should be considered to correct the acid imbalance since this is difficult to treat in utero.

Even though fetal and maternal complications are infrequent, it is the physician's responsibility to be aware of the potential dangers inherent in FHR monitoring. The invasive internal monitoring procedures predispose the fetus and mother to the hazards of having to rupture the membranes beforehand, including prolapse of the umbilical cord and infection. Superficial scalp wounds resulting from the direct application of the electrode on the fetal skull, may become infected with the mother's normal vaginal bacteria. In addition, pathogenic organisms may be introduced into the woman's uterine cavity if equipment such as an intrauterine pressure-sensing instrument is not sterile. Assuring the sterility of all instruments and limiting the number and frequency of vaginal examinations in women who are monitored, may help offset the risk of infection imposed by rupturing the membranes and placing an indwelling catheter inside the uterus for a prolonged time.

The obstetrician must also guard against trauma during internal monitoring. Perforations of the uterus, as well as punctured fetal blood vessels may occur following the insertion of the pressure-recording catheter. Injuries may also result when the baby's scalp is incised to obtain a blood sample for pH analysis. The three major complications of this procedure, namely infection, blade breakage, and bleeding, can all be prevented with the proper technique.

The known dangers of external monitoring are more minimal than those of internal monitoring since the former is not an invasive procedure. The primary concern is the hazard of keeping the woman on her back during most of the examination. Although this position ensures that the external detectors remain attached to her abdomen, it is not ideal because it hinders her blood flow after a while and may consequently impede the fetal oxygen supply as well.

In summary, based on continuous FHR monitoring, acute fetal distress *during labor* is related to the stress of the uterine contractions and the resultant decreased blood flow and oxygen transfer to the fetus. Since brain damage or death may occur if the fetus experiences a prolonged oxygen deficiency, early detection of the tell-tale FHR patterns characteristic of fetal distress is crucial. When incurable, recurrent, late decelerations of any severity or recurrent, variable decelerations lasting more than one minute (when the FHR has fallen to 50 bpm or less) occur, the obstetrician can assume that fetal asphyxia is present. On the other hand, when there are no abnormalities in the FHR or rhythm, and when there are no responses to uterine contractions other than early decelerations, fetal distress is not present.

Although conventional fetoscopic auscultation has been greatly overshadowed by the recent growth and popularity of electronic instrumentation, it is not an outdated procedure. The disproportionate amount of time devoted to electronic fetal heart monitoring merely reflects its complexity; it does not indicate that expensive and complicated equipment is always necessary to ensure an optimal neonatal outcome. Properly timed systematic clinical (nonelectronic) monitoring also offers a comparable prognosis for many fetuses. In several standardized studies, trained nurses monitored the FHR every fifteen minutes during the first stage of labor, and every five minutes during the second stage, until the baby was born. If they suspected an abnormality, they examined the heart more often. The nurses also observed the mother continuously, including frequent abdominal palpations, to evaluate her uterine contractions. The results of systematic clinical monitoring revealed that the newborns' Apgar scores were as high as those of their counterparts who were monitored continuously by electronic methods, and the cesarean rate was appreciably lower as well.[8]

The conclusions of the "task force on the predictors of fetal distress" reflect these studies. In 1979, they stated that intermittent fetal surveillance during labor, as described in the preceding paragraph, is an acceptable method of intrapartum monitoring in *low risk* patients. According to their evaluation, electronic fetal heart monitoring has had no apparent impact on the perinatal morbidity and mortality rates in *low risk* patients, so it is safe to conclude that the risks of monitoring do not justify its benefits in these cases. Assuming that

---

[8] Haverkamp, Orleans, Langendoerfor, et al., *A Controlled Trial of the Differential Effects of Intrapartum Fetal Monitoring*, 134 *Am. J. Obstet. Gynecol*, 399 (1979).

such accidents as a prolapsed umbilical cord and premature separation of the placenta are properly managed, the healthy fetus is not in danger of dying during delivery. However, as the maternal and fetal risks increase, electronic fetal heart monitoring may indeed have a beneficial effect upon the intrapartum and neonatal morbidity and mortality rates, since it can detect life-threatening abnormalities before the onset of labor while treatment is still possible.[9]

The task force goes on to state that a normal FHR pattern during continuous electronic monitoring indicates a greater than 95 percent probability of fetal well-being.[10] The converse is not always true, however. Although fetal hypoxia is consistently associated with deviations in the FHR tracings, abnormal patterns may also occur in the absence of fetal distress. Since a one-to-one correlation does not necessarily exist, these investigators propose that intermittent and continuous heart monitoring be used as a screening rather than a diagnostic technique. When FHR data indicate fetal distress, the physician should support this finding with other clinical and laboratory information (including fetal scalp blood pH), especially before intervening surgically to alleviate the hypoxia. Relying solely on FHR tracings may lead to inappropriate management of the patient. Likewise, evaluation of the heart rate should be an ongoing process because few conclusions can be drawn from the fetal response to a single contraction.

A final point to remember is that *maternal* heartbeats, which may also be picked up during conventional or electronic heart monitoring, must always be differentiated from fetal heartbeats, otherwise erroneous conclusions will be made about the fetal status. This is more likely to occur when the FHR is slow or absent. To prevent such mistakes, the obstetrician should always simultaneously measure the mother's pulse rate while listening to the fetal heart.

§ 10.19   Radiography

While passing an x-ray beam through a pregnant woman's abdomen, the physician is able to photograph the desired region of either the maternal pelvis or the fetal skeleton, and obtain a permanent picture of these anatomical structures. By delineating anatomical features which would not be possible to evaluate on an external examination alone, the procedure known as either

---

[9] J.A. Pritchard, M.D. & P.C. MacDonald, M.D., Williams Obstetrics, 16th ed., 362-63 (Appleton-Century-Crofts, 1980).

[10] *Antenatal Diagnosis*, report of a Consensus Development Conference, sponsored by the National Institute of Child Health & Human Development, NIH Publication Number 79-1973 (U.S. Gov't Printing Office, 1979).

radiography, or roentgenography, enables the obstetrician to predict whether certain problems have developed or are likely to arise during the pregnancy. Although a variety of diagnostic radiologic techniques have been utilized in the past, the widespread trend toward ultrasound has markedly reduced their use, primarily because ultrasound procedures typically provide more precise results without the risks of radiation-induced carcinomas, mutation, or deleterious drug effects.

Roentgenographic studies were typically ordered for the following reasons:

1. Determination of the pelvic dimensions (x-ray pelvimetry)
2. Estimation of fetal maturity
3. Diagnosis of intrauterine fetal death
4. Determination of multiple fetuses and certain fetal abnormalities
5. Placental localization using radionuclide imaging and arteriography.

Today, the use of x-rays and radionuclide imaging are generally contraindicated for pregnant women. With the notable exception of x-ray pelvimetry (and even its use has declined sharply), x-ray studies are rarely performed to obtain the other information listed above, since it is not justifiable to subject a mother and her unborn baby to radiation hazards when safer methods such as ultrasound offer comparable results. Most authorities feel that the risks are only warranted in locations where ultrasound is still not available, or as in the case of x-ray pelvimetry, where the procedure provides information critical to the welfare of the mother or fetus.

Currently, x-ray films are primarily ordered to measure the critical dimensions of the mother's pelvis, a set of parameters which can reveal whether a relative disproportion exists between the size of her child with respect to the size of her pelvis. By evaluating her pelvic contours and pelvic capacity, the obstetrician is able to predict whether the fetus will be able to descend freely through the birth canal during vaginal delivery, or whether a cesarean delivery will have to be performed to prevent birth trauma resulting from the disproportion. Cases in which a cesarean section is likely to be done despite the roentgenographic findings do not warrant x-ray pelvimetry.

Most clinicians stress that pelvimetry is not an end in itself, for regardless of how large the pelvis is, a very large baby may have difficulty passing through it. Conversely, a small or unfavorable pelvis may pose no problem for a tiny infant. As these examples illustrate, the baby's size is also a key factor affecting the outcome of delivery, as are the position and presentation of the fetus, the flexion and malleability of its head, the efficiency of the uterine contractions, and the state of the membranes. Yet, the size of the fetal head is the only other factor besides the dimensions of the maternal pelvis which can be studied radiographically. Therefore, unless the entire clinical picture is considered, conclusions drawn solely from pelvimetry films are likely to be erroneous.

In the majority of pregnancies, manual estimation of the pelvic dimensions (also referred to as clinical or digital pelvimetry) is often adequate even though it does not provide as accurate measurements as x-ray pelvimetry. It is especially advantageous because, unlike x-ray pelvimetry, it does not expose the fetus and the radiation-sensitive reproductive organs of the mother to the deleterious effects of the x-ray beam. To prevent the adverse consequences of the indiscriminate use of x-ray pelvimetry, the procedure is restricted to patients who are likely to have a contracted pelvis or a difficult labor, since precise measurements may be invaluable in managing these deliveries. The most frequently cited indications for x-ray pelvimetry are:

1. Failure to progress satisfactorily during labor regardless of the manual measurements; for instance, if a primipara is in early labor and the fetal head fails to engage, there is a 25 percent chance of fetopelvic disproportion, which must be investigated.

2. Abnormal fetal presentations such as breech, face, brow, and transverse presentations, especially in a nulliparous woman.

3. A history of fetopelvic disproportion, traumatic vaginal delivery, or an unexplained stillbirth.

4. An excessively large fetus or a clinically small, borderline, or unfavorable pelvis.

5. A pelvis distorted by previous injury or disease.

6. Unproven pelvic adequacy prior to induction of labor of oxytocin.

If x-ray pelvimetry is indicated, it should be done at term, or preferably, in early labor when the manifestations of fetopelvic disproportion typically become evident. An important exception to this rule is made for a fetus in the breech presentation. Awaiting the onset of labor before obtaining the pelvic measurements is not suggested in breech pregnancies, particularly if the mother has never been pregnant before, because the course of her labor and its variations may develop rapidly, without forewarning the obstetrician of impending disproportion at an early enough stage. However, under normal circumstances, once a woman is in active labor, x-ray pelvimetry not only accurately assesses her pelvic capacity, but it also uncovers any unsuspected malpresentations of the fetal head, which may have been caused by a contracted pelvic inlet, and may be responsible for delays or difficulties in the progress of labor.

In order to clearly delineate the areas of pelvic narrowing, the x-ray films must provide the three-dimensional picture of the entire pelvis, including the critical diameters of the pelvic inlet, midpelvis and pelvic outlet; the slope of the sidewalls; the prominence of the ischial spines and the station of the fetal head when the mother is standing. There is one technique which fulfills all of these requirements and is available to all x-ray departments. It consists of a series of three films, including a lateral view, an inlet view, and a film of the suprapubic arch. Regardless of the technique chosen, accurate measurements are only possible if the patient is correctly positioned so the proper reference points and planes can be x-rayed.

The probability of fetopelvic disproportion can be assessed using the x-ray pelvimetry guidelines. See **Table 10-1**. Difficulties during labor and delivery are likely to occur when the mother's measurements are less than these critical values and when the fetus is average-sized or larger.

Table 10-1

X-RAY PELVIMETRY GUIDELINES[11]

Anteroposterior Diameters		Transverse Diameters
Pelvic Inlet	10.0 cm	12.0 cm
Mid-Pelvis	11.5 cm	9.5 cm
Pelvic Outlet	11.5 cm	10.0 cm

Before the advent of ultrasound, radiologic studies were often ordered to estimate the extent of fetal development, especially when early delivery was contemplated. Positive identification of the distal femoral epiphyses and the proximal tibial epiphyses (the bony centers of the leg) are considered reliable indicators of fetal maturity, appearing radiographically about the 36th and 38th week of gestation, respectively. On the other hand, an absence of these diagnostic features on the x-ray films does not necessarily indicate fetal immaturity because other factors may affect the picture. For instance, it is sometimes impossible to visualize these bony landmarks because the fetus may move and blur the image, the film may have been incorrectly exposed, or the maternal bones or soft tissue shadows overlie and obscure the fetal limbs.

Compared to the distal femoral and proximal tibial epiphyses, all other radiographic signs are not considered important determinants of fetal maturity. Radiographic measurements of the fetal crown-rump length and the fetal skull are of no value because the relationship of the fetal head to the x-ray beam as

---

[11] L.M. Helman, M.D. & J.A. Pritchard, M.D., Williams Obstetrics, 14th ed., 313 (Appleton-Century-Crofts, 1971).

well as the distance of the head from the x-ray films cannot be controlled, resulting in varying degrees of magnification. Since an ultrasonic estimate of the biparietal diameter of the fetal skull is free of magnification, it is a more accurate and more widely used means of assessing fetal maturity. Radiologic methods are further limited since they possess intrinsic inaccuracies due to variations in the fetal growth rate and skeletal maturation.

§ 10.20   —Diagnosis of Fetal Death

Because radiographs of dead fetuses sometimes appear normal, the most reliable x-ray signs of fetal death are those which eliminate the possibility of death by proving that the fetus is still alive. Blurring of the fetus without blurring of the maternal anatomy suggests that the fetus has moved during the exposure, thereby ruling out intrauterine death. Certain abnormal fetal postures may also indicate the fetus is severely affected or already dead.

An extremely reliable sign of death is the presence of gas on the x-ray film. It is usually observed in the fetal heart or blood vessels. Overlapping of the skull bones and abnormal angulation of the spine strongly suggest fetal death, unless the mother is in active labor. Although these radiologic manifestations of intrauterine fetal death, were valuable in the past, they are much less important now that a more rapid and more accurate diagnosis is possible with ultrasound, or serum estriol analyses.

The presence of twins or multiple fetuses can be diagnosed by radiography. In addition, certain fetal abnormalities such as achondroplasia and osteogenesis imperfecta can occasionally be diagnosed by intrauterine x-ray examinations. Gross skeletal malformations such as ancephaly and marked hydrocephaly can usually be identified during the third trimester.

Although placental localization, using both radionuclide imaging and arteriography, was used to locate the placenta in the past, they are now best avoided in pregnant women. Delineation of the placenta can be obtained with great precision by ultrasound techniques, without infusing large quantities of radioactively labeled pharmaceuticals into the patient's bloodstream and organs as in radionuclide imaging, or without exposing the mother and fetus to high radiation doses as in arteriography. Arteriography is dangerous because a considerable amount of time is needed to position the arterial catheter, and numerous x-ray films are required to display the detailed filling rates of the placental blood vessels.

§ 10.21   —Safety

Whenever x-ray studies are ordered, the obstetrician must carefully weigh their diagnostic benefits against the potential damage they may cause in the mother, the fetus, and unborn generations. Studies have shown that an irradiated fetus has a greater risk of developing leukemia and other malignant disorders after birth, as well as an increased likelihood of mutations. Many fear that serious genetic defects may result from these mutations, showing up either in the baby's lifetime or that of its offspring.

Despite the concern over the harmful effects of x-ray examinations, the experts seem to concur that these studies are justified when they provide information critical to the welfare of the mother or fetus that cannot be obtained as accurately or safety by other methods. As with any potentially dangerous procedure, all women of childbearing age should be informed of the risks of x-ray studies beforehand.

State and federal regulatory agencies have outlined the minimum requirements for the safe use of diagnostic radiation in all branches of medicine. In addition, a number of guidelines have been proposed by various authorities to minimize the harmful effects of radiation, especially in women of reproductive age. Because radiation of the reproductive organs is likely to be more hazardous than radiation of other parts of the body, the physician should strive to avoid the pelvic region or at least limit the amount of pelvic radiation.

The following safeguards and technical principles should always be followed during x-ray examinations. Whenever possible, a lead apron should be placed on the mother's abdomen to shield the developing fetus as well as her reproductive organs from stray x-ray beams. Using the smallest film possible with the proper coning and shield also ensures that only the specific area under study is irradiated. Furthermore, positioning of the x-ray machinery should be perfected to avoid reexposures, and the films should be taken as near to term as possible.

Though some institutions perform a routine chest x-ray on all pregnant women, some physicians suggest postponing it until after delivery unless there is a clinical suspicion of chest disease. It is also wise to defer radiologic studies of nonpregnancy related maternal disorders until the baby is born, especially if the area to be filmed places the fetus in the primary x-ray beam. Intravenous pyelograms, plain abdominal x-ray barium enemas, and x-rays of the pelvis and the lumbosacral spine are examples of studies which place the fetus in the path of the primary x-ray beam.

Whereas some physicians claim that it is safer to x-ray women of child bearing age during the first half of their menstrual cycle (the time before the egg is released into the uterus), others contend that scheduling abdominal x-rays in relation to the menstrual cycle is of little clinical value. Arguing that the developing ovum is at risk prior to ovulation as well as after it is released into the uterus, they believe it is erroneous to assume that one time is safer to be exposed to radiation than another.

§ 10.22 Amniography and Fetography

Amniography is a radiologic technique involving the injection of a *water*-soluble radiopaque contrast medium through the uterine wall into the amniotic sac. An abdominal x-ray is then taken, clearly displaying certain characteristics of the amniotic fluid, the placenta, and the fetus on the x-ray film after the contrast medium has infiltrated these structures.

The primary indication for amniography arises when a fetus suffering from severe hemolytic disease requires an intrauterine blood transfusion to save its life. In order to inject the new red blood cells into the fetal peritoneal cavity, the physician must first locate this structure with an amniogram. Amniograms may also be ordered to reveal hydatidiform moles (they often produce a diagnostic honey-comb pattern on the x-ray), abnormal volumes of amniotic fluid, soft tissue deformities of the fetus, placental location, fetal position, and multiple fetuses. The status of the fetus is readily demonstrated by observing its ability to swallow the contrast medium, after which time any obstructions or malformations of the fetal gastrointestinal tract can then be easily visualized. If the fetus does not ingest the contrast medium after an hour, the possibility of fetal distress or death must be considered.

Fetography is a radiological technique almost identical to amniography, involving the injection of a *lipid*-soluble contrast medium into the amniotic sac. Because the lipid is able to adhere to the outer skin covering of the near-mature fetus, it may outline its body much more vividly than the water-soluble radiopaque agents used in amniography, thereby facilitating the diagnosis of some external soft tissue abnormalities and other pathologic conditions such as the pronounced scalp edema associated with hydrops fetalis.

Since amniography and fetography are both invasive procedures, they predispose the mother and her baby to several hazards. For example, puncture or laceration of the placenta may occur and can occasionally lead to premature delivery. Even the contrast media themselves may initiate early labor. Most significantly though, there is the risk of harmful radiation generated by the abdominal x-ray. All of these inherent dangers can be avoided by the use of ultrasound. When it is carefully performed, an ultrasound examination is a simple procedure which usually provides comparable information without having to mechanically penetrate the amniotic sac, inject potentially harmful chemical contrast agents, or expose the mother and fetus to x-rays. Therefore, most physicians no longer consider amniography the procedure of choice to identify the majority of the previously mentioned maternal and fetal characteristics and conditions. The one exception to this generalization is its important role in intrauterine transfusions.

§ 10.23   Bibliography and Recommended Readings

Freeman, R.D., M.D. & Garite, T.J., M.D., *Fetal Heart Rate* (Williams & Wilkins, 1981).

Hon, Edward H., M.D., *An Introduction to Fetal Heart Rate Monitoring* (Harty Press, Inc., 1975).

Iffy, Leslie, M.D. & Kaminetzky, Harold A., M.D., *Principles and Practice of Obstetrics & Perinatology*, vol. 1 (John Wiley & Sons, Inc., 1981).

CHAPTER 11

THE EVENTS OF LABOR AND DELIVERY

§ 11.1   Changes Observed in the Fetal Head during Delivery

Since the bones surrounding the vault of the skull are loosely connected, they can overlap each other and consequently decrease their original diameter when a particular pelvic region is too narrow to permit the baby's head to pass through without obstruction. This ability of the fetal skull to adapt its shape in response to the changing pelvic contours is called *molding*. Although in typical labors little molding is necessary for an average sized fetus to traverse through a normal pelvis, if the pelvis is contracted, the degree to which the head is capable of molding (in conjunction with efficient uterine contractions), may make the difference between a safe vaginal delivery and the need to perform a cesarean section.

The bones composing the vault are separated from one another by sutures and fontanels. Palpating their fairly distinctive arrangement prior to delivery allows instant determination of the position of the head unless labor is prolonged, in which case, the scalp may be too swollen to differentiate the various sutures and fontanels. Swelling of the fetal scalp, called *caput succedaneum*, is another common reaction to the pressures of labor in vertex presentations, and it disappears entirely several days after birth. The caput is usually only a few millimeters thick in normal labors, and therefore, does not generally obscure the diagnostic landmarks of the skull.

§ 11.2   The Mechanism of Normal Labor

Every time the uterus contracts, the fetus is pushed a little farther down the irregularly shaped birth canal. At each of its constantly changing contours and dimensions, the descending fetal presenting part is forced to rotate slightly, thereby altering its original attitude and position to ensure that the best diameters of its body will pass through the various pelvic regions without obstruction. This gradual advancement normally involves a sequence of seven passive movements—engagement, descent, flexion, internal rotation, extension, external rotation, and expulsion—referred to as the mechanism of labor. Since the mechanism differs somewhat depending on the presentation, the reader should realize that the following discussion specifically applies to fetuses in the vertex (head down) presentation. See § 9.7 on terminology of fetal orientation in the womb.

The term *engagement* signifies that the biparietal diameter (BPD) of the fetal skull (its widest transverse diameter) has passed through the pelvic inlet, providing confirmatory evidence that the inlet is adequately proportioned for the head. Engagement usually occurs in primigravidas (with normal pelves) during the last few weeks of pregnancy, but this important step ordinarily does not begin in multiparas until after the onset of labor.

Descent is a continuous process whereby the force of the uterine contractions propels the fetal presenting part downward through the birth canal. Whereas it typically occurs rather slowly but steadily in nulliparas during the second stage of labor, descent may be very rapid in multiparas, especially those of high parity.

Flexion of the fetal head occurs as soon as the skull meets resistance from the cervix, pelvic walls, or pelvic floor. By causing the chin to tuck inward on the chest, the presenting diameters of the head are significantly reduced, allowing a smaller and more favorable circumference of the head to pass through the narrower pelvic regions.

Internal rotation, extension, and *external rotation* are all mechanisms which progressively alter the fetal position so the fetus can move safely and efficiently through the different sized crevices of the lower pelvic canal. *Expulsion* is the final step of the birth process, occurring when the uterine forces rapidly extrude the rest of the fetus's body after its shoulders have been delivered.

Since no two pelves are exactly the same, the optimal mechanism for each pelvis may differ entirely from the "normal" mechanism of labor. Precise knowledge of each patient's pelvic structure and its associated mechanism of labor is therefore essential in order to expeditiously manage any complications that may develop during delivery. For example, the downward progress of the fetal head may unexpectedly stop if flexion of the head is not adequate or the uterine contractions are not strong enough, and in such circumstances, the obstetrician may decide that the baby must be delivered by forceps. If so, traction on the instrument must be applied in the proper pelvic diameter and without undue resistance or else the baby could be killed, and the mother could be seriously injured.

Besides being influenced by the pelvic dimensions, the mechanism of labor is also affected by the quality of the mother's uterine contractions, the size of the baby, and the ability of its head to mold and flex. If any of these factors are inadequate or abnormal, the anticipated mechanism of labor may be altered, in which case delivery may be prolonged until the problem is resolved. The only time the head can advance freely and independently without regard for the particular pelvic configuration is when the baby is small, and the birth canal is comparatively large. Otherwise, as the dissimilarity in size diminishes, the head is forced to turn and rotate in order to negotiate the changing pelvic contours, and its successful descent depends on the adequacy of the four factors just mentioned.

Unlike the characteristic movements observed in cephalic presentations, the mechanism of labor in breech presentations differs due to the inverted orientation of the fetal body. It consists of three separate parts: the mechanism of the buttocks, the mechanism of the shoulders, and the mechanism of the aftercoming head. Although this sequence of movements also prepares the smallest diameter of the fetus for passage through the various pelvic regions, more problems are liable to beset these births. An even more difficult mechanism of labor is associated with the mentum (chin) posterior position. Regardless of the pelvic configuration, it is an extremely formidable position, and as with brow presentations, cesarean section is usually the preferable solution.

§ 11.3 Prelabor: Signs and Preparatory Changes

In the period called prelabor, certain signs and preparatory changes occur, alerting the physician that labor is approaching. Among the first of these changes is lightening, or the movement of the fetal presenting part from the upper uterus to the lower uterus. Regardless of whether it occurs gradually over the course of a few days or with an almost imperceptible thud, the pregnant woman is usually aware of the resultant downward shift in the fetal weight because the pressure on her diaphragm is reduced, allowing her to breathe more easily. However, in exchange for this comfort (she reports a feeling of lightness in her upper abdomen), she may begin to experience increased pressure in her lower pelvis. Occurring generally two to four weeks before labor in a primigravida, but sometimes not until after labor has already started in a multigravida, lightening is readily observed during an abdominal examination since the shape of the patient's abdomen is different, and the fetal presenting part is palpated at a lower level than on previous examinations.

A second sign of approaching labor is a uterine tightening known as *Braxton Hicks contractions*. In the first pregnancy, Braxton Hicks contractions generally become painful about an hour before the onset of true labor, but with each additional pregnancy, the painful contractions are likely to begin at progressively earlier periods. Since they may be different to distinguish from the pains accompanying true labor, Braxton Hicks contractions are often called false labor pains in retrospect, though a careful examination usually reveals the differences. Whereas the contractions of true labor occur at regular intervals that gradually become shorter and more intense, Braxton Hicks contractions are irregular in frequency, duration, and/or intensity. Another difference is that the contractions of true labor do not become less painful in response to medications. Perhaps the most definitive way to differentiate the two pains is to measure their effect on the cervix; the contractions of true labor cause the cervix to dilate, whereas Braxton Hicks contractions have minimal, if any, effect. Yet despite these differences, complaints of relatively infrequent, brief, and painful contractions should not be casually dismissed because false labor may convert to the contractions of true labor rapidly and without apparent forewarning.

A third preparatory change of prelabor is shortening and thinning of the cervical canal, referred to as *cervical effacement*. It is generally evident in both primigravidas and multigravidas about a month before term, and is usually accompanied by a slight dilatation of the cervix.

As long as neither a rectal nor a vaginal examination have been performed in the preceding 48 hours, another rather dependable sign of approaching labor is a small, often blood-tinged plug of mucus called the *show*, or bloody show. Once this mucus is discharged from the cervix (where it closes off communication between the uterine cavity and the vagina throughout pregnancy), spontaneous labor often ensues within hours to a few days.

In addition to the major signs and preparatory changes just mentioned, several other conditions are customarily observed in the days or weeks preceding labor. They include a loss of one to three pounds (a water loss resulting from shifts in the pregnant woman's electrolyte balance), frequent urination, increased vaginal secretions, extreme congestion of the vaginal mucous membranes, and increased backache and sacroiliac discomfort.

§ 11.4   Admission to the Hospital

Recommendations for the timing of admission are based on the frequency of uterine contractions, parity, antenatal risk factors (such as diabetes or hypertension), previous duration of labor, and transit time to the hospital. The usual rule of thumb is for nulliparas to report to the hospital when contractions occur every five minutes and for multiparas to come when they recur every eight to ten minutes. Upon arrival at the hospital, the woman's condition should be promptly assessed since the frequency of her contractions largely determines how thoroughly the admitting procedure should be followed. If frequent contractions and other outward signs indicate that labor is clearly imminent, the typical admission routine should be postponed (or interrupted if the woman goes into labor during the questioning), and while preparations are being made for immediate delivery, the obstetrician should verify the diagnosis with a pelvic examination. As long as the patient is not in labor, the obstetrical nurse should obtain the following information from her upon admission:

1. Her name
2. Her obstetrician's name
3. Parity
4. Estimated due date
5. Frequency of uterine contractions
6. Presence or absence of bleeding
7. Status of the membranes (ruptured or intact)
8. Medical disorders
9. Allergies, drug sensitivities and current medications being taken
10. Time when solid food was last eaten (part of the preanesthetic evaluation)
11. The use of contact lenses or removable dentures (these must be removed before analgesia is administered)
12. Any special warnings or instructions the patient may have received during pregnancy.

The woman's temperature, blood pressure, pulse rate, and respiratory rate should be checked for any abnormalities. A blood sample should also be drawn to measure the hematocrit, and a urine specimen should be examined for sugar and protein.

The next part of the protocol involves the history and the physical examination. Comprehensive evaluations are only necessary for women who have not received prenatal care, and therefore, lack a complete antenatal record containing the relevant background and information. Those who have visited obstetricians regularly during the antenatal period should have their records transferred to the obstetrical ward once they are admitted so the attending physician(s) can review them. Careful scrutiny of the birth weights of previous babies, the length of previous labors, the complications of past pregnancies or deliveries, and the condition of the infants at birth is advisable because prior abnormalities may predispose the present pregnancy to similar problems. After the records have been reviewed, they should be updated, legibly entering any new problems or risks that developed since the last clinic appointment. A specific inquiry should be made about heart disease, tuberculosis, recent respiratory infection, hypertension, toxemia and abnormal pain, and the estimated gestational age should also be reevaluated at this time.

Provided that the patient has received proper antenatal care, many clinicians just perform a limited general physical examination oriented toward problems that commonly develop in pregnancy or labor. Only if edema or bruises are found on the patient's body or if problems are discovered while examining her nose, throat, heart, lungs, and legs, do they perform further check-ups. However, other physicians claim that all women should receive a complete physical examination regardless of their past medical care.

An obstetrical examination is typically begun after the history and physical examination. It consists of an abdominal (external) examination and a pelvic (internal) examination.

§ 11.5 Abdominal Examination

Unless labor is extremely active, the abdomen should be examined first, checking the external scars and intra-abdominal abnormalities such as enlarged liver or spleen, or ovarian cysts. Afterwards, the obstetrician should measure the fundal height and then, using the four manuevers of Leopold (see **§ 9.7**), should systematically palpate the appropriate abdominal regions in order to determine the presentation, attitude, and station of the fetus. Since the size of the fetus provides important information regarding its development and the ease or difficulty of delivery, an estimate of its weight should also be made. Besides recognizing prematurity, detailed abdominal studies also facilitate the diagnosis of multiple gestations, malpresentations, intrauterine growth retardation, macrosomia (large body size), and abruptio placenta.

Another essential part of the abdominal examination is ascultation of the fetal heart. Particularly during labor, meticulous monitoring is of utmost importance in order to evaluate the fetal vital signs and detect any deviations from the normal range of 120-160 heartbeats-per-minute. Gross changes in the heart rate or rhythm, especially if they are more pronounced during uterine contractions, are usually indicative of fetal hypoxia or distress. Although the clinical significance of meconium (the fetal feces, varying from shades of greenish black to light brown) in the amniotic fluid, when observed together with substantial variation in the fetal heart tones, is controversial, some physicians believe it is an important warning sign in cephalic presentations.[1]

§ 11.6 Pelvic Examination

An internal pelvic examination, done either rectally or vaginally, should be performed after the abdominal examination. It is important to withhold the vaginal examination until the patient's perineum is checked for fluid suggestive of ruptured membranes as well as any past or current evidence of exces-

---

[1] R.J. Bolognese, R.H. Schwartz, & J. Schneider, Perinatal Medicine, 203 (Williams & Wilkins, 1982).

sive vaginal bleeding. Although a small amount of blood is normally lost when the cervical mucous plug (the show) is expelled, blood clots or unusually large amounts of blood are abnormal and should be further evaluated before performing the pelvic examination. However, as long as the mother's condition permits it, the following information should be obtained during the first in-hospital pelvic examination:

1. The state of the membranes (ruptured or intact);

2. The position, length (effacement), consistency, and dilatation of the cervix. These are the four main physiologic changes observed as the cervix adapts to approaching labor; by observing their rate of change in the weeks and days preceding delivery, the obstetrician is able to confirm the diagnosis of labor and evaluate its course;

3. The station of the presenting part;

4. Whether the presenting part fits snugly against the cervix and lower uterine segment. Lack of a tight fit suggests that something (for example, the placenta) is positioned between the cervix and the presenting part, or that a condition such as a short or entangled umbilical cord or pelvic inlet disproportion is preventing the presenting part from descending;

5. The pelvic capacity as well as the shape and position of the lower sacrum;

6. The distensibility of the vagina and the firmness of the perineum;

7. Whether there is much fecal material in the rectum. Whereas some physicians recommend giving a routine cleansing enema early in labor to remove fecal material from the lower bowel and thereby minimize subsequent fecal contamination during delivery, others believe that its routine use is not warranted. Even its advocates agree that enemas may sometimes have undesirable consequences, so they should not be used if there is, or has been, recent bleeding since it may aggravate the bleeding. If labor is extremely active or delivery is imminent since the enema may be difficult to expel and may unduly stimulate contractions; if analgesics have already been given since the patient may be too anesthetized to expel it; and if the pregnancy is several weeks preterm and the onset of labor is uncertain, again no enema should be given because nothing that might stimulate labor should be given;

8. The presence of arterial pulsations. Although pulsations matching the maternal heartbeat are not troublesome, pulsations in synchrony with the fetal heartbeat are an ominous sign because they are due to prolapse of the umbilical cord or vasa previa.

In the following section, some of the important cervical and pelvic concepts will be explained in more detail.

§ 11.7 —Dilatation

In sole response to the uterine contractions, the opening of the cervical canal progressively widens or dilates to permit the passage of the fetal presenting part. Since the diameter of the flexed head of an average sized fetus is between 9-10 cm, dilatation is not considered to be full or complete until the cervix is 10 cm wide. Smaller diameters will impede fetal descent.

During the course of labor, the cervical diameter is first assessed from the number of fingers the obstetrician is able to insert into the cervical canal, and this value is then converted into its approximate equivalent in centimeters. Estimating the extent of dilatation at the peak of a uterine contraction instead of between contractions is a more accurate method of predicting the course of labor, especially for multiparas, whose dilatation may differ by as much as 3 cm during the active and quiescent phases of the contraction cycle.

§ 11.8 —Effacement

Whereas dilatation describes the change in the width of the cervical canal that occurs as labor draws nearer, effacement (also called obliteration or taking up) describes its change in length. It is reported as the percentage by which its length has been reduced or shortened. Therefore, the normal 2 cm-long cervical canal is uneffaced, a 1 cm-long canal is 50 percent effaced, a 0.5 cm-long cervix is 75 percent effaced, and a completely flattened out, paper thin cervix is 100 percent effaced.

§ 11.9 —Presentation and Position

When the cervix is adequately dilated, the obstetrician can touch the lowermost section of the fetus and directly identify its position and presenting part. Even while the membranes are intact, gentle palpation between contractions provides very accurate information and rarely causes the membranes to rupture. By correlating the location of the fetal heart tones with the findings of the abdominal and pelvic examinations, the physician can usually make a definite diagnosis of the presentation.

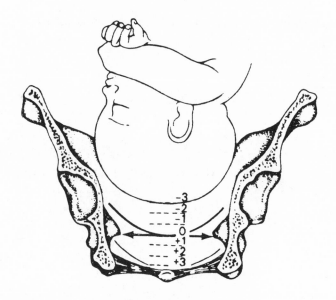

Figure 11-1. Stations of the fetal head. © Permission to reprint granted. Sharon J. Reeder, R.N., Ph.D., Luigi Mastroianni, Jr., M.D., & Leonide L. Martin, R.N., Maternity Nursing, 15th ed., 478 (Philadelphia: J.B. Lippincott Co., 1983).

§ 11.10 —Pelvic Capacity

If the pelvic size was considered borderline during the antenatal physical examination, or if the fetus appears to be large, manual pelvimetry should be repeated during the admission work-up. Comparing the size of the fetal head with the size of the pelvis is important because it can sometimes reveal whether cephalopelvic disproportion exists, and therefore, warn the obstetrician of complications liable to occur if the fetus were to descend through an inadequately sized birth canal. Another way of evaluating the pelvic adequacy is to observe the degree to which the fetal head descends when gentle fundal pressure is applied. If the top of the head can be pushed to station zero or lower, disproportion at the pelvic inlet probably does not exist.

§ 11.11 —Station

This term, which simply refers to the precise location of the fetal presenting part in the pelvis, is commonly used to describe the downward progress of the fetus during delivery. The ischial spines of the pelvis (also called mid-pelvis) have been designated as the zero station because they are located about half-way between the pelvic inlet and the pelvic outlet. Using them as a reference point, the distance between the ischial spines and the pelvic inlet is then divided into five levels or stations (-5, -4, -3, -2, -1, 0), each differing from the adjacent level by about 1 cm. Accordingly, if the fetal presenting part is palpated at the uppermost level (the pelvic inlet) during a pelvic examination, it is reported to be at the -5 station, whereas if it has already descended three-fifths of this distance, it is reported to be at the -2 station. The distance between the mid-pelvis and the pelvic outlet (the lowermost pelvic region) is similarly divided into five stations ($+1$, $+2$, $+3$, $+4$, $+5$).

Instead of dividing the pelvis into 10 levels and measuring its length in centimeters as just described, it can also be divided into sixths and measured by fingerbreadths. According to this older convention, also used in the United States, the corresponding stations are -3, -2, -1, 0, $+1$, $+2$, $+3$. See **Figures 11-1**. In either case, unless distortions in the shape and size of the head are taken into account, errors may be made while evaluating the station, since exceptional molding or extensive swelling of the skull may make it appear that the important diameters of the head (such as the biparietal diameter, which is used to determine when engagement occurs) have descended lower into the pelvic canal than is actually the case.

§ 11.12   The Three Stages of Labor

Labor is essentially the process by which the mother's uterine contractions progressively expel the fetus from her uterus and vagina into the outside world. As the force of the actively contracting upper uterine segment causes the lower uterine segment and the cervix to dilate, a greatly expanded, thinned out, muscular tube is formed to facilitate descent and eventual birth. Since the contractions of the uterine muscles are painful, they are commonly called labor pains in laypersons terminology.

Ordinarily, the transition into labor is gradual, but in some cases it may start abruptly. Although its exact time of onset may be difficult to pinpoint, particularly if it is preceded by a period of regular, forceful, and painful contractions that have no influence on the cervix (Braxton Hicks contractions), a patient is generally considered to be in labor when contractions of good quality have occurred at regular intervals of six minutes or less, for at least one hour. For the purpose of clinical management, the continuum of events which take place during labor has been divided into three stages:

First Stage = Stage of Cervical Dilatation: From the onset of regular uterine contractions until complete cervical dilatation;

Second Stage = Stage of Expulsion: From complete cervical dilatation until delivery of the entire fetus;

Third Stage = Placental Stage: From delivery of the fetus until delivery of the placenta.

§ 11.13   Normal Duration of Labor

Due to such diverse factors as the woman's parity, the size of the fetus relative to the size of the pelvis, the fetal presentation and position, the types of medications prescribed, the efficiency of the uterine contractions, and the condition of the membranes, wide variations are observed in the normal progress of labor. Yet despite this large number of variables, it is still possible to determine whether delivery is proceeding normally or abnormally by constructing a graph called the Friedman curve. Based on the information gathered during each pelvic examination made at the time of labor, the obstetrician plots the extent of *cervical dilatation* (0-10 cm) and the *fetal station* (-5 to $+5$)—the two primary indicators of the progress of labor—against the *duration of labor* (in hours). She can then quickly evaluate whether the length of labor is normal, and if not, which factor is responsible for prolonging it. Other signs of progress, though not as reliable or as able to reveal abnormalities as the cervical dilatation and fetal station, include increasing frequency, duration and intensity of uterine contractions; rupture of the membranes; discharge of bloody mucus; bearing down; and perineal bulging and anal dilatation. The latter two suggest that delivery is rapidly approaching.

The following principles, which were derived from the Friedman curve, have been recognized as important rules of labor since the late 1950s:

1. The average rate of cervical dilatation in active labor is 1.2 cm per hour for primiparas, and 1.5 cm for multiparas.

2. Shortly before full cervical dilatation, the fetal presenting part should begin to descend, proceeding at a minimum rate of 1 cm per hour. Lack of adequate fetal descent during progressive cervical dilatation or slower than normal rates of dilatation strongly suggest the possibility of cephalopelvic disproportion.

3. Delivery should occur within a few hours but definitely no more than 8-10 hours later. Markedly prolonged labor, or a second stage lasting two hours or more, is deleterious to the fetus' health, and the risk is further compounded if other obstetrical complications such as premature rupture of the membranes or prolapse of the umbilical cord exist.

The data of another prominent obstetrician named Hellman demonstrated that the chances of fetal survival decline rapidly when active labor exceeds 12-14 hours, as indicated by exponential increases in the perinatal mortality rate when this time limit is surpassed. Therefore, if any deviations from the above patterns are found, the cause must be investigated immediately and then a prompt decision must be made concerning whether a vaginal delivery can ensue safely, or whether a cesarean section is needed to avert birth trauma.

Although the data for the Friedman curve is obtained from pelvic examinations performed during labor, there are no fixed rules specifying how many vaginal or rectal examinations should be made. Some physicians claim that the decision varies considerably, depending on the woman's parity, the rate of progress of labor, and the stage of labor.[2] Manual pelvic examination should be performed approximately every two to three hours during the latent phase of the first stage, once an hour during the active phase of the first stage, and at least every 30 minutes during the second stage. Other clinicians believe that limiting the number and frequency of pelvic examinations may help decrease the inherent risk of maternal infection associated with the internal manipulations used to assess the cervical dilatations, and the station and position of the fetal presenting part.[3] This practice is particularly important if the patient's membranes are already ruptured. In such instances, vaginal examinations are actually contraindicated until the patient is in good labor, because they carry an appreciable risk of infection.

§ 11.14   Danger Signs in Labor

In addition to evaluating the progress of labor, the status of both the mother and fetus must be continually observed and appraised since no labor can be called normal until it is completed. **Table 11-1** lists a summary of the danger signs to watch out for during labor along with their possible significance.

---

[2] Louis M. Hellman, & Jack A. Pritchard, Williams Obstetrics, 14th ed., 405 (Appleton-Century-Crofts, 1971).

[3] J.A. Pritchard, M.D. & P.C. MacDonald, M.D., Williams Obstetrics, 16th ed., 408 (Appleton-Century-Crofts, 1980).

Table 11-1

DANGER SIGNS IN LABOR

Observation or Finding	Possible Significance
Rapid, slow or irregular fetal heart tones	Fetal hypoxia (fetal distress)
Greenish-brown amniotic fluid (vertex presentation)	Fetal distress
Port-wine colored amniotic fluid	Ruptured vasa previa; premature separation of placenta
Unengaged presenting part	Disproportion or malpresentation
Failure of progress in dilatation	Prolonged labor with increasing danger of perinatal loss
Failure of presenting part to descend after full dilatation	Disproportion or error in estimate of dilatation
Bleeding (liquid or clots)	Separation of placenta; torn maternal tissue
Rising blood pressure	Preeclampsia
Low blood pressure	Shock; postural hypotension; reaction to drug
Fever	Amnionitis; extrauterine infection
Maternal tachycardia	Impending shock
Foul or purulent vaginal discharge	Amnionitis (eventual fetal pneumonia or sepsis)
Abnormal abdominal pain and tenderness	Separation of placenta; rupture of uterus; abdominal condition necessitating surgery
Uterine tetany (failure of uterus to relax between contractions)	Intrauterine bleeding due to premature separation of placenta
Excessive complaint of pain	Hysteria; undetected abnormality; reaction to medication
Prolapsed cord	Without instant action by attendant, perinatal death
Contractions getting further apart, weaker and more irregular	Uterine inertia; too much medication
Unconsciousness	Eclampsia; shock; hysteria; heavy sedation; epilepsy
Pallor; cool damp skin; air hunger	Bleeding; shock
Cyanosis	Aspiration of vomitus; cardiac failure

§ 11.15   Care of the Fetus and the Mother

Monitoring of the fetal heart rate is essential throughout labor in order to detect changes indicative of fetal distress. If any abnormalities have been discovered, the heart rate must be checked more frequently than usual. Under normal circumstances, it should be evaluated every 15 minutes during the first stage of labor, and every 5 minutes during the second stage; and immediately after a contraction in both instances, since that is when the most ominous cardiac patterns develop. Continuous electronic fetal heart monitoring is currently recommended when the fetus is at high risk (for example, in the presence of diabetes, post-maturity, toxemia, cardiac failure, and prolonged labor) or when there are signs of fetal distress such as a heart rate less than 100 beats-per-minute. On the other hand, auscultation of the fetal heart rate by fetoscope is generally adequate for a low risk pregnancy. In both situations, the fetal heart activity and the maternal pulse rate should be measured simultaneously to avoid mistaking maternal tachycardia for a normal fetal heart rate, since the normal adult heart rate of 72 beats-per-minute is considerably slower than the normal fetal heart rate of 120-160 beats-per-minute.

Compared to the fetus, many more tests of the maternal status are required during the intrapartum period. The tone of the mother's uterus should be checked carefully in the interval between contractions, a period which gradually diminishes from about 10 minutes, at the onset of the first stage of labor, to as little as one minute in the second stage. If her uterus fails to relax completely between contractions, its uninterrupted movement may interfere with the placental blood flow sufficiently enough to produce fetal hypoxia.

During active labor, the mother's temperature and respiratory rate should be checked at least every four hours (some say every one to two hours), and just prior to delivery. Her blood pressure and pulse rate should be measured at least every hour. The optimal time to check these vital signs is *between* uterine contractions in order to avoid the unrepresentative, transient increases that occur in the blood pressure, pulse rate, and respiratory rate *during* a contraction. Furthermore, if the mother's membranes have been ruptured for many hours before the onset of labor, or there has been a borderline elevation in her temperature, hourly temperature readings should be obtained to quickly detect whether an infection has developed. Infections, which are typically accompanied by temperature increases, are especially common following prolonged rupture of the membranes. As this example illustrates, abnormalities in the patient's vital signs are frequently the first clues of newly arising medical disorders, and the faster these problems are discovered and treated, the better the prognosis for both the mother and fetus.

Besides assessing the patient's physical health, it is equally important to observe her emotional status. Physicians, nurses, and all other medical personnel should strive to be patient and gentle with the pregnant woman since she often enters the hospital worried about the health of her unborn child, and fearful of the pain of delivery.

Although the patient should be permitted to assume the position she finds most comfortable, she should be discouraged from lying flat on her back. In that position, the weight of her gravid uterus compresses her major blood vessels, and consequently, diminishes the blood flow to the fetus.

In almost all circumstances, solid food should be withheld, and liquids should be limited immediately prior to, and during, active labor since the stomach's normal emptying ability is markedly prolonged at this time. As a result, any food and most medications that are ingested remain in the stomach without being absorbed, and are liable to be vomited-up; a rather common occurrence following the first stage of labor, during the induction of general anesthesia, and after delivery. This is very dangerous because if the vomitus is aspirated, it may lead to a condition called *aspiration pneumonitis*, a major cause of maternal mortality. To prevent such unnecessary deaths, whenever the woman is hungry or thirsty just prior to labor and during long labors, she should be given an intravenous infusion of 5 percent dextrose in water, rather than solid food and oral liquids.

Even when fluid is restricted during labor, urine continues to accumulate. If precautions are not taken to prevent overdistension of her bladder, the fluid-filled sac may obstruct the progress of labor, become paralyzed (losing its function for a week or more), and predispose the woman to a urinary tract infection. Therefore, whenever the abdominal examination reveals a distended bladder, the patient should be asked to urinate, and if she is unable to, catheterization should begin to drain the urine. There is currently a trend away from the previous practice of *routine* catheterization because the danger of introducing an infectious organism into the bladder from the catheter itself may be greater than the danger of a full bladder.

At some point during the first or second stage of labor, the membranes usually rupture spontaneously, though they may sometimes rupture *before* the onset of labor, or in rare instances, not until the head is being born. Although rupture is easily diagnosed when amniotic fluid gushes forth after the obstetrician slightly elevates the fetal head during a pelvic examination, a firm diagnosis may be difficult to make if the fluid is not seen or felt by either the patient or her physician. To complicate matters, none of the tests devised to detect the state of the membranes (for example, the nitrazine test and the Nile blue stain test) are completely reliable.

Whenever the membranes rupture, the fetal heart rate should always be checked immediately, and if the fetal head was not previously engaged, a pelvic examination should also be performed without delay to assess the station. In addition, it is important to enter the date and time of rupture in the patient's medical record along with the amount and color of the amniotic fluid which escaped, because in many cases the subsequent management of labor depends on whether the membranes are intact or ruptured. For instance, if the membranes rupture prematurely (an event which has been broadly defined by different authorities as rupture occurring from 1-12 hours prior to the onset of labor), but delivery is prolonged for two or more hours, serious intrauterine infection is liable to develop and eventually harm the fetus, even though its mother may be receiving prophylactic antibiotics. Consequently, if spontaneous labor does not begin within a fixed number of hours after the membranes have ruptured, some clinicians recommend inducing labor (as long as the fetus is not premature) to prevent the danger of maternal and fetal infection. The longer the latent period prior to the onset of labor, the greater the incidence of intrauterine infection.

At the other extreme, the membranes may remain intact until delivery is completed. When this happens, the portion covering the baby's skull, referred to as the caul, must be removed as soon as its head emerges or else the newborn will not be able to breathe. Sometimes intact membranes may actually retard the fetal descent, in which case certain physicians contend that they should be ruptured artificially, or by a procedure called amniotomy. Although the ability of amniotomy to speed up the progress of labor has not been clearly established, it is definitely known to be hazardous at specific times, and it is therefore contraindicated whenever the fetus is at a high station, and before its presenting part is well-applied to the cervix. In these two situations, the force generated by the escaping amniotic fluid (which gushes out once the membranes are severed) frequently causes the umbilical cord to prolapse, a condition associated with a very high fetal mortality rate even if immediate delivery by cesarean section is performed. The impact of the surging amniotic fluid can be reduced by only severing the membranes in the interval between contractions, providing that amniotomy is judged to be necessary and there are no contraindications to its use.

Amniotomy is also considered dangerous because if labor does not ensue soon after the procedure, an ascending infection is once again likely to develop and adversely affect maternal and fetal health. Furthermore, if it is done too early, the fetus loses the protective benefits of the intact membranes and the shock-absorbing amniotic fluid it contains, thereby exposing its head to unnecessary trauma during descent through the pelvic canal.

Most analgesics and anesthetics administered in the intrapartum period not only tend to delay the progress of labor, but also affect the health of the fetus as a result of their ability to cross the placenta. Since atypical electroencephalogram (EEG) patterns and behavioral changes have been observed for several days after birth following their use, analgesics should not be prescribed before carefully weighing their potential to cause neonatal depression along with their ability to relieve pain. The effectiveness of the chosen anesthetic agent should then be tested, and if necessary, an alternate type of anesthetic should be administered. Anesthetic agents should ideally exert their maximal effect just before delivery, and persist until after the woman's incisions are sutured.

§ 11.16   Preparations for Delivery

With the onset of the characteristic symptoms of the second stage of labor, such as bearing down and the urge to defecate, a pelvic examination should be performed to reevaluate the position and station of the presenting part, and the extent of cervical dilatation. A multigravida is not generally brought to the delivery room until her cervix is already 6-8 cm dilated. A nulligravida, however, is usually transferred there earlier, for example, when the fetal head advances to the point where it causes her perineum to bulge during contractions, when inhalation anesthesia is to be administered to assist her bearing down or pushing efforts, and when there is evidence of fetal distress in the second stage of labor. Despite these initial differences, all patients must be attended in the delivery room until the baby is born, and if they have received analgesics, the attendant must not turn her back on them for an instant.

Although a detailed discussion of the recommended sterile techniques is beyond the scope of this book, suffice it to say that the objective of all the painstaking aseptic preparations is to prevent the woman and newborn from acquiring an infection during delivery.

§ 11.17   Delivery of the Fetus

Since most women are able to deliver spontaneously, obstetrical intervention is usually not necessary unless there are maternal or fetal indications for forceps delivery. Obstetricians stress that the goal of intrapartum care should be intensive observation and minimal intervention. The physician's function during the course of a spontaneous delivery includes promoting slow emergence of the head, preventing umbilical cord complications, assisting with the slow delivery of the shoulders if necessary, clearing the baby's air passages, encouraging it to breathe, assessing its condition, clamping and cutting the umbilical cord, minimizing maternal blood loss, ensuring that the placenta is delivered appropriately, checking the woman's reproductive tract after delivery, and suturing any wounds or incisions.

The following discussion of the normal sequence of events during the first and second stages of labor applies almost exclusively to fetuses in the vertex presentation. Except for a separate section on breech presentations, the details of the birth process and the specific obstacles encountered in the other less common or abnormal positions and presentations are quite lengthy and are not covered in this book.

In vertex presentations, the fetal head is the first part of the baby to emerge. As soon as it crowns (when the largest diameter of the head is visibly encircled by the external vaginal opening), it can be delivered readily, either spontaneously, or by applying slight pressure on the fundus. However, if anesthesia has been given, crowning may not occur, or if it does, the head may then recede. If slight fundal pressure does not easily advance the head in these instances, forceps should be employed. Regardless of what technique is used, adequate control of this phase of delivery is of paramount importance in order to avoid maternal perineal lacerations and trauma to the delicate fetal head.

Immediately following the birth of its head, the baby's neck should be palpated to make sure the umbilical cord is not wrapped around it. This occurs approximately 25 percent of the time, ordinarily causing no harm as long as the proper steps are taken to correct it when it is first discovered. If the cord is loosely coiled, it should be carefully slipped over the baby's head to facilitate delivery and avoid cord laceration. However, if numerous or tightly wound loops are found, the umbilical cord must be doubly clamped, cut between the clamps, and then unwound from around the fetal neck. Because tightly wrapped segments of the umbilical cord obstruct the uteroplacental blood flow, the baby may not have received adequate supplies of oxygen during descent and will, therefore, probably try to breathe immediately after its chest is born, so the obstetrician must clear its airway promptly.

Clearing the mouth and throat of mucus and foreign debris should be done for all infants before their thorax is delivered in order to enable them to breathe freely and independently when the time comes. A considerable quantity of the foreign material can be removed by simply scooping it out with the examining finger, or even more thoroughly, with a soft rubber suction bulb. Though bulb suction is considered adequate in most cases, some physicians claim that in the presence of meconium, deep suction is indicated to remove the meconium-stained amniotic fluid before the chest is delivered.[4]

In addition to clearing the air passages, a number of clinicians recommend stimulating the baby's gag reflex. By inducing it to vomit-up the fluid in its stomach under controlled supervision, the obstetrician can minimize the risk

---

[4] D.N. Danforth, Ph.D., M.D., Obstetrics and Gynecology, 4th ed., 652 (Harper & Row Publishers, Inc., 1982).

of vomiting after delivery, a dangerous event because it may lead to aspiration of the vomitus while no one is watching.

The baby's shoulders emerge after its head and, in most cases, they are born spontaneously. Occasionally, however, a delay occurs and immediate extraction may be necessary. If so, excessive force must be avoided since it can lead to serious fetal injury. Failure to deliver the shoulders spontaneously or using the recommended manipulations constitutes an obstetrical emergency called *shoulder dystocia*.

When coordinated with the uterine contractions, the delivery of the rest of the body requires little, if any, assistance. The obstetrician should simply cradle the infant along her forearm, keeping the baby's head lower than its body to prevent it from aspirating any of the remaining contents of its hypopharynx. If there is a prolonged delay in the birth of the body, moderate traction on the head and pressure on the uterine fundus may hasten the descent. During these accessory procedures, the physician must refrain from hooking her fingers in the baby's axillae, since this may injure the neighboring nerves, and thereby cause a transient or even permanent paralysis of the child's upper extremity. Immediately after the infant is born, there is usually a gush of amniotic fluid, often tinged with blood, though not grossly bloody.

Unless the cord was cut earlier to prevent it from choking the fetus, the newborn remains attached to its mother by the umbilical cord after delivery. The optimal time to sever the connection depends on the infant's condition. By holding the baby at or below the level of the vaginal opening while the cord is still intact, as much as 100 ml (milliliter) of iron-rich blood can be transferred from the placenta to the infant. Whereas this blood is beneficial for the healthy baby and would have gone to waste if its umbilical cord was clamped before it was held in the position described, the additional placental blood is sometimes detrimental. For example, babies born with a blood group incompatibility such as Rh-disease are actually endangered by added quantities of incompatible maternal blood, just as babies who are already depressed from having received inhalation anesthetics (administered to their mothers) may become further depressed if the cord is not promptly clamped to prevent more of the anesthetic from entering their circulation. For these reasons, the majority of physicians clamp and then sever the umbilical cord as soon as possible (for instance, right after clearing the airway), and only a minority wait until the cord stops pulsating.[5]

Before examining the umbilical cord for anomalies and sending a sample of the cord blood to the laboratory for ABO/Rh (blood group typing), the obste-

---

[5] J.A. Pritchard, M.D. & P.C. MacDonald, M.D., Williams Obstetrics, 16th ed., 423 (Appleton-Century-Crofts, 1980).

trician should check the uterus to make sure that a second, undiagnosed fetus is not present. Care of the newborn will be discussed in **Chapter 23**.

§ 11.18   —Delivery of the Placenta

The placenta normally remains attached to the uterine wall until a few minutes after the baby is delivered. Then, the sudden diminution in size of the uterine cavity spontaneously forces it to separate from the wall, at which time sufficiently strong uterine contractions can expel it from the vagina. At no time must the obstetrician ever induce expulsion before the placenta is completely separated from the uterine wall, since downward pressure on a relaxed uterus and excessive umbilical cord traction can lead to acute inversion of the uterus, a serious emergency.

Most authorities seem to agree that awaiting spontaneous separation (signaled by an increased volume of vaginal bleeding, protrusion of the umbilical cord from the vagina, and a change in uterine shape from discoid to globular) is normally beneficial because it decreases the chances of a retained placenta, traumatic injury, feto-maternal transfusion, and unnecessary maternal discomfort.[6] However, this policy of watchful waiting is only recommended when the uterus is rising and hard (this indicates that the placenta has separated and a contraction is occurring). If it is rising and soft, immediate action must be taken because these characteristics may be the result of intrauterine bleeding. In either this case or when fresh vaginal bleeding is actually seen, gentle massage of the fundus is begun to induce a contraction to help stop the bleeding. On the other hand, when the uterus is firmly contracted but the placenta fails to separate spontaneously, a series of gentle uterine manuevers coupled with moderate traction on the umbilical cord may be attempted. If these efforts are unsuccessful, manual removal of the placenta is indicated to avoid excessive blood loss. Since the risks of manual separation and delivery of the placenta outweigh its advantages in many circumstances, it should only be performed when hemorrhage clearly threatens or has already occurred.

The critical hour immediately following placental delivery has been designated by some obstetricians as the fourth stage of labor. At this time, the placenta should be carefully sponged of blood clots and then inspected on the fetal and maternal surfaces to determine whether it has been completely delivered. If an obvious gap or placental defect is found, the uterus should be manually explored to retrieve the missing piece since retained fragments frequently cause bleeding several days after delivery. Occasionally, an internal

---

6 *Id.* at 425.

injury may be responsible instead, as is often indicated by continual profuse vaginal bleeding despite a firmly contracted uterine fundus. The blood loss from such vaginal lacerations can usually be controlled with sutures.

During the critical fourth stage of labor, the uterus normally contracts and retracts, thereby mending the tears in the surrounding blood vessels and preventing further bleeding from the placental implantation site, the major sources of maternal blood loss. Yet despite the natural ability of the uterine contractions to repair the damage, there is still a high risk of postpartum hemorrhage immediately after delivery and up to several days later (accounting for appreciable maternal morbidity and a leading cause of maternal death), making this the most hazardous phase of labor for the mother.

Inadequate contractions of the uterine muscles or any circumstances that hinder their ability to control the bleeding such as overdistension of the uterus, deep anesthesia, or attempts to deliver the placenta before it has separated, all increase the probability of developing postpartum hemorrhage. This condition, which is particularly dangerous because blood can accumulate in the uterus without external evidence of bleeding, can be prevented by periodically measuring the mother's vital signs, and frequently palpating her uterus to ensure that it remains hard and round, and does not become relaxed and atonic. At the slightest sign of relaxation, her uterus should be massaged until it stimulates a contraction to help stop the bleeding. The vaginal and perineal regions of her body should also be inspected often to detect excessive bleeding.

Oxytocic drugs (the most common of which is oxytocin and is commercially available in the United States as Pitocin and Syntocinon) provide another means of controlling hemorrhage related to uterine atony since they artificially stimulate uterine contractions. At the present time there is a wide range of opinions concerning the best time to begin an oxytocin infusion, with some clinicians favoring early administration (in the second stage of labor while the baby is being delivered) to decrease the average blood loss, and others preferring to await placental delivery.[7] The latter group contends that earlier administration may injuriously or fatally entrap an undiagnosed second fetus in the uterus, as well as hinder manual delivery of the placenta and uterine exploration when indicated. Still other physicians choose to observe the mother's uterus after delivery before routinely administering oxytocic agents during the placental phase. Unless the woman is predisposed to postpartum hemorrhage because of her age (35 or older), a history of hemorrhage, prolonged or dysfunctional labor, increased volumes of amniotic fluid, many past pregnancies or previous twins, the third and fourth stages of most uncomplicated vaginal deliveries can generally be conducted with only a reasonably small blood loss without resorting to oxytocics.

---

[7] *Id.* at 429.

It is important to distinguish the potentially dangerous use of oxytocin prior to the onset of spontaneous labor, with the safer administration of the drug after the fetus is out of the uterus. In the first case, the uterus is so sensitive to oxytocin that even a weak intravenous infusion of the drug may cause the pregnant uterus to contract so violently that it ruptures and/or kills the fetus right before it is born.

§ 11.19   —Episiotomy

Episiotomy is often used synonymously with perineotomy to describe a surgical incision of the perineum. It is commonly performed when three to four centimeters of the baby's head are visible during a contraction because after that time, the perineum is extremely thin and almost at the point of rupture with each contraction. Therefore, a properly timed episiotomy not only prevents undue perineal stretching, but it also promotes easier repair and better healing of the maternal wounds by substituting a straight, neat incision for the ragged laceration that frequently results otherwise. Since there is an extraordinary increase in the number and size of the blood vessels supplying the lower reproductive tract during pregnancy, the magnitude of blood loss is substantially greater when the tissues are torn, so a procedure that can improve the repair and healing process is quite beneficial. In addition, episiotomy spares the fetal head from pounding against the perineum, which could cause intracranial injury. The procedure is also advantageous if the pelvic floor is not sufficiently elastic to permit the obstetrician to perform the vaginal or intrauterine manipulations that may be necessary as labor progresses.

One of two incisions is generally used, the *midline episiotomy* or the *mediolateral episiotomy*. Because of its numerous advantages, the midline incision is preferred unless the fetus is large, is in the breech presentation, or has been delivered by a mid-forceps procedure. A mediolateral episiotomy would then be favored since it tends to reduce the high incidence of rectal tearing (the one disadvantage of the midline incision) observed when a midline episiotomy is used in these three situations. Repair of the episiotomy is most commonly deferred until after the placenta has been delivered. At this time, the obstetrician should also examine the woman's reproductive tract for any lacerations, and repair them if present.

§ 11.20　Immediate Postpartum Care of the Mother

Before moving the mother to the recovery room, her condition must be stable, and then once she is transferred, she must remain under constant supervision for a minimum of two hours. At intervals of at least every 15 minutes for the first hour and every 30 minutes for the second hour, her pulse, blood pressure, and uterine height and consistency should be measured, and the amount of uterine bleeding should be estimated. The obstetrician should not leave the patient until her vital signs are within normal limits, her uterus is firm and well-retracted, and she shows no signs of convulsions or active bleeding. If she is bleeding excessively, immediate action must be taken to prevent the insidious and precipitious development of hemorrhagic shock. If the woman received general anesthesia during delivery, the physician should stay until she is fully reacted. Unlike the previous examples of potentially serious problems, chills are frequently reported and are considered a normal sensation following delivery.

§ 11.21　Bibliography and Recommended Readings

Danforth, D.N., Ph.D, M.D., *Obstetrics and Gynecology*, 4th ed. (Harper & Row Publishers, Inc., 1982).

Iffy, Leslie, M.D. and Kaminetzky, Harold A., M.D., *Principles and Practice of Obstetrics & Perinatology*, vol. 2 (John Wiley & Sons, Inc., 1981).

Niswander, K.R., M.D., *Obstetrics, Essentials of Clinical Practice* (Little, Brown & Co., Inc., 1981).

Oxorn, Harry A., B.A., M.D., *Human Labor and Birth* (Appleton-Century-Crofts, 1980).

Pritchard, J.A., M.D., MacDonald, P.C., M.D., Gant, N.F., M.D., *Williams Obstetrics*, 17th ed. (Appleton-Century-Crofts, 1985).

Willson, J. Robert, M.D., Beecham, Clayton T., M.D. and Carrington, Elsie Reid, M.D., *Obstetrics and Gynecology* (The C.V. Mosby Co., 1975).

CHAPTER 12

OBSTETRICAL TRAUMA AND BIRTH INJURIES

§ 12.1   Introduction

The probability that a fetus will be injured while descending through the birth canal is directly and indirectly related to the difficulties encountered during labor and the methods used to resolve them. Although injuries may occur during the uncomplicated labor and delivery of a normal-sized infant, the likelihood of birth trauma is substantially increased by the following adverse factors: fetopelvic disproportion (due to a contracted pelvis, excessive-sized fetus or both), unfavorable fetal positions and presentations, fetal distress, prolonged labor, forcep deliveries (excluding the low forcep type), and operative breech deliveries. In addition, failure to recognize and/or properly manage high-risk conditions that threaten the fetus's life in utero (such as diabetes, intrauterine growth retardation, preeclampsia, premature rupture of the membranes and post-maturity), may also result in iatrogenic (physician induced) trauma or death. Despite the inherent dangers of the birth process, most obstetricians point out that the majority of birth injuries can be prevented by properly managing high risk pregnancies throughout the antepartum and intrapartum periods, avoiding premature deliveries whenever possible, and anticipating high risk neonatal situations well in advance so that optimal care can be provided for both the mother and her baby during labor, and immediately afterwards.

§ 12.2   Cerebral Injuries

A large percentage of perinatal deaths and serious injuries occur because the baby's brain is traumatized during the delivery process. Direct injury of the head, severe hypoxia (see § 12.3), or a combination of these two factors, may lead to intracranial hemorrhage—one of the most common types of cerebral injuries. It is most apt to develop in a small or a very large infant. Even if the baby is fortunate enough not to succumb to severe intracranial hemorrhage in utero, its prognosis after birth is usually not very favorable either, as evidenced by the fact that such infants are often born in a state of asphyxia and receive poor Apgar scores (4 or less) at one minute and at five minutes.

§ 12.3   Hypoxia

Approximately 25 percent of all intrauterine deaths are due to insufficient oxygenation; and about 4 percent of all live-born, premature infants die as a direct or indirect result of intrauterine hypoxia. Any of the following conditions may be responsible: reduced blood flow through the maternal arteries and veins (due to hypertension, hypotension, or forceful, rapidly recurring or prolonged uterine contractions), reduced oxygen content of the maternal blood (resulting from hemorrhage or chronic anemia), and impaired fetal circulation (due to abnormal cardiac function, compression of the umbilical cord, or premature separation of the placenta).

The length of time the fetus was deprived of oxygen largely determines its fate. Whereas prolonged periods of oxygen deprivation often lead to intrauterine death, shorter periods of hypoxia are usually not fatal, but have been linked to such diverse health disorders as abnormal bleeding, constriction of the pulmonary blood vessels, interruption of surfactant production (a substance necessary for lung expansion), respiratory depression, acidosis, hypoglycemia, and cell-tissue damage. Hypoxia is especially damaging to the sensitive tissues of the central nervous system, inducing lesions responsible for cerebral palsy, mental retardation, epilepsy, and the syndrome of minimal brain dysfunction. Afflicting an estimated three million Americans, the last syndrome describes those infants, children, and adolescents with behavorial disorders (often accompanied by learning disabilities, reading inability, hyperactivity and motor disturbances) or abnormal neurologic findings and electroencephalographic (EEG) irregularities.

> Among term infants, the effects of asphyxia on the central nervous system represent the most serious problems. Studies in institutions have shown that among patients with cerebral palsy (except those with congenital defects, malformations, and postneonatally acquired disease) 80 percent have histories of severe perinatal asphyxia.[1]

Since these serious handicaps often develop despite outstanding efforts to revive the newborn, a number of physicians believe that the resuscitative procedures may invariably be started too late to save the life of or prevent irreversible brain damage in babies who did not receive adequate oxygenation. Contending that this bleak outlook can be improved by eliminating the actual causes of antepartum and intrapartum asphyxia, they stress the avoidance of conditions or procedures known to interfere with the fetal blood supply, such as prolonged or violent labor, the inappropriate use of oxytocic drugs, and undue pressure on the umbilical cord or fetal head during delivery.[2] In the rare cases in which hypoxia and asphyxia cannot be prevented, the subsequent effects can at least be minimized by knowing which factors prolong the asphyxiated newborn's recovery, including prematurity, intrauterine growth retardation, certain analgesic and anesthetic agents given prior to delivery and exposing the naked infant to room temperature. The two most important factors are certain analgesic and anesthetic agents which are given prior to delivery. Therefore, the obstetrician should select only those methods of analgesia and anesthesia known to allow adequate oxygenation of the maternal blood, and attempt to avoid premature deliveries whenever possible. He should also refrain from performing difficult vaginal deliveries in light of the evidence that the infants most liable to develop serious mental disabilities are those which are small for gestational age (associated with a poorly functioning placenta) who have undergone such difficult forcep deliveries.

---

[1] Leslie Iffy M.D. & Harold A. Kaminetzky, M.D., Principles and Practice of Obstetrics & Perinatology, vol. 2, 1609 (John Wiley & Sons, Inc., 1981).

[2] M.E. Avery, & H.W. Taeusch, Schaffer's Diseases of the Newborn, 5th ed., 100 W.B. Saunders Co. 1984).

§ 12.4   Peripheral Nerve Injuries

Peripheral nerve injuries most commonly involve the brachial plexus and the facial nerve. Consisting of the fifth, sixth, seventh, and eighth cervical nerve roots, plus the first and second thoracic nerve roots, the complex known as the brachial plexus may be damaged if extreme lateral traction is applied to the head (for example, when the shoulders do not emerge easily) or if downward traction is applied to the shoulders themselves while attempting to deliver the aftercoming head of a baby in the breech presentation. The facial nerve is usually traumatized by pressure from the tip of the forceps blade.

Depending on which of these vulnerable nerve roots is damaged, the new-born's eye, mouth, upper arm (Erb's palsy), forearm, or hand (Klumpke's paralysis) will become paralyzed. Respiratory problems may also develop since the fifth cervical nerve of the brachial plexus supplies the diaphragm. Fortunately, the majority of the peripheral nerve injuries either resolve spontaneously, or respond well to therapy when they are diagnosed and treated promptly.

§ 12.5   Spinal Cord and Brain Stem Injuries

If an infant is having difficulty taking its first breaths, the obstetrician should consider the possibility of damage to the spinal cord or brain stem, especially if any of the following predisposing conditions are also present: prematurity, precipitous or forceful delivery, or breech deliveries. Unlike peripheral nerve lesions, spinal cord and brain stem injuries are life-threatening injuries which generally are not amenable to treatment. Consequently, the baby typically dies within a few hours after birth.

§ 12.6   Bony Injuries

True skull *fractures* are rare in modern obstetrics, but skull *depressions* (often confusingly called depressed fractures) may occur if the fetus's head is compressed either by incorrectly applied forceps, or by the prominent bony regions of the maternal pelvis during spontaneous vaginal delivery. Although these injuries usually cause no symptoms and require no treatment, surgery may occasionally be necessary in order to decompress the affected area.

Separation or fracture of the vertebrae may result when strong traction is applied to the fetal head or shoulders during delivery. Even more serious than the fracture itself is the accompanying damage to the exposed spinal cord which is no longer protected by an intact vertebral column.

The clavicle is a frequent site for fractures to occur. The clavicle is most frequently fractured when the obstetrician has trouble delivering the shoulders of a large infant, or when excessive force is used to facilitate delivery. Although treatment is usually not needed, if displacement is evident on x-ray films, restraining bandages or splints can be applied to ensure good healing. Recovery is generally good, even without treatment.

The humerus (arm bone) and femur (thigh bone) are the most common sites of limb fractures. Limb fractures are commonly associated with breech deliveries, and in and of themselves, do not constitute any negligence on the part of the obstetrician. However, fractured limbs often are seen in cases where excessive force or other mismanagement is evident. As long as bones are set properly, they generally heal within a few weeks.

§ 12.7   Soft Tissue Injuries

Although trauma to the skin and subcutaneous tissues may be alarming at first sight, marks left by abrasions, bruises, and forcep blades are usually insignificant. They require no treatment aside from applying antibiotic ointment where the skin is broken.

§ 12.8   Encephalomalacia

One form of brain damage that occurs particularly frequently in premature infants is one of periventricular encephalomalacia. Essentially, this condition consists of bilateral, but not necessarily symmetrical, necrosis, having a periventricular distribution. What the word means is basically, softening of the brain. The lesions found suggest inadequate circulatory profusion and infarction of the vascular border zones between the middle and posterior cerebral artery. Episodes of serious cardio-respiratory insufficiency and hypotension can be documented in most of these infants, and could account for these lesions.

§ 12.9   Perinatal Trauma

Physical damage to the brain while contributing significantly to mortality during the neonatal period is a rare cause for persistent major neurologic deficits.

These are far more commonly the outcome of hypoxia. However, gross traumatic lesions to the brain stem and spinal cord are produced by traction of the fetal neck during labor or delivery. This form of birth trauma is more likely to be encountered in breech deliveries. Laceration of the cerebellar area of the brain accompanied by a local brain stem hemorrhage is a sequel of stretch injuries to the brain stem associated with breech extractions. Though it is possible to have direct damage to the brain from a breech delivery, it is rarely the sole cause of long-term disability absent the hypoxia.

When the fetus or child is exposed to prolonged partial asphyxia, it develops high PCO_2 (elevated carbon dioxide) levels and mixed metabolic and respiratory acidosis. The metabolic acidosis is a result of metabolism occurring without oxygen and releasing lactic acid. Respiratory acidosis is the result of abnormally high carbon dioxide PCO_2 levels. This is accompanied by marked brain swelling. The relative significance of the three variables (hypoxia, PCO_2, and acidosis) in the induction of cerebral edema is still unclear. However, cerebral edema can cause pressure on the blood vessels, thus decreasing circulation to the brain tissue. Brain swelling compresses the small blood vessels. This results in shock and a drop of systemic blood pressure, and leads to failure of cerebral profusion and a number of lesions. These can be microscopic lesions and/or evidencing as encephalomalacia.

Disordered cerebral circulation caused by shock acting as a sole factor is probably an uncommon cause of brain damage, but when present with hypoxia and acidosis, may result in edema and damage to the brain directly.

In contrast to extra-cerebral hemorrhages, intracranial hemorrhages can occur which result not only from direct trauma to the brain, but also from anoxia. There are two major types of lesions encountered: (1) intraventricular, and (2) subarachnoid.

Intraventricular hemorrhage is encountered in up to 15 percent of all premature births and, subject to autopsy, is a common cause of death. The cause of intraventricular hemorrhage is not fully understood; however, it is predominantly seen in males. This is associated with perinatal and postnatal hypoxia and particularly with respiratory distress syndrome. The following factors are thought to play a role in the production of this condition:

1. Acidosis
2. Impaired response to hypoxia and hypercarbia (high CO_2)
3. Prolonged PT, a blood clotting factor
4. Low temperature, and
5. Increased concentration of the serum by excessive administration of sodium bicarbonate (excess concentration is termed hyperosmolarity).

The bleeding usually does not occur at the time of delivery, but rather the second or third day of life. It originates from the capillaries, the small veins and arteries in the walls of the lateral ventricles. The extent of hemorrhage varies from slight oozing to massive bleeding. The extent of bleeding can bear on the prognosis of the infant as determined by CAT-scan. The blood usually clears rapidly from the subarachnoid spaces; however, it may induce a fibrous reaction and cause hydrocephalus by occluding the flow of cerebral spinal fluid through the ventricle spaces and ducts.

Subarachnoid hemorrhage, the second type of hemorrhage seen, can be seen in both the premature and full-term infant, and is caused by hypoxia. It accounts for approximately 3 percent of all hemorrhages in the newborn. The bleeding is fairly well-contained and a relatively minor occurrence. Occasionally, you can have hemorrhage into the brain substance itself, secondary to anoxia, which is relatively rare.

Thus, direct trauma, anoxia, and circulatory disturbances (shock and decreased profusion due to edema) play an important part in the production of the brain lesions associated with perinatal trauma. There is no doubt that premature infants have faulty maturation of the nervous system and thus have greater vulnerability to perinatal trauma and anoxia. There is a very high incidence of these two conditions in premature infants.

§ 12.10   Hyperbilirubinemia

Bilirubin is a normal by-product of the breakdown of red blood cells. Bilirubin is metabolized through the liver and results in becoming bile. However, the fetal and newborn liver is immature and cannot handle excessive amounts of bilirubin. Prior to birth, the placenta and maternal systems undertake this function for the child; however, after birth the newborn's liver must take over this process. The problem that arises when there is excessive bleeding such as an intracerebral hemorrhage is that there is a large breakdown of red blood cells, and a great deal of bilirubin being released into the blood. The fetal liver is very slow in breaking down these products; however, damage is unlikely to occur until the bilirubin reaches 15 points.

The excessive bilirubin becomes deposited in the skin tissue, resulting in jaundice; and when reaching high levels in the body, begins to deposit in the brain tissue, which is termed *kernicterus*. This is yellow staining by bilirubin of the brain stem and cerebellum (the part of the brain associated with coordination) and can cause hearing loss, impaired control of the eye muscles, and athetosis (a condition marked by constant, slow, and voluntary withering movements of the hands, fingers, and sometimes feet).

Clinical manifestation of the jaundiced infant developing kernicterus is that he becomes drowsy on the second to fifth day of life, and begins to nurse poorly. He then develops a fever, his cry becomes monotonous, and the moro reflex becomes unattainable. By two weeks of age, there is hypertonia and extensor spasms, and about 10 percent of the infants develop clonic convulsions. Over the next few months, the child becomes hypotonic and at four years of age, the full syndrome of kernicterus is evolved. The great majority of these children are mentally retarded, and athetosis is almost invariably present with rigidity and tremors. Auditory problems may take the form of hearing loss or receptive aphasia, or a combination of both. Thus, in the premature infant, exchange transfusions ought to be undertaken whenever the bilirubin level exceeds 15 mg per dl (milligrams per deciliter), or whenever it has risen about 10 in the first 24 hours of life, especially if there is also evidence of active hemolysis (such as in bleeding).

§ 12.11   Bibliography and Recommended Readings

Aladjem, Silvio, M.D., *Risks in the Practice of Modern Obstetrics* (The C.V. Mosby Co., 1975).

Arias, Fernando, M.D., Ph.D., *High-Risk Pregnancy and Delivery* (The C.V. Mosby Co., 1984).

Burrow, G.N. M.D. & Ferris, T.F., M.D., *Medical Complications During Pregnancy* (W.B. Saunders Co., 1975).

Coleman, Mary, M.D., *Neonatal Neurology* (University Park Press, 1981).

Courville, Cyril B., M.D., *Birth and Brain Damage* (Margaret Farnsworth Courville, 1977).

Iffy, Leslie, M.D. & Kaminetzky, Harold A., M.D., *Principles and Practice of Obstetrics & Perinatology,* vol. 2 (John Wiley & Sons, Inc. 1981).

Menkes, John H., M.D., *Textbook of Child Neurology* (Lea & Febiger, 1980).

Merritt, H.H., M.D., *A Textbook of Neurology* (Lea & Febiger, 1979).

Volpe, Joseph J., M.D., *Neurology of the Newborn* (W.B. Saunders Co., 1981).

CHAPTER 13

PLACENTAL ABRUPTION

§ 13.1   Premature Separation of the Placenta

Premature separation of the placenta, which occurs in approximately 1 percent of all deliveries,[1] refers to the partial or complete detachment of a normally implanted placenta (in the upper uterine wall) at any time *before* the fetus is born. Developing most commonly in the third trimester of pregnancy, this unpreventable syndrome is also known as placental abruption, abruptio placentae, or ablatio placentae.

Unlike the varying degrees of premature placental separation which inevitably occur in placenta previa as a result of the abnormally low implantation site, premature detachment in abruptio placentae is not due to an unnatural anatomical relationship. Instead, spontaneous rupture of the placental blood vessels is thought to gradually tear the placental membranes from the uterine wall, which not only progressively destroys the organ's ability to transport

---

[1] D.N. Danforth, Ph.D., M.D., *Obstetrics and Gynecology*, 4th ed., 449 (Harper & Row Publishers, Inc., 1982).

oxygen and the essential nutrients to the fetus, but also results in potentially life-threatening maternal hemorrhage. The released blood typically flows out through the woman's vagina (external bleeding), or it may be completely trapped between the detached placenta and the uterine wall (concealed hemorrhage), or a combination of the two may exist simultaneously. Since the extent of the hemorrhage is difficult to recognize and adequately treat whenever some portion of the blood is trapped inside the uterus, the presence of a concealed hemorrhage is a particularly dangerous complication.

Generally, the clinical findings and their significance correspond to the degree of detachment, which may range from just a few centimeters to complete separation of the placenta from the uterine wall. For example, a marginal separation producing few, if any, symptoms, is clinically insignificant and may not even be detected until after delivery, when the placenta is routinely inspected. In sharp contrast, complete detachment may be rapidly fatal if its sequelae are not treated at once. As a result of these diverse clinical pictures, premature separation of the placenta is classified as mild, moderate, or severe. See §§ 13.2 through 13.4.

Although the precise etiology of premature separation of the placenta is unclear, it is known to develop most frequently in multiparas (especially those who have given birth to five or more children), women over the age of 35, patients with diabetes mellitus or one of the hypertensive disorders in pregnancy, and those who have been exposed to external abdominal injury or obstetrical trauma. In addition, this syndrome has a high incidence of recurrence in subsequent gestations.

§ 13.2   —Mild Abruption

Since mild premature placental separation is only associated with a minimal blood loss, 50-150 ml (milliliter), it usually does not cause the maternal shock or the fetal distress (here, the fetal heart tones remain strong and regular) that characterize the more severe forms of the disorder. Sometimes, the scant amount of vaginal bleeding is the obstetrician's only clue of the disease process, though various other symptoms such as lower abdominal tenderness and discomfort may also be present. Although such findings rarely require special action, if uterine irritability develops, the patient must be closely watched for any further signs of placental separation.

Unlike the severe forms of placental abruption which are generally marked by classic diagnostic signs and symptoms, the *milder* states of the syndrome are often asymptomatic, making them difficult to detect clinically. Consequently, the diagnosis is often made by trying to exclude the other likely causes of third trimester bleeding such as placenta previa, uterine rupture, or cervical or vaginal lesions. The *indirect* diagnostic tests (the abdominal and vaginal examinations, as well as ultrasonic placental localization) should be performed for this purpose when the gestation is less than 37 weeks' duration, the external bleeding is not profuse, and uterine irritability is absent or minimal. If the previously mentioned cause of hemorrhage can be ruled out, it is appropriate to *passively* await the spontaneous onset of labor, or the appearance of new clinical findings, before intervening since the lives of neither the mother nor her unborn child are endangered.

The protocol is quite different, however, when the gestation is over 37 weeks' length. At this stage of pregnancy, a *direct* examination (the manual pelvic examination) should be conducted in an operating room in order to determine the source of the bleeding. As long as placenta previa is not implicated, delivery should be *actively* induced by rupturing the patient's membranes, and if necessary, administering an oxytocin infusion as well. These techniques are also recommended if the woman is about to go into labor since in both cases, rupturing the membrances usually accelerates the birth process and thereby reduces the blood loss. However, if the bleeding persists, if the fetus is in distress, if the uterus fails to relax between contractions, or if labor does not begin within a reasonable period of time, a cesarean section will have to be performed instead.

§ 13.3   —Moderate Abruption

Moderate premature separation of the placenta implies that one-fourth to two-thirds of the placental surface is separated from the uterine wall. The onset of symptoms may either be gradual (beginning with a mild degree of separation), or abrupt (appearing with continuous abdominal pain followed by an outflow of dark red vaginal blood). Depending on the extent of the hemorrhage— which is usually moderate at first, but may be much more severe by the time the woman is seen by her physician—there may be evidence of shock (cold, clammy skin, an increased pulse rate, and a decreased blood pressure) and fetal distress. In addition, the patient's uterus is quite tender and irritable, and of major diagnostic importance, it fails to completely relax between contractions—a reaction which strongly suggests the development of premature separation of the placenta regardless of any prior or accompanying signs. If labor is not already in progress, it usually ensues within a couple of hours.

Due to the fact that a patient with moderate premature separation of the placenta will continue to bleed until either her baby is delivered or until she is dead, the onset of hemorrhage is regarded as an acute emergency which must immediately be treated by restoring her diminished circulatory fluids and promptly inducing delivery is mandatory because as long as the uterus is distended by the fetus, it cannot contract sufficiently to close off the torn blood vessels and prevent further hemorrhage.

§ 13.4   —Severe Abruption

Occurring with brief warning signs, if any, the classic clinical picture in severe premature separation of the placenta is one of tetanic (stone intensity) uterine contractions, uterine tenderness and rigidity, excruciating abdominal pain, and an absence of fetal heart sounds since the baby is frequently already dead. Although over two-thirds of the placenta is detached from the uterine wall, the external blood loss is not necessarily excessive because the hemorrhage may be concealed behind placenta. In any event, shock usually ensues with astonishing speed due to the overall decrease in the blood volume; unless the hemorrhage is promptly brought under control, serious renal and coagulation problems may also arise in the mother.

§ 13.5   —Treatment

The following two therapeutic guidelines are considered invaluable for determining the amounts and kinds of fluids needed to replenish the decreased blood volume caused by obstetrical hemorrhage, irrespective of the source.

1. Lactated Ringer's solution (a solution resembling the blood in its salt constituents) and whole blood should be given in such proportions that the uterine flow is at least 30/ml-per-hour (and ideally approaches 60/ml-per-hour) and the hematocrit is 30 percent or slightly higher. Diuretics should not be prescribed while these studies are being conducted because their effect on urine output invalidates the test results.

2. If these initial measures do not promptly restore the woman's urine flow, her central venous pressure (CVP) should be measured in order to evaluate the blood flow back to her heart, and to determine the ability of her circulatory system to withstand further transfusions, since additional fluids will have to be administered.[2]

---

[2] J.A. Pritchard, M.D. & P.C. MacDonald, M.D., Williams Obstetrics, 16th ed., 492 (Appleton-Century-Crofts, 1980).

According to most obstetricians,[3] when the diagnosis of moderate placental abruption with actual or impending shock is made, the following measures (based, in part, on the previous guidelines) should be instituted at once:

1. At least four units of whole blood should be cross-matched for possible transfusion, and an additional supply of fresh, whole blood should be available in case a severe clotting problem develops. This precautionary measure is intended to prevent the physician from underestimating her patient's need for whole blood, a common problem in the management of this sydrome. In addition, precious minutes can be saved by keeping one of the woman's arm veins open with a large gauge needle through which an infusion of lactated Ringer's solution is temporarily flowing. With the apparatus already in place, the Ringer's solution can quickley be replaced with the desired number of blood packs as soon as a transfusion becomes necessary.

2. A vaginal and a pelvic examination should be performed to estimate the amount and source of the bleeding as well as the condition of the patient's cervix in preparation for the impending delivery. Regardless of whether she is in shock and regardless of which route of delivery is anticipated, her membranes should be ruptured in order to quickly stimulate labor, and an oxytocin infusion should be started if active labor does not ensue shortly after the rupture. Under these circumstances, the benefits of inducing labor with oxytocin override its risks, provided that care is taken not to overstimulate the uterus, espcially in women of high parity and those with fetopelvic disproportion. In the not so distant past, delivery within six hours was advocated to ensure the best maternal outcome; though now, many clinicians believe that the prognosis depends more on the rapidity and adequacy of fluid replacement (particularly blood) than on the time that elapses after the membrances are ruptured.

3. The fetal heart rate should be continuously monitored since the baby faces a high risk of intrauterine hypoxia and death as a result of its mother's hemorrhage and tetanic uterine contractions. If the fetus is found to be in distress, it must be delivered immediately. In such cases, a cesarean section is nearly always required in order to maximize the baby's chances of survival. Conduction anesthesia should not be ensued for the surgery because it may induce a dangerous blood pressure decrease in patients with appreciable hemorrhage.

---

[3] D.N. Danforth, Ph.D., M.D., *Obstetrics and Gynecology*, 4th ed., 452 (Harper & Row Publishers, Inc., 1982).

4. The expectant mother's condition should be constantly observed and evaluated. Besides analyzing her blood for its hemoglobin content, hematocrit, and number of red blood cells, a fibrinogen level should also be obtained. This test, which enables the obstetrician to evaluate the clotting ability of the patient's blood, must be repeated at frequent intervals until she is out of danger of a coagulation derangement. Although clotting deficiencies should ideally be corrected before performing surgery, early operative intervention may become necessary if the woman is losing blood rapidly

5. If shock is present or if it appears imminent, the patient's central venous pressure should be monitored, and her urinary output should be assessed using an indwelling bladder catheter.

The procedures outlined for the treatment of moderate premature separation of the placenta are also applicable for severe premature separation of the placenta, with the following exceptions: there is a greater need for blood replacement, the clotting derangement is far more serious and therefore requires much closer vigilance, and consideration of the fetus is rarely necessary since it is almost always dead by this advanced stage of syndrome. A dead fetus, or one whose viability is doubtful, should be delivered vaginally unless its mother's hemorrhage is rapid and uncontrollable, or other existing complications contraindicate the procedure, in which case a cesarean delivery is required. Aside from these last two possibilities, a cesarean section is only resorted to in severe premature separation of the placenta, if there is still a reasonable chance that the distressed fetus will survive, and if there is little likelihood that vaginal delivery will ensure promptly.

§ 13.6 —Complications

Maternal complications, which result either from the treatment of premature separation of the placenta or from the disease itself, vary tremendously in incidence and nature, depending primarily on the extent of placental detachment. As mentioned earlier, minimal areas of separation cause few, if any, problems, whereas total placental detachment is responsible for the most serious complications. These include diffuse intravascular coagulation, postpartum hemorrhage, renal failure, impaired uterine contractility, acute cor pulmonale, transfusion hepatitis, and fetal hypoxia or death.

Early treatment of premature separation of the placenta is of utmost importance, particularly in view of the fact that many of the serious complications are much more likely to develop the longer the disease manifestations go un-resolved. A prime example is the onset of diffuse intravascular coagulation. This life-treatening condition occurs most frequently within the first few hours after the onset of pain and bleeding due to the fact that unusually large quanti-ties of the essential blood clotting factors (mainly fibrinogen and platelets) are used to plug the numerous broken blood verssels in the uterus and placenta. A severe deficit of coagulation factors therefore arises, rendering the body in-capable of repairing any further leaks or tears. As a consequence of this and other related problems, the woman begins to manifest heavy uterine bleeding and/or spontaneous bleeding from other areas of her body.

In order to detect the early signs of a diffuse intravascular coagulation (DIC) clotting deficiency and thereby prevent the dangerous development of DIC and hemmorrhage, the patient's fibrinogen level must be continually monitored from the time of her hospitalization until her baby is delivered (in women afflicted with premature separation of the placenta, the process of in-travascular coagulation ends once the infant is born), but it can be life-threat-ening. Although both the thrombin time test and the clot observation test provide accurate information, the fact that the body's consumption of fibrino-gen may occur quite quickly, may sometimes make it preferable to perform the fast and simple bedside clot observation test rather than to await the re-sults of the relatively time-consuming laboratory-performed thrombin time test. If so, every hour, a 5 ml aliquot of freshly drawn blood should immedi-ately be placed inside a clean, dry test tube (kept at the patient's bedside) and observed for the information of a clot and its subsequent dissolution. Failure to clot within 5-10 minutes, or dissolution of a formed clot by gently shaking the tube, constitutes proof of a coagulation derangement that is almost surely the result of a lack of fibrinogen and platelets.

Usually within eight hours of the onset of symptoms, the concentraton of fibrinogen (which is normally 375-700 mg/100 ml at term) may fall to well below the critical level of 100 mg/100 ml that is required to clot the blood. Depending on the extent of the clotting deficiency, the amount of active bleed-ing, and the anticipated route of delivery, one or more of the following modes of treatment will be needed to replenish the depleted coagulation factors, and thereby stop the hemorrhage: *fresh* whole blood, cryoprecipitate packs, plate-let packs, and as a last resort, fibrinogen itself. The use of heparin to prevent the development of diffuse intravascular coagulation in patients with prema-ture separation of the placenta is condemned because, in the vast majority of cases, the drug actually increases the blood loss.

Postpartum hemorrhage is another serious complication that should always be anticipated, especially in severe forms of premature separation of the pla-centa. If conservative measures (correction of the clotting defect, bimanual compression of the uterus and administration of oxytocic drugs) do not effectively stop the bleeding, the ultimate means of treatment involves ligating the hypogastric arteries or performing a hysterectomy.

Renal failure, which may be precipitated by shock, vascular spasm, intravascular clotting or combinations of these conditions, occurs most frequently in the moderate and severe degrees of placental abruption. Inadequate renal blood flow is reflected by a urinary output that does not improve after the blood volume has been restored. In order to prevent this rare, though potentially fatal complication, the obstetrician must be sure to treat shock and infection in their early stages, adequately replace the lost fluids, and terminate the pregnancy as soon as possible. These measures are believed to forestall serious kidney failure even when diffuse intravascular coagulation complicates the clinical picture.

When the uterine blood cannot easily escape through the vagina, it may infiltrate the amniotic sac of the fetus. It may also infiltrate the mother's uterine muscles, causing them to harden and lose their ability to contract and expel the fetus. In the latter condition, called uterine apoplexy or the Couvelaire uterus, the womb turns a blue-purple color.

When the placenta is completely, or almost completely, detached from the uterine wall, fetal hypoxia and death are virtual certainty. On the other hand, the degree of fetal distress in the less severe forms of separation varies according to how extensively the placental circulation is impaired by the mother's diminished blood flow or her tetanic uterine contractions. On the rare occasions in which the newborn has anemia, a promptly administered blood transfusion usually brings about a dramatic improvement in its condition.

§ 13.7   —Prognosis

The maternal prognosis can be improved by careful monitoring of the patient until her pregnancy is terminated and her bleeding is controlled; by totally replacing her lost fluids and blood to prevent severe decreases in her blood volume; by early recognition of clotting deficiencies; and by early delivery of the fetus. As of now, most of the maternal deaths are caused by hemorrhage—either from the site of the placental separation or from the onset of diffuse intravascular coagulation—or cardiac or renal failure.[4]

Although the fetus's chances for survival vary greatly with the severity of its mother's disease process, the astoundingly high mortality rate of 30-50 percent clearly reveals how dismal the fetal outcome generally is.[5] Even among

---

[4] Barry *Accidental Hemorrhage or Abruptio Placentae Clincial Features*, 70 J. Obstet. Gynecol. Br. Cwith., 708 (1963).

[5] F. Arias, M.D., High Risk Pregnancy and Delivery, 278 (The C.V. Mosby Company, 1984).

infants who are lucky enough to survive, the adverse effects of intrauterine hypoxia, birth trauma, and prematurity (due to the need for early delivery) also result in a high rate of neonatal morbidity.

§ 13.8   Placenta Previa—Diagnosis

The normal site of placental implantation (attachment) is high, and on the anterior wall of the uterus. However, for reasons still unclear, in about 0.5 percent of all deliveries, the placenta attaches to the lower segment of the patient's uterus instead,[6] giving rise to the condition called *placenta previa*. As the name suggests, the placenta is located in front of the fetal presenting part rather than behind or alongside it, and as a consequence of this abnormal anatomical relationship, it lies over the cervical outlet. Depending on how much of the cervix is covered, placenta previa is classified as:

1. Total—the placenta covers the entire cervix
2. Partial—the placenta only covers part of the cervix, or
3. Marginal—the placenta is implanted in the lower uterine segment and extends to, but does not cover, any part of the cervical opening; also referred to as a low-lying placenta.

As more of the cervix is obstructed, the probability of hazardous complications progressively increases because the abnormally positioned placenta not only interferes with the descent of the fetus through the birth canal, but more seriously, it also causes appreciable hemorrhage when it is inevitably stripped away from the uterine wall.

Women over the age of 35, multiparas, patients carrying multiple fetuses, and those with healed uterine scars (particularly one resulting from a low cervical cesarean section incision), appear to be predisposed to placenta previa. In addition, women who have had the disorder once are likely to have it again in subsequent gestations.

The onset of painless vaginal bleeding in the third trimester of pregnancy is the cardinal sign of placenta previa. Even though the expectant mother may notice spots of blood on her underwear during the first and second trimesters, the initial episode of hemorrhage usually begins after the 28th week of gestation, and is characterized by the sudden appearance of a rather large quantity of fresh, bright red blood. This color readily distinguishes the typical hemor-

---

[6] J.A. Pritchard, M.D. & P.C. MacDonald, M.D., Williams Obstetrics, 16th ed., 508 (Appleton-Century-Crofts, 1980).

rhage of placenta previa from that of menstruation or placenta abruption, since in the latter conditions, the escaping blood is generally a dark burgundy color, the sign of an older specimen.

Fortunately, the initial hemorrhage is rarely so profuse as to induce shock or death. In fact, it usually ceases spontaneously as long as the woman gets plenty of rest and her physician does not probe the area. The main danger is that severe bleeding may recur without warning, especially during late pregnancy when the mother's lower uterus and cervix begin to expand, dilate, and elongate in preparation for the upcoming birth. These anatomical adaptations stretch the abnormally implanted placenta and inevitably tear it from the uterine wall, which results in the characteristic hemorrhage of this syndrome.

As the number one cause of maternal mortality,[7] hemorrhage must be dealt with seriously whenever it develops. It is, therefore, an obstetrical maxim to immediately hospitalize all patients with third-trimester vaginal bleeding, regardless of the severity, in order to expeditiously stop the blood loss and determine its cause.

Upon admission, the expectant mother should be confined to bed and at least two tubes of her blood should be drawn. The first specimen is tested for its hemoglobin content, hematocrit, and number of red blood cells in order to provide an estimate of the extent of the woman's hemorrhage; the second specimen is typed (according to its ABO/Rh group) and then cross-matched to ensure that compatible units of donor blood are readily available in case a blood transfusion is necessary. While awaiting the laboratory results, the fetus's status should be evaluated by monitoring its heart rate and activity.

Once the bleeding subsides, the obstetrician can concentrate on ascertaining its source and cause. This entails performing a complete physical examination of the patient, with the notable exception of the pelvic portion of the examination which, because of its high probability of provoking life-threatening hemorrhage, must be withheld until specific conditions are satisfied. These will be thoroughly discussed later in this section.

Upon palpating the abdomen of a woman with placenta previa, the obstetrician will characteristically find it to be soft, nontender, and of normal tone. She will also discover that the fetus, if it is in either the cephalic or the breech presentation, is situated higher in the abdomen than expected as a result of the underlying placenta. Some physicians believe that the abnormally implanted placenta may also be responsible for the high incidence of *abnormal* fetal presentations, which occur in as many as one third of the patients with this syndrome.

---

[7] D.N. Danforth, Ph.D., M.D., *Obstetrics and Gynecology*, 4th ed., 443 (Harper & Row Publishers, Inc., 1982).

Unlike the pelvic examination, a carefully performed examination of the patient's vagina with a speculum carries little risk of inducing hemorrhage because the instrument is only inserted into the vagina, so there is no danger of it penetrating either the cervix or the vulnerably low placenta. The procedure is therefore permitted to rule out local sources of vaginal bleeding such as, lesions or infections of the external or internal genitalia, placental abruption, cancer, or uterine rupture.

If placenta previa still cannot be eliminated as a cause of bleeding *and* if immediate delivery is not indicated, the exact site of placental implantation should be determined by one of the noninvasive methods. Ultrasonic placental localization is considered the procedure of choice because besides being simpler, safer, and more precise than any of the other identification techniques, it has the added advantage of being able to simultaneously assess the biparietal diameter of the fetal skull, an important determinant of fetal maturity. Since it is often advantageous to defer delivery until the fetus reaches maturity, the ultrasound scan (especially in conjunction with the abdominal and vaginal findings), enables the obstetrician to make a tentative diagnosis of placenta previa without performing the hazardous pelvic examination. In these cases, continued hospitalization of the expectant mother is recommended because, with the ever present threat of recurrent hemorrhage, she is unquestionably safer in a setting where medical personnel and life-saving equipment are immediately accessible.

Despite the usefulness of the previous diagnostic techniques, the *definitive* diagnosis of placenta previa can rarely be established without directly palpating the placenta during a pelvic examination. Unfortunately, as was already alluded to, this procedure is extremely dangerous due to the fact that even the gentlest sort of manual probing can induce rapid, life-threatening hemorrhage. For this reason, every obstetrical textbook emphatically reiterates that both of the following conditions must be satisfied before undertaking a pelvic examination: the patient must be in an operating room that is fully prepared for an immediate blood transfusion(s) and cesarean section in case uncontrollable bleeding is precipitated; and delivery of the fetus must either be desirable or mandatory because, in the event that profuse hemorrhage develops, there will be no other way of preventing intrauterine hypoxia and death. Listed are the current indications and contraindications to the procedure:

1. A pelvic examination may be performed when the fetus is mature, as evidenced by a pregnancy of at least 37 weeks' duration and a fetal size (estimated by ultrasound) that correlates well with the length of gestation. Although the obstetrician might be inclined to postpone the procedure in order to allow the fetus additional time to grow in utero, this policy is not justified since the number of neonatal deaths attribu-

table to prematurity—the major fear when the examination induces profuse hemorrhage—does not decline significantly at this late stage of gestation. If the diagnosis of total or partial placenta previa is established, the pregnancy should be terminated by a cesarean delivery.

2. Regardless of the duration of the pregnancy, a pelvic examination is indicated when the patient is in active labor and is bleeding persistently or profusely. In this case, the obstetrician must quickly determine the source of the hemorrhage so that the appropriate measures can be taken to control the blood loss during the impending delivery.

3. A pelvic examination is contraindicated when circumstantial evidence, such as profuse hemorrhage in combination with an abnormal fetal presentation and a soft uterus, is sufficent to diagnose placenta previa. With such classic signs, attempting to confirm what is already a virtual certainty not only needlessly intensifies the blood loss regardless of its source, but also delays delivery.

4. The procedure should be withheld if the fetus is still premature (estimated weight of less than 2,500 grams and pregnancy of less than 37 weeks' duration), and the mother is neither in active labor nor is bleeding heavily. The purpose of this conservative approach, called *expectant therapy*, is to give the fetus more time to develop in utero, since every day that the gestation is prolonged (up until about 37th week of pregnancy), the perinatal survival rate increases dramatically.

    Expectant therapy is also advisable from the standpoint of the mother's health. Since these women are not in immediate danger of hemorrhage, it is much safer to confine them to bed for 48 hours and closely evalute their status, than to risk the possibility of precipitating profuse bleeding and early delivery by performing a pelvic examination. Under these circumstances, the diagnostic information can be sufficiently pieced together from the indirect findings of the ultrasound scan, and the abdominal and vaginal examinations. If placenta previa cannot be ruled out, the patient must be managed as though it were present, which means remaining under close observation until the fetus reaches maturity, at which time a pelvic examination may be performed if necessary. However, even when the fetus is not yet mature, expectant therapy must be abandoned if spontaneous labor begins, or if heavy bleeding recurs and cannot be brought under control.

§ 13.9   —Delivery of the Fetus

Delivery of the fetus is indicated when one or more of the following conditions are present: the onset of spontaneous labor (there is always a chance that it may ensue shortly after hemorrhage develops, even weeks or months before the expected due date), the persistence or recurrence of severe hemorrhage, or the discovery of placenta previa during a pelvic examination performed in accordance with the recommended guidelines. The choice between a cesarean delivery or a vaginal delivery depends on the clinical findings of each patient.

Since the conditions required to induce a safe vaginal delivery are rarely favorable in women with placenta previa, these patients are practically always delivered by cesarean section. Particularly when the syndrome is associated with violent bleeding, as in total placenta previa and most degrees of partial placenta previa, rapid delivery is required because the normal uterine mechanism of counteracting fatal hemorrhage, namely contraction of the uterine muscles against the broken blood vessels, seems to be ineffective while the fetus is inside the womb. In such emergency situations, there is no spare time to await the rather lengthy process of vaginal delivery. For the same reasons, unless vaginal delivery is imminent, a cesarean section is recommended when the fetus's heart rate, which must be monitored throughout the intrapartum period, indicates that it is in jeopardy.

Before performing the operation, the patient's diminished blood volume should be corrected by administering intravenous fluids and blood transfusions. Not only will the mother be better protected, but the compromised fetus will also recover more quickly in utero than if delivered while its mother is still in shock.

Vaginal deliveries are usually reserved for patients with mild forms of the syndrome such as marginal placenta previa, or for women with a total or partial placenta previa when there is little or no prospect of saving the baby's life. In the former group, permitting the fetus to continually compress the detached placenta and its broken blood vessels against the uterine wall during its descent through the birth canal is often an effective way of stopping the hemorrhage. If not, a cesarean section is indicated.

The pediatric staff should be notified as far in advance as possible to expect a high risk infant so they can make the appropriate preparations for its specific needs. After delivery, the newborn's hemoglobin should be measured to detect whether it, too, suffered significant blood loss, a likely event if the placenta was accidentally incised during the cesarean section. If the baby's hemoglobin concentration drops to 12 gm/dl (grams per deciliter) within 3 hours, or to 10 gm/dl within 24 hours, a blood transfusion is urgent.

Before the availability of blood transfusions and the more liberal use of cesarean sections, the hemorrhage caused by placenta previa was treated as a

life-threatening emergency. Today, however, the former policy of immediately terminating the woman's pregnancy, regardless of its duration, in order
to control her blood loss and thereby save her life, is no longer exclusively
advocated because less dramatic means of management have been shown to
offer a better fetal and maternal prognosis, especially when the fetus is still
premature and the hemorrhage can be controlled. Under these circumstances,
the current recommendations include hospitalization of the patient until the
fetus is mature, prolonged bed rest, careful evaluation of her hematologic status and the well-being of her fetus, and blood transfusions as indicated. This
therapy should be continued until intervention is forced by the onset of labor,
persistent or recurrent hemorrhage, or adequate fetal maturity.

§ 13.10   Prognosis

According to the optimistic predictions of some clinicians, the combination of
expectant therapy plus the immediate performance of a cesarean section when
severe hemorrhage develops can be expected to reduce the maternal death rate
to near zero.[8] At the present time, maternal mortality and morbidity primarily result from the hemorrhage and shock induced by placenta previa, from
the treatment of the syndrome, or both. The complications associated with
treatment include severe hemorrhage due to the pelvic examination, blood
transfusion reactions, serum hepatitis, infection, embolism, and operative
trauma to the reproductive tract (during a cesarean section).

   As far as the fetus is concerned, its health is generally not affected by the presence
of an abnormally implanted placenta unless the oxygen transfer to the placenta
is compromised by maternal shock due to extensive blood loss, a detached placental
fragment, or a prolapsed or compressed umbilical cord during delivery. Unfortunately, these events occur with increasing frequency as larger percentages of
the cervix are obstructed by the placenta, placing the developing fetus at a high
risk of intrauterine hypoxia and death. To prevent the occurrence of these disasters,
the obstetrician is often forced to deliver the fetus long before the due date, which
has ironically caused prematurity to become the greatest threat to perinatal survival.

---

[8] J.A. Pritchard, M.D. & P.C. MacDonald, M.D., Williams Obstetrics, 16th ed., 514 (Appleton-Century-Crofts, 1980).

§ 13.11 Bibliography and Recommended Readings

Danforth, D.N., Ph.D., M.D., *Obstetrics and Gynecology*, 4th ed. (Harper & Row Publishers, Inc., 1982).

Iffy, *Contribution to the Etiology of Placenta Previa*, 83 Am. J. Obstet. Gynecol., 969 (1962).

Iffy, Leslie, M.D. & Kaminetzky, Harold A., M.D., *Principles and Practice of Obstetrics & Perinatology*, vol. 2 (John Wiley & Sons, Inc., 1981).

Niswander, K.R., M.D., *Obstetrics, Essentials of Clinical Practice* (Little, Brown & Co., Inc., 1981).

Pritchard, J.A., M.D., MacDonald, P.C., M.D., & Gant, N.F., M.D., *Williams Obstetrics*, 17th ed. (Appleton-Century-Crofts, 1985).

CHAPTER 14

HYPERTENSIVE DISORDERS IN PREGNANCY

§ 14.1   Introduction

The physiologic changes accompanying pregnancy may induce hypertension in women who did not previously have high blood pressure, or intensify it in those who already have the disease. In either case, generalized edema and/or proteinuria (protein in the urine) often occur in conjunction with the hypertension, and convulsions and coma may also develop, especially if the syndrome is not detected and treated in its early stages. For many years, the disorders characterized by these abnormalities (most notably preeclampsia and eclampsia) were called the toxemias of pregnancy, a term that is still used despite the more recent recommendations of the American College of Obstetricians and Gynecologists. See their more accurate definitions and classifications in §§ 14.2 through 14.7.

§ 14.2 —Hypertension

During pregnancy, hypertension is defined as:

1. A diastolic blood pressure of 90 mm Hg (millimeters of mercury) or more; or,
2. A systolic blood pressure of 140 mm Hg or more; or,
3. A rise of 15 mm Hg or more above the prepregnancy diastolic level, or a rise of 30 mm Hg or more above the prepregnancy systolic level.

The diagnosis should only be made when these abnormal levels are manifest on at least two occasions, six or more hours apart, and are compared with previous blood pressure readings. These specifications are necessary because physical activity, psychological stress, and hormonal changes frequently elicit transient fluctuations in the arterial blood pressure, thereby making it unlikely for a single measurement to reflect the patient's actual condition.

§ 14.3 —Preeclampsia

One of the few syndromes that occur exclusively during pregnancy, preeclampsia is characterized by hypertension, proteinuria, edema, and sudden, excessive weight gain. It typically develops after the 20th week of gestation, though it may appear earlier in association with certain diseases. Since it is seen predominantly in primigravidas, the diagnosis of preeclampsia should be made cautiously in multigravidas, who may have other vascular disorders which coincidentally present with similar clinical findings.

§ 14.4 —Eclampsia

When preeclampsia progresses to its most advanced stages, convulsions occur, signaling the official onset of eclampsia. By definition, the convulsions may not be induced by other underlying neurologic disorders such as epilepsy, encephalitis or cerebral hermorrhage, or a toxic response to anesthetic agents.

The worldwide perinatal mortality rate associated with eclampsia may be as high as 30-35 percent,[1] making it one of the most dangerous complications of modern obstetrics.

---

[1] Gilstrap, Cunningham, & Whalley, *Management of Pregnancy-Induced Hypertension in the Nulliparous Patient Remote from Term,* 2 Semin. Perinatology 73–79 (1978).

Besides facing the same dangers as she did throughout preeclampsia, the eclamptic patient is also liable to seriously injure herself during the course of a convulsion, which is essentially a period of violent, uncontrollable muscular contractions. After her seizure subsides, the woman usually lapses into a coma. As long as the convulsions do not occur very often, she usually regains some degree of consciousness following each attack, but if they recur frequently, she is likely to die.

The life of the fetus is also endangered during convulsive attacks, primarily because the muscular contractions of the mother's body temporarily reduce the uterine blood flow and thereby limit the fetal oxygen supply. If the seizures last for a long time or if the interval between successive seizures is short, the fetus is liable to die as a result of intrauterine hypoxia. Its chances for survival are also threatened because labor usually begins spontaneously shortly after the onset of convulsions, and progresses to such a rapid completion that skillful, obstetrical management is required to prevent serious birth trauma or death.

Fortunately, convulsions can almost always be prevented by properly caring for preeclamptic patients as soon as the syndrome is diagnosed. As previously mentioned, many obstetricians prophylactically administer magnesium sulfate to women with severe preeclampsia in order to forestall the convulsions, prevent intracranial hemorrhage, or serious damage to other vital organs, and increase the probability of delivering an infant who will thrive. Yet even though the physician dutifully adheres to this protocol, he must still be prepared for the development of fulminant convulsions by always having the necessary anticonvulsive medication and equipment available.

Frequent examinations of preeclampic patients, another crucial step in the prophylaxis of eclampsia, should include regular measurements of the blood pressure, auscultation of the chest, testing of the deep tendon reflexes, and observation for hyperactivity or other evidence of impending convulsions. The presence of any of the following signs and symptoms in a preeclamptic woman indicates that eclampsia is imminent;

1. A sharp increase in blood pressure,
2. Marked hyperreflexia (especially transient or sustained ankle clonus),
3. A sharp increase in proteinuria,
4. A urinary output of less than 30 ml per hour,
5. Epigastric pain,
6. Visual problems,
7. Drowsiness, or
8. Severe headaches.

Continuous monitoring of the fetus's status is mandatory since its heart rate commonly decreases following convulsions, indicating that it may be in serious distress. Some clinicians report improved fetal outcome when the convulsions are controlled and oxygen is administered to the mother, because these measures allow the woman (and in turn, her baby) to overcome the hypoxia and acidosis precipitated by the attack.[2] They advocate this conservative therapy instead of a quickly performed cesarean section. Cesarean deliveries, which should be undertaken in a patient who is comatose or who is continuing to have convulsive attacks since the stress of the surgery may be lethal, should only be considered when the coma or seizures have subsided for at least 12 hours and the status of the cardiovascular and pulmonary systems has stabilized.

After delivery, the first sign of recovery is often an increased urine output. Conversely, pulmonary edema, cerebral hemorrhage, cyanosis, a rapid heart rate, and a sharp fall in blood pressure are grave prognostic signs, often occurring shortly before the mother's death. Oxygen therapy should be initiated immediately in a patient who exhibits any of these signs. Eclampsia resembles preeclampsia in that the pathologic changes completely disappear after delivery, leaving no neurologic deficits or vascular diseases as long as no underlying disorders were responsible for its onset.

§ 14.5 —Superimposed Preeclampsia or Eclampsia

Superimposed preeclampsia or eclampsia refers to the onset of preeclampsia or eclampsia in a patient with chronic hyptertensive vascular or renal disease.

§ 14.6 —Chronic Hypertensive Disease

Regardless of the cause, chronic hypertensive disease is defined as the presence of a continually elevated blood pressure before pregnancy, prior to the 20th week of gestation, or persisting six or more weeks after delivery.

---

[2] Gant, Chand, Worley, et al., *A Clinical Test Useful for Predicting the Development of Acute Hypertension in Pregnancy*, 120 *Am. J. Obstet. Gynecol.* 1 (1974).

§ 14.7 —Gestational Hypertension

Gestational hypertension is hypertension precipitated by the state of pregnancy in a patient who did not previously have high blood pressure. Developing during either the latter half of gestation or the first 24 hours following delivery, this syndrome is not accompanied by the other classic signs and symptoms of preeclampsia or hypertensive vascular disease, and it disappears within 10 days after delivery.

Although the etiology of the hypertensive disorders in pregnancy is still unknown, research has shown that the disease complex is accompanied by spasms in the mother's arteries which are ultimately responsible for the poor fetal and maternal prognosis. The deleterious sequence of events occurs because the spasms reduce the diameter of the arteries and thereby cause a decrease in the blood flow to the woman's vital organs, as well as to the developing fetus in her uterus, and a rise in her blood pressure in order to compensate for the circulatory derangement. These problems become increasingly more ominous toward the end of gestation.

Since the fetus is completely dependent on its mother's bloodstream for nutrients and oxygen, it faces a high risk of malnourishment, growth retardation, mental deficiencies, and death whenever her circulation is impaired. Yet efforts to spare the child from these adverse intrauterine conditions by delivering it before term often result in the birth of a premature baby who is too underdeveloped to survive, even in an intensive care unit. Nonetheless, most obstetricians believe that the lesser of the two evils is prematurity because with proper medical assistance, at least some of these newborns will eventually be able to overcome the difficulties of their inadequate organ development and lead normal lives, an impossibility if intrauterine hypoxia is allowed to take its full course. The fate of the fetus depends to a large extent on the severity of its mother's disorder.

From the standpoint of the mother's health, the hypertensive disorders in pregnancy are also very dangerous because in addition to the metabolic derangements, there is also the likelihood of concurrent or subsequent cardiac failure, stroke, violent episodes of convulsions, and impaired renal and pulmonary function. Another potentially disastrous complication that is frequently observed with this disease complex is premature separation of the placenta (abruptio placenta). Like the other sequelae, it too endangers the lives of both the mother and her unborn child. See **Chapter 13** for a discussion of placental abruption.

Despite the fact that the hypertensive disorders in pregnancy are one of the leading causes of mortality in obstetric patients (ranking third after hemorrhage and infection), many clinicians claim that the death toll can be almost entirely eradicated by recognizing and treating the early signs and symptoms of these disorders before their life-threatening complications arise.[3] The obstetrician's efforts are especially well-rewarded in preeclampsia since the pure form of this disorder appears to be completely reversible after delivery, regardless of its severity. The only long-term effect is a hereditory predisposition to preeclampsia in daughters of women who suffered from the syndrome.

§ 14.8   Signs and Symptoms

One of the earliest and most important warning signs of impending or actual preeclampsia is a weight gain of two or more pounds in any given week, or six or more pounds in a month, particularly during the third trimester. Whereas a gradual weight increase of about one pound per week throughout the last two thirds of gestation is considered normal and healthy, a *sudden, excessive weight* gain usually indicates an abnormal retention of sodium and water. Generally, the weight gain occurs before the more visible signs of edema, such as swollen eyelids, fingers, ankles, or feet appear.

Another telltale sign is a substantial rise in the blood pressure (see § **14.2**) or an upward trend in the diastolic blood pressure despite the fact that the value is still in the normal range. The last stipulation is necessary because the hemodynamic changes associated with a normal gestation usually cause a 10-15 mmHg drop in the prepregnancy diastolic blood pressure during the second trimester, presumably because a portion of the mother's blood supply is channeled to the placenta. Consequently, hypertension may be masked and easily overlooked unless the obstetrician makes a point of checking for suggestive patterns in the patient's previous blood pressure results. The midpregnancy physiologic alterations also explain why the blood pressure measurements of preeclamptic women do not tend to be extremely high, except in severely affected patients and those with preexisting hypertensive vascular disease.

Proteinuria, which is typically the last of the three major signs to appear, may be minimal or even absent in the early stages of preeclampsia, but as the disorder progressively worsens, the concentrations of protein rise. Due to the appreciable diurnal and hourly variation in the urinary excretion of protein, a 24-hour specimen is required for accurate quantitation. A concentration of greater than 300 mg-per-liter in 24 hours is defined as proteinuria, though even smaller amounts of protein are considered abnormal and should not be disregarded.

---

[3] R.J. Bolognese, R.J. Schwartz, & J. Schneider, Perinatal Medicine, 2nd ed., 351 (Williams & Wilkins, 1982).

The importance of early and continual prenatal care for all pregnant wo-men cannot be emphasized enough. Only by routinely weighing each patient, measuring her blood pressure, and analyzing her urine at every prenatal visit can the obstetrician hope to detect the three cardinal signs of incipient or mild preeclampsia before the syndrome becomes so severe that it threatens the lives of the mother and fetus. These simple evaluations are particularly impor-tant in view of the fact that hypertension and proteinuria are both asymptom-atic, so the woman is typically unaware of the early progress of the disease until she develops headaches, epigastric pain, and visual disturbances (ranging from a slight blurring of vision to blindness), by which time preeclampsia is already very advanced. Nevertheless, the obstetrician must instruct each ex-pectant mother (at her first prenatal examination) to immediately report the onset of these more obvious signs and symptoms instead of dangerously wait-ing for her next scheduled appointment, which could be anywhere from one to four weeks away.

In addition to the standard obstetrical protocol, especially close observation is required for women known to be predisposed to preeclampsia. Included in this group are nulliparas, particularly those under 17 or over 35 years of age; women carrying multiple fetuses; patients with a family history of preeclamp-sia or eclampsia; or those who have diabetes mellitus, chronic hypertensive or renal disease, hydatidiform mole, fetal hydrops, an increased volume of amni-otic fluid, or a history of stillborns.

Recently, another category of high risk patients has been discovered. Using a procedure known alternatively as the roll over test or supine pressor test, researchers have demonstrated that a blood pressure change can be instantly induced by having the woman lie on her side for about 15 minutes, and then roll over onto her back (the supine position). Over 90 percent of normotensive nulliparas who later developed pregnancy-induced hypertension showed at least a 20 mmHg elevation in their diastolic blood pressure between the 28th and 32nd weeks of gestation following the position change. Conversely, al-most the same percentage of those who did not develop pregnancy-induced hypertension did not exhibit such an increase in blood pressure in response to the position change.[4] Many clinicians believe this simple procedure has great promise for use in identifying susceptible patients so they can be carefully watched and treated as soon as the disease manifestations arise.[5]

---

[4] J.A. Pritchard, & P.C. MacDonald, Williams Obstetrics 16th ed., 682 (Appleton-Century-Crofts, 1980).

[5] D.N. Danforth, Ph.D., M.D., Obstetrics and Gynecology, 4th ed. 470 (Harper & Row Pub-lishers, Inc., 1982).

§ 14.9 Prevention and Treatment

Despite the fact that the cause of preeclampsia is still unknown, experience has shown which measures are likely to prevent its occurrence. Of prominent importance is a well-balanced diet consisting of an ample daily intake of protein, vitamins, and minerals. There is no evidence that restricting the normal average salt consumption of 4-6 grams per day prevents preeclampsia, though foods with a particularly high sodium content should be avoided during pregnancy since *excessive* salt intake can aggravate the disease process by causing the patient to retain additional water. Low calorie diets are also not recommended because they do not appear to affect the cause of sudden, excessive weight gains (namely water retention, rather than fat accumulation), and may actually be detrimental to the fetus's growth. Similarly, diuretic medications, once a highly acclaimed method of managing sodium and water retention in incipient, mild, and in some cases, severe preeclampsia, were not only found to be ineffective but even potentially harmful due to their disruption of the optimal electrolyte balance and impairment of other bodily functions. Consequently, instead of imposing strict low calorie diets, limiting the salt intake, and prescribing dangerous diuretics such as the thiazide compounds, patients predisposed to preeclampsia are currently managed by long periods of bed rest. Encouraging the woman to lie on her left side is advisable because that position improves the blood flow to her uterus and kidneys, resulting in enhanced fetal oxygenation and increased urine output without the need for diuretic drugs.

Sedatives are often given to enforce bed rest in ambulatory patients and in hospitalized patients who are not expected to give birth right away. Phenobarbital is the standard choice, though the possibility of its adverse fetal effects must always be taken into account.

Many physicians consider magnesium sulfate to be the most important single agent in the management of severe preeclampsia and eclampsia due to its ability to prevent convulsions and control their recurrence.[6] Despite its unquestionable value when administered in the therapeutic range of 6-8 mEq/L (milliequivalents per liter), serious toxicity (the woman's knee jerk reflex disappears and cardiorespiratory failure ultimately develops) results when the blood levels of the drug climb to 10-15 mEq/L. In order to prevent potentially lethal overdoses, it is mandatory to test the patient's knee, ankle, and biceps reflexes before and after injecting magnesium sulfate, and to have a vial of 10 percent calcium gluconate (an antidote which instantly reverses the toxic effects) available for use at all times. A repeat dose of magnesium sulfate

---

[6] *Id.* at 470-71.

is contraindicated by a very sluggish or nonexistent knee-jerk reflex, a respiratory rate below 16 breaths-per-minute, and a urinary output of less than 100 ml in the preceding four hours.

In addition to potential maternal toxicity, magnesium sulfate may also be toxic for the newborn. Infants who have very slow respirations or decreased reflex activity may need an exchange transfusion in order to replace their tainted blood with healthy blood.

At the present time, the consensus is that antihypertensive medications have no effect on the underlying mechanisms of the hypertensive disorders.[7] Therefore, they are only recommended if the patient's diastolic blood pressure exceeds 110 mm Hg because under these circumstances, the severe hypertension must be treated in order to prevent the development of a stroke. Hydralazine is preferred over diazoxide since the latter is known to cause a steep blood pressure decrease, which dangerously diminishes the blood flow to the woman's vital organs as well as to the developing fetus in her uterus.

The following regimens are recommended by most obstetricians for managing the different stages of preeclampsia.[8]

Incipient Preeclampsia.   The patient with incipient preeclampsia (excessive weight gain with ankle edema; elevated blood pressure, but below 140/90 or less than 30 mm Hg systolic and 15 mm Hg diastolic above the prepregnancy levels; no proteinuria) may be tentatively managed at home as long as neither her health nor that of her fetus's decline. Examinations should be performed twice a week, thoroughly checking for any changes in the maternal or fetal conditions which might necessitate hospitalization. Included among the prophylactic measures are:

1.   A high-protein diet (1.5 grams of protein for each kilogram of body weight) with no salt restriction if the syndrome is discovered before the 32nd week of gestation

2.   Bed rest for 12 hours each day

3.   Phenobarbital, 30-60 mg given three times per day

4.   Hospitalization, if preeclampsia is diagnosed.

Mild Preeclampsia.   All patients with preeclampsia should be hospitalized. In the mild stages (blood pressure is less than 170/100 or systolic/diastolic

---

[7] R.J. Bolognese, R.J. Schwartz, & J. Schneider, Perinatal Medicine, 2nd ed., 360 (Williams & Wilkins, 1982).

[8] J.A. Pritchard, & P.C. MacDonald, Williams Obstetrics 16th ed., 690-92 (Appleton-Century-Crofts, 1980).

blood pressure is not greater than 40/20 mm Hg above prepregnancy or early pregnancy levels; urine protein is less than 5 grams per 24 hours; edema is not massive), the following regimen is suggested to correct the specific manifestations of the disease and prevent it from becoming worse:

1. A high-protein diet
2. Bed rest with bathroom privileges
3. Daily weighing
4. Evaluation of the fetal heart rate every 4 hours
5. Phenobarbital, 30-60 mg every 6 hours while patient is awake
6. Evaluation of the fetal maturity and condition of the maternal pelvis and cervix in case delivery is needed.

Severe Preeclampsia. The management of the woman with severe preeclampsia (blood pressure is above 170/100 or systolic/diastolic blood pressure is greater than 60/30 mm Hg above prepregnancy or early pregnancy levels; urine protein exceeds 5 gms in 24 hours; urine output is 500 ml or less in 24 hours; massive generalized or pulmonary edema) is symptomatic rather than preventative. The requirements are:

1. Absolute bed rest
2. Close observation
3. Magnesium sulfate to suppress hyperreflexia
4. Determination of fluid intake and output
5. Continuous fetal monitoring until delivery is completed
6. Delivery of the baby after adequately sedating the mother.

Eclampsia. The regimen for eclamptic patients include:

1. Absolute bed rest in a perfectly quiet, darkened room
2. Constant observation
3. Hourly determination of urinary output
4. Hourly monitoring of the fetal heart rate
5. Having equipment available to maintain a patent airway and prevent trauma to the woman's tongue and lips if another seizure occurs
6. Magnesium sulfate
7. Morphine sulfate to maintain deep sedation

8. Intravenous sodium diphenylhydantoin if seizures persist in spite of the treatment above

9. Delivery as soon as the seizures are controlled

Further management of the patient depends on the severity of her syndrome, its immediate response to treatment, and the precise gestational age of the fetus. As long as preeclampsia is mild and the therapeutic regimen corrects, or at least stabilizes, the woman's altered physiology, her pregnancy is allowed to continue—though under close observation and only until the fetus is mature enough to survive outside the uterus. In contrast to normal gestations, when the hypertensive disorders complicate a pregnancy, the obstetrician is obliged to rely on frequent tests of the placental function and fetal well-being in order to select the most favorable time of delivery since awaiting spontaneous labor is considered too dangerous. In fact, some clinicians never allow the gestation to continue past 37 weeks, claiming that the single risk of prematurity is far outweighed by the hazards of preeclampsia and its sequelae.[9]

When mild cases of preeclampsia cannot be brought under control within 24-48 hours following therapy, or when the syndrome is severe to begin with, termination of the pregnancy is mandatory in the best interests of the mother and the fetus. Postponing delivery in order to give the fetus additional time to mature in utero is not advisable in the advanced stages of preeclampsia due to the adverse effects of the diminished utero-placental blood flow. Many physicians believe that even an underweight and underdeveloped fetus has a greater chance of survival in a neonatal intensive care unit than in an oxygen deficient uterus. Besides the threat of intrauterine growth retardation and death, there is the ever-present danger that the expectant mother may develop convulsions, in which case the lives of both the woman and her unborn child are in serious jeopardy. To guard against this outcome, most obstetricians routinely administer magnesium sulfate throughout labor and during the first 24 hours after delivery, the critical periods during which seizures are liable to develop, particularly in patients who have already had such attacks.[10]

Induction of labor, which is almost always preferrable to a cesarean delivery, may be attempted by infusing oxytocin and/or rupturing the membranes. However, if active labor does not ensue within six hours of the start of the oxytocin infusion, or if immediate delivery is needed to save the baby's life, a cesarean section is the procedure of choice.

---

9 Leslie, Iffy, M.D. & Harold A. Kaminetzky, M.D., Principles and Practice of Obstetrics & Perinatology, vol. 2, 1286 (John Wiley & Sons, Inc., 1981).

10 J.A. Pritchard, & P.C. MacDonald, Williams Obstetrics 16th ed., 691 (Appleton-Century-Crofts, 1980).

Regardless of the route of delivery, continual monitoring of the fetal heart rate and frequent evaluation of the mother's blood pressure, fluid intake, urinary output, and uterine contractions are mandatory. The reason why regular blood pressure measurements are essential during the intrapartum and immediate postpartum periods is because preeclamptic and eclamptic women have a lower blood volume than normal pregnant women, making them less able to tolerate the typical blood loss accompanying the birth process. If their blood pressure falls abruptly during labor, it is usually indicative of severe hemorrhage or shock, and must therefore not be mistakenly interpreted as the immediate relief of their hypertension. The recommended treatment consists of blood transfusions and lactated Ringer's solution.

Anesthetics must also be carefully chosen due to the preeclamptic patient's poor vascular condition. Inhalation anesthesia is favored over spinal, caudal, or lumbar anesthetics because the latter preparations may produce sudden, severe hypotension.

Despite years of extensive research, delivery of the fetus is the only known care for preeclampsia. As long as no underlying diseases were responsible for triggering the syndrome, not only does the mother's health return to normal after she gives birth, but the characteristic signs and symptoms of preeclampsia completely disappear and do not recur in future pregnancies. Even when a predisposing condition does exist, high quality obstetrical care can prevent the onset of preeclampsia in most of the subsequent gestations.

§ 14.10   Chronic Hypertension

The disease state known as chronic hypertension, which is characterized by a *continually* elevated blood pressure, may cause damage to any region of the vascular system. Although it most frequently complicates the gestation of older women and obese women, any pregnant patient with chronic hypertensive disease is at a high risk of developing cardiac failure, stroke, premature separation of the placenta, or superimposed preeclampsia.

Bed rest during the latter months of gestation is crucial for these women because besides improving their poor blood flow, it may also help prevent the dangerous development of preeclampsia. In addition to restricting their activity, the obstetrician should avoid administering spinal or epidural blockade anesthetics to chronically hypertensive patients since these agents are likely to induce harmful decreases in their blood pressure.

During labor, the blood pressure of hypertensive patients, particularly those with superimposed preeclampsia, is likely to rise suddenly, so it must be checked frequently. However, the value of *routinely* administering antihypertensive medication to them during the intrapartum or antepartum periods is still controversial.[11] Women who were taking antihypertensive drugs *prior to* pregnancy, are usually maintained on the same medications during pregnancy, though their dosages must be closely regulated (reducing it in midpregnancy and generally increasing it in the last trimester) in accordance with the known gestational blood pressure fluctuations. For those who develop hypertension *during* the course of their pregnancies, antihypertensive medication is only indicated when their blood pressure dangerously persists over 100 mmHg. In mildest cases, it might also be theoretically beneficial to prescribe these drugs to lower the patient's blood pressure, but this advantage must be carefully weighed against the further reduction in the already compromised uteroplacental circulation which would result, and be likely to endanger, the fetus's life.

One of the most common and most feared complications in pregnant women with chronic vascular diseases, is the onset of preeclampsia. Developing in 10-30 percent of the patients,[12] the syndrome is apt to occur relatively early and explosively in gestation, manifested by a sudden rise in blood pressure (the systolic pressure often exceeds 130 mm Hg) and almost always associates with substantial proteinuria, decreased urine output, and the retention of toxic nitrogenous compounds. Extensive hemorrhages and exudates may be seen in the retina, and eclamptic convulsions and coma may also be present. Because the maternal and fetal status rapidly deteriorates when preeclampsia becomes superimposed on essential hypertension, and because the disease complex is much more difficult to manage than preeclampsia alone, the patient should be hospitalized as soon as the diagnosis is made. Prompt termination of the pregnancy is required in order to prevent maternal and fetal death when the diastolic blood pressure persists above 110 mm Hg, when significant proteinuria develops, when the cardiac or renal function becomes impaired, or when the tests of fetal well-being are unfavorable.

In order to detect the almost inevitable episodes of fetal distress in gestations complicated by chronic hypertension (either with or without concurrent preeclampsia), complete intrauterine evaluation of the fetal status, especially fetal heart monitoring, is essential during the antepartum and intrapartum periods. The increased incidence of life-threatening complications resulting from either the effects of the impaired uteroplacental circulation, or the need to deliver these fetuses prematurely, makes it mandatory to alert the neonatal intensive care staff of these births so they can arrange for the proper care of the compromised newborns.

---

[11] *Id.* at 696.

[12] *Id.* at 697.

§ 14.11   Bibliography and Recommended Readings

Arias, Fernando, M.D., Ph.D., *High-Risk Pregnancy and Delivery* (The C.V. Mosby Co., 1984).

Danforth, D.N., Ph.D., M.D., *Obstetrics and Gynecology*, 4th ed. (Harper & Row Publishers, Inc., 1982).

Gant, N.F., Worley, R.J., Cunningham, F.G., & Whalley, P.J., *Clinical Management of Pregnancy Induced Hypertension*, in 21 Clinical Obstetrics & Gynecology 397 (Harper & Row Publishers, Inc., June, 1978).

Greenhill, J.P., M.D. & Friedman, Emanuel A., M.D., *Hypertensive States of Pregnancy* in Biological Principles and Modern Practice of Obstetrics (W.B. Saunders Co., 1974).

Haesslein, Hanns C., M.D. & Niswander, Kenneth R., M.D., *Fetal Distress in Term Pregnancies*, 137 Am. J. Obstet. Gynecol. 245 (1980).

Iffy, Leslie, M.D. & Kaminetzky, Harold A., M.D., *Principles and Practice of Obstetrics & Perinatology*, vol. 2 (John Wiley & Sons, Inc., 1981).

Lindheimer & Katz, *Pathophysiology of Preeclampsia*, 32 Ann. Rev. Med. 273-89 (1981).

Niswander, K.R., M.D., *Obstetrics, Essentials of Clinical Practice* (Little, Brown & Co., Inc., 1981).

Pritchard, J.A., M.D., MacDonald, P.C., M.D., & Gant, N.F., M.D., *Williams Obstetrics*, 17th ed. (Appleton-Century-Crofts, 1985).

Queenan, John T., M.D., *Management of High-Risk Pregnancy* (Medical Economics Co., 1980).

Studd, J., *Preeclampsia*, 18 Br. J. Hosp. Med., 52 (1977).

DIABETES MELLITUS

§ 15.1 Introduction

Diabetes mellitus is characterized by an abnormally high concentration of glucose in the bloodstream, which typically develops when the body's insulin mechanism is impaired. Inability to regulate the normal blood glucose levels is particularly dangerous for a pregnant diabetic because the deleterious effects of the disease not only further strain her poor health, but also subject her unborn child to profound risks during gestation and labor. Unless her abnormal glucose levels are carefully controlled by diet and/or insulin therapy, the fetus is likely to die in utero. Or, if it survives within the womb, it is prone to birth injuries as a result of its characteristically large body size relative to the dimensions of its mother's pelvis. Also, the placenta is known to age prematurely, and thus at term, placental function is diminished. Since early diagnosis and prompt initiation of insulin therapy will dramatically improve this bleak fetal outlook, routine antepartum screening to detect diabetes mellitis is essential.

Diabetes mellitus, which complicates approximately 1 percent of all pregnancies,[1] should be suspected in women with the following background or clinical symptoms:

1. A family history of the disorder;

2. A previous baby who weighed more than 4,000 grams;

---

[1] D.N. Danforth, M.D., *Obstetrics and Gynecology*, 4th ed., 526-27 Harper & Row Publishers, Inc., (1982).

3. A previous unexplained intrauterine fetal death near term;

4. A previous fetal deformity;

5. Sugar in the urine;

6. An increased volume of amniotic fluid or urine;

7. Excessive weight gain or obesity.

Suspicion of diabetes is also intensified upon discovering retinal and neurological disorders, impaired kidney function, or unexplained vascular disturbances, since these conditions frequently result from the diabetic disease process.

A variety of stressful situations such as obesity, infection, and pregnancy may trigger the onset of diabetes. Because the physiologic changes associated with pregnancy progressively impair the action of insulin, a woman who was not diabetic either before she became pregnant, or in the early months of gestation, may suddenly develop the disorder in the latter half of her pregnancy. To prevent overlooking these cases of pregnancy-induced or gestational diabetes, all women should be screened in the first trimester. If they are normal, they should be retested later in pregnancy to ensure that their glucose levels have not abruptly risen.

To distinguish their different clinical pictures, diagnostic features, and methods of treatment, diabetes mellitus is generally divided into two basic categories—the overt form and the chemical form. Overt diabetes is diagnosed when two or more fasting blood sugar tests (a morning blood specimen assayed for glucose before the patient eats or drinks) are elevated, and when the typical symptoms of the disease are also present. A glucose value of 105 mg/dl (milligram per deciliter) or higher is considered abnormal for pregnant diabetics, as compared to a value of 120 mg/dl or higher for their nonpregnant counterparts.[2]

Unlike overt diabetes, chemical or gestational diabetes is a mild, *asymptomatic* disorder in which the patient has a normal fasting blood sugar, and only demonstrates abnormal responses when her system is stressed by the high sugar intake of a glucose tolerance test. To find out whether this diagnostic reaction can be elicited, a two-hour post-prandial blood sugar test (which some suggest as a routine screen for all pregnant women), or more preferably, a three-hour oral glucose tolerance test is performed. In the latter, the patient is placed on a high carbohydrate diet (100-300 grams of carbohydrate per day) for three days. On the morning of the fourth day, the woman's blood is drawn to measure her overnight fasting blood sugar concentration. Next, she is given

---

[2] Gilmer, Beard, Brooke, & Oakly, *Carbohydrate Metabolism in Pregnancy* 3 *Br. Med. J.* 399 (1975).

a special glucose solution to drink and is then instructed not to eat or drink any sweetened beverages during the procedure. Her response (tolerance) to the high glucose load is measured by drawing her blood one, two, and three hours after she has finished the solution. In normal individuals, the excess sugar is promptly removed from the bloodstream by the insulin mechanism, thereby restoring the physiologic level of glucose, but since this metabolic pathway is impaired in diabetics, the glucose levels remain elevated for a longer period than is ordinarily expected. Chemical diabetes can therefore be diagnosed when two or more of the following glucose results equal or exceed the established values.

Fasting—105 mg/dl
1 hour—190 mg/dl
2 hour—165 mg/dl
3 hour—145 mg/dl

Since any laboratory results differ somewhat depending on the technologist and the specific procedure used, the table of glucose values should not be regarded as an absolute, but rather as a representative guideline for understanding how the diagnosis is made.

The oral glucose tolerance test may sometimes be difficult to interpret if the glucose levels are not blatantly abnormal, in which case other clinical signs and symptoms may be helpful.

Another point to remember is that the results of repeated tests in the same patient may differ because glucose metabolism varies with the length of gestation. Since the incidence of gestational diabetes far exceeds that of the overt form, its potential impact on perinatal outcome for a defined population may be more significant. It has been estimated that in 1973, as many as 4,500 pregnancies in the United States resulted in perinatal death from undiagnosed or untreated gestational diabetes.[3] Therefore, the importance of screening for abnormal glucose tolerance during pregnancy must be reemphasized.

The rate of perinatal mortality in insulin-dependent diabetics has increased markedly over the past five decades.[4] This is due to improvement in the control of diabetes as well as better obstetric and neonatal care. Before these advances, reduction of perinatal mortality required delivery at about 36 to 37 weeks by cesarean section or induction of labor. It was well known that the fetus of a diabetic gravida could die suddenly at any time in the third trimes-

---

[3] O'Sullivan, Charles, Maham, et al., *Gestational Diabetes and Perinatal Mortality Rate*, 116 *Am. J. Obstet. Gynecol. 901 (1973)*.

[4] Schwartz, & Fields, *The Management of the Pregnant Diabetic*, 26 *Obstet. Gynecol. Surv.* 277 (1971).

ter, or during labor. The pathologic findings are nonspecific and appear to relate to hyperglycemia and hyperinsulinemia on the one hand, and to mild, chronic hypoxia on the other. None of these explain fully the events leading to sudden fetal death. Babies with macrosomia (4,000 grams or more) tend to have severe neonatal hypoglycemia about 30 minutes after birth, just about the time the glucose received from the maternal circulation has been dissipated.

Adashi and colleagues have suggested that a neonatal blood-glucose level of 30 mg percent or less defines hypoglycemia in babies weighing 2,500 grams or more, whereas a level of 20 mg percent or less should be used to define this condition in those weighing less.[5] Many authorities ascribe to the theory that inadequate control of maternal hyperglycemia, during the second half of gestation, lends to fetal macrosomia.[6] It is reasonable to assume that strict control of maternal blood sugar might reduce macrosomia and neonatal hypoglycemia, consequent to the fetal hyperinsulinism.

It has been suggested that in pregnancies complicated by maternal diabetes, an intrauterine environment of mild hypoxia exits. This is thought to be due to alterations in placental hemodynamics.

Hydramnios is common in insulin-dependent diabetics; however, the pathogenesis is unknown since the controlling factors for amniotic volume have not been defined.

Regardless of the severity of their disease, all diabetic patients require close supervision and management of their condition by experienced physicians throughout their pregnancies. As long as no unusual circumstances arise, biweekly examinations are recommended for the first six months, and at least weekly after that time. The obstetrician's primary objective is to maintain the woman's blood glucose in the normal physiologic range, since control of maternal hyperglycemia (high blood sugar) is an important factor governing the outcome of the pregnancy. This is achieved by measuring the glucose concentration at each visit, and either initiating insulin therapy if necessary, or adjusting the existing insulin dose to the appropriate level. At the same time, the carbon dioxide (CO_2) content and urea nitrogen (BUN) concentration of the woman's blood should also be quantitated. Complete blood counts (CBC), urinalysis, and renal function tests should be performed regularly, and the fetal condition should be frequently assessed as well. If the patient has high blood pressure, her cardiovascular status should be evaluated.

Regulation of the glucose concentration is so essential that even between appointments, the woman must ensure that her metabolism always remains

---

[5] Adashi, Pinto, & Tyson, *Importance of Maternal Euglycemia for Fetal Outcome in Diabetic Pregnancy*, 133 Am. J. Obstet. Gynecol. 263 (1979).

[6] Coustan, & Lewis, *Insulin Therapy for Gestational Diabetics*, 51 Obstet. Gynecol., 306 (1978).

normal. Since the amount of sugar and acetone (ketone) in the *urine* reflect the *blood* glucose levels, measurement of these two urinary constituents enables the patient to continually monitor her delicate metabolism while she is at home. By dipping a color-coded plastic stick into her urine specimen and then comparing the two colors to a standardized chart, the patient can easily and accurately measure and keep a daily record of her sugar and acetone levels. If any marked fluctuations occur, she should be instructed to notify her obstetrician immediately.

The diet and insulin dosage must also be judiciously regulated. Pregnant diabetics should be advised to eat a well-balanced, high-protein diet and carefully distribute their food intake throughout the day, so as to avoid wide swings in blood glucose levels. The normal pregnancy weight gain of about 25 pounds should be the goal. Chemical or gestational diabetics are typically treated by dietary management alone, but if that regimen does not maintain the physiologic blood glucose level, insulin should be prescribed. The majority of women need to begin insulin therapy or increase their original dosage by the second trimester because the body requires progressively increased amounts of insulin as the pregnancy advances. The insulin requirements may also increase if any type of infection develops. On the other hand, it may decrease if the woman is vomiting, or it may vary in response to other complications. Established trends, as well as unpredictable fluctuations in the insulin requirements during pregnancy, make management of the diabetic woman extremely difficult.

Bedrest is also essential, particularly for patients with underlying vascular disease. Some suggest hospitalizing these women for most of the third trimester, or at least one week before the probable due date, to ensure adequate bedrest and allow ample testing time to detect any life-threatening fetal or maternal problems.[7] Hospitalization is mandatory for *all* diabetics when complications such as infection, toxemia, or difficulty controlling the diabetes arise, especially when they develop between the 30th and 35th week of gestation. Respiratory or urinary tract infections, fairly common occurrences during pregnancy, can rapidly precipitate a serious acid imbalance called ketoacidosis in a diabetic. This condition not only endangers the mother's life, but may adversely affect the neurological development of her unborn child as well.

With the advent of tools for antenatal monitoring of fetal health (ultrasonography, electronic fetal heart monitoring, estriol level determinations, etc.),

---

[7] Gabbe, Mestman, Freeman, Goebelsmann, Lowensohn, Nochimson, Centrulo & Quilligan, *Management and Outcome of Diabetes Mellitus, Classes B-R,* 129 Am. J. Obstet. Gynecol. 723 (1977).

it is usually not necessary to hospitalize the patient prior to the 35th week of gestation.

An important piece of evidence regarding fetal well-being is the mother's perception of fetal activity. She must be counseled to notify the obstetrician if she fails to feel motion for 16 hours or more, or if there is diminution in activity for two to three days. These changes frequently precede fetal death by as many as two to five days.

Even if no complications have occurred, some clinicians routinely admit their diabetic patients to the hospital around the 35th week of pregnancy, where they stay until the baby is born.[8] During the hospitalization, the woman is thoroughly examined and the fetus's heart rate is monitored to assess its condition and decide whether early delivery is necessary to avoid the risks of sustained intrauterine life. Dr. Danforth even recommends that every diabetic be hospitalized when she first becomes pregnant so her health and the extent of her vascular damage can be determined in detail and treated accordingly.[9] Dramatic improvement in the perinatal mortality rate has been reported when the appropriate prophylactic measures are begun in the earliest stages of gestation.[10]

Also, the majority of serious problems in the diabetic gravida usually occurs during the third trimester of pregnancy. The main clinical problems that arise are hydramnios, superimposed preeclampsia, and renal impairment with a nephrotic syndrome. Hydramnios itself is no cause for alarm, since most diabetics exhibit it to a certain degree. There are no data supporting the idea that the rate of perinatal mortality is correlated with the degree of hydramnios. Superimposed preeclampsia should be diligently sought and agressively treated. See § 14.5. The nephrotic syndrome, with or without a moderate degree of uremia, should be treated conservatively as long as the fetal health indicators and the maternal conditions are satisfactory.

Respiratory distress syndrome (RDS) in the infant has been a major cause of morbidity and mortality as a result of premature delivery often due to errors in gestational dating.[11] Thus, a critical determinant of the outcome of the diabetic pregnancy is the timing of delivery. The risk of intrauterine death increases as term approaches; on the other hand, the infant delivered preterm is exposed to the risks of prematurity, particularly that of respiratory distress, which may result in neonatal loss.

---

[8] D.N. Danforth, M.D., Obstetrics and Gynecology, 4th ed, 530 (Harper & Row Publishers, Inc., 1982).

[9] *Id.* at 531.

[10] *Id.* at 528.

[11] Leslie Iffy, M.D. & Harold A. Kaminetzky, M.D., Principles and Practice of Obstetrics & Perinatology, vol. 2, 1432 (John Wiley & Sons, Inc., 1981).

The combined use of daily monitoring by serial estriol measurements and periodic fetal heart rate monitoring provides the opportunity for following the fetal condition carefully while awaiting the development of functional lung maturity. Fetal biparietel diameter measurements by ultrasound have proven useful in determining fetal age and growth, particularly when an initial examination is performed early in gestation. This assists the physician in removing some of the uncertainties of pregnancy-dating, associated with irregular menses in the diabetic woman, and late macrosomia in her fetus. See §§ **10.6** through **10.8** for further discussion on ultrasound.

Since the major consequence of premature birth is respiratory distress syndrome (RDS), fetal pulmonary functional maturity is the most critical objective of current care. Biochemical estimations of this maturity can now be obtained from the analysis of amniotic fluid. The most popular biochemical method to evaluate fetal lung development is the measurement of amniotic fluid phospholipids as a direct reflection of fetal pulmonary surfactant.[12] The initial report on amniotic fluid lecithin to sphingomyelin (L/S) ratios was in 1971 by Louis Gluck and co-workers.[13] A mature L/S ratio of greater than 2:1 predicts the absence of RDS in newborns with 98 percent accuracy. Most of the infants who develop RDS but have mature L/S ratios are born to mothers with Class A to C diabetes mellitus, Rh isoimmunization, or fetuses who are severely asphyxiated.[14] Because physicians need more predictive information for managing complicated pregnancies, the lung profile was developed. The profile includes the L/S ratio and percentages of disaturated (acetone-precipitated) lecithin, phosphatidyl inositol (PI), and phosphatidyl glyceryl (PG) found in surfactant. Information from the lung profile will help obstetricians separate infants who will have a favorable neonatal respiratory outcome from those likely to develop neonatal pulmonary complications.[15] These determinations afford the physician an important new dimension in the management of the pregnant diabetic, particularly when maternal blood sugar control has been good, and a normal physiologic milieu has been approximated.

The application of current technology thus provides the clinical team with the means of minimizing both fetal death in utero, and preventable neonatal

---

[12] R.J. Bolognese, R.H. Schwartz, & J. Schneider, Perinatal Medicine, 26d ed. 200 (Williams & Wilkins Co., 1982).

[13] Gluck, Kulovich, Borer, Brenner, Anderson, & Spellacy, *Diagnosis of the Respiratory Distress Syndrome by Anmiocentesis*, 109 Am. J. Obstet. Gynecol. 440 (1971).

[14] Kulovich & Gluck, *The Lung Profile: II, Complicated Pregnancy*, 135 Am. J. Obstet. Gynecol. 57 (1979).

[15] Kulovich, Hallman, & Gluck, *The Lung Profile: I, The Normal Pregnancy*, 135 Am J. Obstet. Gynecol. 57 (1979).

morbidity and mortality from the hazards of prematurity. Together with intensive control of maternal blood glucose, the technology of fetal surveillance offers the possibility of normalizing perinatal outcomes in large groups of diabetic pregnancies.

§ 15.2 Delivery

Selecting the optimal time of delivery in diabetic pregnancies is particularly difficult because after 37 weeks of gestation, the intrauterine environment may actually be hazardous for the fetus, and an early delivery may be required to save its life. Nonetheless, the decision to deliver the baby before the due date in order to prevent intrauterine death must be carefully considered along with the equally dangerous possibility of delivering a premature infant who will not be adequately developed to survive outside the uterus. Previously mentioned attempts to resolve this dilemma have produced various opinions concerning which group of tests and physiologic signs best determine when a diabetic mother should give birth. According to one group of investigators, when delivery prior to the 37th week seems advisable, the fetal well-being and the probable effects of labor on the fetus should be evaluated by weekly contraction stress tests and frequent urinary estriol studies, beginning at 36 weeks of gestation in women with mild diabetes, and earlier in patients with severe diabetes, vascular disease, or a history of stillbirth.[16] Preterm delivery is often not necessary in patients with chemical diabetes, as long as the contraction stress test is normal, and the estriol excretion does not fall to low levels. But if either of these tests suggest fetal distress, or if the clinical picture warrants early delivery, the degree of fetal maturity must then be assessed. By measuring the lecithin to sphingomyelin (L/S) ratio of the anmiotic fluid, the obstetrician can determine the maturity of the fetus's lungs, an important factor governing the newborn's ability to survive outside the uterus. A normal L/S ratio indicates that the fetal lungs are developed, strongly suggesting that the baby can be safely delivered without the risk of developing respiratory distress syndrome, a potentially fatal lung disorder associated with premature infants. On the other hand, if the pulmonary system is not adequately developed and the clinical situation allows a delay before inducing labor the fetal heart rate must be continuously monitored so the physician will immediately be alerted to a deteriorating intrauterine environment. Sometimes, even where there is a high probability of developing respiratory distress syndrome, it may still be more advantageous to deliver the immature fetus and attempt to sustain its life

---

[16] D.N. Danforth, M.D., Obstetrics and Gynecology, 4th ed., 531 (Harper & Row Publishers, Inc. 1982).

outside the womb, rather than allow it to remain in a rapidly deteriorating environment inside the uterus. Other investigators agree, stressing that the fetus is not in serious jeopardy as long as it is growing in utero and there are no other complications, such as maternal hypertension or grossly large quantities of amniotic fluid.[17]

According to another group of clinicians, delivery prior to 18-24 days before the estimated due date is seldom appropriate because it carries such a high fetal mortality rate as a result of prematurity.[18] They believe that intervention is only justified at an earlier time when adverse factors (such as untreatable acidosis, a severely edematous fetus, or a previous fetus who died in utero before the 37th or 38th week) threaten continued intrauterine fetal life so seriously, that the risk of prematurity is the lesser of two evils.

§ 15.3 Method of Delivery

When unfavorable intrauterine conditions do not dictate the method of delivery, the choice between a vaginal birth and a cesarean section is determined by parity, pelvic size, cervical dilation, station, presentation and position of the fetus, and the estimated fetal size. Large fetuses require special vigilance because their size predisposes them to mechanical problems with resultant birth trauma as they rotate and descend through the pelvis during vaginal delivery. Doubts about the adequacy of the pelvic canal in these cases can be confirmed by x-ray pelvimetry. See § **10.19**.

Vaginal delivery is preferred in healthy, well-controlled diabetics provided that fetopelvic disproportion is not present, and *if* a short, productive labor is expected, and *if* the woman is physiologically ready for labor. However, if (as in the majority of diabetic pregnancies) these conditions cannot be met, or if other complications arise, the baby should be delivered by cesarean section. Also, another frequent cause of neonatal morbidity in infants of diabetic mothers is neurologic and/or orthopedic damage secondary to shoulder dystocia during vaginal delivery. Therefore, the physician must provide a careful evaluation of pelvic and fetal size, and the progress of labor must be carefully evaluated so as to prevent the occurrence of this complication.

Since a diabetic woman's metabolism is so sensitive, elective cesarean sections should be scheduled in the early morning; so she is not forced to fast for a long period prior to the operation. She should stick to her typical diet and

---

[17] J.A. Pritchard, M.D. & P.C. MacDonald, Williams Obstetrics, 16th ed., 745 (Appleton-Century-Crofts, 1980).

[18] D.N. Danforth, M.D., Obstetrics and Gynecology, 4th ed., 530 (Harper & Row Publishers, Inc., 1982).

receive her usual insulin dose the day before surgery. On the morning of the operation, the obstetrician's major concern is to assure that the woman receives adequate glucose and insulin during the procedure so she will not develop acidosis and hypoglycemia. Except for atropine, the routine premedications for cesarean section are generally withheld.

Independent of the method of delivery, the heart rate of the fetus should be monitored during labor. Conduction anesthesia (either local or regional) is usually administered for both vaginal and abdominal deliveries because it is superior to inhalation anesthesia. An intravenous infusion of the appropriate amount of insulin in a 5 percent dextrose solution is begun, carefully controlling the drip rate to maintain the desired glucose concentration of 100-150 mg/dl (milligrams per deciliter). Both during labor and after the baby is born, the woman's diabetes should be evaluated based on the results of hourly *urine* analysis for glucose and acetone. If only acetone is present, additional dextrose should be given; and if both acetone and glucose are detected, more insulin should be administered. At this time, the presence of only glucose in the urine is not treated.

The insulin requirement is generally markedly reduced after the baby is born, and the woman's glucose tolerance is highly variable.[19] The insulin requirement gradually rises and finally stabilizes at its prepregnancy levels approximately 7-10 days after delivery.

§ 15.4   Management of the Newborn

A pediatrician should be notified of a diabetic pregnancy as long before delivery as possible, and she should keep in contact with the attending obstetrician during the last few weeks of gestation. A number of authorities believe it is desirable for the pediatrician to be present at the time of birth, since special care is frequently required to manage the special hazards which threaten the survival of the newborn infant of a diabetic mother.

Following the normal routine of clearing the baby's naso-pharyngeal passages, resuscitation, postural drainage, and aspiration of the stomach contents if the baby was delivered by cesarean section, the infant should promptly be placed in an incubator with humidified compressed air for 24-48 hours, depending on its respiratory condition. If supplemental oxygen is required, the concentration should not exceed 40 percent.

Samples of the umbilical cord blood should immediately be analyzed for the pH content and the concentrations of glucose, sodium, bicarbonate, potas-

---

[19] *Id.* at 531.

sium, and calcium to determine whether hypoglycemia, hypocalcemia, shock, and heart failure have developed, since these conditions are more common in these infants. Neonatal hypoglycemia often ensues because the fetus, whose body was accustomed to producing extra insulin to offset the increased levels of glucose it received from its mother, cannot abruptly shut this mechanism off at birth, even though the elevated sugar concentrations are no longer present. If the baby's blood glucose level falls below 50mg/dl, glucose should be administered by slow intravenous drip in the delivery room, and then supplemented with frequent oral feedings of glucose in water once the infant is brought to the nursery. Current evidence indicates that adequate amounts of blood glucose augment the newborn's resistance to hypoxia.

If tremors or convulsive movements develop, calcium-gluconate should be given if the results of the calcium test are not available. It is also equally important not to be misled by a robust-looking baby who may physically appear mature because of a typically larger than normal body size, but who may actually be functionally premature and require appropriate treatment. Constant nursing supervision and supportive care during the first 24-36 hours may be vital to ensure the survival of infants born to diabetic mothers.

When optimal care is provided, the perinatal mortality rate for pregnancies complicated by chemical diabetes is no higher than that of the general obstetric population. However, if the disorder intensifies as the gestation progresses, both the fetal and perinatal prognoses become much worse. The outcome for severe diabetes primarily centers around control of the maternal blood sugar levels thoughout pregnancy, though it is also influenced by placental function and the presence of complications such as preeclampsia, premature labor, acidosis and vascular disease. In general, the degree of vascular damage the mother has sustained as a result of the pathologic diabetes disease process directly influences the perinatal death rate, which has been reported to be at least 50 percent when significant maternal microvascular disease is present. Similarly, fetal growth retardation is seen more frequently when the mother has underlying vascular disorders, a markedly different finding from the excessively large infants typically born to diabetic women who do not have vascular disease.[20] The large and often edematous bodies of these newborns predispose them to birth injuries if they are delivered vaginally, or to the inherent risks of a cesarean delivery.

The primary *fetal* hazard during gestation is anoxia, often resulting when the diabetic mother develops preeclampsia or keto-acidosis late in the pregnancy, since these conditions limit the fetus's oxygen supply and threaten its continued intrauterine survival. Ironically, attempts to avert the fatal conse-

---

[20] *Id.* at 528.

quences of anoxia by early delivery sometimes end in respiratory distress syndrome, the primary *neonatal* risk of diabetic pregnancies.

Respiratory distress syndrome, which may be fatal if the newborn's lungs do not function adequately, is more likely to develop if intrapartum asphyxia or maternal bleeding occurred, and it is more commonly seen in premature and low birth weight infants.

The fetuses and newborns of diabetic pregnancies are also more susceptible to other problems. Particularly during the last few weeks of gestation, there is an increased likelihood of unexplained fetal death. Infection also occurs more frequently and is likely to be more severe in diabetic women. For example, extreme preeclampsia may lead to placental disruption (abruptio placenta), which poses a grave hazard to both the woman and fetus. Finally, there is also a three to four fold increase in serious congenital deformities, which is usually associated with increased volumes of amniotic fluid.[21]

As an aside, oral contraceptives are generally contraindicated in women with overt diabetes because they are likely to intensify the disorder.[22] Since the birth control pill has been implicated in precipitating vascular disease in nondiabetic women, it may further compound the already high incidence of vascular disorders to which diabetics are predisposed.

§ 15.5   Bibliography and Recommended Readings

Arias, Fernando, M.D., *High-Risk Pregnancy and Delivery* (The C.V. Mosby Co., 1984).

Cornblath, Marvin, M.D. & Schwartz, Robert, M.D., *Disorders of Carbohydrate Metabolism in Infancy*, 2d ed. (W.B. Saunders Co., 1976).

Iffy, Leslie, M.D. & Kaminetzky, Harold A., M.D., *Principles and Practice of Obstetrics & Perinatology*, vol. 2 (John Wiley & Sons, Inc., 1981).

Pritchard, J.A., M.D., MacDonald, P.C., M.D., & Gant, N.F., M.D., *Williams Obstetrics*, 17th ed. (Appleton-Century-Crofts, 1985).

Queenan, John T., M.D., *Management of High-Risk Pregnancy* (Medical Economics Co., 1980).

---

[21] *Id.*

[22] J.A. Pritchard, M.D. & P.C. MacDonald, M.D., Williams Obstetrics, 16th ed., 748 (Appleton-Century-Crofts, 1980).

CHAPTER 16

INTRAUTERINE GROWTH RETARDATION

§ 16.1   Introduction

Fetal development is characterized by sequential patterns of tissue and organ growth and maturation that are determined by the maternal environment, uteroplacental function, and the inherent genetic growth potential of the fetus. When circumstances are optimal, none of these factors has a rate-limiting effect on fetal growth and development. Thus, the healthy fetus should achieve complete functional maturity and somatic growth, with the anticipation of an uncomplicated intrapartum course, and thus, a smooth neonatal cardiopulmonary and metabolic adaptation to extrauterine life.

However, fetal growth and development do not always occur under optimum intrauterine conditions. Those neonates who are subjected to aberrant maternal, placental, or fetal circumstances that restrain growth are a high risk group, and are categorized as small for gestational age (SGA). The cumulative effects of both adverse environmental conditions and aberrant fetal growth (intrauterine growth retardation, IUGR) threaten continued intrauterine survival; and labor, delivery, and neonatal adaptation become increasingly hazardous. Similarly, postneonatal growth and development may be impaired as a result of intrauterine growth retardation and the subsequent problems encountered during the neonatal period.

The following conditions predispose to impairment of fetal size:

1. Small mother: little women are more likely to give birth to small infants.

2. Poor maternal weight gain.

3. Vascular disease: chronic vascular disease, especially when further complicated by superimposed preeclampsia, commonly causes growth retardation.

4. Chronic renal disease: chronic renal disease with appreciably reduced renal clearance is commonly accompanied by retarded fetal growth.

5. Chronic hypoxia: fetuses of women who reside at high altitudes are much more likely to weigh less than those of women who live at lower altitudes.

6. Maternal anemia.

7. Smoking: tobacco smoking impairs fetal growth; the more cigarettes smoked, the greater the impairment.

8. Hard drugs: the use of heroin (and almost certainly other hard drugs) during pregnancy impairs fetal growth.

9. Alcoholism: the chronic consumption of appreciable amounts of alcohol by the mother during pregnancy results in growth retardation of the fetus, often accompanied by physical malformation and subsequent intellectual impairment.

10. Abnormalities of placenta and cord.

11. Multiple fetuses.

12. Previous birth of a growth retarded infant.

13. Fetal infections: cytomegalic inclusion disease, rubella, and other chronic infections of the fetus can cause growth retardation.

14. Fetal malformation: in general, the more severe the malformation, the more likely the fetus is to be small for gestational age.

15. Prolonged pregnancy. The longer the pregnancy endures beyond term, the greater the likelihood of the fetus appearing undernourished and chronically distressed.

16. Extrauterine pregnancy. Commonly, the fetus who is not housed in the uterus is growth retarded.

When aberrant fetal growth is identified during the gestation, it is commonly referred to as intrauterine growth retardation (IUGR); following delivery, the neonate is classified as small for gestational age (SGA).

Studies have revealed that approximately one-third of all infants whose birth weight is less than 2,500 grams are not truly premature, but rather, small for gestational age. The SGA infant is almost as much risk as the premature infant. In fact, the fetal death rate is higher in the SGA group than the premature group; conversely, the premature infant has a higher neonatal mortality rate over the SGA infant.[1] Death from intrapartum asphyxia alone is 10 times greater in SGA's, than it is for appropriately grown infants, with a rate of 14 percent of all still births, and 6 percent of all deaths occuring in those infants whose birth weights are below the third percentile for gestational age.[2]

These infants are more frequently born with cogenital anomalies, the incidence of which is any where from 5-7 percent higher in this group.[3] Compromised physical as well as neurodevelopmental growth appears to be common in many of these infants.

Normal intrauterine growth for body weight and organ weights progress in systemic fashion between 28-38 weeks. From about 38 weeks onward, growth of the fetus and placenta departs from this previous pattern.

Two major factors influence fetal growth: (1) the inherent growth potential of the fetus, and (2) the growth support it receives through the placenta from the mother.

Fetal factors which can influence the growth potential include: genetically determined dwarfs, fetal infections, chromosomal syndrome, severe congenital anomalies, and some inborn errors of metabolism.

Fetal growth retardation can also be caused by impaired support while intrauterine, which implies either a placental or maternal origin. During the first and second trimesters of pregnancy, the support and supply of nutrients far exceeds the needs of the fetus for growth, and therefore, growth is determined by the inherent fetal potential. However, by the third trimester, the adequacy of the maternal fetal blood supply becomes the determining factor of growth. After approximately 32 weeks of gestation, abnormalities of fetal growth are common and become more prominent as the pregnancy continues past term. The placental reserves, so abundant in early pregnancy, become insufficient.

§ 16.2 Fetal Complications

The development of chronic fetal distress with growth retardation depends upon the duration of intrauterine life beyond the time of optimal placental function. This situation is commonly referred to as *placental insufficiency* and

---

[1] Schlesinger & Allaway, *The Combined Effect of Birth Weight and Length of Gestation on Neonatal Morality among Single Premature Infants*, 15 Pediatrics, 698 (1955).

[2] Lugo & Cassady, *Intrauterine Growth Retardation: Clinicopathologic Findings in 233 Consecutive Infants*, 109 Am. J. Obstet. Gynecol. 615 (1971).

[3] Avery, Gordon (ed.), *Neonatology*, 2d ed., 263 (J.B. Lippincott Co., 1981).

is commonly associated with pregnancies complicated by postdatism, hypertension, and IUGR.

Although rare, there are a wide variety of anatomic abnormalities of the placenta which can contribute to impaired fetal growth. Placental infarctions, hemangiomas, aberrant cord insertions, single umbilical artery, or umbilical vascular thrombosis are some of the more common placental abnormalities. An unfavorable intrauterine environment is likely to affect placental as well as fetal development. Therefore, it is not surprising that small babies have small placentas.

Maternal factors which may affect the fetus by affecting a reduction in uteroplacental blood flow include: living at high altitudes and teratogens such as irradiations, smoking, low socio-economic class, low maternal age, primiparity, grand multiparity, and low prepregnancy weight. These factors are thought to contribute to fetal growth retardation.

When there are not congenital anomalies present, most studies demonstrate normal I.Q. results in children who were SGA at the time of birth. Major neurologic problems have been infrequent in SGA infants. Therefore, all current available data clearly demonstrates that an infant is not permanently damaged merely by virtue of being SGA. Further, it can be stated that the degree of impairment in fetal growth has no correlation in subsequent child development. However, recent studies have shown that severe perinatal asphyxia plays a major role in the outcome of the SGA infants. This is due to the IUGR infant's precarious state of existence during labor. These infants do not tolerate labor and delivery well, and thus, fetal distress, aspiration of meconium, and intrapartum deaths are more likely. Small for gestational age infants also frequently experience hypothermia because of their inability to conserve heat. Hypoglycemia (low blood sugar) is another common problem. Hypoglycemia occurs because the infant's depleted glycogen stores occur just as the infant's energy requirements are at their peak. Fetal distress during labor mobilizes all available stores of glycogen (the state glucose is stored) so that immediately following delivery, the infant is left with virtually nothing in reserve. Therefore, when hypoglycemia is present, glucose must be supplied promptly after birth, otherwise central nervous system (CNS) damage can occur in the neonate.

§ 16.3   Hypoglycemia

The SGA neonate has an increased susceptibility for developing clinically significant hypoglycemia, primarily because he must produce up to four times the adult amount of glucose in order to maintain a stable blood sugar concentration. This is because the newborn's brain is a prominent glucose-utilizing organ as compared to the adult's, and the neonate has a higher brain to body ratio than the older infant or child. Therefore, brain size is a major determinant of corporeal glucose needs. Thus, at a time when glucose turnover is extraordinary, the newborn's ability to produce glucose may also be impaired.

The pathogenesis of brain damage due to hypoglycemia is predicated on the assumption that neuronal (brain cell), glucose deprivation specifically damages cerebral nerve cells. Thus, untreated hypoglycemia may result in severe brain damage or death.

The key to treating hypoglycemia is to administer sufficient glucose to raise the blood sugar level; however, the administration of hypertonic (high concentrations) solutions is theoretically hazardous, since the hypertonic solutions can cause intracellular dehydration (due to increased kidney filtration) and, if abruptly discontinued, rebound hypoglycemia. The preferred way to treat hypoglycemia is to administer constant intravenous glucose infusion that mimics the endogenous glucose production rate (approximately 8 mg/kg per minute).[4]

Because of the increased risk of hypoglycemia in the SGA infant, Dextrostick monitoring must begin shortly after birth. The Dextrostick is a simple test used to screen the infant's blood sugar. This test should be carried out in the delivery room as soon as possible following delivery. It is a quick and simple test which only requires a drop of blood from a heel stick. Labor and delivery room nurses should be familiar with the proper techniques for Dextrostick screening. Whenever the result of the Dextrostick is abnormal, an immediate blood glucose must be obtained.

Dextrostick monitoring should be initiated whenever an infant's weight is at the 10th percentile or less for the gestational age, or is two or more standard deviations less than the length.

Neonatal hypoglycemia may be associated with very poor outcomes including mental retardation, severe seizure disorders, disturbances in gait, spastic paraplegia, and ataxia.

The clinical symptoms of hypoglycemia are nonspecific, but the frequent clustering of symptoms should put one on notice that hypoglycemia may be present. Convulsions are present in 20–25 percent of neonates with hypoglycemia. Numerous other clinical symptoms are associated with hypoglycemia:

---

[4] Volpe J., *Neurology of the Newborn*, 317 (W.B. Saunders Co., 1981).

1. Tremors
2. Irritability
3. Apneic spells
4. Cyanotic spells
5. Convulsions
6. Limpness
7. Hypothermia
8. Lethargy
9. High-pitched or weak cry
10. Eye rolling
11. Cardiac arrest
12. Cardiac failure
13. Refusal to feed
14. Sweating

Symptomatic hypoglycemia has almost three times more serious resultant sequelae than does asymptomatic hypoglycemia.[5] The infant who convulses from hypoglycemia incurs the risk for poor outcome. Early detection and aggressive management of low blood sugar in the newborn will reduce the risk for significant neurological dysfunction.

The definitions of the level of blood glucose that should be considered too low is difficult, inpart, because the newborn does not have the neural capacity to demonstrate, by overt symptomatology, when a critical lower limit has been passed. In few areas of neonatal neurology, other than hypoglycemia, has the mistaken concept persisted so firmly that a serious disturbance of the neonatal central nervous system is unlikely in the absence of overt neurological signs.[6] In essence, what is known is that the critical lower limits of blood glucose for maintenance of neonatal neutral integrity in various clinical circumstances are unknown. In addition, and of greater importance, these lower limits probably diminish considerably with concommitant insults that are deleterious to the central nervous system (e.g., hypoxemia and ischemia), accompanying the hypoglycemia. This concept of the additive and potentiating role of hypoglycemia in the production of brain injury in the sick newborn, is the most critical neurolgoical aspect of neonatal hypoglycemia.

According to Joseph Volpe,[7] the most widely accepted definition of significant hypoglycemia is a whole blood level of below 20 mg/dl (below 25 mg/dl of serum or plasma) in the SGA neonate, and below 30 mg/dl (35 mg/dl of serum or plasma) in the full size or full term neonate.

§ 16.4   Polycythemia

Small for gestational age infants are also frequently polycythemic (increase in the number of red blood cells in the blood) on the basis of intrauterine hyp-

---

[5] *Id.* at 316.

[6] *Id.* at 301.

[7] *Id.* at 312.

oxia. Polycythemia is said to occur whenever the hematocrit is above 65, or the hemoglobin greater than 22, during the first week of life. The elevation of the hematocrit potentially increases blood viscosity, which interfers with vital tissue perfusion. The altered viscosity adversely affects neonatal hemodynamics and results in abnormal cardiopulmonary and metabolic postnatal adaptation, producing hypoxia and hypoglycemia.

Placental insufficiency is thought to be a contributing factor in polycythemia. Chronic intrauterine hypoxia results in an erythropoietin—stimulated, increased red cell mass which increases the risk of polycythemia/hyperviscosity syndrome.

In the event polycythemia is present (central hematocrit greater than 65 percent), appropriate therapy should be directed at correcting hypoxia and hypoglycemia while a partial exchange transfusion to reduce blood viscosity and improve tissue perfusion is carried out.

§ 16.5   Hypothermia

The small for gestational age neonate is also vulnerable to hypothermia due to diminished subcutaneous fat, which leads both to reduced insulation, and to a reduction in readily available calories. The normal core temperature of a neonate is from 36.5 degrees to 37.5 degrees centigrade. If body temperature falls, heat production is increased several times the basal level, resulting in a more rapid depletion of energy stores. Hypothermia also contributes to hypoglycemia since the neonates consumption of glucose is increased when hypothermia is present.

The idealized setting has been referred to as *neutral thermal environment*, and is an environment in which a baby can maintain a normal body temperature while producing only the minimum amount of heat generated from basal, life-sustaining, metabolic processes.

Prevention of heat loss is often best achieved by simple methods applied with knowledge born from common sense. Since heat loss requires the presence of a thermal gradient, it is important to avoid exposing the baby to a cold environment by either warming the environment or covering the baby. In utero, a fetus is warmer than the mother. Born wet, warm and naked into the usual delivery room environment, the newborn loses heat rapidly. Therefore, the infant should be dried with warm towels, and every attempt should be made to minimize evaporative heat loss.

The resuscitation of a newborn should not interfere with thermal protection. If, during resuscitation, access is needed to some body surface, then only that body surface, and no other, should be exposed.

It is reasonable to back-up the protection of swaddling by using a radiant heater to add extra warmth. Radiant heaters, when combined with swaddling, provide a superb method of protection.

§ 16.6   Bibliography and Recommended Readings

Adams, Grandy & James, *The Influence of Thermal Factors upon 0_2 Consumption of the Newborn Human Infant*, 66 J. Pediatrics 495 (1965).

Arias, Fernando, M.D., Ph.D., *High-Risk Pregnancy and Delivery* (The C.V. Mosby Co., 1984).

Avery, Gordon B., M.D., Ph.D., *Neonatology-Pathophysiology and Management of the Newborn* (The J.B. Lippincott Co., 1981).

Behrmans Neonatal-Perinatal Medicine, edited by Avory A. Fanaroff & Richard J. Martin, 3d ed. (The C.V. Mosby Co., 1983).

Bolognese, Ronald J., M.D., Schwartz, Richard J., M.D., & Schneider, Jan, M.D., *Perinatal Medicine*, 2d ed. (Williams & Wilkins, 1982).

Cornblath, Marvin, M.D. & Schwartz, Robert, M.D., *Disorders of Carbohydrate Metabolism in Infancy*, 2d ed. (W.B. Saunders Co., 1976).

Klaus, Marshall H., M.D. & Fanaroff, Avroy A., M.B., *Care of the High-Risk Neonate*, 2d ed. (W.B. Saunders Co., 1979).

Resuscitation of the Newborn Infant, 3d ed., edited by H. Abramson (The C.V. Mosby Co., 1973).

Scipien G., R.N., B.S., M.S., et al., *Comprehensive Pediatric Nursing* (McGraw-Hill, 1975).

Shnider, Sol M., M.D. & Levinson, Gershon, M.D., *Anesthesia for Obstetrics* (Williams & Wilkins, 1979).

VanLeeuwen's Newborn Medicine, edited by Charles L. Parson, M.D. (Yearbook Publishers, 1979).

Volpe, Joseph H., M.D., *Neurology of the Newborn* (W.B. Saunders Co., 1981).

CHAPTER 17

TERATOGENIC AGENTS

§ 17.1 Introduction

§ 17.2 Risk/Benefit Assessment

§ 17.3 Bibliography and Recommended Readings

§ 17.1 Introduction

A teratogenic agent is a drug, chemical, virus, physical agent (such as x-rays), or maternal metabolic imbalance which, if present during pregnancy, alters the morphology or subsequent function of the fetus. Showing up immediately at birth or remaining dormant until a later stage of the child's life, the severity of the resulting deformities makes it imperative for all physicians who treat women of reproductive age, to be well-informed of the latest findings and recommendations concerning teratogenic pharmaceuticals and diagnostic procedures.

With rare exception, most medications used during pregnancy cannot be considered absolutely safe because, besides remedying the mother's disorder, they are also able to cross the placental barrier and affect the course of fetal growth and development. The specific effects are determined by the type and dose of the drug, and most importantly, when it is taken during pregnancy. Medications given in the critical first trimester, when the fetus's organs are developing and are most susceptible to drug-tissue interactions, are known to cause a higher incidence of congenital deformities than when they are given in the last two trimesters. To complicate matters, many women may not yet be aware that they are pregnant in the very early stages of gestation, such as during the crucial first month to month-and-a-half of fetal growth. So, before inadvertently prescribing potentially harmful drugs for these women, every physician, obstetrician, and internist alike, must routinely inquire whether her patients of childbearing age might indeed be pregnant, or plan to conceive in the near future.

The obstetrician should also try to discourage the expectant mother from treating her own ailments with over-the-counter remedies or with prescription pharmaceuticals she has used in the past or may receive from concerned friends and relatives. Prescription medications must be dispensed cautiously following a thorough examination, not after just listening to the patient's complaints over the telephone, and only if the drug is vital to the mother's health and is not just ordered to alleviate minor symptoms. Thus, while it might be essential for an epileptic woman to take barbiturates in early pregnancy, it would not be appropriate for a nonepileptic patient to take them to calm nerves. Similarly, anticonvulsants, such as Dilantin, are justified to prevent seizures in pregnant epileptic women because their ability to save the mother's life overrides their potential for teratogenicity. As these examples point out, the maternal benefits of a particular drug or diagnostic test must always be balanced against the risks of fetal side effects.

§ 17.2 Risk/Benefit Assessment

Table 17-1 provides a risk/benefit assessment of various drugs administered to women in the critical first trimester of gestation. By referring to this chart, the physician is not only able to avoid prescribing dangerous teratogens, but she can also select the least toxic form of treatment when several suitable drugs are available. For instance, if a patient acquires a bacterial infection during the first trimester, penicillin is a much safer choice than tetracycline, provided that both antibiotics can successfully combat the disease.

Table 17-1

TERATOGENIC AND FETOTOXIC DRUGS

Maternal Medication	Fetal or Neonatal Effect
Established teratogenic agents	
Alcohol	Fetal alcohol syndrome (growth retardation, increase in anomalies)
Anticoagulants (dicumarol, warfarin)	Optic atrophy, mental retardation, hydrocephalus
Anticonvulsants (phenytoin, trimethadione)	Mental and growth retardation, microcephaly
Antineoplastics	Multiple anomalies, abortion
Alkylating agents (cyclophosphamide)	
Folic acid antagonists (methotrexate, aminopterin)	

Table 17-1 (Continued)

TERATOGENIC AND FETOTOXIC DRUGS

Hormones	
Estrogens, progestins	Anomalies involving vertebrae, anus, cardiovascular system, trachea, esophagus, renal system, and limbs (VACTERL)
Diethylstilbestrol	Genital anomalies, late development of clear cell carcinoma of the vagina
Androgens	Masculinization of female fetus
Isotretinoin (Accutane)	Multiple anomalies involving central nervous system
Organic mercury	Central nervous system anomalies
Possible teratogens	
Lithium carbonate	Cardiac defects
Sulfonylurea derivatives	Anomalies
Tranquilizers	
Benzodiazepines	Facial cleft deformities
Meprobamate	Multiple anomalies
Fetotoxic drugs	
Analgesics, narcotics	
Heroin, morphine	Neonatal death or convulsions, tremors
Salicylates (excessive)	Neonatal bleeding
Antithyroid drugs	
Radioiodine	Destruction of fetal thyroid
Propylthiouracil, methimazole	Fetal goiter
Sedatives, hypnotics, tranquilizers	
Phenobarbital (excessive)	Neonatal bleeding
Phenothiazines	Hyperbilirubinemia
Tetracyclines	Dental Discoloration and abnormalities
Thiazides	Thrombocytopenia
Tobacco smoking	Undersized babies
Vitamin K (excessive)	Hyperbilirubinemia

© Permission to reprint granted. Krupp, M.A., M.D., Chatton, M.J., M.D., & Werdegar, D., M.D., *Current Medical Diagnosis & Treatment-1985*, 488 (Los Altos: Lange Medical Publications, 1985).

Besides these considerations, the timing of drug administration with respect to the mother's health is also important. If she is suffering from low blood pressure, dehydration, or other related conditions which tend to increase the permeability of the placenta to various medications, then a therapeutic dose of a muscle relaxant that is normally unable to enter the fetal circulation would consequently be able to cross the placenta, and possibly paralyze the fetus.

The probability of drug interactions must also be taken into account when more than one medication is prescribed; a likely event if several physicians are involved in the patient's care.

During the prenatal period, the obstetrician should explain to her patient the importance of restricting the ingestion of coffee, tea, and alcoholic beverages and discontinuing smoking, or at least cutting down on the number of cigarettes smoked. In excess, these habits are potentially hazardous, especially in the early months of pregnancy, giving rise to premature or low birth weight infants, liver damage, and blood clotting deficiencies. Women who habitually take hallucinogens, stimulants, and depressants (including alcohol and narcotics) often have a tendency to be malnourished, and as a result, also give birth to a disproportionate number of underweight infants. In addition to impairing fetal growth, the ability of the drugs themselves to cross the placental barrier may cause passive neonatal drug addition, in which case the baby will face an unpleasant or even fatal period of withdrawal.

One of the worst disasters in modern obstetrics was the discovery that the drug thalidomide interfered with the development of fetal limbs, causing infants to be born without arms or legs. Following that incident, it became mandatory to test the teratogenicity of all drugs in pregnant laboratory animals before dispensing them to humans. Yet, many authorities question the effectiveness of these investigations, claiming that it is difficult to apply the results to humans when drug metabolism differs in individual strains of the same laboratory species, let alone within a given litter of the experimental animal.

Furthermore, even the fact that a laboratory-tested and approved drug is used extensively without immediate adverse fetal or neonatal consequences does not guarantee its safety, since its detrimental effects may take months, or possibly years, to surface. The diethylstilbestrol story exemplifies such a delayed drug response. Although no side effects were observed during their childhood, vaginal cancer began to develop in a large percentage of young women whose mothers received diethylstilbestrol during those pregnancies, on the average of 18-25 years after a drug was taken.

Now that greater numbers of women have entered the work force, there is also growing concern about the biologic consequences of environmental chemicals which they may be exposed to on the job. Even those who are not employed outside the home are subject to the toxic effects of agricultural and industrial chemicals and their waste products, as the following case illustrates. When pregnant women unknowingly ingested mercury—an established human teratogen—on chemically treated grains or in contaminated fish, their children were often born with severe central nervous system damage.[1]

---

[1] Gordon B. Avery, M.D., Ph.D., *Neonatology-Pathophysiology and Management of the Newborn* 1164 (J.B. Lippincott Co., 1981).

X-ray irradiation of the pregnant abdomen is also known to be teratogenic, including fetal malignancies, central nervous system abnormalities, and chromosomal breakage in the unfertilized egg cells of the mother's ovaries. Long-term genetic defects such as Down's syndrome, a common type of mental retardation, are liable to result when the chromosones are altered or damaged. In order to minimize the incidence of radiation-induced anomalies, the obstetrician should only order diagnostic x-rays when they are absolutely essential for a pregnant patient's treatment, and whenever possible, defer them until at least the second trimester; again because the fetal organs are particularly sensitive to excessive irradiation during the first three months of development.

§ 17.3   Bibliography and Recommended Readings

Avery, Gordon, B., M.D., Ph.D., *Neonatalogy-Pathophysiology and Management of the Newborn* (J.B. Lippincott Co., 1981).

Avery, Mary Ellen, M.D. & Taeusch, H. William, Jr., M.D., *Schaffer's Diseases of the Newborn*, 5th ed. (W.B. Saunders Co., 1984).

Brenner, Edelman, et al., *A Standard of Fetal Growth for the United States of America*, 126 Amer. J. Obstet. Gynecol. 555 (1976).

Iffy, Leslie, M.D. & Kaminetzky, Harold, M.D., *Principles and Practice of Obstetrics & Perinatology* (John Wiley & Sons, Inc., 1981).

Pritchard, Jack A., M.D., MacDonald, Paul C., M.D. & Gant, Norman F., M.D., *Williams Obstetrics*, 17th ed. (Appleton-Century-Crofts, 1985).

CHAPTER 18

OBSTETRICAL ANESTHESIA

§ 18.1   Introduction

Labor may subject the nulliparous woman to the most pain that she has ever experienced. Fortunately, it often proves to be the most rewarding. The relief of pain in labor presents special problems which may be best appreciated by reviewing the several important differences between obstetric and surgical anesthesia and analgesia:

1. In surgical procedures, there is but one patient to consider, whereas in parturition, there are at least two, the mother and the fetus-infant.

The respiratory center of the infant is highly vulnerable to sedative and anesthetic drugs, and since these agents (if given systemically) regularly traverse the placenta, they may jeopardize respiration after birth.

2. In major surgery, anesthesia is essential to the safe, satisfactory, and humane execution of the technical procedures. Whereas anesthesia is mandatory in many abnormal deliveries, it is not absolutely necessary in spontaneous vaginal delivery because the baby can be born satisfactorily without any medication, although some mothers may suffer severe pain.

3. Surgical anesthesia is administered for the duration of the operation which lasts, in most cases, for not more than an hour or two. Efficient pain relief in labor must cover not only the delivery (obstetric anesthesia), but also a preceding period from one to twelve hours or longer (obstetric analgesia).

4. In both obstetric analgesia and anesthesia, it is important that the agents that are used exert little deleterious effect on uterine contractions and maternal voluntary expulsive efforts. If they do, the progress of labor may stop, or if uterine contractility is depressed immediately after delivery, postpartum hemorrhage is likely to occur.

5. In the majority of surgical operations, there is ample time to prepare the patient for anesthesia, especially by withholding food and fluids for 12 hours. Since most labors begin without warning, obstetric anesthesia is often administered within a few hours after a full meal. Moreover, gastric emptying is likely to be delayed appreciably during labor, especially after analgesics for pain relief. Vomiting with aspiration of gastric contents is, hence, a frequent threat and a major cause of morbidity and mortality in obstetric anesthesia.

Because of these inherent difficulties, no completely safe and satisfactory method of pain relief in obstetrics has yet been developed. It is, therefore, sometimes falsely alleged that the hazards of pain relief in labor offset its advantages. On the contrary, vast experience has shown that obstetric analgesia and anesthesia (when judiciously employed by skilled personnel) are, in general, beneficial rather than detrimental to both baby and mother. Pain relief forestalls the importunities of the parturient and her family for premature operative interference. Formerly, premature and injudicious operative delivery so provoked constituted a common cause of trauma to both mother and infant. Such injuries were occasionally fatal to the mother and frequently so to the baby. The relief of pain itself, however, although desirable, does not justify the use of anesthetic procedures that are potentially lethal if administered by poorly trained individuals, or with inadequate equipment.[1]

The Joint Commission on Accreditation of Hospitals has urged that skilled personnel and appropriate equipment be immediately available to provide obstetric anesthesia: "obstetric anesthesia must be considered as emergency anesthesia demanding a competence of personnel and equipment similar to or greater than that required for elective procedures."[2] The societal benefits to be derived from modifying existing priorities for utilization of trained anesthesia personnel were stated succinctly: "Young women with babies are far more important to society than old people with irreversible disease. If we cannot do justice to both, then we should concentrate on the obstetrical patients."[3]

A reduction in perinatal mortality and morbidity is, in part, dependent on the quality of obstetric anesthesia and analgesia. These procedures require close, continuing cooperation between obstetricians, anesthesiologists, and neonatalogists.

Three essentials of obstetric pain relief are preservation of fetal homeostasis, simplicity, and safety. Fetal homeostasis must not be impaired by the analgesic or anesthetic method. Most important is the transfer of oxygen, which is dependent on the concentration of inhaled oxygen, transfer of oxygen across maternal alveoli, uterine blood flow, transfer of oxygen across the placenta, and umbilical blood flow. Impaired fetal oxygenation most often is the consequence of either compression of the umbilical cord, or prolonged or repeated falls in placental perfusion. Prominent causes of reduced placental perfusion include hypertonic uterine contractions, severe pregnancy induced hypertension, hemorrhage, premature separation of placenta, and hypotension from spinal or epidural anesthesia.

The woman who receives any form of analgesia requires constant surveillance. If left alone and under heavy sedation, she may throw herself out of bed or against a wall, or she may vomit and aspirate the gastric contents. Numerous injuries and a few deaths as a result of such negligence are on record. Similarly, safe spinal and epidural anesthesia demands assiduous attention to the blood pressure and anesthetic levels.

---

[1] J.A. Pritchard, M.D. & P.C. MacDonald, M.D., Williams Obstetrics, 16th ed., 436 (Appleton-Century-Crofts, 1980).

[2] *ACOG National Study of Maternity Care Survey of Obstetric Practice and Associated Services in Hospitals in the United States*, a report of the Committee on Maternal Health, The American College of Obstetricians and Gynecologists (Chicago 1970).

[3] Jacoby, *Anesthesia for Normal Vaginal Delivery*, 1 Anes. Rev. 11 (1974).

§ 18.2   Pharmacologic Analgesia and Anesthesia

The pharmacologic techniques that are used to relieve pain during labor and delivery fall into four general categories:

1. Systemic medication with narcotics, sedatives, tranquilizers, and amnesiacs. See § 18.3.
2. Inhalation analgesia with subanesthetic concentrations of inhalation drugs. See § 18.5.
3. General anesthesia. See §§ 18.7 through 18.11.
4. Regional or conduction anesthesia (i.e., nerve block with local anesthetics). See §§ 18.12 through 18.16.

§ 18.3   —Systemic Medication

Systemic medications, given intravenously or intramuscularly, are frequently used to decrease pain and anxiety of the first stage of labor. In the past, this form of pain relief was selected because it is simple to administer. Small doses of systemic medication can be used with relative safety for the mother, although certain aspects of newborn neuro-behavior may be modified for several days following their use in labor.

Narcotics or analgesics are the keystone of systemic medications. In general, equal analgesic doses of various narcotics produce equal amounts of depression in both mother and newborn. The major difference among the various narcotics is in the duration of their action. Knowledge of the duration of action allows the rational selection of the appropriate narcotic. If prolonged duration is desired, for example, in early labor, narcotics such as meperidine (Demerol) or morphine are indicated. If narcotics are administered late in labor, when only a short duration of action is desired, short acting narcotics such as fentanyl (Sublimaze) or nisentil are appropriate.

Fear has been expressed by some that administration of Demerol to provide obstetric analgesia might, at times, prolong or even arrest labor. Certainly, with the doses usually used for analgesia, there is no convincing evidence that this occurs; for example, the effects of Demerol on labor have been evaluated, and there was observed not a decrease, but a slight increase in uterine activity following their injection.[4]   However, all narcotics are rapidly transferred

---

[4] Riffel, Nochimson, Paul, & Hon, *Effects of Meperidine and Promethazine During Labor*, 42 Obstet. Gynecol. 738 (1973).

across the placenta and are capable of producing neonatal respiratory depression and changes in neurobehavioral status. With most narcotics, the maximum neonatal depression of Apgar scores occurs in newborns delivered two to three hours after maternal intramuscular administration.[5]

Demerol is the most popular narcotic currently used in obstetrics. The usual dosage is 50 to 100 mg intramuscularly, or 25 to 30 mg intravenously. The peak analgesic effect occurs 40 to 50 minutes after intramuscular injection, and 5 to 10 minutes after intravenous administration. The duration of action is three to four hours.

Demerol reaches the fetal circulation within 90 seconds of intravenous administration to the mother, and the fetal and maternal concentrations achieve equilibrium within six minutes.

Maternally administered Demerol may produce neonatal depression as evidenced by decreased Apgar scores, lower oxygen saturation, decreased minute volume, respiratory acidosis, and abnormal neurobehavioral examinations. These effects are related to the dose and to the time interval between maternal administration and delivery of the infant. In a study of a group of parturients with no medical or obstetric complications, if Demerol was given intramuscularly within one hour of birth, there was no statistically significant difference in the incidence of depressed babies compared to a controlled, unmedicated group. This was found even when the mother received up to 100 mg of drug. However, there was a significant increase in the percentage of depressed babies born during the second hour after intramuscular drug administration. This was true even if mothers had received only 50 mg of Demerol. Increased doses tended to prolong the period in which significant neonatal depression was observed. The addition of a barbiturate not only prolonged the period, but also increased the percentage of neonatal depression.[6]

Neonatal depression after Demerol may be prolonged. Oxygen saturation is significantly depressed for at least 30 minutes after birth in full term babies of mothers who receive 100 mg of Demerol, two to four hours before birth.[7]

Nisentil is another synthetic narcotic which has achieved great popularity in many obstetric units because of its rapid onset and short duration. The peak analgesic effect occurs five to ten minutes after subcutaneous, and one to two minutes after intravenous administration. The duration of action is one to

[5] Kuhnert, Kuhnert, & Rosen, *Meperidine and Normeperidine Levels in the Mother, Fetus and Neonate Following Meperidine Administration During Labor*, Annual Meeting, Society for Obstetric Anesthesia and Perinatology, Memphis, 1978, at 58.

[6] Shnider & Moya, *Effects of Meperidine on the Newborn Infant*, 89 Am. J. Obstet. Gynecol. 1009 (1964).

[7] Taylor, von Fumetti, Essig, et al, *The Effects of Demerol and Trichlorethylene on Arterial Oxygen Saturation in the Newborn*, 69 Am. J. Obstet. Gynecol. 348 (1955).

two hours. Recommended use is "initially 40 to 60 mg subcutaneously after cervical dilatation has begun, repeated as required at two hour intervals."[8] However, many authorities feel the above dosage is excessive and advocate that Nisentil be given in doses no greater than 20 to 30 mg subcutaneously, or 10 to 20 mg intravenously—and repeated if necessary.[9]

Morphine is no longer popular in obstetrics. When used, it is usually administered in doses of 5 to 10 mg intramuscularly, or 2 to 3 mg intravenously. The peak analgesic effect is one to two hours after intramuscular administration. The duration of action is four to six hours. In equilanalgesic doses, morphine produces more respiratory depression of the newborn than does Demerol. Because of the delayed onset and prolonged duration of action in the mother, coupled with the greater sensitivity of the newborn's respiratory center to morphine, Demerol has replaced morphine as an obstetric analgesic.

Scopolamine produces an inhibition of acetylcholine which results in decreased salivary secretions and gastric motility. Placental transfer is rapid; after intravenous administration (0.3 to 0.6 mg), fetal tachycardia and loss of beat-to-beat variability are produced within 10 to 25 minutes and last 60 to 90 minutes. Scopolamine crosses the blood-brain barrier and produces profound amnesia and mild sedation, presumably by its anticholinergic actions on the central nervous system. Amnesia does not occur until at least 20 minutes after intravenous administration. Scopolamine does not possess analgesic properties, and like most sedatives, will result in severe agitation, marked excitement, and loss of inhibitions in the presence of severe pain. Hallucinations and delirium are common if a parturient in active labor is given scopolamine without adequate narcotics. "Twilight sleep," once a popular analgesic-amnesic technique, consisted of the administration of a single dose of morphine and scopolamine during labor, followed by later injections of scopolamine only. Maternal amnesia for labor and delivery was intense, neonatal narcotic depression was common, and the parturient was difficult to manage. Scopolamine, per se, has adverse effects on the progress of labor, or significant respiratory depressant effects on the neonate. Today, most authorities believe that scopolamine has little place as a sedative during labor because maternal amnesia is no longer desired by most parturients.[10]

---

[8] Physicians Desk Reference, 32d ed., 1407 (Medical Economics, 1978).

[9] S.M. Shnider, & G. Levinson, Anesthesia for Obstetrics 84 (Williams & Wilkins, 1979).

[10] Id. at 87.

§ 18.4 —Narcotic Antagonists

Narcan is currently the preferred narcotic antagonist. Unlike the earlier narcotic antagonists, Narcan produces no cardiorespiratory or central nervous system depression in and of itself.

Narcotic antagonists have been administered in three ways: (1) to the mother with each dose of narcotic; (2) to the mother 10 to 15 minutes before delivery; and (3) to the neonate immediately after delivery.

The rationale for administering a narcotic and a narcotic antagonist simultaneously is to provide maximum analgesia with minimal respiratory depression. Numerous studies have proved that the antagonists will reverse the analgesia as well as the respiratory depression, and therefore, offer no advantage.[11]

The rationale for administering Narcan just before delivery is to allow placental transfer and intrauterine reversal of narcotic depression in the fetus and neonate. Many consider this approach inadvisable because removal of maternal analgesia immediately before delivery is unfair to the mother. It may result in an uncontrollable and difficult delivery, and is usually unnecessary insofar as the neonate is concerned.

The rationale for administering Narcan routinely to all neonates whose mothers have received narcotics within four hours of delivery, is that even apparently vigorous babies will have some central nervous system depression and alteration of neurobehavioral status. The objection to this approach is based on the lack of documentation of long-term safety of Narcan. The short-term safety of Narcan is well documented. Even when administered in excessive doses, no adverse effects are found.[12]

It should be emphasized that adverse neonatal effects of Narcan have never been demonstrated and the drug should not be withheld when indicated. Parturients who receive an absolute or relative overdose of narcotics, as evidenced by obtundation or hypoventilation, should receive Narcan. Depressed infants who have a high probability of being narcotized and do not respond to routine resuscitation with oxygenation, ventilation, and tactile stimulation, should also receive Narcan.

In adults, the usual initial dose is 0.4 mg intravenously. The neonatal dose is 0.01 mg/kg (milligram per kilogram) either intravenously or, if perfusion is good, intramuscularly. Effects are seen within minutes, and last one to two hours. Because of the relatively short duration of action of Narcan, the narcotically overdosed mother or neonate must be observed carefully. Repeat

---

[11] Teleford & Keats, *Narcotic - Narcotic Antagonist Mixtures*, 22 Anesthesiology 465 (1961).

[12] S.M. Shnider & G. Levinson, Anesthesia for Obstetrics 89 (Williams & Wilkins, 1979).

doses of the antagonist should be administered, if necessary. Narcan should not be used in narcotic addicts or their neonates because acute withdrawal symptoms may be precipitated.

§ 18.5 —Inhalation Analgesia

Inhalation analgesia requires that the mother breathe subanesthetic concentrations of inhalation anesthetics. If the analgesia is administered properly, the mother remains conscious, yet has profound analgesia. Numerous inhalation anesthetic drugs have been used including chloroform, ether, nitrous oxide, ethylene, cyclopropane, Trilene, methoxyflurane (Penthrane), and more recently in this country, Ethrane. Today in the United States, the two most commonly used inhalation drugs to produce analgesia in obstetrics are nitrous oxide and methoxyflurane.[13]

Inhalation analgesia may be administered in the first stage of labor. Because of its potency, methoxyflurane (Penthrane) is usually administered in air in concentrations between 0.2 percent to 0.6 percent. The drug may be self-administered through a calibrated vaporizer such as the Duke Inhalor or the cyprane inhalor, held in the mother's hand and set at the desired concentration. A disposable inhalor is also available for use with methoxyflurane. When the contraction begins, the mother breathes through the vaporizer until the contraction ends. After two to three contractions, an adequate blood level is maintained to provide profound analgesia in a conscious patient who remains responsive and cooperative. This analgesia may be continued through delivery of the newborn, delivery of the placenta, and the immediate postpartum examination. The total amount of Penthrane administered throughout labor and delivery should not exceed 15 ml of liquid to avoid renal toxicity secondary to its breakdown in both the mother and the newborn to inorganic floride.[14]

Since nitrous oxide is a gas at atmospheric conditions, it is stored under pressure in sealed gas cylinders, and must be administered through a calibrated anesthesia machine with oxygen by a trained physician or nurse. As 30 percent to 50 percent nitrous oxide is required to produce analgesia, it is given in a mixture of 50 percent to 70 percent oxygen.

---

[13] *Id.* at 134.

[14] *Id.* at 128.

§ 18.6   —Advantages and Disadvantages

Inhalation analgesia provides profound but not complete analgesia for labor and delivery. Used alone, it often produces adequate pain relief for labor, and uncomplicated vaginal delivery without episiotomy. If an episiotomy is to be performed and repaired, or use of forceps is anticipated, the obstetrician should supplement inhalation analgesia with local infiltration of the peritoneum, or a bilateral pudendal block. In addition to analgesia, inhalation analgesia often provides amnesia, particularly for painful events.

If inhalation analgesia is properly administered, it has many advantages and is extremely safe for mother and newborn. Maternal and newborn depression is not produced in measurable degree by subanesthetic concentrations of inhalation drugs, regardless of the duration of their administration. The mother remains awake with upper airway reflexes intact and is protected from catastrophe of pulmonary aspiration of gastric contents without the need for intubation. The mother's reflex-urge and ability to bear down in the second stage of labor are little affected. The onset of inhalation analgesia is rapid, and the degree of analgesia can be altered quickly by changing the inspired concentration of the inhalation drug. It can be given safely to nearly every parturient and may be used to supplement other forms of analgesia, particularly regional or conduction anesthesia.

Despite its advantages, however, inhalation analgesia does have drawbacks. The amount of inhalation drugs required for adequate analgesia varies from mother to mother, and indeed, from the same mother throughout the various phases of labor. She may pass from the stage of analgesia and amnesia (first stage anesthesia) into the stage of delirium and excitement (second stage of anesthesia), or even into the stage of surgical anesthesia (third stage of anesthesia) with loss of protective airway reflexes, subjecting her to the danger of pulmonary aspiration, and her fetus to newborn anesthetic depression. *It is imperative that a fully trained nurse or physician always be present when inhalation analgesia is used.* Inhalation analgesia does not produce complete analgesia. Except for the uncomplicated vaginal delivery, it must be supplemented. Even then, adequate analgesia and patient cooperation may not be satisfactory. Increasing the concentration of the inhalation drug often results in excitement and activity, or general anesthesia with its attendant problems. When a patient receiving inhalation analgesia is delerious and uncooperative, this is often an indication that too much inhalation drug is being administered; this can be corrected rapidly by decreasing the concentration of the inhalation drug.

§ 18.7   General Anesthesia

General anesthesia is rarely, if ever, indicated for uncomplicated vaginal delivery. Indeed, most vaginal deliveries are more safely performed with other forms of analgesia or anesthesia. Obstetricians today are coming to realize that vaginal delivery with general anesthesia is fraught with many serious complications.[15] Fortunately, women of the child-bearing age are less inclined to request that they be put to sleep for delivery. Rather, they want to take part in the delivery and frequently wish the baby's father to be present in the delivery room to share the joy of birth. These changing attitudes deserve to be encouraged and supported by all those involved in the care of the mother-to-be.

The disadvantages of general anesthesia in obstetrics are many. General anesthesia prevents the mother from participating in the birth of her baby and relating with her newborn at birth. When used for vaginal delivery, it cannot be administered until the baby is deliverable because it immediately stops the bearing-down reflex of the second stage of labor. In addition, the newborn, like the mother, is depressed by the anesthetic. Despite occasional statements to the contrary,[16] controlled settings indicate that neonatal depression, following general anesthesia for delivery, is directly proportional to the depth of anesthesia and the length of the interval from induction of anesthesia to the delivery of the baby.[17] While this depression from general anesthesia is usually rapidly overcome by ventilatory support of the newborn, it may compound depression from other sources. If the interval from the induction of anesthesia to the delivery of the newborn is kept to less than 10 minutes with light anesthesia, newborn depression from well-administered general anesthesia is minimal.

§ 18.8   —Aspiration during General Anesthesia

Pneumonitis from inhalation of gastric contents has been the most common cause of anesthetic death in obstetrics. For example, a survey in Great Britain identified inhalation of gastric contents to be associated with at least one-half

---

[15] Leslie Iffy, M.D. & Harold A. Kaminetzky, M.D., Principles and Practice of Obstetrics & Perinatology, vol. 2, 1005-1006 (John Wiley & Sons, Inc., 1981).

[16] F. Moya, *General Anesthesia,* in Obstetrical Anesthesia: Current Concepts and Practice 88 (Williams & Wilkins, 1969).

[17] Moya, *Violatile Inhalation Agents and Muscle Relaxants in Obstetrics,* 25 Acta Anaesth. Scand. (Suppl) 368 (1966).

of all obstetric deaths.[18] The aspirated material from the stomach may contain undigested food, and thereby cause airway obstruction that (unless promptly relieved) may prove rapidly fatal. Fasting gastric juice is likely to be free of particulate matter but extremely acidic, and thereby capable of inducing a lethal chemical pneumonitis. The aspiration of strongly acidic gastric juice is probably more common, and perhaps more dangerous, than is the aspiration of gastric contents that contain particulate matter, but are buffered somewhat by the food.

§ 18.9   —Prophylaxis to Prevent Aspiration

Important to effective prophylaxis are (1) fasting for 12 hours before anesthesia, (2) use of agents to reduce gastric acidity during the induction and maintenance of general anesthesia, (3) skillful endotracheal intubation accompanied by pressure on the cricoid cartilage to occlude the esophagus, and (4) at completion of the operation, extubating with the mother awake and lying on her side with her head lowered.

Withholding food for 12 hours should rid the stomach of undigested food but not necessarily of acidic liquid. If general anesthesia is necessary soon after eating, the stomach contents may be emptied by provoking emesis. Many consider such prophylactic treatment to be cruel, yet it may protect the life of the mother and the fetus. Unfortunately, use of apomophine to induce vomiting may cause respiratory depression; and use of a nasogastric tube with suction to empty the stomach of particulate matter is unpleasant, time consuming, and not totally effective.

Ingestion of antacids shortly before induction of anesthesia can appreciably reduce the acidity of the gastric juice.[19] It is essential that the antacid disperse promptly throughout all of the gastric contents to neutralize the hydrogen ion effectively. It is equally important that the antacid, if aspirated, not incite comparably serious pulmonary pathologic problems. A number of antacids are now being used. Magensium hydroxide (milk of magnesia) is an effective neutralizer. The usual dose of 30 ml of magnesium hydroxide suspension given up to one-half hour before the anticipated time of induction of anesthesia.

The woman who aspirates may develop evidence of respiratory distress immediately, or as long as several hours after aspiration depending, in part, upon

---

[18] Crawford, *A Critical Account of the "Confidential Enquiries" Report*, 67 Proc. R. Soc. Med., 905 (1974).

[19] Wheatley, Kallus, Reynolds, & Giesecke, *Milk of Magnesia in an Effective Pre-Induction Antacid in Obstetrical Anesthesia*, 50 Anesthesiology 514 (1979).

the material aspirated, the severity of the process, and the acuity of the attendants. Aspiration of a large amount of solid material causes obvious signs of airway obstruction. Smaller particles without acidic liquid may lead to patchy atelectasis and later to bronchopneumonia.

When highly acidic liquid is inspired, tachypnea, bronchospasm, rhonchi, rales, atelectasis, cyanosis, tachycardia, and hypotension are likely to develop. At the sites of injury in the lungs, protein-rich fluid containing numerous erythrocytes exudes from capillaries into the lung interstitium and alveoli to cause decreased pulmonary compliance, shunting of blood, and severe hypoxemia. X-ray changes may appear relatively late and be quite variable. Therefore, chest x-rays alone should not be used to exclude aspiration of a significant amount of strongly acidic gastric contents.

In recent years, the methods recommended for treatment of aspiration have changed appreciably, indicating that previous therapy was not very successful. Suspicion of aspiration of gastric contents demands very close monitoring of the patient for evidence of any pulmonary damage.

As much as possible of the inhaled fluid should be immediately wiped out of the mouth and removed from the pharynx and trachea by suction. If large particulate matter is inspired, prompt bronchoscopy is indicated to relieve airway obstruction. Otherwise, bronchoscopy not only is unnecessary, but may contribute to morbidity and mortality.

Although of questionable value,[20] corticosteroids such as Solu-Medrol, are usually administered intravenously in an attempt to maintain cell integrity in the presence of strong acid.

Oxygen delivered through an endotracheal tube in increased concentration by intermittent positive pressure, is often required to raise and maintain the arterial oxygen level. Frequent suction is necessary to remove secretions including edema fluid. Mechanical ventilation that produces positive and expiratory pressure may prove lifesaving by preventing, on expiration, the complete collapse of the now surfactant-poor lung, and by retarding the outpouring of protein-rich fluid from pulmonary capillaries into the microscopic airways.

General anesthesia predisposes the parturient to the dreadful complication of pulmonary aspiration of gastric content. Every parturient is at risk of this catastrophe because her stomach is rarely empty—the gastroespohageal junction may not function as a result of changes in gastric position caused by the enlarged uterus, and the gravid uterus and lithotomy position increase intragastric pressure. General anesthesia for any women in the third trimester of pregnancy necessitates intubation with a cuffed endotracheal tube. The endotracheal tube should be inserted either before induction or immediately after a

---

[20] Chapman, Downs, Modell, et al., *The Ineffectiveness of Steroid Therapy in Treating Aspiration of Hydrochloric Acid*, 108 Arch. Surg. 858 (1974).

rapid induction, during which cricoid pressure (pressure on neck so as to occlude esophagus) is applied from the time of the loss of consciousness, until
intubation. General anesthesia for the parturient without endotracheal intubation is unacceptable anesthetic practice today.[21]

§ 18.10   —Indication for General Anesthesia

Despite the numerous disadvantages and problems associated with the use of
general anesthesia for delivery, its proper use with rapid induction by a skilled
anesthetist may result in the delivery of a healthy baby, and prevention of
maternal morbidity and mortality. In certain circumstances, general anesthesia is the only form of anesthesia that can provide adequate conditions for the
obstetrician to deliver the newborn rapidly and safely. The immediate availability of a skilled anesthetist, who is provided with proper equipment and
assistance in the obstetrical suite, is a primary requirement for good obstetrical
care. The indication for general anesthesia for vaginal delivery includes the
following:

1. Fetal distress, which demands immediate delivery and which can be
    safely accomplished by the vaginal route; often the use of inhalation
    analgesia is supplemented by local infiltration of the perineum or pu-
    dendal block which provide satisfactory conditions for such a delivery.
2. The parturient becomes uncontrollable after delivery.
3. A parturient refuses regional or other forms of analgesia or anesthesia,
    or when these forms of pain reliever are contraindicated.
4. The need for rapid depression of uterine activity.

Depression of uterine activity may be indicated to abolish a tetanic uterine
contraction, which is usually the result of too large a dose of oxytocin given
during induction or augmentation of labor. It may also be required to allow
intrauterine manipulation for the extraction of a distressed second twin or removal of a retained placenta. Although ether and all of the halogenated inhalation anesthetic drugs can depress uterine activity, halothane (given
initially in a 2 percent concentration), or enflurane (given initially in a 3 percent concentration), is usually favored because the onset of its effect is rapid
and its action is predictable.

---

[21] S.M. Shnider, & G. Levinson, Anesthesia for Obstetrics 298 (Williams & Wilkins, 1979).

§ 18.11 —Techniques for General Anesthesia

While the scope of this section does not allow a discussion of techniques of general anesthesia, the following points concerning its use should be emphasized:

1. Patients in the third trimester of pregnancy, who require general anesthesia, need to be intubated during anesthesia to protect against the risk of pulmonary aspiration of gastric contents. The time interval from the last ingestion of food, or the onset of labor, to the time of induction of general anesthesia, is of no value in determining the risk of aspiration. The use of oral antacids during labor does not lessen the need for intubation when general anesthesia is used.

2. The extent of newborn depression is directly proportional to the induction to delivery interval. General anesthesia is induced only when the obstetrician is ready. Delivery should be accomplished as rapidly thereafter as is in keeping with good obstetrical principles. Nothing is gained by delaying delivery after induction to allow the drug to be removed from the fetus. Such delay only exposes the fetus to more depressant anesthetic drugs.

3. The plane of anesthesia sought before delivery is that which provides maternal analgesia and amnesia. Favorable surgical conditions and prevention of movement are provided by the use of minimal amounts of skeletal muscle relaxant such as succinylcholine and curare. If used in large doses, nondepolarizing relaxants such as curare may cross the placenta in amounts sufficient to depress newborn skeletal muscle activity.

4. Oxygen should make up more than 50 percent of the inspired maternal anesthetic mixture before birth to assure more vigorous and better oxygenated newborns. To insure maternal analgesia and amnesia, the addition of low concentrations of potent inhalation drugs such as 0.5 percent halothane, 0.75 percent to 1 percent enflurane, or 0.2 percent to 0.5 percent methoxyflurane added to 30 percent to 40 percent nitrous oxide as required.

5. While adequate maternal ventilation is to be assured, marked maternal hyperventilation as regulated by the anesthetist must be avoided until birth of the newborn, since hyperventilation is associated with decreased uterine blood flow and fetal acidosis.

6. Left uterine displacement must be maintained at all times until the birth of the newborn to avoid aorta-caval compression with its associ-

ated hypotension and decreased maternal cardiac output, and hence, depressed uterine blood flow.

7. Following delivery, the depth of maternal anesthesia may be increased by increasing the concentration of nitrous oxide and giving narcotics. The concentration of the potent inhalation drug should not be increased because this may cause depressed uterine contractions, and may be associated with increased maternal blood loss.

8. The same quality of anesthetic care must be available to the parturient as it is to the surgical patient. This includes adequate monitoring during anesthesia and adequate postoperative observation.

9. When general anesthesia is required in an emergency, it is usually in the mother's interest to wait until qualified anesthesia personnel are available, or to proceed with an alternative form of anesthesia. Nurses and physicians who are not fully trained and competent in anesthesia should not attempt to administer general anesthesia.

§ 18.12   Regional Anesthesia

Regional or conduction anesthesia is ideally suited to vaginal delivery. If the complications of hypotension and a local anesthetic toxicity are avoided, it is associated with minimal newborn depression and a mother who is awake and free from pain, and capable of relating to her newborn baby immediately following birth. Awake, she is unlikely to aspirate gastric contents and can cooperate with the obstetrician. Except when uterine relaxation is required, regional analgesia can provide complete pain relief and suitable conditions for both vaginal and abdominal delivery. The most common forms of regional anesthesia are spinal, lumbar, epidural, caudal, paracervical, pudendal, and local perineal infiltration. Each technique has a specific application and can be used to block some or all of the nerves carrying the pain impulses.

Uterine pain, resulting from dilatation and effacement of the cervix from uterine contractions, is conveyed by small nerve fibers which pass from the cervix diffusely through the pelvis, join the sympathetic chain at L-2 to L-5, and enter the spinal cord at T-10 to T-12. These pain fibers can be blocked effectively by a paracervical block. Vaginal and perineal pain associated with the second and third stages of labor, is mediated primarily through the pudendal nerve originating from S-2 to S-4. There is additional perineal innervation from the genitofemoral, ilioinguinal, and lateral femoral cutaneous nerves. Pudendal nerve block, true saddle block (subarachnoid or spinal block), and low caudal epidural block alleviates most of the vaginal and perineal pain. A combination of blocks or a subarachnoid, lumbar epidural, or caudal epidural block provides relief from all pain during labor and delivery.

Before performing any regional block in obstetrics, the physician must be prepared for the management of possible complications. The most serious life-threatening complications are severe hypotension, local anesthetic convulsions, total spinal anesthesia with respiratory arrest, and vasopressor-induced hypertension.

Any room in which anesthesia is performed should have the following items immediately available before starting the block: apparatus for monitoring blood pressure, oxygen with positive pressure breathing apparatus and mask, suction with a wide-bore suction catheter, oral and nasal airways, a laryngoscope and endotracheal tubes, thiopental or valium to stop a convulsion, and ephedrine to treat hypotension. Prior to placing any block, an intravenous route should be established. The bed should be capable of being placed in the Trendelenburg position (head-down) rapidly. The suggested contents of a mobile resuscitation cart should include the following:

1. Positive pressure breathing apparatus
2. Oxygen supply
3. Laryngoscope, adult and infant blades
4. Endotracheal tubes, adult and infant
5. Nasal airways
6. Suction catheters
7. Board for closed chest massage
8. Drugs:
   a. Ephedrine
   b. Calcium chloride
   c. Sodium bicarbonate
   d. Atropine
   e. Dopamine
   f. Thiopental or valium
   g. Succinylcholine
   h. Curare
   i. Narcan
9. Nasal-gastric tubes
10. Intravenous supplies, plasma expanders and electrolyte solution, syringes, needles, plastic indwelling catheters.

Each labor room should contain an oxygen supply, suction, and bed capable of rapid Trendelenburg position. An ECG monitor and defibrillator should be readily available. The cart should be checked prior to starting any type of regional anesthesia.

Despite its many advantages, regional anesthesia has disadvantages and requires constant observation of the mother if it is to be safe and effective.

The newer amide local anesthetics, xylocaine, carbocaine, nesacaine, and marcaine, have a prolonged half-life in maternal and neonatal blood due to their slow metabolism by the liver. This causes no difficulty in routine use, as levels usually remain well below toxic levels. However, repeated injection of these drugs, as in the case of continuous lumbar and caudal epidural anesthesia, can result in increasing blood levels in both mother and fetus.

Local anesthetics administered during labor may decrease fetal heart rate beat-to-beat variability, making fetal heart rate evaluation more difficult. This action of local anesthetics has not been associated with deleterious effects on the newborn and is shared by other drugs including narcotics, tranquilizers, and anticholinergics.

Hypotension remains the most common side effect of major regional anesthesia for vaginal delivery. The incidence and severity of hypotension depend on the height of the block, maternal position, the addition of epinephrine to the local anesthetic, the physical status of the parturient, and the prophylactic means taken to avoid hypotension. Measures to reduce the incidence of hypotension include the administration of fluids prior to the block, left uterine displacement, and prophylactic administration of ephedrine. If hypotension occurs, more left uterine displacement should be applied, the patient placed in Trendelenburg, and intravenous fluids administered rapidly. If blood pressure is not restored within 30 to 60 seconds, ephedrine 10 to 15 mg should be given intravenously and oxygen administered by face mask.

The use of regional anesthesia in the obstetrical patient requires a constant monitoring during labor, delivery, and in the postpartum period by a trained maternity nurse. An accurate record of maternal vital signs must be kept. A reliable intravenous infusion must be maintained at all times. The personnel and means to assure a clear airway and apply positive pressure ventilation with oxygen—and the ability to treat local anesthetic reactions, high levels of block, and maternal hypotension—must be immediately available if serious problems to both mother and fetus are to be avoided. Continuous recorded electronic monitoring of fetal heart rate and uterine contractions should be considered when regional anesthesia is used in the first stage of labor. Such monitoring is indicated in the high risk pregnancy, or when regional anesthesia is used for the mother receiving oxytocin stimulation.

§ 18.13 —Paracervical Block

Paracervical block is produced by injection of small quantities of local anesthetic solution into the parametrium at sights in the cervix of 3:00 and 9:00, or 4:00 and 8:00. It provides rapid and complete relief of uterine pain with minimal maternal side effects. Paracervical block does not affect vaginal and perineal sensation, and therefore, does not interfere with the bearing-down reflex of the second stage of labor. Unfortunately, paracervical block has been associated with fetal bradycardia, fetal acidosis, and even fetal death.[22] These untoward fetal effects are thought to be caused by the local anesthetic passing rapidly through the placenta to the fetus, secondary to absorption through the uterine artery. There is also evidence that proximity of the local anesthetic to the uterine artery may result in vasoconstriction of the uterine artery with decreased uteroplacental perfusion. The danger to the fetus can be minimized by using minimal doses of the less toxic local anaesthetic, such as Nesacaine, and by injecting them superficially in the parametrium. The use of paracervical block is a good indication for continuous electronic fetal heart monitoring. Paracervical block is best avoided in the premature fetus and the fetus at high risk.

§ 18.14 —Pudendal Block

Of all the regional anesthetic blocks for vaginal delivery, bilateral pudendal nerve block is perhaps the safest and one of the most useful available. Although pudendal block provides no relief of uterine pain and no analgesia for cervical or uterine manipulations, it does alleviate most of the vaginal and perineal pain associated with delivery. It produces adequate analgesia for episiotomy and repair, and allows most uncomplicated outlet forceps deliveries. When supplemented with inhalation analgesia, it usually produces adequate analgesia for other types of forceps deliveries. Since pudendal block does not completely anesthetize the perineum, it does not completely abolish the bearing-down reflex of the second stage of labor. It is relatively painless to administer, and when local anesthetic toxicity is avoided, it has essentially no ill effects on the mother or her newborn. Pudendal block is not associated with maternal hypotension and is the only technique of conduction anesthesia that does not affect autonomic innervation of the uterus.

---

22 D.H. Ralston & S.M. Shnider, *The Fetal and Neonatal Effects of Regional Anesthesia in Obstetrics*, 48 Anesthesiology 34 (1978).

The pudendal nerve runs just lateral to the tips of the ischial spines, the obstetric landmarks which determine the station of the presenting part. It may be blocked from either the transvaginal approach, most commonly used in obstetrics, or from the transcutaneous route. A bilateral block requires only 10 ml to 20 ml of a dilute local anesthetic solution such as 1 percent xylocaine, and is usually administered by the obstetrician who is delivering the baby.

§ 18.15   —Spinal Anesthesia

Subarachnoid, or spinal block, is one of the most useful blocks for obstetrics and is technically easy to administer. The amount of drug needed is less than that required for any other block used in obstetrics—about one-fifth that required to produce the same level of anesthesia by the epidural route. Thus, local anesthetic toxicity in both the mother and the fetus is not a problem. Onset of anesthesia is very rapid, usually complete within five minutes. Essentially, every obstetric procedure not requiring depression of uterine activity can be accomplished with subarachnoid block. Later in labor, a true saddle block of the perineum (S-1 to S-5) allows forceps delivery and repair of episiotomy. If a modified saddle block (T-10 to S-5) is produced, both uterine as well as perineal discomfort are completely abolished. Long-acting local anesthetics such as tetracaine (Pontocaine) with epinephrine, produce three hours of pain relief when injected into the subarachnoid space, permitting elimination of all pain in the latter part of labor, and for delivery. Increasing the level of block to T-4 or higher, produces satisfactory anesthesia for cesarean birth.

The major disadvantages of subarachnoid block are its potential for causing maternal hypotension, total spinal block, postspinal headache, the abolishment of the reflex urge to bear down in the second stage of labor, and early relaxation of the perineal musculature, which can result in persistent occiput posterior presentation, and prolong the second stage of labor.

As previously mentioned, severe and sudden maternal hypotension which leads to fetal distress and maternal cardiovascular collapse due to vasodilation, secondary to sympathetic block, is still a significant cause of maternal mortality. Prophylaxis includes left uterine displacement (manually pushing the uterus to the left side of the mother's abdomen which relieves the pressure on the aorta) and hydration with a liter or more of balanced salt solution administered intravenously 15 minutes to 30 minutes before the block is instituted. Treatment of hypotension includes these two steps as well as the use of a central acting vasopressor, such as ephedrine (10 to 25 mg given intravenously), and the administration of high concentrations of oxygen. Potent peripheral vasoconstrictors such as norephinephrine (Levophed), phenylephrine

(Neo-synephrine), and methoxamine (Vasoxyl), rapidly correct maternal hypotension; but they are to be avoided because they cause further decline in uterine perfusion, resulting in additional fetal distress.

Total or dangerously high levels of subarachnoid block usually result when the subarachnoid injection is made just before or during a uterine contraction, or when too large a dose of local anesthetic is used. The same level of block can be obtained in the obstetric patient with only two-thirds of the amount of drug required to produce a given level in her nonpregnant counterpart. Treatment of a high block consists of immediate correction of hypotension, support of maternal ventilation with positive pressure oxygen and, if necessary, protection of the upper airway with a cuffed endotracheal tube. With proper therapy, a high or total spinal need not delay delivery and should not be associated with increased maternal or fetal morbidity or mortality.

The incidence of postspinal headache is highest in the postpartum patient. An incidence of over 40 percent can be expected when the subarachnoid space is entered with a 20-gauge or larger bore needle.[23] The headache usually occurs within 24 hours to 72 hours of the subarachnoid block, may last a few days to several weeks, and can be mild to incapacitating. The headache inevitably resolves. It is positional, and is characteristically exacerbated in the upright position and relieved by assuming the supine position, or by increasing abdominal pressure. It is caused by a loss of cerebral spinal fluid through the holes made in the dura (protective covering of the spinal canal) from the spinal needle. Steps to prevent post-spinal headaches include using small gauge needles (25 gauge or less), adequate hydration during the postpartum, and using a tight abdominal binder when the patient is in the upright position. Treatment consists of appropriate analgesics, bedrest (preferably in the prone position with head down), hydration, a right abdominal binder, and reassurance. When the headache is incapacitating, epidural blood patch (which consists of sealing the hole in the dura by injecting the patient's own nonanticoagulated blood into the epidural space) can result in a dramatic cure.

Abolishment of the reflex urge to bear down in the second stage of labor results from the complete perineal analgesia produced by spinal block. It does not prevent the patient from bearing down voluntarily with each contraction. In cases of occiput posterior presentation, the tone in the muscles of the perineum causes the occiput to rotate to the anterior presentation. As spinal block does produce profound relaxation of the perineum, an increased incidence of persistent occiput posterior presentations can be expected with its use. Since perineal relaxation occurs, the occiput can usually be easily rotated manually, or delivery can be accomplished in the occiput posterior position.

---

23 Abouleish, de la Vega, Blendinger, et al., *Long Term Follow-up of Epidural Blood Patch*, 54 Anesth. Analg. 459 (1975).

§ 18.16   —Epidural Anesthesia

Epidural anesthesia is carried out by introducing anesthetic agents into the epidural space. The epidural space is a potential space filled with loose fatty tissue and a marked plexus of veins. It is the space in the vertebral canal that is surrounded by the ligamentous and bony structure of the vertebral canal on the outside, and the dura containing the cerebrospinal fluid and the spinal cord on the inside. The uppermost limits of the epidural space is the foramen magnum at the base of the skull; interiorly it ends at the sacral hiatus at the base of the sacrum. It may be entered at any of the intervertebral spaces from the cervical area C 1-2 to the L 1-S 1 interspace, or through the sacral hiatus. As the nerve roots leave the spinal cord, they pass through the epidural space, and hence, are exposed to a local anesthetic injected in the epidural space.

Injection of local anesthetic through the sacral hiatus is referred to as caudal epidural block. Because the sacral hiatus is located low in the vertebral column, the anesthetic agent reaches the sacral nerves first, resulting in perineal anesthesia initially. In order to provide relief during contractions, additional amounts of agent must be introduced at the level of the lumbar and low thoracic nerves.

When the anesthetic agent is introduced at the lumbar level, the technique is referred to as lumbar epidural anesthesia. Lumbar epidural anesthesia has largely replaced caudal epidural anesthesia in obstetrics. The latter is technically more difficult to perform, requires three to four times as much anesthetic agent, and cannot reliably be extended to provide adequate analgesia for cesarean birth. Using a continuous catheter technique, a segmental block with an upper level of T-10 can be established with the onset of painful contractions, and then maintained throughout the first stage of labor. In the second stage of labor, the block can be extended to give perineal anesthesia. If a cesarean section becomes necessary, the level of the block can be elevated to T-4. Thus, as with subarachnoid block, lumbar epidural block can provide adequate anesthesia for all obstetrical procedures not requiring depression of uterine activity. Its use allows a pain-free labor and an alert and cooperative mother who will require no additional medications for pain.

§ 18.17   Bibliography and Recommended Readings

Danforth, David N., Ph.D., M.D., *Obstetrics and Gynecology*, 4th ed. (Harper & Row Publishers, Inc., 1982).

Iffy, Leslie, M.D. & Kaminetzky, Harold A., M.D., *Principles and Practice of Obstetrics & Perinatology*, vol. 2 (John Wiley & Sons, Inc., 1981).

Intrauterine Asphyxia and the Developing Fetal Brain, edited by Louis Gluck, M.D. (Year Book Medical Publishers, Inc., 1977).

Klaus, Marshall, M.D. & Fanaroff, Avroy, M.D., *Care of the High-Risk Neonate*, 2d ed. (W.B. Saunders Co., 1979).

Niswander, K.R., M.D., *Obstetrics, Essentials of Clinical Practice* (Little, Brown & Co., 1981).

Resuscitation of the Newborn Infant, 3d ed., edited by H. Abramson (The C.V. Mosby Co., 1973).

Scipien, G., R.N., B.S., M.S., et al., *Comprehensive Pediatric Nursing* (McGraw-Hill, 1975).

CHAPTER 19

INDUCTION OF LABOR

§ 19.1   Introduction

From the standpoint of obstetrics, the term induction refers to a *preplanned* method of *artificially* stimulating labor. This procedure is indicated when either the patient's uterine contractions are not strong enough to push the fetus through the birth canal, or when her pregnancy must be terminated early in order to prevent the fetus from succumbing to deteriorating intrauterine conditions. Induction is most commonly done (1) mechanically by stripping or rupturing the membranes, or (2) chemically by using specific pharmaceuticals to induce uterine contractions.

§ 19.2   Simple Corrective Measures

Before resorting to mechanical or chemical induction, some of the simpler and less precarious methods of stimulating labor should be attempted. For example, if the bladder is over-distended late in the first stage of labor, simply removing the excess fluid (by asking the patient to urinate or inserting a urinary catheter if she is unable to do so) often hastens the completion of cervical dilatation, and encourages further descent of the fetus.

As long as no contraindications exist, an alternate way of stimulating uterine contractions is to give the pregnant woman an enema. Altering her position may also improve the nature of her contractions. Generally, contractions occur less frequently when the patient is lying on her side than when she is lying on her back, though they tend to be better coordinated and more intense in the former position. Labor occasionally resumes with increased vigor if the woman is permitted to walk around or sit up in a chair, but for safety's sake, this should only be allowed if her membranes have not yet ruptured, and the fetus's head is deeply engaged.

As helpful as these simple measures may be, the obstetrician must realize their limitations and not delay the initiation of additional treatment if conditions do not change. Depending on the urgency of the situation, it may be appropriate to induce labor by mechanical or chemical means, or consider a cesarean section when those procedures are contraindicated or unsuccessful, or when delivery must be carried out promptly.

§ 19.3   Mechanical Induction

The amniotic sac, also referred to as the bag of waters because it contains the amniotic fluid in which the fetus is suspended throughout pregnancy, is enclosed by a thin covering called the amniotic membrane, or simply the membranes. The mechanical methods of induction are based on the fact that disrupting the integrity of the membranes usually causes labor to begin soon afterwards.

In the technique known as *stripping* the membranes, the obstetrician can stimulate labor by inserting her finger through the patient's cervix, and gently separating the membranes from their point of attachment on the lower uterine wall. However, before doing so, the obstetrician must determine exactly where the placenta is located. Without prior knowledge of whether it is situated closer to the cervix than the fetus is (a condition called *placenta previa* which contraindicates this procedure, see §§ **13.8** and **13.9**), the placenta might be accidentally stripped away from the uterine wall along with the membranes, a potentially catastrophic event for the fetus.

Another way of mechanically inducing labor involves *rupturing* the membranes using a technique called amniotomy. Done more frequently in combination with the drug oxytocin than alone, its success rate depends on the physician's ability to select the proper patient and the proper time since a large percentage of complications occurs when mechanical procedures are attempted before the woman's body has prepared itself for delivery. The known hazards can be avoided by first performing a thorough vaginal examination, checking for whether the cervix is soft, effaced, adequately dilated, and situated in the middle of the vagina. If so, it is usually possible to initiate labor, whereas when the cervix is firm, uneffaced, and located in the posterior region of the vagina, induction is dangerous.

Although the cervix provides one of the best indications of whether induction is likely to be successful, the station of the fetus is also an important factor, so it too must be evaluated during the pelvic examination. If the fetal presenting part has not descended well into the pelvis when amniotomy is performed, the sudden release of amniotic fluid may cause the umbilical cord to prolapse. In these cases, it is usually preferable to leave the membranes intact and induce labor with an oxytocic drug instead.

§ 19.4   Chemical Induction

Ordinarily, when the pituitary hormone called oxytocin is released into the bloodstream at the end of pregnancy, it stimulates the woman's uterus to contract. Contractions are essential because they are the force responsible for triggering the chain of anatomic and physiologic responses needed to expel the fetus from the womb. If for some reason these natural events either do not begin on time or are ineffective, synthetic analogues of oxytocin, marketed as Pitocin and Syntocinon, are often administered to the patient because in the proper concentration, they are capable of inducing contractions equivalent to those normally accompanying spontaneous labor (meaning contractions that occur every two to three minutes and last 40 to 50 seconds).

§ 19.5   —Prerequisite for Oxytocin Administration

Not intended for normally progressing full-term labors, oxytocin should only be used to induce early labor or treat abnormal progress of labor (including dysfunctional labor and uterine inertia). Under these circumstances, artificial stimulation of labor may be less hazardous to the mother and her baby than the usual alternative, waiting until labor begins spontaneously. For example, induction of labor before the due date may save the fetus's life if deteriorating intrauterine conditions threaten its ability to survive inside the womb, as may happen when complications such as hemolytic (Rh) disease, diabetes, hypertensive disorders, bleeding problems, maternal infection, or premature rupture of the membranes cannot be treated and controlled medically. Oxytocin induction may also be indicated to augment weak uterine contractions, or to convert an abnormal pattern of uterine contractility to a normal one since uncorrected cases of uterine inertia, predispose the mother to infection and the fetus to periods of distress, and ultimately death.

It is important to remember that a legitimate medical indication is not the sole criterion for safe induction. Carefully evaluating the entire clinical picture is essential because in certain instances, even *normal* uterine contractions may cause traumatic or lethal maternal and/or fetal injuries. These needless additions to the morbidity and mortality statistics can be prevented by assuring that all of the following conditions are satisfied before oxytocin is administered.

1. The progress of labor must definitely be slowing down. Administering oxytocin to simply speed-up a normally advancing labor is potentially dangerous.

2. There must be no mechanical obstacles to labor. Conditions such as an unfavorable pelvic shape, a pelvic abnormality, fetopelvic disproportion, tumor obstruction, and previous uterine surgery (including cesarean sections) are contraindications to oxytocin administration because they may subject the fetus to inadequate oxygen supplies and intracranial hemorrhage during delivery, in addition to predisposing the mother to uterine rupture.

3. A well-flexed head should be the presenting fetal part. An extended head is a relative contraindication, and transverse lie, face, or brow presentations are unequivocal contraindications to oxytocin. Oxytocin stimulation is hardly ever used in breech presentations. See § **9.7** for a discussion of fetal orientation in the womb.

4. The fetus should be mature and in good condition, as evidenced by the appropriate maturity tests and a normal heart rate. See §§ **10.2, 10.7,** and **10.10**. If the fetus is distressed, a cesarean section is generally preferable because the baby can be delivered much faster than during induction, an important consideration in such emergencies.

5. The mother must not be carrying more than one fetus. She also must not be older than 35 nor have given birth to six or more children, since

women of advanced reproductive age or those of such high parity have a greater incidence of uterine rupture following oxytocin induction.

6. The mother must not have veneral disease. If so, there is a high probability that her child will acquire the disease during its descent through the infected birth canal.

7. The mother must not have cardiac disease.

A good rule of thumb to remember is that whenever normal labor would be dangerous for the mother or the fetus, mechanical or chemical induction is contraindicated. If prompt delivery is indicated before the prerequisites are met, cesarean section should be considered.

§ 19.6   —Routes of Administration

Oxytocin can be administered by one of three routes, intramuscularly, orally, or intravenously. The intramuscular method may be used *after* the baby is born in order to stimulate the expulsion of the placenta, or control blood loss during the postpartum period.[1]

Opting for the convenience of placing a 200 I.U. (international units) tablet of oxytocin in the patient's mouth instead of preparing an intravenous solution of the drug to infuse through her veins, the advocates of the controversial oral route contend that it is a satisfactory method of induction when only a small amount of uterine stimulation is required.[2] Although this point is still contestable, most clinicians agree that complete control of the effects of oxytocin (provided only by an intravenous infusion) assumes vital importance if a prolonged period of stimulation is anticipated.[3] The oral route is contraindicated in these instances: breech presentations, twin pregnancies, and in women who have given birth to six or more children.

Dissolving usually within one hour, the effect of an oxytocin tablet can supposedly be stopped by merely removing it, and then asking the patient to rinse her mouth out with water. No more than one tablet should be taken at a time, and additional doses should not be given until at least 30 minutes later.[4]

---

[1] J.A. Pritchard, M.D. & P.C. MacDonald, M.D., Williams Obstetrics, 16th ed., 426 (Appleton-Century-Crofts, 1980).

[2] Chalmers & Moorhouse, *Further Experience With Buccal Oxytocin*, 73 J. Obstet. Gynecol. Br. Cwlth. 59 (1966).

[3] Theobold G.W., *Research Project on Buccal Pitocin* Brit. Med. J. 190 (1965).

[4] Newman & Hon, *Induction of Labor With Transbuccal Oxytocic*, 21 Obstet. Gynecol. 3 (1963).

Others say 20 minute intervals are acceptable until a maintenance level simulating adequate labor is achieved.[5] If inhalation anesthesia is to be used, the tablet should be removed beforehand.

A constant intravenous infusion of oxytocin is considered the procedure of choice, being the safest and most efficient way of chemically inducing uterine contractions.[6] If a constant infusion pump is not available, a simple alternative is to add an oxytocin ampule to a 1 liter bottle of 5 percent glucose, and then allow the solution to drip into the patient's vein, counting the number of drops per minute. Regardless of which method is used, controlling the effects of oxytocin as it enters the bloodstream is of utmost importance, because the uterus becomes increasingly responsive to oxytocin as pregnancy progresses into the third trimester, and it is exquisitely sensitive to extremely small doses at term.

The dosage required to stimulate normal uterine contractions is quite variable from patient to patient, ranging from as low as 0.5 mU/min (milliunits per minute) to 10.0 mU/min. Occasionally, 20.0 mU/min of the drug may be indicated and rarely an even larger dose may be needed, though such high levels should not be necessary in *term labors*. For patients requiring *preterm* induction, it is advisable to first reassess their pelvic adequacy and previous progress of labor before increasing the infusion rate beyond 20.0 mU/min.

If the recommended dose range is exceeded, or if the uterus is excessively responsive to low doses, the contractions will become much more forceful and the interval between successive contractions will be shortened, leading to fetal injury and/or uterine rupture. Since one of the primary dangers associated with oxytocic drugs is the inability to determine in advance just how responsive the uterus will be to them, a trial run of a very dilute oxytocin solution (.05-1.0 mU/min) is advisable to minimize the serious risks. Generally, the drug takes effect rapidly, so if the trial dose is sufficient, uterine contractions will typically occur within 2-4 minutes after the infusion is started, and will reach their peak about 15 minutes later.

Measuring the mother's vital signs and the fetus's heart rate about three to five minutes after the initial test dose allows the obstetrician to quickly detect signs of mild pituitary shock or other evidence of sensitivity, findings which contraindicate this class of pharmaceuticals. But as long as no abnormal signs or symptoms develop and no appreciable increase in uterine activity is observed, it is customary to gradually increase the dosage of oxytocin to 1-2 mU/min 15-20 minutes following the trial infusion. If the contractions are

---

5 Maxwell, *A Comparison of Buccal and Intravenous Oxytocin*, 71 J. Obstet. Gynecol. Br. Cwlth. 37 (1964).

6 J.A. Pritchard, M.D. & P.C. MacDonald, M.D., Williams Obstetrics, 16th ed., 790 (Appleton-Century-Crofts, 1980).

still inadequate after another 20-30 minutes, the flow rate may be slowly increased at regular intervals until contractions lasting approximately 35 seconds and recurring every 3 minutes are induced.

Once regular and efficient uterine contractility is achieved, the amount of oxytocin should be stabilized, and the progress of labor should be evaluated. Some obstetricians conduct the remainder of the delivery with a very small dose of oxytocin to prevent uterine inertia from recurring.[7] The latter group often suggest leaving the infusion needle in the patient's vein so the flow of the oxytocin solution can be reinitiated without delay if it becomes necessary at a later time. This measure allows optimal control of uterine contractility during delivery and in the immediate postpartum period.

Another important, though not unanimously agreed upon issue, is how long to run the intravenous infusion. Some physicians feel it may be necessary for up to six to eight hours,[8] whereas others call the procedure a failure when the cervix does not dilate appreciably, and labor does not start after just a few hours.[9] They claim that not only are the chances for successful therapy minimal when oxytocin does not improve the uterine contractions in a short time, but more importantly, fetal and maternal complications may even arise if induction is continued for too long without good results.

Regardless of which route or method of oxytocin administration is chosen, the fetus's heart rate must be checked regularly in the interval between contractions, and the mother's blood pressure, pulse rate, and uterine activity must be evaluated. The frequency, intensity, and duration of her contractions, as well as the uterine tone between contractions, must not exceed the values observed during normal spontaneous labor. If at any time her contractions become tetanic, recur too frequently (more than three in ten minutes; others say less than two minutes apart), or last too long (greater than one minute); or if the fetal heart rate decelerates, or is irregular, the infusion must be stopped immediately. The adverse effects of oxytocin should disappear soon afterwards because oxytocin breaks down rapidly in the bloodstream.

Only constant diligence and careful regulation of the dosage will minimize the number of injuries and deaths attributed to oxytocin induction. For this reason, the obstetrician must remain in the labor and delivery room throughout the entire period of induction. It is her responsibility to be fully aware of the prerequisites, contraindications, and techniques of administration, as well

---

[7] D.N. Danforth, Ph.D., M.D., Obstetrics and Gynecology 723, 4th ed. (Harper & Row Publishers, 1982).

[8] Friedman & Sachtleben, *Dysfunctional labor*, 21 Obstet. Gynecol. 13 (1963).

[9] Fernando Arias, M.D., Ph.D., High-Risk Pregnancy and Delivery 308 (The C. V. Mosby Co., 1984).

as to be prepared to adjust the oxytocin levels if conditions change during labor.

Considered an important therapeutic agent when properly administered for legitimate medical reasons, oxytocin can have deleterious or even fatal consequences if the recommended guidelines are not strictly followed. The potential dangers of oxytocin induction, believed by many to be avoidable and inexcusable, include:

1. Delivering a premature infant
2. Water intoxication
3. Uterine rupture
4. Excessive uterine contractility.

In addition to the recognized dangers of oxytocin induction, no one knows what, if any, direct effect oxytocin or the combination of oxytocin with other pharmaceuticals has on the newborn.

§ 19.7 —Delivering a Premature Infant

Unless a maternal disorder necessitates early intervention, and a continuation of intrauterine life jeopardizes the fetus's chances for survival more than the risks of prematurity, induction should be deferred until the appropriate fetal maturity tests indicate that the baby is adequately developed to live outside the womb.

§ 19.8 —Water Intoxication

When large doses of oxytocin are intravenously administered in salt-free solutions for long periods of time, an electrolyte imbalance is created. It not only causes the mother to retain water, but depending on the severity of her condition, she may also develop water intoxication, edema, and convulsions. Some clinicians have even reported convulsions in newborns delivered to mothers who received such infusions.[10] To prevent these dangers, it is mandatory to accurately record the patient's fluid intake and fluid output (urine flow) during oxytocin administration, and as a further precautionary measure, when relatively high rates of oxytocin (over 20 mU/min) need to be infused for a

---

[10] J.A. Pritchard, M.D. & P.C. MacDonald, M.D., Williams Obstetrics, 16th ed., 427 (Appleton-Century-Crofts, 1980).

prolonged period, it is preferable to increase the concentration of the drug in the existing solution rather than increase the flow rate of a more dilute solution.

§ 19.9   —Uterine Rupture

Multiparas, especially those who have given birth to six or more children, are very susceptible to uterine rupture, as are all patients with an overdistended uterus (including women carrying twins or triplets). Uterine rupture may also occur when oxytocin is given to patients with scarred uteri, when it is used to stimulate uterine activity in the presence of fetopelvic disproportion, or when it is prescribed in doses exceeding the physiologic range.

§ 19.10   —Excessive Uterine Contractility

Excessive uterine contractility, a condition, which almost always results from an excessive dose of oxytocin, seriously endangers the fetus's life. Because the blood flow to the placenta essentially stops while the uterus is contracting, any medication or procedure which inappropriately lengthens or strengthens the nature of the contractions is liable to cause substantial fetal oxygen loss during delivery. Contractions which are too intense (the labor is described as tumultus) also subject the fetus's head to increased pressure—a particularly hazardous situation if the membranes are already ruptured since they can no longer protect the child from internal trauma.

§ 19.11   —Sparteine

Sparteine, though not a synthetic analogue of oxytocin like Pitocin and Syntocinon, produces similar effects on the pregnant uterus and is therefore said to have oxytocic properties. A popular intramuscular method of inducing labor in the 1960s, sparteine is no longer recommended because its action is too unpredictable.[11] Sometimes it actually worsens the contraction pattern and it is not safer than the other oxytocics, causing many of the same complications as they do.

---

[11] Louis M. Hellman & Jack A. Pritchard, Williams Obstetrics, 14th ed., 846-47 (Appleton-Century-Crofts, 1971).

§ 19.12 —Postpartum Use of Oxytocin Agents

Even *after* the baby has been delivered, adequate uterine contractions are still of vital importance in order to expel the placenta and reduce the maternal blood loss. Although some obstetricians routinely administer oxytocic drugs at this stage as preventative measure, others believe that these pharmaceuticals should only be given to patients who are predisposed to postpartum hemorrhage, or to those who are actively bleeding, since the normal uterine contractions are generally able to regulate the blood loss without assistance.

Next to oxytocin, the alkaloids ergonovine maleate (Ergotrate) and methylergonovine maleate (Methergine), are the most commonly used oxytocic agents in the postpartum period. Whether given intravenously, intramuscularly, or orally, these two powerful uterine stimulants produce strong, long-lasting contractions which effectively control, or even prevent, excessive blood loss and hemorrhage. However, the intensity and duration of their effects are so great, that they should never be given to an undelivered patient, and unlike oxytocin, are strictly limited to the postpartum period.

§ 19.13   Bibliography and Recommended Readings

Aladjem, Silvio, M.D., *Risks in the Practice of Modern Obstetrics* (The C.V. Mosby Co., 1975).

Aladjem, Silvio, M.D., Brown, Audrey, K., M.D., Sureau, Claude, M.D., *Clinical Perinatology*, 2d ed. (The C.V. Mosby Co., 1980).

Danforth, D.N., Ph.D., M.D., *Obstetrics and Gynecology*, 4th ed. (Harper & Row Publishers, Inc., 1982).

Iffy, Leslie, M.D. & Kaminetzky, Harold A., M.D., *Principles and Practice of Obstetrics & Perinatology*, vol. 2 (John Wiley & Sons, Inc., 1981).

Newman, J.W., M.B. & Hon, Edward H., M.D., *Induction of Labor with Transbuccal Oxytocic*, 21 Obstet. Gynecol. 3 (1963).

Niswander, K.R., M.D., *Obstetrics, Essentials of Clinical Practice* (Little, Brown & Co., 1981).

Oxorn, Harry, B.A., M.D., *Human Labor and Birth*, 4th ed. (Appleton-Century-Crofts, 1980).

Pritchard, J.A., M.D., MacDonald, P.C., M.D., & Gant, N.F., M.D., *Williams Obstetrics*, 17th ed. (Appleton-Century-Crofts, 1985).

Reeder, Sharon J., R.N., Ph.D., Mastroianni, Luigi, Jr., M.D., & Martin, Leonide, L., R.N., *Maternity Nursing*, 15th ed. (J.B. Lippincott Co., 1983).

Vasicka, Alois, M.D. & Hutchinson, Harry T., M.D., *Fetal Response to Induction, Augmentation, and Correction of Labor by Oxytocin*, 85 Am. J. Obstet. Gynecol. 1054 (1963).

CHAPTER 20

FORCEPS

§ 20.1 Introduction

Obstetric forceps are designed to extract the fetus from the birth canal, or to rotate its head within the vagina. If the instrument is accurately applied to the fetal head and traction is made in the proper diameters of the maternal pelvis, considerable force may be exerted without injuring the mother or her baby. However, even the slightest misuse of force may damage the fetal skull, since its bony framework is still delicate and pliable, and therefore unable to resist excess compression and traction. The risk of permanent brain damage is so serious that all obstetricians must learn the principles of forceps extraction before attempting the procedure.

§ 20.2   Description of Forceps

Obstetric forceps vary somewhat in size and shape, but they all basically consist of two steel branches that cross each other like scissors. Each branch is composed of a handle, shank, lock, and blade. The blades have two curves: (1) the *cephalic curve*, which conforms to the contours of the fetus's head, and (2) the *pelvic curve*, which approximates the curve of the mother's pelvic canal.

The blades are designated left and right according to their position in the mother's pelvis after application. "The rule of the forceps is 'left blade, left hand, left side of the pelvis,' "[1] and vice versa. Following this guideline, the left blade is held in the operator's left hand and is inserted into the left side of the pelvis. Using the right hand, the right blade is then placed separately in the right side of the mother's pelvis.

Presently, over 600 types of forceps have been invented, the majority of which are called classic forceps. A smaller percentage of instruments are considered specialized forceps. Two large categories of classic forceps exist, easily distinguished by the configuration of their shanks. *Simpson-type forceps* have separated shanks, whereas *Elliot-type forceps* have overlapping shanks.

Selection of the appropriate instrument depends on the degree of molding anticipated, the shape of the pelvis, and the development of any special problems. Generally, a Simpson-type forceps is recommended for the well-molded, elongate head resulting from a long labor, especially in a nullipara. One of the Elliot-type forceps is suggested for the relatively unmolded, rounded head which is more commonly seen in a multipara after a short labor.[2]

---

[1] D. N. Danforth, Ph.D., M.D., Obstetrics and Gynecology, 4th ed., 653 (Harper & Row Publishers, Inc., 1982).

[2] Leslie Iffy, M.D. & Harold A. Kaminetzky, M.D., Principles and Practice of Obstetrics & Perinatology vol. 2, 1498 (John Wiley & Sons, Inc., 1981).

§ 20.3   Function of Forceps

Forceps primarily provide a means for traction and rotation. The objective of traction is to mimic the natural birth process in the amount, direction, and intermittent nature of the force applied.

Although some compression of the fetal head is inevitable when forceps are applied, it should be minimized. To prevent the maximal force from compressing the head, the handles of the articulated forceps must not be squeezed together. In addition, the operator should sit with his arms flexed and elbows held closely against his chest, since he must be careful not to apply his body weight during the traction.

Although traction is the principle function of forceps, they can also be used as a rotator to reposition the fetal head. Transverse and posterior positions of the occiput can often be successfully managed by rotation. However, rotation with forceps is risky, and irreparable damage to the supporting structures may follow unskillful efforts. For this reason, rotation should never be combined with pendulum, corkscrew, or twisting motions.

§ 20.4   Prerequisite for the Use of Forceps

Before the availability of adequate blood-banking facilities and the more liberal use of cesarean sections, it was often the lesser of two evils to deliver a fetus with forceps, regardless of the neonatal outcome. This reasoning is no longer valid. In fact, in addition to a well-defined indication for forcep delivery, all obstetric textbooks emphasize that the following conditions must also be satisfied, otherwise the procedure will be unjustifiably dangerous for the mother and baby:

1. The operator must be thoroughly familiar with the mechanism of labor, and be trained to recognize the different types of forceps, their advantages, and intended uses.

2. There should be no disproportion between the size of the head and the size of the midpelvis or pelvic outlet. Before considering a forceps extraction, the anatomic characteristics and capacity of the maternal pelvis must be evaluated to assure that it is large enough to permit the delivery of an untraumatized fetus. In borderline cases of cephalopelvic disproportion, a trial forceps procedure is permitted. This situation is discussed in § 20.9.

3. The fetal position and presentation must be precisely determined. Otherwise, the proper application of the forcep blades and accurate extraction and rotation in the appropriate direction are impossible.

4. The fetus must present either by the vertex or by the face, with the chin anterior. The head must be large enough to be grasped by the blades. If it is too large, forceps are contraindicated and another procedure should be chosen. The use of forceps is not intended for transverse lie, brow, or breech presentations; except for the application of forceps to the aftercoming head in breech deliveries. It is worth emphasizing that forceps should only be applied to the infant's head, and never to any other part of its body.

5. The head must be engaged, preferably deeply engaged; that is, the biparietal diameter of the fetal head is well-*below* the pelvic inlet. Its exact location can be determined by pelvic and x-ray examination. Application of forceps when the head is moveable above the pelvic inlet is absolutely indefensible in modern obstetrics. Even when the presenting part is already deep in the vagina, if the blades are applied before the head has reached the perineal floor, it is common to find the head significantly higher than the rectal or vaginal examination has indicated. This misleading situation is more apt to occur following vigorous labor, when elongation of the fetal head resulting from a marked degree of molding and caput formation create the erroneous impression that the head is engaged, even though the biparietal diameter has not yet passed through the pelvic inlet. See § 9.7.

6. The cervix must be completely effaced and dilated. Even a small rim of cervix may offer great resistance when traction is applied, causing extensive cervical lacerations that may also involve the lower uterine segment. Some clinicians feel that if the cervix is completely dilated but not completely retracted (as occurs frequently with an occiput posterior presentation), it may be gently pushed back manually, provided that the head is well-engaged in the pelvis. Others consider this maneuver too risky and conducive to cervical laceration.

   The presenting part usually remains relatively high in the pelvis until the cervix is completely dilated, and labor should be allowed to continue until this point. If prompt delivery is required before complete cervical dilation occurs, cesarean section is generally preferable.

   There is some controversy concerning the propriety of using the forceps themselves to aid in dilating the cervix. Many obstetricians are strictly opposed to this practice. However, some believe that in certain life-threatening situations, a properly performed Duhrssen's incision (multiple radial incisions in the cervix) may be justified to complete a partial cervical dilation. Delivery is then brought about by either forceps or breech extraction, depending on the presentation.

7. The membranes must be ruptured. If left intact, traction on the membranes might detach an edge of the placenta, causing premature placental separation. There is also the risk of the forceps slipping, since the blades cannot adequately grasp the fetal head.

8. The patient's bladder and rectum must be empty in order to reduce trauma to adjacent maternal structures.

9. Anesthesia must be adequate for the procedure.[3]

Except in rare, extenuating circumstances, if any of these prerequisites cannot be met, the use of forceps is contraindicated.

§ 20.5   Indications for Forceps Delivery

Fetal indications for forceps delivery include failure of labor to progress, rotatory arrest, certain abnormal presentations, and some instances of fetal distress. The majority of indicated forceps operations are now done to correct the first two situations. Failure of the fetus to descend (also known as failure of labor to progress, or simply, arrest of progress) is usually associated with insufficient uterine contractions and expulsive forces, excessively resistant or inelastic perineal tissues, a slightly enlarged fetal head, or a malposition or malpresentation. Likewise, inability of the fetus to rotate is often seen in abnormal positions.

The use of forceps is frequently the best method of managing breech presentations (restricting the application of forceps to the aftercoming head) and face presentations. Face presentation by itself is not an indication for forceps delivery, though help is often required in this and other cases of deflexion because labor may be delayed. The position of the chin is critical. Since atraumatic delivery cannot be expected unless anterior rotation of the chin (at least to the transverse diameter of the pelvis) has occurred, forceps should not be applied before this movement has occurred. For a more thorough discussion of the specific ways to manage each position and presentation, the interested reader should refer to a major obstetrical textbook. Selected books including this subject are listed at the end of this chapter.

Forceps delivery is also justified when fetal distress is caused by prolapse of the umbilical cord, premature separation of the placenta, maternal anoxia, and

---

[3] J.P. Greenhill, M.D. & E.A. Friedman, M.D., Biological Principles and Modern Practice of Obstetrics, 769 (W. B. Saunders Co., 1974).

pressure exerted on the head due to prolonged perineal arrest. Similarly, the procedure may be indicated if the obstetrician detects changes in the cardiac rhythm and the passage of meconium in vertex presentations when none had been present before. Despite these indications, the relative risks of the forceps procedure must always be weighed against those of other methods of delivery, such as a cesarean section, particularly when the prerequisites have not yet been fulfilled. Further delay of labor to allow more optimal conditions to evolve for either a spontaneous delivery, or less hazardous forceps delivery, should also be considered, as should the danger of the condition for which immediate forceps delivery is indicated.

Systemic diseases which complicate pregnancy and weaken the mother provide additional indications for forceps delivery, as long as the risk of interference is less than the risk of waiting for spontaneous delivery. Assuming that the prerequisites have been satisfied, the use of forceps is justified to eliminate the perineal phase of labor in certain patients with heart disease and pulmonary tuberculosis, and to shorten labor in others with toxemia of pregnancy or hemorrhage. Other maternal indications include eclampsia, acute pulmonary edema, certain neurologic disorders, intrapartum infection, or maternal exhaustion.

§ 20.6   Application and Technique

The use of obstetric forceps should be restricted to a delivery room equipped with all of the necessities of an operating room, including adequate lighting and resuscitative and anesthesia facilities. A sterile field must always be maintained.

The forceps procedure consists of five maneuvers:

1. Applying the blades
2. Checking the application
3. Adapting, adjusting and locking
4. Extracting the head
5. Removing the instrument.

Before the forceps are inserted into the vagina, it is very helpful to make a "phantom" application. After determining the location of the occiput, the articulated forceps are held close to the perineum, simulating the position in which they should rest after correct application.

It is essential that the forceps be applied directly to the sides of the fetal head along the occipitomental diameter, also referred to as the cephalic, biparietal, or bimalal application. A cephalic application should always be employed instead of a pelvic application (the blades are applied to the side of the maternal pelvis without regard to the position of the fetal head), because the latter exposes the fetus to harmful stresses.

Unless the exact position of the head is determined, a proper cephalic application is impossible. The biparietal diameter of the fetal skull should be located, since it corresponds to the greatest distance between the blades. A perfect grasp of the head can only be achieved when the long axis of the blades corresponds to the biparietal diameter, with the tips of the blades lying over the cheeks while the concave margins of the blades are directed toward either the sagittal suture or the face. Following this technique, the cephalic curve of the forceps should be large enough to grasp the head firmly without compression, but not so large that the instrument slips.

Cephalic application of the forceps along the occipitomental diameter is possible in several different situations, including the occiput anterior, occiput transverse, and occiput posterior positions; as well as in face presentations. It may also be used for the aftercoming head in breech presentations.

Once both blades are in place, they are articulated and the application is carefully checked for accuracy before traction is applied. If the shanks are not perpendicular, the instrument is not aligned with the head. Similarly, difficulty in locking the forceps, or failure of the head to advance when traction is tested, indicates a faulty application. In all of these cases, the forceps should be removed and the application reevaluated.

The physician must make sure that nothing lies between the forceps and the fetal head. By inserting a finger into the birth canal, the physician can determine if there is more than one fingertip of space beneath the heels of the forceps (the part nearest the shank). If so, it is likely that either the forceps are too long or too tapered for the head, or that the distal end of the blades is anchored behind the zygomas. Both of these errors are serious because slippage is likely, resulting in appreciable trauma.

When properly applied, the blades usually fall into the correct position by their own weight. Pressure must never be exerted to advance the blades, or severe damage may occur. "Tentative" traction is a useful means of detecting a difficulty before excessive force is applied.

Once the blades are locked, the fetal heart sounds should be auscultated. If they suddenly become faint or slow, the umbilical cord may be compressed by the forceps. The blades must then be unlocked immediately. By pushing one or two fingers up along the back of the fetal neck, it is possible to feel if the umbilical cord is encircling the neck.

§ 20.7   Extracting the Head

During birth of the head, spontaneous delivery should be simulated as closely as possible. Therefore, traction, like the uterine contractions which they mimic, should be intermittent. To relieve the pressure on the fetus's head, the forceps are loosened following each traction, but the handles should not be separated too far. The forceps are then retightened when the next traction is made.

The condition of the fetal heart is monitored by auscultation in the intervals between contractions. In addition, the descent and rotation of the head are evaluated by frequent examination. The head should only be allowed to recede very slowly during the intervals between contractions. Regardless of the original position of the head, delivery is brought about by exerting traction forward and downward (not straight out), following the curve of the pelvic canal until the occiput appears at the vulva. Except when urgently indicated, as in fetal distress, delivery should be slow, deliberate, and gentle enough to enable the pelvic tissues to gradually stretch.

§ 20.8   Removing the Instrument

The forceps are removed when the widest diameter of the fetal head is about to pass the vulvar ring. Delivery may then be completed in several ways. The forceps may be kept in place in order to maintain the greatest control over the advance of the head. However, the likelihood of maternal laceration is increased when the blades remain in place and keep the vulva distended. In these cases, the forceps can be removed and the delivery can be completed more naturally.

§ 20.9   Classification and Selection of Forceps Operations

Forceps operations are defined according to the station and position of the head in the pelvis at the time the instrument is applied. The American College of Obstetricians and Gynecologists currently recognizes three procedures:

Low Forceps Operation: The forceps are applied to the fetal skull when the scalp is easily visible at the introitus during a contraction; in addition, the skull has reached the pelvic floor and the sagittal suture is in the anteroposterior diameter of the pelvic outlet. See § **20.10**.

Mid-forceps Operation: The instrument is applied when the head is engaged, but before the above criteria for a low forceps operation have been met; by definition, any procedure in which the occiput is not anterior, and artificial rotation is required before traction is applied, is considered a mid-forceps operation, regardless of the station from which extraction is begun. See § **20.11**.

High Forceps Operation: The forceps are applied before the fetal head is engaged. See § **20.12**.[4]

A final technique, trial forceps, is included here because like the previous three procedures, it is also a method of forceps delivery. Trial forceps is a modern concept of attempted vaginal delivery in borderline instances of cephalopelvic disproportion. See § **20.13**.

Regardless of the method chosen, a record should be made of the position and stage of the head when delivery is begun. A description of the various maneuvers used, and any difficulties encountered in the forceps operation, should also be recorded.

§ 20.10   —Low Forceps Operation

The purpose of this procedure is to supply the final force required to deliver the fetal head. Usually, the major obstacle to delivery in these cases is insufficient expulsive forces (that is, inadequate uterine contractions) or abnormal perineal resistance. To overcome these difficulties, DeLee recommended the "prophylactic forceps operation," more commonly called "elective low forceps."[5] This liberal procedure is considered prophylactic for three reasons. First, the delivery is controlled by the physician, rather than depending on the unpredictable voluntary effort of the mother, whose uterine contractions are sometimes unable to expel the fetus. Secondly, since the fetal head is lifted out over the perineum, it is spared from any cerebral damage that might have occurred if it were allowed to press against an excessively rigid perineum for a prolonged period of time. Finally, injury to the maternal soft tissues is minimized if the procedure is combined with an episiotomy. Episiotomy is usually performed when traction on the head begins to distend the perineum. As a result of these steps, the mother is spared from the strain of the last 15-30 minutes of the second stage of labor.

---

4 Hughes E.C. (ed.), Obstetric-Gynecologic Terminology (F. A. Davis Co., 1972).

5 J.B. DeLee, *The Prophylactic Forceps Operation*, 1 Amer. J. Obstet. Gynecol. 34 (1920).

In a prophylactic forceps operation, the obstetrician chooses to intervene, realizing that it is not absolutely necessary since spontaneous delivery can normally be expected within about 15 minutes. Although it is usually not a definite indication for the use of forceps, prophylactic forceps procedures account for the vast majority of such operations in the United States. One reason for its increased incidence is that all methods of anesthesia interfere, to a certain extent, with the mother's voluntary expulsive efforts, and obliterate her perineal reflex. Consequently, the low forceps operation actually becomes necessary in order to deliver the fetus.

For the maximal safety of both mother and infant, forceps should not be used electively until the criteria for a low forceps operation is fulfilled. Under these circumstances, forceps delivery preceded by an episiotomy is generally considered a relatively simple and safe operation, requiring only gentle traction. However, the results of Emanuel Friedman's studies challenge this assertion.[6] His findings show that even low forceps procedures significantly increase the perinatal mortality rate, regardless of whether the operation is performed electively, or based on specific indications.

§ 20.11 —Mid-Forceps Operation

Because the use of forceps at this level entails a considerable risk, it is generally contraindicated, unless a clear-cut reason to terminate labor exists, and an experienced obstetrician is present. According to Danforth,[7] before undertaking mid-forceps delivery, regardless of the indication, the physician must be able to unequivocally conclude that he can perform a safe vaginal delivery *and* that this method of delivery is less dangerous to the mother and the baby than cesarean section.

Most mid-forceps deliveries are performed because the orderly progress of the second stage of labor ceases. In other words, the fetus does not continue to spontaneously rotate and descend as expected. If this occurs when the mother has been in the second stage of labor for two hours, and when the fetal head is deep in the transverse diameter of the pelvis, the condition known as deep transverse arrest of labor has developed. Forceps delivery should be considered, provided that there are normal uterine contractions, and no significant disproportion. However, even when the delay in labor is a result of uterine inertia, a trial of oxytocin stimulation is usually preferable to immedi-

---

[6] E.A. Friedman *Patterns of Labor as Indicators of Risk*, 16 Clin. Obstet. Gynecol. 172 (1973).

[7] D.N. Danforth, Ph.D., M.D., Obstetrics and Gynecology, 4th ed., 696 (Harper & Row Publishers, Inc. 1982).

ate forceps extraction. If effective uterine activity can be restored with oxytocin, the labor may terminate spontaneously, or at least progress until a safer, low forceps extraction is possible. On the other hand, if the cause of deep transverse arrest of labor is cephalopelvic disproportion, vaginal delivery should not be attempted.

Cesarean section is usually recommended instead of a difficult mid-forceps delivery. As illustrated in the preceding example, when there is a definite cephalopelvic disproportion, cesarean delivery is the best solution. This may also be true if the presenting part cannot be rotated to a favorable position for extraction, or if the presenting part has not descended below the "plus one" station. If the fetal head has not rotated to an anterior position, it can often be rotated manually, or with forceps. However, the application of the blades and the extraction itself, are much more difficult when the fetus is in the tranverse or posterior position.

Delivery from a plus one station has become contraindicated because it is now understood that the higher the application of forceps, the greater is the likelihood of fetal mortality.[8] Whenever the instrument is applied too early, it tends to pull and compress the fetal head excessively. Furthermore, forceps extraction from a high station, especially in primigravidas, often result in deep soft tissue lacerations as the fetal head is drawn through the unprepared vagina.

It is generally agreed that patients with heart disease and preeclampsia should be spared the bearing-down efforts of the second stage of labor, if at all possible. But such efforts may actually be less harmful than a difficult mid-forceps extraction.[9] Unless the fetal head is in a favorable position for an easy forceps delivery, the risks of the procedure are significantly higher than that of patiently waiting for the descent of the head by the natural forces of labor.

Similarly, according to some obstetricians, forceps extraction should even be deferred in fetal distress if the infant's skull is not close to the perineal floor.[10] Although the fetal heart rate may be suggestive of hypoxia, they feel it may still be judicious to allow more time for the head to descend, rather than superimpose the trauma of a difficult mid-forceps operation on an infant who is already distressed. More infants are reported to have been killed by forceps operations to relieve fetal distress, than have been saved.[11]

In summary, except for situations in which the fetal head has arrested in the mid-pelvis because of maternal exhaustion or intractable inertia, it is best to

---

[8] *Id.*

[9] L.M. Helman & J.A. Pritchard, Williams Obstetrics, 14th ed., 1123 (Appleton-Century-Crofts, 1971).

[10] *Id.*

[11] *Id.*

wait until a low forceps operation is possible, even in the presence of maternal disease or fetal distress. If prompt delivery is mandatory, but easy vaginal delivery without delay is not expected, cesarean section is preferable.

§ 20.12   —High Forceps Operation

Many years ago, when cesarean section was a very dangerous operation, high forceps extraction was performed. However, it is an extremely difficult procedure, often causing brutal trauma to the maternal tissues, and the death of a large percentage of babies.[12] Today, it is rarely justified, and is usually only mentioned in textbooks to condemn it. When delivery must be started before the head is engaged, cesarean section is almost always preferable.

§ 20.13   —Trial Forceps

In this procedure, vaginal delivery with forceps is attempted in questionable cases of cephalopelvic disproportion, knowing in advance that the operation may not succeed. The physician waits until the fetal head is engaged and the cervix is fully dilated, and he then tries to accurately apply the forceps. In spite of these efforts, disproportion, incomplete cervical dilatation, or malposition of the fetal head often makes it impossible to extract the head. If the disproportion can be overcome, or the position can be corrected without using force, the delivery can be completed successfully. However, when forceps extraction is impossible or too hazardous, cesarean section should be performed.

The term *failed forceps* generally implies that repeated, desperate attempts have failed to deliver the infant when the physician fully expected the forceps extraction to succeed. Since these efforts are usually forceful, the fetus or maternal soft tissues may be seriously injured. If this occurs, the forceps should be removed, and the cause of the failure should be determined.

§ 20.14   Vacuum Extraction

Designed to be used in place of forceps, the vacuum extractor combines suction and traction in one instrument. It is considered effective and easy to use. The device consists of a round, metal cup with an attached hose and pump.

---

[12] J.R. Willson, M.D., C.T. Beecham, M.D., & E.R. Carrington, M.D., Obstetrics and Gynecology, 5th ed., 5109 (The C.V. Mosby Co., 1975).

When the cup is pressed against the fetal scalp, air is pumped out of the instrument, creating a partial vacuum which causes the cup to adhere to the scalp. At this point, traction on the hose can be applied with sufficient force so the head can be pulled through the birth canal. As the scalp is sucked into the cup, a huge artificial caput succedaneum is produced. The lesion is often quite marked, and although it is only temporary and not dangerous, it may be a disconcerting sight to the infant's parents.

Before considering the use of vacuum extractor, certain conditions must be present, many of which are similar to the prerequisites for the use of forceps. The fetal head must be engaged, the mother's bladder must be empty, and her cervix must be completely dilated. Maternal injury should not occur if the instrument is applied after the cervix is fully dilated. However, if it is applied too early, cervical lacerations and undesirable pulling on the pelvic ligaments may occur.

The vacuum extractor should not be used when there is evidence of cephalopelvic disproportion, nor when the fetus is at a high station. Before attempting traction, the operator should allow sufficient time for the development of an artificial caput succedaneum. Then, the traction should be applied intermittently *during* uterine contractions, never between them. Also, negative pressure must be applied gradually. Finally, the maximum length of time for traction should be limited to 30 minutes (that is, approximately 10-15 contractions). Trauma to the scalp is common if the vacuum is applied rapidly, or maintained for excessively long periods of time (that is, longer than 30 minutes).

The main indication for the vacuum extractor is dysfunctional labor in the absence of cephalopelvic disproportion. Abnormal presentations and positions can also be corrected using this device, and it may even accelerate labor and delivery.

Despite some initial enthusiasm for the vacuum extractor in this country, it is not used extensively here, partly because of numerous reports of fetal injury (including scalp lacerations, cephalhematomas and intracranial hemorrhage), as well as some instances of fetal death.[13] Unlike the Americans' reluctance to use the instrument, it has been well-received in many other parts of the world.[14] Physicians in some of these countries also report a lower maternal and fetal morbidity and mortality rate than their American colleagues.

---

[13] Leslie Iffy, M.D. & Harold A. Kaminetzky, M.D., Principles and Practice of Obstetrics & Perinatology, vol. 2, 1517 (John Wiley & Sons, Inc., 1981).

[14] *Id.* at 1518.

§ 20.15   Complications

Selection of the proper instrument along with the application of the correct tractive forces will minimize the serious injuries induced by the forceps operations. The main immediate danger to the mother is from hemorrhaged lacerations which may become infected. If the supporting structures of her pelvic organs are traumatized, cystocele, rectocele, and uterine prolapse may develop later. Forceps may also cause extensive perineal tears if a proper episiotomy is not performed. Vaginal and perineal injuries from forceps operations are directly related to the level of the fetal head when the procedure is started. The higher the fetal head is in the pelvis, the greater the damage to the maternal tissues, and the greater the possibility of serious fetal injury.

Traumatic fetal lesions resulting from forceps delivery include paralysis of the facial nerve (seventh nerve palsy), skull fracture, intracranial hemorrhage, soft tissue laceration, and compression of the brain. Injury to the seventh cranial nerve may follow forceps application to a long, molded head if the toe of the blade strikes, or a mid-forceps rotation of the blade slips, and lands right in front of the ear. When the newborn is examined in the delivery room, the affected side will remain stationary while the infant is smiling or crying. Most seventh-nerve palsies regress spontaneously, but it may take months to do so completely.

A basilar skull fracture may be suspected if otoscopic examination reveals an eardrum bulging with blood. In addition, subdural hematomas often do not become evident until 48-72 hours after birth, by which time the caput formation has disappeared. A skull x-ray should be taken to rule out fracture in such instances.

A more significant complication is intracranial hemorrhage due to compression of the pliable fetal skull. Although the volume of the head is reduced only slightly when extraneous force is applied, even this is dangerous because compression of the head adversely effects the brain. Circulation may be impaired, causing asphyxia and hemorrhage in addition to direct injury to the cranial bones and vessels, as well as the brain itself. Computer-assisted tomography or ultrasonography may help make this diagnosis in a newborn who is experiencing respiratory distress following forceps delivery.

§ 20.16   Prognosis

The perinatal mortality associated with forceps delivery depends on the condition of the fetus, and the station of the head when the operation is performed. There should not be any fetal death if the head is allowed to reach the perineum before the forceps are applied. Specialized forceps have inherent risks of their own which must also be carefully evaluated beforehand.

§ 20.17   Bibliography and Recommended Readings

Danforth, D.N., Ph.D., M.D., *Obstetrics and Gynecology*, 4th ed. (Harper & Row Publishers, Inc., 1982).

Laufe, L.E., *Obstetric Forceps* (Holber, 1968).

Marin, *A Review of the Use of Barton's Forceps for the Rotation of the Fetal Head from the Transverse Position*, 18 J. Obstet. Gynecol. 234 (1978).

Pritchard, J.A., M.D., MacDonald, P.C., M.D., & Gant, N.F., M.D., *Williams Obstetrics*, 17th ed. (Appleton-Century-Crofts, 1985).

Reeder, Sharon J., R.N., Ph.D., Mastroianni, Luigi, Jr., M.D., Martin, Leonide, L., R.N., *Maternity Nursing*, 15th ed. (J.B. Lippincott Co., 1983).

Thompson, James P., M.D., *Forceps*, in Principles and Practice of Obstetrics & Perinatology, vol 2 (John Wiley & Sons, Inc., 1981).

CHAPTER 21

BREECH PRESENTATION

§ 21.1   Introduction

In a breech presentation, the fetus is usually positioned in the womb so that its buttocks emerge first, instead of the typical head-first, or vertex presentation. However, in some instances, part of one or both legs may enter the birth canal before (or together) with the buttocks. The different interrelationships of the fetus's extremities to its body result in three varieties of breech presentation.

1. Frank or Single Breech: the legs are fully extended upward on the thorax so that the feet lie against the face, and the buttocks descend first; this occurs in about two-thirds of all breech deliveries.
2. Complete or Double Breech: the feet present along with the buttocks because the hips and one, or both knees, are flexed.
3. a. Single or Double Footling: either one or both feet descent through the birth canal *ahead* of the buttocks because the hips and knees are partially extended downward.
    b. Knee: one or both knees descend through the birth canal *ahead* of the buttocks, because the knees remain flexed.

Since the infant mortality and maternal morbidity are significantly higher in breech presentations than in vertex presentations, they are considered potentially abnormal and deserving of special attention. The cause of the condition is unknown, but many hypotheses have been offered. For instance, breech deliveries occur more frequently in multiparas than primiparas, probably because the experienced uterus is more relaxed, enabling the fetus to move about relatively freely. This uninhibited movement is especially evident during the second trimester and early part of the third trimester, but as the due date approaches in a *normal* pregnancy, the fetus tends to accommodate to the shape of the uterine cavity. The baby usually assumes a vertex presentation, lying longitudinally with its own head down. This position is favored because the fetal buttocks are bulkier than the head; and they generally fit better in the roomier, upper uterine segment, than in the smaller, lower uterine segment.

However, this tendency may be offset by prematurity or atypical uterine configurations. If, for example, the fetus is premature or small in comparison to the size of the uterine cavity, it is not forced to conform to the uterine dimensions, and breech presentation is much more likely. Similarly, uterine anomalies, hydramnios, hydrocephalus, and multiple fetuses may also interfere with normal accommodation, and may therefore increase the likelihood of breech and other abnormal presentations. In contrast to these abnormalities, in as many as 30-40 percent of twin pregnancies, one of the fetuses may be in the buttocks-down position.

§ 21.2 Diagnosis

Since the fetal risk in breech deliveries is so high, evaluation of the woman with a breech presentation should be made *before* the onset of labor. Under normal circumstances, the diagnosis can usually be made by external abdominal examination alone, using the four maneuvers of Leopold and Sporlin. See § 9.7. Instead of palpating a hard, round head over the pelvic inlet as would be expected in a vertex presentation, the soft and irregular buttocks can be felt there. There, the physician can feel the head in the upper uterus (the fundus). The fetal heart tones are loudest on the side of the mother's abdomen where the fetal back lies, and are always heard above the level of the umbilicus, unless the breech lies deep in the pelvis.

The abdominal evaluation may be complicated if labor is advanced and the contractions are strong and frequent, since the uterus may be too rigid to palpate. Similarly, if the uterus is tender or irritable, if the abdominal wall is too thick or if the fetus is too large, the abdominal examination may not be informative. Several other studies can then be done to confirm the existence of a breech presentation.

The condition can often be diagnosed based on a rectal examination, but a vaginal examination is recommended for verification. In a frank breech presentation, the buttocks resemble a soft mass of bumps and depressions when palpated from within the birth canal. If the cervix is partially dilated and if the presenting part has descended far enough, the irregular bony portions of the baby's lower pelvic can also be identified. In footling presentations, one or both feet can be palpated; in complete breech presentations, the feet can be felt alongside the buttocks. If the obstetrician's finger entered the fetus's anus during the examination, fresh meconium may be seen on his glove when he withdraws his hand. Care must be exercised during the procedure, otherwise the physician may injure the fetus's anus or genitals.

As long as the vaginal examination is performed soon after the membranes rupture, the diagnosis will not be difficult. However, if several hours have elapsed, the buttocks may become so swollen that many of the landmarks of the breech may be confused with those of a face or shoulder presentation. These mistakes can be avoided by locating the bony orbits of the face and the sucking action of the mouth, which are indicative of a face presentation, or the scapula and ribs, which are suggestive of a shoulder presentation. On the other hand, the diagnosis of the breech position and variety can be established most accurately by locating the sacrum and its spinous process.

If the abdominal or vaginal examinations still leave questions or doubts about the fetal position during early labor, an x-ray examination is advisable. To ensure a precise classification of the breech presentation, the radiologic examination must include the entire maternal abdomen so the physician can rule out a multiple gestation, fetal hydrocephalus, or hyperextension of the fetal head on the spine.

§ 21.3   Procedures to Consider

Certain clinicians believe that the fetal mortality can be substantially reduced if the obstetrician tries to *prevent* breech presentations whenever possible.[1] Consequently, these physicians advocate the *external cephalic version* for all breech babies during the prenatal period. As the name implies, the manipulations are only made through the external abdominal wall, their purpose being to turn the fetus from a breech-first to a head-first position, by continually pushing the buttocks upward and away from the pelvic inlet, while gently pulling the head downward, toward the pelvis. The obstetrician should hold the fetus in its new position for five minutes, and should listen to its heart tones after each step. Alterations in the cardiac rhythm indicate that something is interfering with the fetal oxygen supply, such as a compressed, or twisted umbilical cord. If these complications develop, if the uterus is irritable, or if the manipulations are painful, the physician should stop the maneuvers and return the fetus to its original position. To ensure that the manipulations are gentle and atraumatic, external cephalic version is conducted without anesthesia. Although external cephalic version may be readily accomplished in multiparas with lax abdominal walls, it is more difficult to perform in primigravidas, since their abdominal and uterine muscles are more apt to be tense.

It is important to realize that the incidence of breech presentations in *mid* pregnancy is about 25 percent, but most of these fetuses *spontaneously* shift to vertex presentations by the 34th week, and seldom revert to their initial buttocks-down position. Therefore, external cephalic version is usually attempted around the 34th week of pregnancy, since most spontaneous versions will have already occurred.

Even if a successful manipulation is performed after this time, fetuses will return to their former breech-first positions, especially if there is an anatomic reason for its occurrence, or if the presenting part is not fixed in the pelvis. The failure rate of the procedure increases as the end of the pregnancy approaches, with a marked rise after the 36th week. Since reversion is so likely, many physicians believe that external cephalic version does not offer a satis-

---

[1] J.A. Pritchard, M.D. & P.C. MacDonald, Williams Obstetrics, 16th ed., 804 (Appleton-Century-Crofts, 1980).

factory solution to the problems posed by breech presentations. This view-point, coupled with the dangers of the manuever, explains why many obstetricians are opposed to it.[2] Even its adherents admit that the procedure has intrinsic risks, including injury to the uterus, partial or complete separation of the placenta, and kinking or prolapse of the umbilical cord, all of which may adversely affect the fetus.[3]

External cephalic version is dangerous and should be prohibited if the fetal membranes have ruptured, if there is a marked fetopelvic disproportion, or if the presenting part has already descended into the pelvis. In addition, it should not be attempted when there is a risk of placental disorders or uterine rupture due to overdistention, excessive thinning, or a previous cesarean section.

Unlike external cephalic version, digital and x-ray pelvimetry are unanimously recommended to evaluate the architecture of the maternal pelvis.[4] Whenever vaginal delivery is contemplated, x-ray pelvimetry is crucial. It is particularly important for a primgravida (since her pelvic capacity has never been tested by a previous pregnancy) and a woman with a suspicious past history of pregnancies. Neither clinical pelvimetry nor prior successful vaginal deliveries provide adequate and reliable information about the pelvic size and morphology. Unless the radiologic pelvic measurements correspond to the average normal dimensions, breech delivery will be very risky.

Radiologic evaluation is also essential to determine the precise position of the fetal head in order to detect any change which might complicate its delivery, such as deflexion, hyperextension, or hydrocephalus. In addition, the size of the fetal head might be compared to that of the maternal pelvis to determine whether vaginal delivery is feasible. Unfortunately, this data is not as easy to obtain as in a vertex presentation, because simple manual palpation of the biparietal dimensions of the skull cannot be done accurately when the head is located in the fundus. As a result, the only reliable way to obtain these measurements (to rule out disproportion) is by ultrasonography. It should be done during late pregnancy or early labor.

In contrast to vertex presentations, the possibility of a vaginal breech delivery cannot be tested by a trial labor in questionable cases of fetopelvic disproportion. Although the buttocks and body of the fetus may be able to descend through a small pelvis, the head of the breech baby will not be able to pass through atraumatically. If it is allowed to mold and deliver gradually, the infant will probably die of anoxia, because its umbilical cord will be com-

---

[2] *Id.*

[3] *Id.*

[4] Leslie Iffy, M.D. & Harold A. Kaminetzky, M.D., Principles and Practice of Obstetrics & Perinatology, vol. 1, 739 (John Wiley & Sons, Inc., 1981).

pressed between its head and the mother's pelvic brim, cutting off its oxygen supply until its head is born.

Another method of predicting potentially problematic breech cases is the Zatuchni-Andros breech score. Having determined that the outcome of breech deliveries is based on parity, gestational age, estimated fetal weight, previous breech deliveries, cervical dilatation, and fetal station, Zatuchni and Andros devised a system for ranking each of these indices.[5] A value of 0, 1, or 2 is assigned to each factor, depending on how significantly it affects the prognosis. The sum of values is the breech score, and it can be used to determine which method of delivery (vaginal or cesarean) is most suitable.

The lower the breech score, the poorer is the expected outcome. According to this system, the complications of labor and delivery will occur more frequently when the mother is a primigravida, when the pregnancy exceeds 39 weeks, when the fetus weighs 8 pounds or more, when the cervical dilatation is minimal, and when the buttocks are at a high station (about −3) at the onset of labor. Despite these useful indices, the criteria of the breech score are not considered all-inclusive, since they do not take into account such important factors as prematurity, cephalopelvic disproportion, and deflexion of the fetal head.

§ 21.4   Prerequisites for Breech Extraction

Like any delivery procedure, breech extraction should always be done under sterile conditions. The following criteria must also be fulfilled before it is acceptable to perform a breech extraction:

1. The cervix must be completely dilated, retracted, and obliterated.
2. The pelvis must be adequate and free of mechanical obstacles. Cephalopelvic disproportion as well as pelvic contraction can injure or kill the fetus, if not discovered beforehand by x-ray or digital pelvimetry.
3. The uterus must be intact and not excessively thinned, otherwise rupture may occur.
4. The mother's bladder and rectum must be empty.
5. An assistant must be present to aid in the delivery if extraction is required, or if forceps are used, to deliver the aftercoming head.
6. The mother must be anesthetized.

---

[5] Zatuchni & Andros, *Prognostic Index for Vaginal Delivery in Breech Presentation at Term*, 93 Am. J. Obstet. Gynecol. 237 (1965).

7. An episiotomy should be made to prevent the pelvic floor from obstructing the fetus's head.

§ 21.5 Indications for Breech Extraction

Fetal distress, which is commonly seen in all varieties of breech presentation, is the usual indication for breech extraction. Whereas the passage of meconium is indicative of fetal distress in vertex presentations, it is of no significance during breech labors because it is often merely the result of abdominal compression of the baby. In contrast, the rate and regularity of the fetal heart are very important and must be followed meticulously. Before the umbilicus is born, the baby's heart should be auscultated following each uterine contraction. If the heart rate falls below 100 bpm (beats-per-minute), rises above 160 bpm or becomes irregular during the second stage of labor, extraction may be warranted. It is also indicated after the umbilicus is born, if any change in the rate or regularity of the umbilical cord pulsations is observed.

Breech extraction is also legitimate in those rare instances when the mother's condition is such that continuation of the second stage of labor is more dangerous than the breech extraction itself. This may occur if the labor is complicated by heart disease or other systemic disorders.

If the fetus fails to descend after the mother has been in the second stage of labor for two and one-half hours, breech extraction is justified to terminate the labor. Prolongation of the second stage of labor is more common with frank breech than with complete or footling breech presentations.

§ 21.6 Mechanism of Labor

Although the buttocks or the feet are considered poor cervical dilators compared to the well-flexed head, labor usually progresses at a normal rate. A slight prolongation is not uncommon, especially if the uterine contractions are somewhat abnormal. Even in nulliparas, the breech may remain high in the pelvis, not descending until the labor is well-advanced, and cervical dilatation is complete. The fact that the buttocks are not engaged during the first stage of labor is not always suggestive of fetopelvic disproportion, as is failure of the head to engage and descend in vertex presentations. However, during the second stage of labor, the buttocks may sometimes descend rapidly, even though the pelvis is too small to permit the aftercoming head to pass. This illustrates the fundamental difference between delivery in vertex and breech presentations.

In vertex presentations, when the cervix is not fully dilated, it prevents the head (which is usually the larger part of the fetal body) from descending. Since the head is forced to wait until dilatation is complete, it has time to gradually adapt to, and stretch, the birth canal, facilitating its delivery and enabling the rest of the body to follow without difficulty. In contrast, in a breech presentation, successively larger portions of the baby are born. The danger arises because the buttocks, the trunk, and even the shoulders, can pass through a partially dilated cervix, but the head (which is also the least compressible part of the fetus) cannot. Once the umbilicus has been delivered, long delays in the delivery of the aftercoming head may cause anoxia, and may therefore be life-threatening.

§ 21.7   Methods of Labor and Delivery

There are three principle methods of vaginal delivery of a breech baby:

Spontaneous Breech Delivery.   The entire fetus is expelled spontaneously by the mother's natural uterine forces without any traction or manipulation; the obstetrician simply supports the infant as it emerges.

The treatment of the first stage of labor is as usual. When the second stage begins, preparations for an operative delivery should be started in case the conditions worsen. Opinions vary considerably as to whether or not this approach is valuable, or whether the routine use of partial breech extraction is preferable.[6] The most favorable conditions occur when the fetus is premature, or very small, or following rapid labors in a multipara who has a large pelvis.

In the Bracht manuever for breech delivery, the natural mechanism of labor is simulated and the breech is allowed to deliver spontaneously to the umbilicus. The obstetrician simply holds the infant's body and legs together against the mother's symphysis pubis in order to take advantage of gravity to support the breech. Maintenance of this position, added to the effects of the uterine contractions and moderate suprapubic pressure applied by an assistant, often suffices to complete the delivery spontaneously. No traction is made during the birth process. Although the Bracht manuever is popular abroad, it is not widely accepted in the United States.[7]

---

[6] D.N. Danforth, Ph.D., M.D., Obstetrics and Gynecology, 4th ed., 709 (Harper & Row Publishers, Inc., 1982).

[7] J.A. Pritchard, M.D. & D.C. MacDonald, M.D., Williams Obstetrics, 16th ed., 1075 (Appleton-Century-Crofts, 1980).

Assisted Breech Delivery or Partial Breech Extraction.   The infant is delivered spontaneously to the umbilicus, at which time the obstetrician actively assists in delivering or extracting the remainder of the body. This approach is often preferred because it results in the lowest perinatal mortality, and is least likely to damage the maternal soft tissues.[8]

Total Breech Extraction.   The entire fetus is extracted by the obstetrician. Of all the obstetrical operations, this is one of the most difficult and potentially traumatic procedures.   Done under deep, general anesthesia, it often involves decomposing or rearranging the fetus's trunk and extremities before the natural forces of labor begin. Though it is supposed to facilitate a complex delivery, it results in unacceptably high perinatal morbidity and mortality rates, even when it is performed by experts.[9] Total breech extraction should therefore be prohibited, unless there are strong indications, and no other alternatives are available.   There are situations that may justify it, including prolapse of the umbilical cord or fetal hypoxia.   However, it should not be initiated until the cervix is fully dilated, and the buttocks are well-descended into the pelvis.   If there are overriding indications for an immediate delivery, cesarean section is far safer for both the mother and fetus.

§ 21.8   Management of Labor and Delivery

Regardless of the method of delivery that is selected, the actual manipulations required to deliver a fetus in the frank breech presentation differ from those needed in a complete, or an incomplete, breech presentation, since each of the various interrelationships has its own peculiarities and hazards. However, the specific rotations and extraction techniques are too lengthy and detailed to cover in this book, though a brief description of their key points and common characteristics will be provided.

Abdominal and vaginal examinations should be performed soon after labor begins to reassess the pelvic capacity, and fetal size and presentation; and to determine the extent of cervical effacement and dilatation, as well as the status of the fetal membranes. The membranes should be left intact as long as possible to diminish the risk of a prolapsed umbilical cord. When they rupture spontaneously, an immediate vaginal examination should be performed to detect a prolapsed cord, even if the fetal heart rate is normal.

---

[8] D.N. Danforth, Ph.D., M.D., Obstetrics and Gynecology, 4th ed., 710 (Harper & Row Publishers, Inc., 1982).

[9] Leslie Iffy, M.D. & Harold A. Kaminetzky, M.D., Principles and Practice of Obstetrics & Perinatology, vol. 2, 1523 (John Wiley & Sons, Inc., 1981).

In *all* varieties of breech presentations, the woman should be transferred to a delivery room, and preparations should be made for an extraction as soon as the buttocks or feet appear at the perineum during a contraction. This is also the optimal time to perform an episiotomy. The incision facilitates all of the manipulations of the delivery, saves time (which reduces the danger of asphyxia), and prevents fetal injury and lacerations of the mother's perineum. Then, depending on the fetal health and the events of labor, the obstetrician will usually decide to perform either a spontaneous, or an assisted, breech delivery.

The condition of the fetus is followed by constant monitoring of its heart rhythm in the interval between uterine contractions. As long as the heart sounds are normal, labor is allowed to continue until the baby's umbilicus is visible. In most breech presentations, delivery to the umbilicus will occur spontaneously, and the obstetrician should refrain from hastening the natural birth process unless the situation warrants intervention. After the umbilicus is born, the umbilical cord is advanced so the physician can monitor its pulsations. If no abnormalities are detected, the rest of the birth can be enhanced by encouraging the mother to bear down with all her force. If her efforts are successful, no obstetrical assistance is necessary aside from supporting the baby's body as it emerges.

However, if the cord pulsations become slow or irregular, assisted breech delivery is indicated. Similarly, if the woman's uterine contractions are not sufficient to deliver the fetus beyond the umbilicus, partial breech extraction is necessary. By wrapping a sterile towel around the baby's hips, the physician can firmly grasp the baby's pelvis in her two hands, and then apply deliberate, but gentle, downward traction to aid the delivery. These motions must be even and smooth; there should be no bending or twisting. In all phases of breech delivery, it is advantageous to coordinate traction with the mother's uterine contractions. It is also important to apply pressure, and make traction on the bones rather than the soft tissues, in order to reduce the possibility of injury.

The fetal back and shoulders follow the umbilicus into the pelvis. If the fetus is large, it is advisable to deliver the arms before the shoulders wedge into the pelvis. The rest of the labor is facilitated if the fetus's arms remain crossed over the chest, and the head stays sharply flexed on the chest. These normal positions are best maintained by avoiding unnecessary traction and fundal pressure that might push the head between the arms. Deflexion of the fetal head is the most dreaded, and most predictable, complication of extraction procedures. Deflexion of the head occurs when the head tips backward with the chin up. This causes the chin to get caught by the pubic bone and prevents further descent of the fetal head.

Piper forceps are frequently recommended to complete the delivery of the aftercoming head once it reaches the pelvic floor, especially when it cannot be delivered quickly following moderate traction.[10] The obstetrician must not be hasty. If the forceps are applied before the head is engaged in the pelvis, or before the cervix is fully dilated, the mother and fetus may be seriously injured. It is also essential that an assistant elevate the fetal body while the forceps are applied to the aftercoming head.

Suspending the infant's body and arms in a sling (easily made with a sterile towel), keeps the arms out of the way, and prevents over-extension of the fetal cervical spine, a complication which could cause spinal cord injury. In addition, traction must never be applied to the fetal *body* when the head is about to be delivered. To do so is analogous to handling the fetus by its neck.

As an alternative to Piper forceps, the head can be delivered by manual manipulation using either the Wigand-Martin or the Mauriceau manuevers.[11] Even if one of these methods is selected, some obstetricians recommend that forceps be ready for immediate use.[12] Regardless of the method chosen, it is crucial to intervene and to help deliver the aftercoming head, otherwise the umbilical circulation will come to a virtual standstill as the cord becomes compressed between the cranium and the pelvic inlet, and it will not be restored until the delivery is completed.

The obstetrician should sponge the mucus from the baby's mouth as soon as it becomes visible at the vulva, and should gently restrain the head from passing through the pelvic floor too quickly. On the other hand, there is not a lot of time to spare. If the head cannot be delivered easily and without delay, resuscitation may be initiated. By inserting a finger in the baby's mouth, the obstetrician can create an airway for the fetus. The infant's nose and mouth can then be aspirated, allowing it to breathe freely. However, if the infant's condition is poor, or if resuscitation is unsuccessful, immediate (but deliberate) extraction of the head is necessary. In light of the grave consequences of oxygen deprivation, every obstetrician who is responsible for breech extractions must be able to provide the essential, lifesaving procedures whenever a complication arises.

---

[10] D.N. Danforth, Ph.D., M.D., Obstetrics and Gynecology, 4th ed., 711 (Harper & Row Publishers, Inc., 1982).

[11] *Id.*

[12] *Id.*

§ 21.9   Anesthesia

In spontaneous deliveries, local anesthesia is ideal because it helps maintain the woman's active cooperation, and preserves her natural expulsive efforts. Similarly, assisted breech deliveries are best accomplished with minimal anesthesia until the umbilicus is born. Then, an anesthetic that produces total muscle relaxation should be administered for the duration of the delivery. Unfortunately, no single agent fulfills these requirements perfectly. The method of choice will be influenced by the mother's ability to bear-down, and by the possibility of further complications in the labor. The final choice should be made by an experienced anesthesiologist, who must always be present for breech deliveries—both to consult with the obstetrician, and in the event that complications develop, and rapid general anesthesia suddenly becomes necessary.

   If the fetus is endangered, precautions must be taken when selecting an anesthetic in order to prevent fetal central nervous system, or cardiovascular, depression. Paracervical blocks (especially lidocaine, mepivacaine, and bupivacaine) should be avoided, since they have been implicated in causing high levels of circulating local anesthetics in the fetal bloodstream, leading to cardiovascular depression and bradycardia. Similarly, evidence of fetal hypoxia prohibits the use of spinal anesthesia, since the anesthesia may cause hypotension, and aggravate the deteriorating situation.

§ 21.10   Complications

There are a sizeable number of factors that can complicate the delivery of the breech baby. They include:

1.   Arrest of the head. See § **21.11**.
2.   Extended arms or nuchal arms. See § **21.12**.
3.   Uterine dysfunction. See § **21.13**.
4.   Hyperextension or deflexion of the fetal head. See § **21.14**.
5.   Premature rupture of the membranes. See § **21.15**.
6.   Prematurity. See § **21.16**.
7.   Miscellaneous complications. See § **21.17**.

§ 21.11   —Arrest of the Head

After the body has been delivered, the head may wedge into the pelvic inlet and be unable to descend, particularly if fetopelvic disproportion exists. Every effort should be made to anticipate atypical descent or dilatation patterns before labor.

Since prompt action is required if the infant's life is to be saved, when arrest of the head develops, a quick examination should be done to determine the cause of the delay. Two common causes of the problem are an unfavorable pelvic shape, or a tight or constricted cervix. In the latter, the cervix can sometimes be manually slipped over the back of the head to rectify the situation. If this should fail, Duhrssen's incisions may have to be made in the cervix, and this is not a simple procedure. It is important to remember that traction on the neck is always condemned.

§ 21.12   —Extended Arms or Nuchal Arms

The fetus's arms normally lie crossed over the chest, and if nothing interferes, they are delivered in this position. However, if the pelvic inlet is contracted, or if an attempt is made to extract the shoulders through an incompletely dilated cervix, one or both arms may extend above or alongside the fetus's head (*extended arms*) or they may even cross behind the fetus's neck (*nuchal arms or nuchal hitch*). If difficulty delivering either arm is encountered, these complications should be considered. Although they can usually be prevented, they pose a serious problem because the arms interfere with the delivery of the head. Delivery of the head should never be initiated before the arms are liberated.

To release the imprisoned arm, the obstetrician should immediately push the fetal body back a few inches. If several such attempts fail, an alternative approach is to rotate the fetal body 180° in one direction to dislodge the first arm, and then 180° in the opposite direction to dislodge the second arm.

§ 21.13   —Uterine Dysfunction

Since the buttocks cannot induce cervical dilatation as well as the head can, cervical dilatation may be more erratic, making uterine dysfunction a common complication. This disorder compounds the fetal risk.

The elective induction of labor, whether by oxytocin, amniotomy, or stripping the amnion from the cervical tissues, should be avoided because the procedures themselves are prone to complications. Furthermore, it is not always possible to detect minor degrees of mechanical obstruction, especially in frank breech presentations. For these reasons, the use of oxytocin to stimulate labor is dangerous and is generally contraindicated.

§ 21.14 —Hyperextension or Deflexion of the Fetal Head

Ordinarily, the breech baby's head is unmolded, and presents in the same shape it had in utero. However, if hyperextension occurred in the uterus, certain changes may be observed after birth. The newborn's head may be flattened on either side or it may be distinctly molded, especially if fundal pressure was exerted on it during delivery.

Hyperextension can be recognized while the baby is still in the uterus by abdominal palpation, or x-ray examination of the fetus. It is not uncommon and it is often not significant, since most cases correct themselves spontaneously during labor. However, if it remains uncorrected and undetected, spinal cord damage, intracranial trauma, or death may occur during vaginal delivery. According to several investigators, the discovery of a hyperextended head warrants cesarean section.[13] Studies from one researcher demonstrated a 21 percent incidence of permanent spinal cord injury among those infants who were delivered vaginally compared to no such injuries in infants delivered abdominally.[14]

Deflexion of the fetal head occurs when the head tips backward with the chin up. This causes the chin to get caught by the pubic bone and prevents further descent of the fetal head. Since deflexion of the fetal head may also produce insurmountable difficulties, it is imperative to maintain flexion of the head during delivery. This is facilitated by the application of gentle, continuous, manual, suprapubic pressure.

§ 21.15 —Premature Rupture of the Membranes

For reasons still unknown, this condition occurs more frequently in breech presentations. Because it is often associated with intrapartum sepsis and prolapse of the umbilical cord, it may substantially influence the fetal prognosis.

---

[13] Leslie Iffy, M.D. & Harold A. Kaminetzky, M.D., Principles and Practice of Obstetrics & Perinatology, vol. 2, 921 (John Wiley & Sons, Inc., 1981).

[14] G.S.Dawes, Fetal and Neonatal Physiology (Year Book Medical Publishers, 1968).

The most common fetal problem related to the cord takes place during delivery of the breech baby's head, since anoxia or asphyxia may occur if the head compresses the cord, or if its delivery is delayed.

As a result of these dangers, the membranes should not be *artificially* ruptured in normal labors. When the membranes rupture naturally (but prematurely), a vaginal examination should be done to ensure that the umbilical cord has not prolapsed.

§ 21.16 —Prematurity

The relatively large head and small body of the premature fetus predispose it to dangerous events during descent. Since the presenting part of the premature breech baby is comparatively small, it may pass through the cervical opening before it is fully dilated. By the time the head (which is less compressible than the body) reaches the partially dilated cervix, the powerful cervical musculature may prevent its delivery for a prolonged period of time. Like all delays, this too is conducive to fetal hypoxia, and the obstetrician's efforts to overcome the cervical resistance is conducive to birth injuries, both of which are especially deleterious for a premature infant because of its more fragile physical structure. Even when the cephalopelvic proportions are favorable, the premature fetus is liable to be excessively stressed.

§ 21.17 —Miscellaneous Complications

Several serious complications often develop in conjunction with footling presentations, the first of which is prolapse of the umbilical cord. Occasionally, the infant's foot may drag the umbilical cord down with it. If the prolapsed cord becomes compressed or entangled around the baby's legs, its life is endangered, and rapid delivery is required.

Secondly, not only is the foot likely to protrude through the vagina before the descent and delivery of the buttocks, but it may even do so before engagement, and often in the absence of total cervical dilatation. Because cervical dilatation must be complete before the fetus can be delivered safely, a hasty extraction initiated solely on the grounds that the foot has descended, may prove fatal. In frank breech presentations, prolapse of the umbilical cord is not as frequent, since the buttocks fit more snuggly into the birth canal than the legs or feet. They therefore block the cervical opening (although not as effectively as the head), leaving little extra space for the cord to prolapse. However, in frank breech presentations, since the legs are extended upward, they may act as splints and interfere with the flexibility of the fetal body, which hinders the delivery of the hips. If this occurs, descent is slowed or impeded, and operative delivery becomes necessary if the fetus stops at station 0 or +1.

§ 21.18   Cesarean Section Versus Vaginal Delivery

The choice between a cesarean section and a vaginal delivery in breech presentations is currently considered judgmental. Many authorities still oppose routine abdominal deliveries, and perform them only when the prognostic signs are poor.[15] They believe a successful spontaneous, or assisted, vaginal breech delivery can be expected under favorable circumstances. Careful prelabor or early labor evaluation will help identify which patients are candidates for a successful vaginal delivery. Among the important factors to consider are age, pelvic size, gestational length, outcome of previous pregnancies, estimated fetal weight, type of breech presentation, station of the presenting part and position of the head when labor begins, and the process of labor itself. Vaginal deliveries should only be attempted by experienced obstetricians. The following personnel must also be present: an assistant (to help with the delivery), an experienced anesthesiologist (to administer the appropriate anesthesia), and a physician qualified to resuscitate the infant, if the need arises.

When a breech extraction does not promise to be an easy, uncomplicated procedure, cesarean section may improve the fetal outcome.[16] In contrast to this conservative viewpoint, some obstetricians advocate a much broader application of cesarean deliveries.[17] Arguing that some degree of umbilical cord compression is inevitable in every vaginal breech delivery, they believe that each fetus's chances for survival are, therefore, jeopardized. As the buttocks are being delivered, they draw the umbilicus and the attached cord into the pelvis, where pressure on the cord reduces the umbilical circulation. This lasts throughout the remainder of the delivery since the umbilical cord is continuously susceptible to compression between the fetal body and the maternal soft tissues, or bones. In order to prevent anoxia, the head must be delivered promptly, usually within eight minutes from the time the umbilicus is visible at the vaginal opening. Unfortunately, this time limit is not easy to meet with vaginal delivery. While some degree of molding may be necessary in order for

---

[15] D.N. Danforth, Ph.D., M.D., Obstetrics and Gynecology, 4th ed., 711 (Harper & Row Publishers, Inc., 1982).

[16] Id. at 709.

[17] Id.

the fetal head to accommodate and successfully negotiate the birth canal, precious time may be lost if the physician awaits these events and delays the delivery in the meantime. On the other hand, if delivery is forced before the fetal adaptations are complete, the brain, spinal cord, and abdominal viscera may be traumatized because of the compression, and/or traction used. The problem is compounded with a premature fetus; the disparity between the size of its head and its buttocks is even greater than with a mature fetus, thereby enhancing the likelihood and consequences of compression.

By eliminating the inherent fetal risks of a breech delivery as well as the grave consequences associated with a breech extraction, cesarean section has become increasingly popular.[18] Although the indications for an abdominal delivery are not always absolute or unanimously approved by obstetricians, the operation is generally performed when potentially adverse conditions prevail.[19] For example, cesarean section is chosen more frequently for the term delivery of a primipara than a multipara, since the former has an untested pelvic capacity, and is likely to have a longer labor. In addition, women who become pregnant for the first time late in their reproductive lives, those who have had difficulty conceiving, and those whose previous pregnancies resulted in the loss or injury of the baby are commonly considered candidates for cesarean section. Any degree of contraction or unfavorable pelvic shapes may also lead to serious trauma, and therefore justifies the use of an abdominal delivery. Even if a moderately contracted pelvis was nonproblematic for the delivery of an average-sized fetus in the vertex presentation, it may be dangerous if the subsequent fetus is in the breech presentation. Round and elliptical pelves are favorable shapes, whereas platypelloid or heart-shaped pelves are not.

Most physicians agree that a large fetus in the breech presentation should be delivered abdominally, since the morbidity and mortality rates for a term fetus delivered vaginally rise with increasing birth weights.[20] Even though the mother's pelvis may appear normal, a fetus weighing more than 3500 grams is believed to benefit from an abdominal delivery because there is a greater likelihood of fetopelvic disproportion due to its size. Cesarean section is indicated whenever any degree of disproportion is documented, since a vaginal delivery under these conditions is usually traumatic. At the opposite end of the spectrum, since premature fetuses are also more prone to traumatic deliveries, some obstetricians advocate cesarean delivery to terminate pregnancies be-

---

[18] J.A. Pritchard, M.D. & P.C. MacDonald, M.D., Williams Obstetrics, 16th ed., 807-09 (Appleton-Century-Crofts, 1980).

[19] Id.

[20] D.N. Danforth, Ph.D., M.D., Obstetrics and Gynecology, 4th ed., 707-10 (Harper & Row Publishers, 1982).

tween 26 and 36 weeks of gestation, provided that the patient is in active labor, or shows evidence of another valid indication for delivery.[21]

Cesarean section should also be considered: if the fetal membranes rupture prematurely, and labor does not ensure promptly and spontaneously; as an alternative to most breech extractions when progress ceases in the second stage of labor because of inadequate cervical dilatation, or uterine dysfunction, or inertia; as an alternative to oxytocin stimulation in most instances of dysfunctional labor; if umbilical cord compression is suspected; in complete or incomplete (particularly the footling variety) breech presentations due to the risk of a prolapsed umbilical cord; if the fetal heart rate is abnormal or if hypoxia is noticed; if the fetal head is hyperextended; and if maternal disorders such as diabetes, preeclampsia, or hypertension complicate the pregnancy.

There is little doubt that the perinatal morbidity and mortality can be reduced by the more liberal use of abdominal deliveries. No matter how carefully the cases are selected, vaginal breech deliveries still appear to increase the fetal risks.[22] Nonetheless, the physician must also weigh the fact that cesarean section, despite the increased safety of the procedure, still involves maternal risks, predominantly from post-operative infection. Ironically though, a serious problem is likely to develop before the contemporary role of cesarean section for breech presentation is defined. Due to the growing trend toward cesarean sections,[23] most training programs in the near future will not be able to provide adequate opportunities for their students to acquire the essential skills needed to perform successful vaginal breech deliveries, so progressively fewer physicians will be capable of performing them.

§ 21.19 Prognosis

Whereas the maternal risks in breech deliveries are only slightly increased, the fetal risks far exceed those encountered in vertex presentations. When all the potentially complicating maternal and fetal factors, except for the breech presentation, are excluded, the fetal problems far exceed those encountered in ver-

---

[21] *Id.*

[22] De Crespigny & Pepperell, *Perinatal Mortality and Morbidity in Breech Presentation*, 53 Obstet. Gynecol. 141 (1979).

[23] J.A. Pritchard, M.D. & P.C. MacDonald, M.D., Williams Obstetrics, 16th ed., 807 (Appleton-Century-Crofts, 1980).

tex presentation.[24]   Those infants who survive a breech birth tend to have lower average Apgar scores than their vertex-birth counterparts.[25]

The principle causes of perinatal morbidity and mortality of breech babies can be divided into four categories:

1.   Anoxia or asphyxia. See § 21.20.
2.   Traumatic deliveries or obstetrical manipulations. See § 21.21.
3.   Unfavorable fetal size. See § 21.22.
4.   Congenital malformations. See § 21.23.

§ 21.20   —Anoxia or Asphyxia

Asphyxic problems (which include prolapse of the umbilical cord, prolonged umbilical cord compression during the descent of the fetus through the pelvis, and aspiration of amniotic fluid prior to the birth of the nose and mouth) occur in approximately 10 percent of all cases of breech presentation.[26]   In one study, all the infants who had sustained permanent injuries to their central and peripheral nervous systems, had experienced moderate to severe hypoxia during vaginal breech delivery.[27]   Because these dangers are so prevalent, close fetal monitoring during labor is crucial.

§ 21.21   —Traumatic Delivery or Obstetric Manipulations

A traumatic delivery can generally be expected when the unmolded fetal head descends rapidly through the pelvis, which usually occurs when the cervix is not fully dilated.   Attempted breech deliveries under these circumstances are a common cause of asphyxia, intracranial hemorrhage, or skull fracture.   However, these complications may even occur after complete cervical dilatation, especially if there is difficulty delivering the aftercoming head.   In addition to

---

[24] Leslie Iffy, M.D. & Harold A. Kaminetzky, M.D., Principles and Practice of Obstetrics & Perinatology, vol. 2, 919 (John Wiley & Sons, Inc., 1981).

[25] De Crespigny & Pepperell, *Perinatal Mortality and Morbidity in Breech Presentation*, 53 Obstet. Gynecol. 141 (1979).

[26] Leslie Iffy, M.D. & Harold A. Kaminetzky, M.D., Principles and Practice of Obstetrics & Perinatology, vol. 2, 920 (John Wiley & Sons, Inc., 1981).

[27] Morley, *Breech Presentation: A 15 Year Review*, 30 Obstet. Gynecol. 745 (1967).

the fetal trauma, the mother may receive deep cervical lacerations, often accompanied by hemorrhage, if the head is extracted through her unprepared cervix. This is apt to result when the cervix is constricted around the baby's neck.

As the manipulations needed to induce vaginal delivery become more complex (increasing in difficulty from spontaneous, to assisted, to complete breech deliveries), the probability of trauma during the extraction increases, and the fetal morbidity becomes progressively higher.[28] In addition, the higher the station of the presenting part when extraction is initiated, the poorer the fetal outcome.[29] The fetopelvic proportions also markedly influence the prognosis. If the fetus is forcibly extracted through a contracted pelvis, depression or fractures of the skull may result. These injuries are usually fatal.[30]

The specific lesions resulting from a traumatic delivery include fractures of the spine, clavicle, humerus, or femur; intracranial or adrenal hemorrhage; hepatic or splenic rupture; brachial plexus injuries; and brain damage due to anoxia. Excess traction on the baby's cervical spine accounts for a large part of the damage and can be avoided by forceps delivery of the aftercoming head. In contrast, fractures of the clavicle and humerus cannot always be prevented when freeing the infant's arms. Similarly, fractures of the femur are particularly apt to occur during difficult frank breech extractions. Many long term follow-up studies of their childhood manifestations of traumatic breech deliveries reveal a high incidence of permanent disabilities, including mental retardation, cerebral palsy, epilepsy, and facial paralysis.[31]

§ 21.22   —Unfavorable Fetal Size

Size is a significant factor among breech babies since the risks of trauma decrease considerably when the fetus weighs less than 3000 grams, and increase approximately ten-fold when it weighs more than 4000 grams, regardless of the pelvic dimensions.[32] A low birth weight may result from prematurity, growth retardation, or both.

---

[28] Leslie Iffy, M.D. & Harold A. Kaminetzky, M.D., Principles and Practice of Obstetrics & Perinatology, vol. 2, 918-19 (John Wiley & Sons, Inc., 1981).

[29] Id.

[30] Id.

[31] Morley, Breech Presentation: A 15 Year Review, 30 Obstet. Gynecol. 745 (1967).

[32] Leslie Iffy, M.D. & Harold A. Kaminetzky, M.D., Principles and Practice of Obstetrics & Perinatology, vol. 2, 919 (John Wiley & Sons, Inc., 1981).

§ 21.23   —Congenital Malformations

The incidence of major congenital abnormalities among breech babies born after a 36 week pregnancy is over twice the expected rate for infants of the same gestational age.[33]

Complications can also be anticipated in the presence of placenta previa, uterine anomalies, multiple fetuses, and cesarean section. Although the fetus is likely to benefit from a cesarean section performed early in labor (if not before), it will be at the expense of a slight increase in maternal morbidity. The maternal morbidity may also be increased by the manipulations, as well as by the deep anesthesia that is sometimes required for delivery.[34] However, according to several obstetricians, as long as the breech presentations are managed properly, the maternal mortality should not be significantly different from the normal rate.[35]

§ 21.24   Bibliography and Recommended Readings

Ballas, *Hyperextension of the Fetal Head in Breech Presentation: Radiological Evaluation and Significance*, 83 Br. J. Obstet. Gynecol. 201 (1976).

Bowes, Taylor, O'Brien, et al., *Breech Delivery: Evaluation of the Method of Delivery on Perinatal Results and Maternal Morbidity*, 135 Am. J. Obstet. Gynecol. 965 (1979).

Langer & Kennedy, *The Passenger*, in Principles and Practice of Obstetrics & Perinatology, vol 2, 747, by Leslie Iffy, M.D. & Harold A. Kaminetzky, M.D. (John Wiley & Sons, Inc., 1981).

Lanka & Nelson, *Breech Presentation with Low Fetal Mortality*, 104 Am. J. Obstet. Gynecol. 879 (1969).

Mayer & Wingate, *Obstetric Factors in Cerebral Palsy*, 51 Obstet. Gynecol. — (1978).

Teteris, Botschner, Ullery & Essig, *Fetal Heart Rate During Breech Delivers*, 107 Am. J. Obstet. Gynecol. 762 (1970).

---

[33] Fernando Arias, M.D., Ph.D., High-Risk Pregnancy and Delivery, 317 (The C. V. Mosby Co., 1984).

[34] R.W. Wilson, C.T. Beecham, & E.R. Carrington, Obstetrics and Gynecology, 489-90 (The C. V. Mosby Co., 1975).

[35] R.W. Wilson, C.T. Beecham, & E.R. Carrington, Obstetrics and Gynecology, 489-90 (The C. V. Mosby Co., 1975).

CHAPTER 22

CESAREAN SECTION

§ 22.1   Introduction

In the surgical procedure known as cesarean section, the fetus is delivered through an incision in its mother's abdominal wall and uterus. Abdominal deliveries are generally performed instead of vaginal deliveries when an underlying disease exists, or an obstetric complication arises which might seriously traumatize the mother or fetus. Since cesarean section is a major operative procedure, it should never be undertaken lightly and without all essential an-

355

cillary support, as well as a thorough evaluation of its justifications and contraindications.

§ 22.2 Indications

The incidence of cesarean section in a given hospital varies with the percentage of complicated pregnancies admitted to its obstetrics ward. In recent years, there has been a marked increase in cesarean sections, due in large part to improved anesthesia, surgical techniques, and the availability of blood transfusions.[1] As a result, the balance between surgical intervention (cesarean delivery) and the natural birth process (vaginal delivery) has tipped in favor of cesarean delivery, though sometimes inappropriately so. Admittedly, the decision is often complex, but it should be based on each patient's clinical data since the indications for cesarean section are usually not absolute. For example, a combination of indications may justify the procedure, whereas the single component factors might not.

With these considerations in mind, the most common single indications for abdominal deliveries are the following:

1.   Fetopelvic disproportion. See § 22.3.
2.   Previous cesarean section. See § 22.4.
3.   Abnormal presentations. See § 22.5.
4.   Tumor obstruction in the pelvis. See § 22.6.
5.   Following certain uterine or vaginal surgeries. See § 22.7.
6.   Certain maternal disorders such as hypertension and diabetes mellitus, but only under specific circumstances. See § 22.7
7.   Fetal distress. see § 22.8.
8.   Elderly primigravida. See § 22.9.

Regardless of the indication, before the possibility of a successful vaginal or cesarean delivery can be accurately assessed, the obstetrician must determine the fetal size, position and presentation, obtain the measurements of the pelvic diameters, evaluate the pattern of labor, and the nature of the uterine contractions. In addition, whenever cesarean section is likely, the number of rectal and vaginal examinations should be kept to a minimum. The rate of amniotitis and post-partum infection following abdominal delivery has been directly

---

[1] D.N. Danforth, Ph.D., M.D., Obstetrics and Gynecology, 4th ed., 769 (Harper & Row Publishers, Inc., 1982).

related to the length of time the membranes are ruptured before the operation, as well as to the number of rectal and vaginal examinations performed during labor.

§ 22.3   —Fetopelvic Disproportion

This condition occurs when there is a disparity between the size of the fetus and the size of the birth canal. If x-ray pelvimetry demonstrates that an excessively-sized infant could be injured if allowed to pass through a pelvis which appears proportionately too small, then cesarean section may significantly reduce the danger to both the fetus and its mother. Similarly, the operation should be performed if disproportion, documented by x-ray pelvimetry, is seen *in association with* secondary arrest of dilatation, a prolonged deceleration phase, an arrest of fetal descent, breech presentation, or a markedly contracted pelvis. Whenever the antero-posterior diameter of the pelvic inlet measures 8 cm or less, a full term fetus cannot be delivered through the pelvis; thus, this constitutes an indication for cesarean delivery.[2]

However, when the results of x-ray pelvimetry do not reveal a clear-cut case of disproportion, a growing number of obstetricians recommend and rely on *trial labor* to determine whether or not a safe vaginal delivery is feasible before resorting to a cesarean delivery.[3] If the patient is given prophylactic anti-microbial drugs beforehand, her health should not be jeopardized by the trial labor. Should the labor be unsuccessful for any reason, cesarean section is then performed. It is important to remember that just because a woman has delivered a normal-sized baby in the past, she is not ensured against fetopelvic disproportion in a future pregnancy if the next fetus is larger.

§ 22.4   —Previous Cesarean Section

The addage "once a cesarean section, always a cesarean section," is losing popularity.[4] Subsequent abdominal deliveries should only be performed if there are new or repetitive indications for the operation. If the initial reason for the previous cesarean delivery no longer exists, *and* if the previous opera-

---

[2] J.R. Willson, M.D., C.T. Beecham, M.D., & E.R. Carrington, M.D., Obstetrics and Gynecology, 5th ed., 512 (The C.V. Mosby Co., 1975).

[3] *Id.*

[4] D.N. Danforth, Ph.D., M.D., Obstetrics and Gynecology, 4th ed., 771 (Harper & Row Publishers, Inc., 1982).

tion was the low cervical type (and not the classic type), then vaginal delivery should be possible. However, the induction of stimulation of labor with oxytocin must be avoided in these cases.

A trial labor is attempted to judge the capability and safety of vaginal delivery. During this time, the patient must be continuously observed, and the physician must be prepared to promptly intervene should there be any sign that the uterine scar has ruptured.

Rupture of the previous uterine scar during future pregnancies, particularly in the final weeks of gestation, is the primary maternal hazard. Therefore, the site of the previous uterine incision should be examined repeatedly throughout the pregnancy for any evidence of thinning. But since it is not always possible to accurately evaluate the strength of the scar, some obstetricians advise elective repeat cesarean sections after the 38th week (as opposed to trial labor) in an effort to minimize the danger of rupture. Other obstetricians believe that if a previous cesarean delivery was complicated by infection, the integrity of the wound should not be trusted, and a repeat cesarean section should be performed before labor begins.[5] However, these decisions must be carefully weighed against the equally hazardous fetal risk of the operation, which is the unanticipated delivery of a premature baby. Prematurity is associated with several serious neonatal disorders which compromise the baby's health, and adversely affect its ability to survive outside of the womb.

Because frequent errors are made when calculating the due date from potentially unreliable menstrual information alone, various guidelines have been established to accurately assess fetal maturity. The gestational age of the fetus is determined by:

1. The date of the mother's last menstrual period
2. Serial uterine (fundal) measurements throughout the pregnancy
3. The date when fetal motion was first detected
4. The date when fetal heart rate was first heard with a fetoscope
5. The estimated size and weight of the infant (a weight of 2500 grams or more reduces the likelihood of delivering a premature infant).

In addition to those criteria, a variety of laboratory parameters are available to determine the maturity of specific fetal organ systems. Opinions vary regarding the most informative and reliable combination of these tests, which include:

---

[5] J.R. Willson, M.D., C.T. Beecham, M.D., & E.R. Carrington, M.D., Obstetrics and Gynecology, 5th ed., 517 (The C.V. Mosby Co., 1975).

1. X-ray of the epiphyseal centers of the long fetal bones (skeletal development)

2. Sonographic measurements of the fetal skull (skull bone size and maturation)

3. Analysis of the amniotic fluid for the lecithin to sphingomyelin (L/S) ratio (pulmonary development), creatinine (kidney maturation), bilirubin (liver maturation) and fat cells (skin lipid maturation).

Ultrasonographic measurement of the fetal head may soon become equal to, or even surpass, other methods of evaluating fetal maturity.

If these tests cannot be obtained, or if they indicate fetal immaturity, it is best to postpone the cesarean section. As long as there are no compelling reasons to delay it, the ideal time to schedule either the *elective* or the *indicated* operations is at, or shortly after, the onset of spontaneous labor. However, if the abdominal delivery must be performed as an emergency procedure, it is more dangerous because of the probability that an operating room will not be available, or that the patient will have eaten recently, and will therefore pose an increased anesthetic risk.

§ 22.5 —Abnormal Presentations

Shoulder and persistent brow presentation are considered unequivocal indications for cesarean section. Other abnormal presentations (particularly brow, transverse lie, and the occasional breech) when associated with some other complication, usually justify abdominal delivery.

Cesarean section is not advocated in all breech presentations. It may be indicated in a primipara, especially if the fetus is large. Because of the high prenatal mortality in complete breech presentations, or in single or double footling-breech presentations, cesarean delivery is often performed, particularly if labor is prolonged or abnormal.

§ 22.6 —Tumor Obstruction in the Pelvis

When ovarian cysts, uterine fibroids, or other tumors lie in the pelvis below the presenting part, they may block the passage of the fetus. The effect may be similar to the case of a contracted pelvis.

Generally, ovarian cysts that are diagnosed during early pregnancy are removed, and the patient can be allowed to deliver vaginally. However, if a tumor is discovered low in the posterior uterine wall or the posterior cul-de-

sac after the 24th week of gestation, cesarean section is almost always necessary. By this time, the uterus is so large that it is virtually impossible to remove without disturbing the pregnancy.

Previous vaginal plastic operations and operative repairs of the cervix or
uterus, such as hysterotomy or unification of a bicornate uterus, are sometimes regarded as absolute indications for cesarean section. Abdominal delivery is supposed to prevent recurrent problems of pelvic tissue relaxation
resulting from the trauma of labor and delivery. Myomectomy patients are
usually managed like those who have had previous cesarean delivery because
of the concern over the possibility of uterine rupture, even though some authors claim that the danger is rare.[6]

§ 22.7 —Certain Maternal Disorders

Currently, the majority of hypertensive disorders are successfully managed by
medical induction of labor, so there is only an occasional need to terminate
these pregnancies with cesarean section. In the case of diabetes mellitus,
cesarean section is indicated when vaginal or rectal findings are unfavorable
for induction (usually as a result of cephalopelvic disproportion), when medical induction fails, or when there is evidence of a high fetal risk due to the
stress and time involved in its birth.

If placenta previa is diagnosed, it is usually safer to deliver viable fetuses by
cesarean section, preferably the low segment operation, because it prevents
lacerations of the lower uterine segment during vaginal delivery. It also increases the fetal survival rate.

Abdominal delivery is recommended for mild, premature separation of the
placenta (abruptio placenta) when it cannot be managed conservatively. It is
also suggested when the cervix is either undilated or considered unfavorable
for induction—indicating that delivery is not imminent. When the fetus is
viable and is estimated to weigh at least 2000 grams, prompt cesarean delivery
is believed to offer a better chance of fetal survival in severe degrees of placental separation, and/or fetal distress. An additional benefit of abdominal delivery is that it may help control maternal blood loss. Premature separation of
the placenta often necessitates an emergency cesarean section.[7]

Although cesarean section is a dangerous method of delivery in the presence of eclampsia, it is warranted if the symptoms progress rapidly despite

---

[6] D.N. Danforth, Ph.D., M.D., Obstetrics and Gynecology, 4th ed., 769 (Harper & Row Publishers, Inc., 1982).

[7] Leslie Iffy, M.D. & Harold A. Kaminetzky, M.D., Principles and Practice of Obstetrics &
Perinatology, vol. 2, 1537 (John Wiley & Sons, Inc., 1981).

treatment, and it appears that convulsions will begin before vaginal delivery occurs. However, the rapid onset of labor and delivery may be accomplished by simply rupturing the membranes artificially. It is frequently necessary to deliver women with severe, chronic hypertensive cardiovascular or renal disease, several weeks before term. Abdominal delivery is usually appropriate in these cases.

§ 22.8   —Fetal Distress

When a prolapsed cord is discovered, fetal survival depends on prompt delivery. If rapid and atraumatic vaginal delivery is not feasible, as in the case of an incompletely dilated cervix, abdominal delivery can save the fetus's life. This also applies if a slow or irregular fetal heart rate and/or the passage of meconium are detected. The one exception to this rule occurs when fetal distress is associated with shock, due to the fact that the mother is in the prone position. In this case, the problem can be resolved by turning the patient on her side.

§ 22.9   —Elderly Primigravida

Because women over the age of 35 are more prone to pregnancies associated with degenerative diseases and obstetric complications, cesarean section is often favored to reduce the risks of vaginal delivery. However, the age factor alone does not justify the more liberal use of abdominal deliveries. A trial of labor is recommended before the operation is attempted.

§ 22.10   Contraindications

With rare exceptions, abdominal delivery is contraindicated if the fetus is dead because vaginal delivery is usually less hazardous to the mother. This applies even in most cases of fetopelvic disproportion. However, if maternally life-threatening circumstances develop, such as serious hemorrhage due to total placenta previa, or abruptio placenta, then cesarean section may be required despite the fact that the fetus is dead.

§ 22.11   Types of Cesarean Section

There are four methods of abdominal delivery:

Classic Cesarean Section: A vertical incision is made in the *upper* uterine segment. See § **22.12**.

Low Segment or Low Cervical Operation: The incision is made either transversely, or vertically transperitoneal in the *lower* uterine segment. See § **22.13**.

Extraperitoneal Operation: By separating the bladder from the uterus, the *lower* uterine segment is reached without entering the peritoneal cavity. See § **22.14**.

Cesarean Hysterectomy: Cesarean section is followed by hysterectomy.

§ 22.12   —Classic Cesarean Section

This was the standard method of abdominal surgery. It is performed less frequently now because better maternal results can be achieved with the low cervical operation.[8]

The primary advantage of the classic method is the ability to operate more rapidly than with the other procedures. In addition, it is the technique of choice when the fetus is in a transverse lie presentation, since extraction is easier and there is not as high a risk of internal version causing fetal distress as there is with the low cervical operation. The main disadvantages of the classic technique are a comparatively increased danger of infection, hemorrhage, and subsequent uterine rupture.

§ 22.13   —Low Segment/Low Cervical Operation

Ever since prophylactic, antibiotic administration minimized the incidence of infections, and thereby improved the safety of trial labors, a larger percentage of low cervical operations were performed. The technique is called the transverse (or Kerr incision) low segment cesarean section. One of its advantages over the classic operation is that it is easier to repair. It also reduces the risk of subsequent rupture (since the uterine scar is stronger); minimizes the inci-

---

[8] D.N. Danforth, Ph.D., M.D., Obstetrics and Gynecology, 773 (Harper & Row Publishers, Inc., 1982).

dence of post-partum, peritoneal infection; diminishes the danger of intestinal adhesions and obstruction; and reduces the rate of hemorrhage. In addition, the patient does not experience as much discomfort post-operatively.

§ 22.14   —Extraperitoneal Operation

This incision is generally more difficult to perform than the others, and a trend has developed away from extraperitoneal operations, toward increased low segment operations instead. Virtually all teaching centers throughout the United States presently share the belief that the indications for extraperitoneal operations are exceedingly rare, even in the case of potential infection.[9]

§ 22.15   Anesthesia

Either conduction or general anesthesia of some magnitude must be administered to the woman undergoing a cesarean delivery. Currently, there are a variety of anesthetic agents and techniques on the market, and each method has its adherents. As of yet, no perfect anesthetic is available that provides the mother with complete pain relief, while at the same time, is free of risk to both the woman and her baby.

Fox suggested some guidelines for selecting the most appropriate form of anesthesia.[10] The primary consideration is the skill and experience of the anesthesiologist. Other important factors include the urgency of the operation, the physical and emotional status of the mother, the condition of the fetus, the pathophysiology associated with the indication for cesarean section, and the skill of the obstetrician.

§ 22.16   Maternal Prognosis

Although there has been a marked decline in maternal deaths associated with cesarean section in the past 50 years,[11] there is still a higher incidence of ma-

---

[9] *Id.* at 772.

[10] Fox, et al., *Anesthesia for Cesarean Section,* 133 Am. J. Obstet. Gynecol., 15 (1979).

[11] Frigoletto, Ryan, & Phillippe, *Maternal Mortality Rate Associated with Cesarean Section: An Appraisal,* 136 Am. J. Obstet. Gynecol. 969 (1980).

ternal mortality following cesarean section than following vaginal delivery.[12] This difference is commonly attributed to the complications necessitating the operation, which in themselves carry risk to the mother, and not entirely to the dangers of the surgery itself. For example, the length of time the woman has been in labor, the number of hours the membranes have been ruptured, and the quantity and quality of vaginal examinations made before the operation may influence the maternal and fetal outcome more than the cesarean section itself.

Abdominal surgery carries the same inherent risks as any major operation, namely infection, shock, hemorrhage, and anesthesia. These factors may be responsible for the woman's death. However, if the proper procedures are followed, and the appropriate emergency measures are instituted immediately as the situation warrants, the experts believe that most of these deaths can be prevented.[13]

§ 22.17   Perinatal Prognosis

Although cesarean section does not guarantee infant survival, statistics demonstrate that the perinatal mortality rate has declined considerably during the past 40 years.[14] Improved pediatric care of the mature and premature infant, avoidance of cesarean delivery for dead or seriously malformed fetuses, and the widespread use of modern techniques for assessing fetal maturity are continuing to lower the perinatal death rate following abdominal delivery.

Presently, most authorities agree that the fetal risk from cesarean section is greater than from vaginal delivery. Studies show an increased mortality associated with the operation, especially when the neonate is undersized, and when the duration of the pregnancy is misjudged.[15] Still other obstetricians claim the fetal survival is directly related to the complication that requires the cesarean section.[16]

---

12 J.A. Pritchard, M.D. & D.C. MacDonald, M.D., Williams Obstetrics, 16th ed., 1083 (Appleton-Century-Crofts, 1980).

13 *Id.* at 1082.

14 U.S. Department of Health, Education and Welfare, *Facts of Life & Death*, Publication No. 79-1222 (1978).

15 D.N. Danforth, Ph.D., M.D., Obstetrics and Gynecology, 4th ed., 771 (Harper & Row Publishers, Inc., 1982).

16 J.A. Pritchard, M.D. & D.C. MacDonald, M.D., Williams Obstetrics, 16th ed., 1082 (Appleton-Century-Crofts, 1980).

§ 22.18   Bibliography and Recommended Readings

Bottoms, Rosen & Sikol, *The Increase in the Cesarean Birth Rate*, 302 N. Eng. J. Med. 559 (1980).

Burchell, M.D., *Cesarean Section*, in Principles and Practice of Obstetrics & Perinatology, vol 2, by Leslie Iffy, M.D. & Harold A. Kaminetzky, M.D. (John Wiley & Sons, Inc., 1981).

Danforth, D.N., Ph.D., M.D., *Obstetrics and Gynecology*, 4th ed. (Harper & Row Publishers, Inc., 1982).

Niswander, Kenneth R., M.D., *Obstetrics, Essentials of Clinical Practice*, 2d ed. (Little, Brown & Co., 1981).

Pritchard, J.A., M.D., MacDonald, P.C., M.D., & Gant, N.F., M.D., *Williams Obstetrics*, 17th ed. (Appleton-Century-Crofts, 1985).

Reeder, Sharon J., R.N., Ph.D., Mastroianni, Luigi, Jr., M.D., & Martin, Leonide L., R.N., *Maternity Nursing*, 15th ed. (J.B. Lippincott Co., 1983).

Sachs, et al., *Cesarean Section—Risk and Benefits for Mother and Fetus*, 250 JAMA 2157 (1983).

CHAPTER 23

IMMEDIATE CARE OF THE NEWBORN

§ 23.1   Introduction

Although most infants make the sudden transition from intrauterine to extra-uterine life without difficulty, the survival of others depends upon prompt recognition and treatment of their life threatening disorders. Yet, instead of waiting until the baby is born to determine whether it requires assistance, the obstetrician should strive to anticipate potential complications well in advance of its arrival, a policy which gives him ample time to plan the best course of intrapartum and postpartum management of the compromised child, and rarely catches him unprepared when a medical emergency arises. Accurate predictions of the expected neonatal status can be made prior to birth by considering the mother's health, the course of labor, the amount and type of analgesia and anesthesia giver prior to delivery, and the delivery procedures themselves, since these variables all influence the fetus's health and eventual outcome.

Following the immediate assessment of the newborn, all efforts must focus on correction of pathophysiologic functions. The problems may be classified as follows:

367

1. Hypoventilation which frequently starts with placental insufficiency which then develops into neonatal depression and apnea.
2. Hypoxia as a result of neonatal asphyxia.
3. Acidosis which is usually a result of insufficient O_2 uptake and CO_2 removal. It is a complex metabolic-respiratory disorder.
4. Hypothermia which is a result of the newborn's inability to maintain its body temperature.

Resuscitation must be provided to help in all these areas.[1]

§ 23.2   Establishing and Maintaining an Adequate Airway

Since the first, and perhaps most critical, challenge facing the newborn is breathing on its own, it is the obstetrician's responsibility to facilitate every child's initial respiratory efforts by establishing and maintaining a patent airway as soon as its nose and mouth emerge; either from the vaginal opening during a vaginal delivery, or from the uterine incision during a cesarean section. Simply wiping the baby's face and then gently aspirating foreign debris (such as blood, mucus, and amniotic fluid) from its nose, mouth, and pharynx with a soft rubber suction bulb will usually suffice to clear the respiratory passages. Keeping the infant's head down and its mouth open throughout delivery is also recommended because this position allows a large quantity of fluid to drain naturally from the trachea, so it too can be removed during aspiration. If the excess fluid and foreign debris which accumulate in the respiratory tract during labor are not promptly removed, they might prevent the lungs from filling up with oxygen, thereby making it much more difficult for the baby to breathe. Once its airway is clear and breathing becomes spontaneous, the infant can be placed on its side (some suggest keeping its neck extended to assure an open airway) in a warm crib or incubator, while awaiting transfer to the nursery.

§ 23.3   Resuscitation

The normal baby cries and begins to respire spontaneously within one minute of its birth, needing no special care other than the routine suctioning of its air

---

[1] Leslie Iffy, M.D. & Harold A. Kaminetzky, M.D., Principles and Practice of Obstetrics & Perinatology, vol. 2, 1595 (John Wiley & Sons, Inc., 1981).

passages as described above. In marked contrast, an infant whose airway is obstructed or who is otherwise unable to breathe spontaneously one minute after delivery, may develop extensive brain damage, or possibly die, unless the obstetrician quickly intervenes and administers oxygen to its lungs. The success of such resuscitative measures depends on well-functioning equipment and well-trained personnel since time is of the essence in managing respiratory emergencies. Even when respiratory problems are not expected, someone trained in newborn resuscitation must be available at each delivery in case complications arise.

The severity of the infant's respiratory depression dictates which method of resuscitation to use. For the moderately depressed baby in whom no airway obstructions are found following aspiration, the physician should attempt to induce breathing by inserting a plastic airway tube into its oropharynx, and then applying intermittent puffs of positive pressure oxygen through a face mask for one to two seconds. Even though the pressure is too low to actually expand the lungs, most apneic infants respond successfully to this procedure, gasping at first and then breathing spontaneously. In such cases, ventilation can be discontinued, but the baby should remain under close observation in a warm, oxygen-enriched environment. Gentle suctioning of its nose and mouth may be necessary from time to time to remove any secretions that have accumulated.

On the other hand, if the newborn is unable to breathe on its own following this treatment, and if its heart rate slows down (which often happens when the initial resuscitative measures do not induce respiration within one to one and one-half minutes after delivery), the emergency life-saving procedure called *endotracheal intubation* is required. Instead of threading the airway tube to the oropharynx as in the previous technique, the physician maneuvers it farther down the respiratory tract until it reaches the trachea, from where he can artifically inflate the lungs themselves. But before doing so, he must clear the nasopharynx and trachea of residual foreign matter or else these substances may be carelessly blown into the child's lungs.

Sometimes, just the stimulus of the endotracheal tube on the tissues lining the respiratory tract is enough to initiate spontaneous breathing. If not, positive pressure ventilation must be applied, either by gently blowing air or oxygen through the tube or by connecting the tube, to a bag of oxygen or an oxygen-enriched gas mixture. While therapy is in progess, the infant's cardiac status must be closely monitored. Although its heart rate typically improves after the first few breaths have been induced, if it remains low (less than 80-100 beats-per-minute) or disappears entirely, cardiac massage must be performed immediately in conjunction with the ventilation.

The baby undergoing endotracheal intubation usually gasps after the first or second application of positive pressure, and then begins to respire on its own.

This response, together with a rise in the upper one third of its chest, an increase in its heart rate, and an improvement in its skin color and muscle tone, indicates that the infant is receiving an adequate amount of oxygen. At that point, the endotracheal tube can be gently removed.

The revived baby can then be placed in an incubator capable of maintaining a constant internal temperature of 37°C (normal body temperature) and supplying the desired concentration of warmed, humidified oxygen (usually 40 percent or less). Cold, dry oxygen or oxygen mixtures should not be used at this time, nor during any of the ventilation procedures since they are liable to damage the mucous membranes of the respiratory tract, in addition to causing thermal stress. Exposure to temperatures below 37°C, whether as a result of cold therapeutic gases or chilly surroundings, *stresses* the newborn by forcing it to needlessly consume its oxygen (which it struggled for so desparately) just to maintain its body temperature at 37°C. Thoroughly drying the infant immediately after birth, and then covering it with a warm blanket, is another important way of dramatically reducing the heat loss and resultant oxygen consumption that occurs when its naked, wet body passes from the warmth of the uterus, to the air-conditioned delivery room.

§ 23.4   Evaluating the Newborn's Physical Status
(Apgar Scores)

The Apgar scoring system is the standard method of quantitating the findings of the preliminary newborn evaluation, and rapidly relating the resultant numerical values to the need for, and extent of, resuscitation. Depending on its condition, the infant is given a score of 0, 1, or 2 (the highest rating) for each of the following easily observable and obtainable parameters: its heart rate and respiratory effort (indicative of the severity and duration of asphyxia), muscle tone and reflex activity (indicative of the status of the central nervous system), and skin color (indicative of cardiopulmonary function). The final score, obtained by adding the five results together, is calculated twice; once, one minute after complete birth, and again, five minutes after birth. See **Table 23-1**.

Whereas the five-minute Apgar score correlates best with survival and neurologic status, the one-minute score determines the need for immediate resuscitation. Most infants are born in excellent condition, as indicated by one-minute Apgar scores of 8-10, and generally begin breathing without assistance. Newborns who are mildly depressed (Apgar score of 7), can usually be roused by gentle stimulation such as slapping the sole of the feet, and blowing oxygen

over their faces. In sharp contrast, much more vigorous resuscitative measures are required for moderately depressed infants (Apgar score of 4-6), who

Table 23-1

THE APGAR SCORING SYSTEM

Sign	0	1	2
Heart Rate	Absent	Slow (below 100)	Over 100
Respiratory Rate	Absent	Slow & irregular, weak cry, hyper-ventilation	Good; accompa-nied by strong crying
Muscle Tone	Limp	Some flexion of the extremities	Active motion; extremities well-flexed
Reflex Activity*	No Response	Grimace	Cry
Skin Color	Blue; pale	Body pink, extrem-ities blue	Completely pink

*Response to stimulating the sole of the foot
© Reprinted with permission. David N. Danforth, Ph.D., M.D., Obstetrics and Gynecology, 4th ed., 844 (Philadelphia: Harper & Row Publishers, Inc., 1982).

may be pale or blue and almost completely limp, one minute after delivery.
Their condition deteriorates rapidly unless positive pressure ventilation is
promptly initiated. If no response is elicited after one to two minutes, endotracheal intubation must be performed immediately.

No time should be lost in clearing the air passages, intubating the trachea,
and establishing positive pressure ventilation for severely depressed babies
(Apgar score of 0-3) who may rapidly develop brain damage if it has not occurred already. These pale, flaccid, and unresponsive newborns may require
three to five minutes of artifical ventilation before gasping spontaneously.

If a premature baby receives a low Apgar score, it is generally due to its
temporarily weak muscle tone and limited overall strength, rather than to a
long-lasting mental or physical abnormality. Since the child typically becomes
stronger as it matures, its Apgar score does *not* reflect its prognosis as accurately as it does for a full term infant, in whom significant improvement is not
expected under the same circumstances.

§ 23.5   External Cardiac Massage

When distant heart sounds, a slow heart rate, or the absence of a heartbeat are
discovered, prompt resuscitative measures are indicated. However, positive

pressure ventilation (either by mask or endotracheal tube) is unlikely to be effective if the newborn's blood pressure is excessively low, unless external cardiac massage is also performed. By manually compressing the heart between the chest wall and the vertebral column, the procedure known as *external cardiac massage* enables the physician to force blood into the major blood vessels of the heart, and together with proper ventilation (the combination of cardiac massage and ventilation is called cardiopulmonary resuscitation or CPR), often allows him to approximate the desirable cardiac and respiratory rates until the baby takes over. CPR is most successful when there is no clinical evidence of fetal distress, and when the fetal heart rate (measured between uterine contractions) is normal throughout the course of labor.

Two important signs of adequate cardiac output are improved skin color and constriction of the pupils. Yet, despite these encouraging reactions, cardiac massage should be continued until a rhythmical heartbeat is readily heard. An electrocardiogram (ECG) should be taken after the procedure.

Ventilation can be discontinued as soon as spontaneous breathing is established. Before transferring the revived child to the nursery, it should be carefully examined, paying particular attention to the warning signs of impending convulsions, a dangerous complication that has been observed in some 12-24 hour old babies who received CPR.

§ 23.6   Correcting Acid-Base Imbalances

As a result of strong uterine contractions, umbilical cord compression, certain maternal disorders, and various other complications which impair the feto-maternal blood exchange during pregnancy and labor, all babies are relatively asphyxiated when they emerge from the womb. *Asphyxia*, which is defined as a combination of hypoxia and acidosis, is considered to be the most common problem faced by newborns.

Unlike healthy, alert babies who are generally able to resolve the acid imbalance on their own after about 24 hours, depressed infants are caught in a vicious cycle. Not only do they have a more serious acidosis which takes longer to correct because of its magnitude, but the high levels of acid also reduce the oxygen uptake of their pulmonary blood vessels, thereby diminishing the effectiveness of resuscitative measures in those who need them the most. The recovery of these newborns depends on prompt medical intervention to restore their normal acid-base equilibrium.

Initially, ventilation technique provides a much more rapid and efficient means of treating acid-base disturbances than infusing alkali (sodium bicarbonate). However, once breathing is established, it is then advisable to administer sodium bicarbonate to correct the remaining acid imbalance, provided that any ventilation procedures which may still be in progress do not have to be interrupted. Such treatment has been shown to increase the recovery rate and responsiveness of the depressed infant, unless it is so severely asphyxiated that its heart rate does not return following CPR. Under these circumstances, alkali infusions are not recommended.

Periodic measurement of the baby's blood pH and blood gas status is necessary in order to evaluate the degree of acidosis, and the effectiveness of the chosen therapy. While treatment is underway, it is crucial to maintain the infant's normal body temperature, since temperatures below 37°C prolong the recovery time from both hypoxia and acidosis.

If depression is due to narcotic agents, then drug antagonists should be administered after assisted ventilation has been established. Nalorane Hydrochloride should be tried in doses of 0.005 mg/kg IM/IV (milligrams per kilogram of body weight either intravenously or intramuscularly).

One must always remember that anytime there is evidence of fetal distress during labor, the presence of a pediatrician or neonatologist in the delivery room to care for the *stressed* neonate will greatly improve the infant's prognosis.

Finally, the sick infant should be transferred from the delivery room to the nursery, or neonatal intensive care unit, as soon as it is safely possible to do so.

§ 23.7 The Neonatal Examination

After the Apgar scores have been calculated and respiration has been well-established, every infant should be carefully checked for life-threatening anatomic or physiologic abnormalities which demand prompt attention. A more thorough examination is not yet appropriate because the baby neither requires, nor easily tolerates, extensive handling and manipulation for the first few hours after birth when it is recovering from the stresses of delivery, and adjusting to the conditions of extrauterine life. Nonetheless, a considerable amount of information can still be obtained in the early neonatal period by simply observing the child's movements and reactions.

A high risk newborn can be quickly identified at this time by correlating its birth weight, length, and head circumference with its estimated gestational age. On the basis of these criteria, the infant is classified as large for gestation age (LGA), appropriate for gestational age (AGA), or small for gestational age (SGA). This simple scheme not only clearly describes deviations from the normal intrauterine growth patterns, but it also provides the obstetrician with a reliable and sensitive method of pinpointing the special problems of each group of babies so they can be properly treated without delay. For instance, LGA infants are known to have an increased risk of birth asphyxia, birth trauma, certain congenital defects, and hypoglycemia. Even though SGA infants are at the opposite end of the size spectrum, they too are predisposed to severe intrapartum asphyxia, mechanical trauma during delivery, and congenital malformations. In addition, they are also prone to nutritional deficiencies and infections. Not surprisingly, the lowest incidence of complications and the lowest predicted mortality rate are found among AGA infants.

Despite the usefulness of these classifications, occasionally a physician may still group newborns as premature, mature, or postmature. In this older system, prematurity is the factor responsible for the majority of high-risk births since the functional and anatomical immaturity of the infant's organs predispose them to infections, metabolic disorders, respiratory distress, and central nervous system hemorrhage.

Once the baby's condition has stabilized, a systemic examination of its entire body must be performed during the first 24 hours, beginning with its skin and moving on to its head and neck, lungs, heart, abdomen, genitalia, back, and extremities. The objective of the first complete physical is to detect the less serious deformities and injuries, and record all of the initial observations and measurements so subsequent physicians will have a foundation from which to evaluate the child's future growth and development.

The color of the skin reveals important information about the status of the heart and lungs. The development of a rosy pink color several minutes after birth usually indicates that the infant is healthy, whereas persistent generalized cyanosis (blue coloration) is often associated with an underlying disease and rapid deterioration of the baby's condition. Therefore, the cause must be determined and treated urgently.

After appraising the skin color, the physician should note the size, shape, symmetry, and general appearance of the head, by closely examining its delicate structures to ascertain whether they were damaged during delivery. If the posterior fontanel is open instead of closed, hydrocephalus should be suspected. Either hydrocephalus or hemorrhage may cause the anterior fontanel to bulge due to the abnormal fluid accumulation. Although the brain swelling may not be apparent immediately following delivery, this serious complication should not immediately be ruled out for awhile because it may still develop several hours later, particularly if it was caused by intrauterine hypoxia.

During the eye examination, the discovery of fixed, dilated pupils is suggestive of severe asphyxia or brain damage. In addition to the routine opthalmic evaluation, the law in most states requires all newborns to receive prophylaxis against maternally acquired gonorrheal infections, since this particular veneral disease may be asymptomatic during pregnancy. If it was not detected, the bacteria inside the mother's vagina might enter the baby's eyes during delivery, causing an infection and eventual blindness. These disorders have been virtually eradicated by placing either one drop of a 1 percent silver nitrate solution, or a squirt of penicillin or tetracycline ointment into both of the newborn's eyes.

To ensure that the infant is breathing evenly, its chest must be observed and auscultated as it moves up and down. Retraction of the sternum or intercostal spaces in mature babies is abnormal, indicating an airway obstruction, or an inability of the lungs to expand completely. This finding, along with rapid breathing, grunting (these sounds are always associated with serious disease) and nasal flaring, are common signs of the respiratory distress syndrome, a serious disorder which must be treated with oxygen, and then closely followed by taking serial chest x-rays of the baby, measuring its blood gas and acid-base status, and frequently monitoring its vital signs.

As the examination progresses, the position of the limbs and their range of movement should be tested. A limply extended arm or leg is suggestive of a nerve injury. Similarly, lack of movement may be the result of a peripheral nerve injury or a fracture. If deformities are discovered, the possibility of a fracture should be investigated by an examination and x-ray study of the area.

A neurologic examination should be performed following the physical examination. Neurologic impairment occurs more frequently among babies who received low Apgar scores and remained limp after respiration was established.

Every few hours, the infant's pulse rate, respiratory rate, blood pressure, temperature, and color should be recorded and evaluated. These measurements and observations provide the information needed to appraise the condition of the vast majority of newborns, with the exception of sick or premature babies who generally require more frequent or continuous monitoring. Premature infants also require warmth, humidity, and oxygen, supplied in a closed environment capable of protecting their undeveloped immune systems from infectious organisms. Regardless of the age or status of the baby, if an infection is suspected, bacterial and/or viral cultures should be obtained and analyzed, and all abnormal laboratory findings (whether bacteriologic, chemical or hematologic) should be reevaluated at frequent intervals.

Healthy infants are typically transferred to the nursery after birth, but those who are not in stable condition, the so-called high risk babies, should be placed in a neonatal intensive care unit. These specially designed facilities enable the medical staff to closely monitor the child's status so that abnormalities can quickly be detected and treated before they cause additional complications or damage. Included among the candidates for intensive care are small or premature babies (those weighing under 2,000 grams or those less than 34 weeks of gestation), infants with respiratory distress, infants who have not yet recovered from asphyxia, babies with congenital anomalies who required specialized nursing care, and those who are liable to develop hypoglycemia (low blood sugar levels).

§ 23.8   Bibliography and Recommended Readings

Danforth, D.N., Ph.D., M.D., *Obstetrics and Gynecology* (Harper & Row Publishers, Inc., 1982).

Iffy, Leslie, M.D. & Kaminetzky, Harold A., M.D., *Principles and Practice of Obstetrics & Perinatology*, vol 2 (John Wiley & Sons, Inc., 1981).

Niswander K.R., M.D., *Obstetrics, Essentials of Clinical Practice* (Little, Brown & Co., 1981).

Oxorn, Harry, B.A., M.D., *Human Labor and Birth* (Appleton-Century-Crofts, 1980).

Pritchard, J.A., M.D., MacDonald, P.C., M.D., & Gant, N.F., M.D., *Williams Obstetrics*, 17th ed. (Appleton-Century-Crofts, 1985).

Willson, J.R., M.D., Beecham, C., M.D., & Carrington, E.R., M.D., *Obstetrics and Gynecology* (The C.V. Mosby Co., 1975).

PART III

MEDICAL BRIEFS: DEPOSITION AND TRIAL PREPARATION

Part II of this book has summarized the medical aspects of a child's birth. We have attempted to meet the dual goal of being comprehensive in the coverage of current medical knowledge and practice, while presenting this information in a form which an attorney having a limited medical background can understand and utilize in preparing a birth trauma case.

Of course, not every birth trauma case is going to involve all of the topics discussed in the medical chapters of this book. In the typical case, the injury to the newborn will be traced to a limited number of errors, usually interconnected to one another.

Although it is useful to an attorney handling a birth trauma case to have a working knowledge of all the medical concepts involved in the birth process, in a particular case, his attention will necessarily focus on the procedures and skills employed in those areas where the malpractice of the defendant is suspected.

In **Chapters 24** through **27** we present examples of case summaries, which are similar to those we prepare in actual birth trauma cases. The summary provides a practical guideline to the attorney as he pursues an individual case. It presents to an attorney a profile of the medical issues which are the focus of litigation. The summary is prepared from several sources: the client interview, the patient's hospital and physician records, the reports of experts, and the independent research of the attorney. (Malpractice attorneys should never rely entirely or exclusively on their experts' reports. An attorney should always conduct his own research into a medical subject in order to be better able to comprehend his experts' reports and to anticipate the defenses and tactics of his opponent). Based upon these sources, the attorney can pull all the facts of the case together, meld these facts into the framework of the salient medical issues, and have at his fingertips a blueprint of the medical aspects of his case. Then, as the case progresses, the attorney can use this blueprint to help him draft interrogatories, to point out the areas needing additional investigation, to prepare for the deposition of the expert witnesses, and to assist in the presentation of proofs at trial. In jurisdictions where a pretrial mediation is a regular part of the litigation process, the case summary provides the best starting point for preparing the mediation brief. In short, the summary serves a multitude of useful purposes, not least of which is to keep the attorney on track with the particular case so that he will not exhaust and squander valuable time and effort on complex irrelevancies, or on the labor of renewing his acquaintance with the file as each new stage in the proceedings is reached.

The summary should be prepared early in the course of litigation, but it is not inflexible. It should be amended and up-dated as necessary as discovery reveals more about the case. Yet, its virtue remains in being concise and incisive; a case summary should only be as long as is necessary to translate the facts and medical issues of a case into a useful prose telling the straightforward story of what should have been done to prevent an injury to the child and what actually occurred in the course of treatment to cause the resulting injury. With such a summary in hand, the attorney can forge an effective and solid case presentation to convincingly persuade the ultimate fact finder when the case reaches trial.

The case summaries in **Chapters 24** through **27** are examples of the attorney's work product to assist him throughout the case. As such, we have written them with very few footnote references. For further information on medical topics with complete references, see **Chapters 9** through **23.**

CASE REVIEW: POST-MATURITY, SMALL FOR GESTATIONAL AGE, NEONATAL HYPOGLYCEMIA, AND HYPOTHERMIA

§ 24.1   Medical Issues

The medical issues in this case involve:

1. Small for Gestational Age
2. Hypoglycemia

3. Hypothermia

4. Polycythemia/Hyperviscosity

5. Hyperbilirubinemia/Kernicterus

Theo Mimar was a product of what was considered to be a full term gestation, based upon a last menstrual period of July 28, 1978 (rendering the estimated date of confinement of May 3, 1979). Delivery transpired on May 4, 1979, one day after the estimated date of confinement. The child has a complex seizure disorder of a mixed type, delayed psychomotor development, and presently exhibits spastic quadriparesis, which has been related to hypoxic brain damage transpiring during the labor as a result of cord compression from a nuchal cord. This stress was evident on the fetal heart monitoring tapes prior to delivery. The combination of meconium stained fluid and severe variable declarations occurred during the labor period. The child also exhibited other problems during the neonatal period, which were related to hypoglycemia and hypoxia. Thus, this case has both obstetric and pediatric negligence.

§ 24.2 Prenatal Care

Mrs. Mimar was seen on three occasions at the outpatient clinic of Barr Hospital. The first examination occurred on March 20, 1979. It was noted that Mrs. Mimar immigrated from Turkey with a student visa in September of 1978. Her husband was a student at a local university. The last menstrual period was noted to be July 27, 1978. At that time, her weight was 137½ pounds and the urine was negative. The blood pressure was 130/90 and the fundal height was 28. The fetal heart tones were 144, and she was considered to be 34 weeks gestation. She was prescribed prenatal vitamins, and told to return to the clinic in one month.

She was seen next on March 17, 1979. Her weight was 138½ pounds and her urine was negative. Her hemoglobin was 12.6 (normal) and her hematocrit was 37.7 (normal). Her blood pressure, at that time, was 120/80 and the fundal height was 34. The presentation of the fetus was vertex, and the fetal heart tones were 138. She was considered to be 38 weeks gestation and doing well. She was instructed to return to the clinic in one week.

At the next clinic visit on May 1, 1979, she weighed 139 pounds, and her urinalysis was negative. Her blood pressure was 120/80 and the fundal height was 32. The presentation was vertex, and the fetal heart tones were recorded as 100. She was considered to be 40 weeks gestation. It was noted that she was doing well. Good fetal movement was noted. The physician's plan was to perform a 24-hour urinary estriol, and she was told to return to the clinic in one week.

It is noted that the urinary estriol was 20, and was reported at 3:50 p.m. on May 4, 1979. The average estriol excretion in a normal pregnancy at 40 weeks gestation is considered 34.49, with a standard deviation of 9.352,[1] which would render the test evidencing possible placental insufficiency. It should be noted, however, that the report was not in the medical record until the next day—two hours after delivery.

§ 24.3 Hospital Admission and Delivery

Mrs. Mimar was admitted at 8:00 a.m. on May 4, 1979, in labor to Barr Hospital. The onset of labor was approximately midnight, with contractions occuring every five to seven minutes. She was first examined at 8:15 a.m., and found to be 3 cm dilated, and had a blood pressure of 150/80. The fetal heart tones were 134, and the contractions were occuring every three minutes. Dr. Kamir was in to examine the patient, and he noted that the abdomen revealed a term vertex presentation with the fetal heart tones at 140 beats-per-minute. The head was in the left lower quadrant, and pelvic examination revealed the cervix 3 cm dilated, and the head -1 to -2 in station, with 50 percent effacement.

At 11:05 a.m., with contractions occurring every three to four minutes, an external fetal monitor was applied. The blood pressure at the time was 90/60, and the fetal heart tone baseline was 120 to 150. Dr. Kamir noted that the labor progressed normally until 11:00 a.m., when variable decelerations were noted with the fetal heart rate dropping to 50 beats-per-minute. At 11:45 a.m., a pelvic exam was done by Dr. Bostic, at which time the membranes were ruptured and an internal monitor was applied. Variable decelerations were noted. At 12:30 p.m., serial decelerations from 42 to 60 beats-per-minute were noted. A pelvic examination revealed thick meconium stained fluid, and fetal heart tones with severe decelerations were noted. The patient was pushing well with the fetus at -2 station.

The nursing note recorded at 12:40 p.m. disclosed that the dilatation was complete, and at the station at +1, and then at +2 (with contractions occurring every two minutes and the fetal heart having a 130 baseline with decelerations at 70, lasting for 10 seconds, with good recovery noted).

---

[1] Iffy, Leslie & Kaminitzky, Harold A., Principles and Practice of Obstetrics and Perinatology, vol. 2, 1787 (John Wiley & Sons, Inc., 1981).

At 1:05 p.m., the patient was transferred to the delivery room, and a saddle block was given by Dr. Bostic. The delivery took place at 1:23 p.m.—a 5 lb. 9½ oz. male was born. The child's Apgar score at one minute was 5, and at five minutes was 7. The presentation of the child was occiput vertex. It is noted that low forceps were used to deliver the infant over a midline episiotomy. It was again noted that at one and one-half hours prior to delivery, the membranes were artificially ruptured and meconium stained. The placenta was considered normal, but small. The cord was considered to be abnormal, since it was collapsed and twisted around the neck once. The anesthesia was spinal (saddle block). A sphincter muscle laceration and a left lateral vaginal-wall laceration were noted. The fetus was noted to be post-mature, approximately one to two weeks.

It should be noted that there was no pathology report on the placenta, just a notation as to it being small but normal appearing.

§ 24.4   Post-natal Care

The infant was held by both his parents in the delivery room and was not admitted to the nursery until 37 minutes of age (at 2 p.m.). This procedure was a violation of the standard of care because based upon the small for gestational age (SGA) status as well as the birth asphyxia the infant should have immediately been transferred to a special care nursery. The nursing assessment notes that he was SGA, and the pediatric resident, Dr. Denton, noted the infant was post-mature (42 weeks). Theo was not examined by his pediatrician, Dr. Donald, until the next morning. No special care, feeding, or tests were ordered despite his stressful birth (evidenced by meconium stained fluid, low Apgars, and SGA appearance).

Stressed, SGA, and post-mature infants are at risk for hypoglycemia. In addition, SGA infants are at risk for hypothermia because of reduced subcutaneous fat stores and are also at risk for the polycythemia/hyperviscosity syndrome. These infants should be (and should have been in 1979) admitted to a special care or transitional nursery for serial destrostix screening, observation for respiratory distress, early feedings, and hemoglobin/hematocrit assessment. Theo was allowed to breast-feed, and received only 15 cc's of glucose water in the first two days of life. This care gave him scant calories and fluids. See §§ **16.3** and **16.5** for a further discussion of hypoglycemia and hypothermia.

Hypothermia was first recorded on May 5, 1979, at 4:00 p.m. with a temperature of 35.8C (T=35.8C) and again throughout the day on May 6, 1979 (T=35.4C, T=35.6C, T=35.2C). Hypothermia leads to acidosis and consumption of glucose; if severe; it may result in cyanosis, persistent fetal circulation (PFC), and hypoglycemia.[2] The care given Theo represents a failure by the nursing staff to deliver ordinary care, and contributed to the development of hypoglycemia, apnea, shock, and persistent fetal circulation.

Jaundice was noted at 7:30 a.m. on May 6, 1979, at 42 hours of age. Despite a markedly elevated bilirubin (Total=16.3, Direct=4.1), it was not treated or further investigated. An elevated bilirubin of 16.8T/4.7D was obtained several hours later, and phototherapy was still not instituted. This represents a serious departure from the standard of care. The failure to appropriately diagnose and treat this child's elevated bilirubin contributed to his overall neurologic defects.

At the time that his jaundice was first noted on May 6, 1979, at 8:00 a.m., a complete CBC (complete blood count) was obtained which was markedly abnormal. The Hgb (Hemoglobin) was 26.6 gms, Hct (hematocrit)=80.9, WBC (white blood count)= 11,200 with polys=59, lymphs=21, bands=14, monos=4 and eos=2. NRBC (normal red blood cells)=3 and reticulocytes=5.1. This was a femoral venous sample. An elevated hemotocrit (greater than 65) requires partial exchange when symptoms occur. Actually, the infant's hemotocrit should have been measured shortly after birth, and prompt therapy given if polycythemia was documented. See § **16.4**.

According to the parents, Theo was noted to be breathing abnormally on May 5, 1979. They requested a doctor examine him, but there is no indication that this was done. Mrs. Mimar also reported that the infant was lethargic, and that he did not breast-feed well on May 5, 1979 in the p.m. No measures were taken to investigate this change in behavior, and no nurses or doctors notes were made until 7:30 a.m. on May 6, 1979. This failure to investigate on the part of the nursing staff represents a serious departure in the standard of care.

Apnea (temporary cessation of breathing) and lethargy are two of the classic symptoms of hypoglycemia. Apnea began on May 6, 1979, shortly after Theo was seen by Dr. Donald at 7:30 a.m. Shortly thereafter, Theo was again noted to be apneic, very cyanotic, lethargic, and to have a sluggish response to stimulation. Despite the fact that these conditions occurred only 15 minutes after Dr. Donald had examined him, the pediatric resident, Dr. Denton not Dr. Donald, responded. Dr. Donald never responded to the infant's increasing deterioration and at 2:00 p.m. on May 6, 1979, the doctor declined to transfer him to a facility with a more extensive neonatal intensive care unit.

At 8:30 a.m., on May 6, 1979, Dr. Denton ordered Theo transferred to the special care nursery in Barr Hospital, where 30 percent oxygen was adminis-

---

2 Klaus, M.H. & Fanaroff, M.B., Care of the High-Risk Neonate 94-108 (W.B. Saunders Co., 1979).

tered by hand. At 9:15 a.m., a lumbar puncture was performed, and the results revealed a cerebral spinal fluid glucose of 5 which is extremely low and indicates profound hypoglycemia. See § **16.3.**

The pediatric resident, Dr. Kenner, was immediately called. Dr. Kenner's progress note of 11:00 a.m. revealed that Theo was:

1. Hypothermic (T=95.4)
2. Dusky
3. Jaundiced
4. Having frequent apneic spells (stops breathing)
5. Having intermittent episodes of cardiac arrhythmia with a heart rate up to 260/min, which respond to gentle occular pressure; during these episodes, he was cyanotic and floppy
6. Laboratory results noted:
   a. Hgb 27.6 (abnormally high)
   b. Hematocrit 82.9 (abnormally high)
   c. Blood glucose 46; Ca 9.2 (normal)
   d. Electrolytes Na 136, K 8.5 (hemolyzed); C1 101, CO_2 14 (normal)
   e. Bilirubin 16.3 Total; 4.1 Direct (elevated)
   f. Capillary blood gases: (in 30% O_2) (abnormal)
      pH 7.18, pCO_2 41, pO_2 50, HCO_2 15
   g. Spinal Tap: Glucose 5 (extremely low)
      Lactate 12, Chloride 118,
      Protein 56, 0 cells

Based upon the above notations, recorded by Dr. Kenner, we know that the treating doctors failed to appreciate the significance of cerebral spinal fluid (CSF) glucose of 5. This failure to diagnose and treat this infant's profound hypoglycemia constitutes a serious violation of the standard of care.

At 2:45 p.m., the nurse notified the nursing office of the deteriorating condition of the infant. This should have alerted the medical personnel that this infant was experiencing problems and should have warranted further investigation.

By 7:00 p.m., the child turned blue and cardiac massage and artificial ventilation had to be instituted. At this point, the nurse finally notified the nursing supervisor. By 7:30 p.m., the child was placed on a respirator. The ongoing hypoglycemia was the most likely cause of this infant's cardiac and respiratory difficulties.

At 7:50 p.m., on May 6, 1979, Dr. Donald was notified by the nurse that the newborn was to be transferred to Sheridan Hospital. There was no order from Dr. Donald nor any other physician for this transfer. It appears that the hospital personnel at Barr Hospital, independent of the treating doctor, decided to transfer the child to a high risk center. This implies that the nursing supervisor went over the pediatrician's head and asked that the infant be transferred. At 8:45 p.m., the newborn was transferred to Sheridan Hospital.

It appears that not one of the treating doctors diagnosed the hypoglycemia while the child remained at Barr Hospital. One physician correctly noted at 11:00 a.m. on May 6, 1979, that the child's blood glucose was 46 and the cerebral spinal fluid glucose was 5. Yet, no correlation was made. The hospital records at Barr Hospital include a report indicating that the cerebral spinal fluid glucose was only 5 mg per dl (milligram per deciliter). The normal range given by the hospital was 40-80. Thus, the doctors should have made the diagnosis of profound hypoglycemia. This information was apparently known to the physician prior to the child's transfer and duly noted in the progress notes; however, nothing was done to treat the hypoglycemia. No one performed a blood glucose test and this, additionally, constitutes a violation in the standard of care.

The failure of the physician at Barr Hospital to diagnose and disclose Theo's hypoglycemia led to a further delay in diagnosis once the child was admitted to Sheridan Hospital. In fact, approximately five hours lapsed after admission to Sheridan Hospital before the hypoglycemia was finally diagnosed and treated.

Further, no attempt was made at Barr Hospital to place an umbilical arterial catheter, obtain any arterial blood gases, or measure blood pressure in an infant with cyanosis, severe apnea, persistent fetal circulation, respiratory arrest, and a near cardiac arrest. This represents *substandard* care and contributed to his current neurological problems.

The significance of the CSF glucose of 5 mg (which is extremely low) was never appreciated at Barr Hospital, and specific corrective and maintenance glucose was not provided. Further, Theo's glucose was not monitored by blood glucose analysis. Hypoglycemia is an important cause of apnea and should have been seriously considered following a CSF glucose of 5 mg, which more closely reflects the glucose status of the CNS (central nervous system) than a blood glucose level. The blood specimen which revealed a normal glucose value of 46 was obtained several hours before the CSF glucose was obtained, and therefore, is not incompatible with a diagnosis of hypoglycemia at the time the lumbar puncture was done. Serial blood sugar values should have been obtained following the extremely low CSF glucose result. This was not performed, and, consequently, adequate glucose was not supplied. Theo suffered a prolonged period of severe, uncorrected hypoglycemia which was not correctly diagnosed until May 7, 1979, at 2:00 a.m. at Sheridan Hospital. Seizure activity was noted shortly after admission to Sheridan Hospital, and quite likely began at Barr Hospital at 2:30 p.m. on May 6th based on the nurses' notes (infant noted to have episodes of crying as if in pain and then apnea).

The discharge diagnosis at Barr Hospital included hypoglycemia; yet the diagnosis, management, and surveillance of that problem were inadequate and ineffective. Similarly, the listed diagnosis of polycythemia was not appropriately confirmed nor was early, aggressive therapy with partial exchange transfusion instituted. The infant had significant hyperbilirubinemia, with a marked direct bilirubin elevation; yet, this was not listed as a diagnosis, nor was it treated or investigated appropriately.

The combination of hypoglycemia, polycythemia, and hyperbilirubinemia all contributed to the neurological damage this infant sustained.

§ 24.5 Research

The normal serum glucose level in an infant at 24 to 40 hours of age is 56, with a range of 30-91 mg per dl (milligram per deciliter).[3] One problem with blood analysis for glucose is that it varies in accordance with the hematocrit value. In addition, neonatal red blood cells contain high concentrations of glycolytic intermediates such as reduced glutathione. This can erroneously reflect on the glucose value in the blood. Thus, whole blood obtained for analysis must be deproteinized with zinc hydroxide before analysis. Further, a large number of enzymatic and chemical methods are currently used for glucose determinations. Those that employ reducing methods may give falsely elevated glucose values since nonglucose reducing substances may range up to 60 mg per dl in newborn blood.

The need for a rapid, simple method of blood sugar determination has led to the development of dextrostix.[4] This is done by placing a drop of the infant's blood on the test strip for exactly one minute, and then washing it with a controlled stream of water. This will quickly give a fair indication of the infant's blood glucose levels. It has been suggested that at least two samples be sent to the lab for blood glucose determination to assure a better laboratory reflection of the infant's blood sugar.

According to the mother, the infant breast-fed well until about 6 p.m. on May 5, 1979. At this feeding, the infant would not nurse. The parents state that the infant was lethargic, and the husband persistently called for a nurse.

---

[3] Cornblath, M. & Schwartz, R., Disorders of Carbohydrate Metabolism in Infancy 218-26 (W.B. Saunders Co., 1976).

[4] Volpe, J., Neurology of the Newborn 311 (W.B. Saunders Co., 1981).

The parents state that they noticed the baby was breathing differently. The parents were aware that the infant did not appear normal. The parents requested that a doctor examine the baby, and were advised that a doctor would be called. A woman, who the parents thought was a doctor, came in with a stethoscope, listened to the infant's heart, and said that the baby was tired. Later, the parents learned that this person was, in fact, a nurse. The morning of May 6, 1979, the Mimars were advised that their baby had stopped breathing, and had been transferred to the intensive care nursery of Barr Hospital.

The feeding problem, lethargy, and abnormal respirations noted by the parents on the evening of May 5, 1979, were symptoms of hypoglycemia. If untrained observers were able to detect a change, why wasn't the medical and nursing staff more responsive, especially in light of the fact that Theo suffered perinatal stress and was an SGA infant, and thus particularly prone to hypoglycemia. The failure of the nursing and medical staff to recognize the symptoms of hypoglycemia constituted a violation of the standard of care.

Evidence that neuronal glucose deprivation damages nerve cells is often difficult to prove since hypoxia, acidosis, and other underlying problems often coexist with severe hypoglycemia.[5]

Untreated hypoglycemia may result in severe neurologic deficit or death. When convulsions occur due to hypoglycemia, there is an increase in central nervous system damage. Research studies reveal that a greater number of hypoglycemic neonates have I.Q. scores below 86 than do the controls, although the mean I.Q. scores were not significantly different. Thus, although treatment resulted in less severe damage, the studies have shown that infants exhibiting signs of symptomatic hypoglycemia should be treated very aggressively to prevent central nervous system damage.[6]

§ 24.6 Hypothermia

The occurrence of hypothermia secondary to hypoglycemia is frequently seen and is a useful clinical sign. Hypoglycemia also may be secondary to hypothermia. The normal core temperature of a neonate is from 36.5 degrees to 37.5 degrees centigrade. If body temperature falls, heat production is increased several times the basal level, resulting in a more rapid depletion of energy stores.

---

[5] *Id.*

[6] *Id.*

§ 24.7   Perinatal Asphyxia

Perinatal asphyxia and its sequelae constitute the most significant problem of
SGA infants. Uterine contractions may add an additional hypoxic stress on
the marginally functioning placenta.

The ensuing fetal hypoxia, acidosis, and cerebral depression may result in
fetal demise or neonatal asphyxia. With repeated episodes of fetal asphyxia or
persistent hypoxemia, myocardial glycogen reserves are depleted, further limiting the fetal cardiopulmonary adaptation to hypoxia. If inadequate resuscitation occurs at birth and Apgar scores are low, both intrapartum and
neonatal asphyxia place the infant in double jeopardy for a continuum of central nervous system insult. The sequelae of perinatal asphyxia include multiple organ system dysfunction (potentially characterized by ischemia–hypoxic
encephalopathy), ischemic congestive heart failure, persistent fetal circulation,
gastrointenstinal perforation, and acute tubular necrosis. Concomitant with
these sequelae, there may be metabolic derangements such as hypoglycemia
and hypocalcemia. Hypocalcemia is due, in part, to excessive phosphate release from damaged cells, acidosis, and its reaction with sodium bicarbonate
and diminished calcium intake. Meconium aspiration syndrome, if managed
inappropriately in the delivery room, may complicate the clinical picture and
further impair respiratory function and oxygenation with the development of
pneumonitis and pneumothorax.

§ 24.8   Hyperviscosity-Polycythemia Syndrome

The plasma volume of SGA infants immediately following birth averages 52
mg/kg (milligram per kilogram of body weight) as opposed to the normal of
42 mg/kg in appropriately grown infants. Once equilibrated at 12 hours of
life, the plasma volume becomes equivalent in the two groups. In addition to
an enhanced plasma space, the circulating red blood cell mass is expanded.
(This is probably a response to the intrauterine stress imposed upon the intrauterine growth retarded (IUGR) infant). Fetal hypoxia may induce red
blood cell production. Alternatively, a placental-fetal transfusion during labor
or periods of fetal asphyxia, may result in a shift of placental blood in the
fetus. Either way, the elevation of the hematocrit potentially increases blood
viscosity, which interferes with vital tissue perfusion (the thickened blood has
difficulty circulating through the very small blood channels). The altered viscosity adversely affects neonatal hemodynamics and results in abnormal cardiopulmonary and metabolic postnatal adaptation, producing hypoxia, and
hypoglycemia. In the event polycythemia is present (central hematocrit

greater than 65 percent) with such symptoms, appropriate therapy should be directed at correcting hypoxia and hypoglycemia, while a partial exchange transfusion to reduce blood viscosity and improve tissue perfusion should be considered. See § 16.4.

§ 24.9   Neutral Thermal Environment

The idealized setting of an optimum thermal environment is called a *neutral thermal environment* and is one in which a baby can maintain a normal body temperature while producing only the minimum amount of heat generated from basal life-sustaining metabolic processes. Maintenance of neutral thermal condition is considered to be of greatest importance in the youngest, most immature infants, whose ability to generate additional heat in a heat-losing environment may be minimal. The ability to increase metabolic rate in these infants may be further hampered by impaired gas exchange in the lungs and/ or restriction of caloric intake.

Prevention of heat loss is often best achieved by simple methods applied with knowledge born from common sense. Since heat loss requires the presence of a thermal gradient, it is important to avoid exposing the baby to a cold environment by either warming the environment or covering the baby.

In utero, a fetus is warmer than the mother. Born wet, warm, and naked into the usual environment of a delivery room, the newborn infant loses heat rapidly. In the delivery room, a large proportion of heat loss is caused by evaporation. Therefore, the skin should be dried by warm towels and evaporative losses severely limited by using plastic bags or other swaddling materials to insulate the skin from the dry room air.

The resuscitation of a newborn should not be allowed to interfere with thermal protection. If, during resuscitation, access is needed to some body surface, then only the body surface and no other should be exposed.

It is reasonable to back up the protection of swaddling by using a radiant heater to add extra warmth. Radiant heaters, when combined with swaddling offer a superb method of protection.

§ 24.10   Temperature Regulation

Following the birth of an infant complicated by uteroplacental insufficiency, the SGA neonate's initial body temperature may actually be elevated. When placental function fails, its heat-eliminating capacity also becomes deficient, resulting in fetal *hyperthermia*. On exposure to the cold environment of the delivery room, SGA infants can increase their heat production (oxygen consumption) appropriately, since brown adipose tissue stores are not necessarily depleted during IUGR. However, their core temperature drops if the cold stress continues, implying that heat loss has exceeded heat production.

Heat loss in these infants is due in part to the large body area exposed to cold, and the deficiency of an insulating layer of subcutaneous adipose tissue stores. The *SGA* infant, therefore, has a narrower neutral thermal environment than full term infants, but a broader one than the premature infant. In SGA infants, hypoglycemia (and/or hypoxia) interferes with heat production and may contribute to the thermal instability of these infants. In all infants, particularly the SGA infant, a neutral thermal environment should be sought to prevent excessive heat loss, and to promote appropriate postnatal weight gain.

As a result, babies are homotherms who attempt to maintain their body temperatures within some narrow range. They respond to heat loss by generating more heat. By attempting to generate more heat the infant uses up its already scarce supply of glucose.

Central nervous system damage, sedation, shock, hypoxia, and drugs may all reduce the metabolic response to cold. This may occur or represent a direct antimetabolic effect, or be due to a blunting of the sensory mechanisms that alert the baby to the stress stimuli. After prolonged stress, depletion of hormonal and energy stores may reduce the ability to further respond.

§ 24.11   Hyperbilirubinemia

It is well recognized that unconjugated bilirubin has the capability of entering the brain cells under certain circumstances, and will cause the death of those cells (kernicterus). This is the reason for the urgency in carefully observing every jaundiced newborn, and in treating neonatal jaundice.

The pathophysiology of kernicterus is, basically, that staining and necrosis of neurons results in bilirubin encephalopathy. The areas of the brain most commonly affected are the basal ganglia, hippocampal cortex, and subthalamic nuclei.

Behrman's Neonatal Perinatal Medicine,[7] states that survivors of neonatal manifestations of bilirubin encephalopathy often demonstrate choreoathetoid cerebral palsy, high-frequency deafness, and less often, mental retardation.

---

[7] Behrmans Neonatal-Perinatal Medicine, edited by Avory A. Fanaroff & Richard J. Martin, 3d ed., 409 (The C.V. Mosby Co., 1983).

Theo Mimar has been diagnosed as having choreoathetoid cerebral palsy and mental retardation.

Behrman also states that certain sequelae (one of which is chocrioathetoid cerebral palsy) are specific for kernicterus. Also, both clinical and laboratory studies[8] have indicated that certain neonatal risk factors which produce brain damage (i.e., hypoxia) also increase the likelihood that kernicterus will develop in the presence of mild to moderate hyperbilirubinemia. Leading among these factors is hypoxia. The relationship between brain hypoxia and kernicterus is so close that some investigators have suggested that kernicterus will not develop in the absence of some degree of central nervous system hypoxia. This relationship may be particularly valid for those clinical situations in which kernicterus develops at relatively low serum bilirubin concentrations (5 to 15 mg/100 ml).

In the pathogenesis of kernicterus, unconjugated bilirubin moves from the plasma pool into the neuron. This movement results either from (1) a reduction in the quantity or quality of binding of bilirubin by the circulating albumin, or (2) a major alteration in a membrane function of the brain cell that normally excludes bilirubin from entry (the so-called, *blood-brain barrier*).

The management of hyperbilirubinemia should be undertaken in infants who become icteric during the first 24 hours of life, or whose bilirubin concentrations exceed 12mg/100 ml thereafter. Skin color cannot be relied on for estimation of serum bilirubin concentrations, and it is essential that serum bilirubin determinations be performed (on every infant at the time jaundice is first observed). In most infants, a repeat determination in four to eight hours will be necessary the first day jaundice is noted, and at least daily thereafter until a clear pattern or decline is observed.

> The method of management chosen for an individual infant will, in part, determine the serum bilirubin concentrations at which therapy is to be instituted. It is essential, therefore, that every newborn nursery and neonatal intensive care unit have established policy regarding the methods to be used and criteria for initiation of therapy.[9]

Serum bilirubin and hematocrit levels should be monitored every four to eight hours in babies with hemolytic disease, and those with bilirubin levels in the range considered *toxic* for the individual infant. Older infants may be monitored every 12-24 hours.

---

8 Volpe, J., Neurology of the Newborn 351 (W.B. Saunders Co., 1981).

9 Behrmans Neonatal-Perinatal Medicine, edited by Avory A. Fanaroff & Richard J. Martin, 3d ed., 409 (The C.V. Mosby Co., 1983).

"Kernicterus is never present at birth and must be regarded as a largely *preventable* disease. Evidence of encelphalopathy in affected infants rarely occurs before 36 hours of age; its appearance in newborn hemolytic disease is most common between the second and sixth day of age."[10]

Frequent monitoring of the serum bilirubin level is essential to prevent the brain damage. Phototherapy (placing a naked baby under fluorescent lights which lowers the serum bilirubin levels slowly over a period of days) or exchange transfusion (immediately lowers the serum bilirubin level) are the preferred methods of treatment.

§ 24.12   Post-Discharge Course

It is highly unlikely that Theo will ever function with any degree of independence, and will require total care for the rest of his life. His life span should not be shortened due to his neurological problems, providing he receives appropriate care.

Theo has had the following problems:

1.   Intrauterine growth retardation
2.   Fetal distress during labor
3.   Postmaturity
4.   Meconium aspiration pneumonia
5.   Neonatal seizures due to hypoglycemia
6.   Respiratory arrest
7.   Symptomatic hypoglycemia
8.   Hyperbilirubinemia requiring phototherapy
9.   Severe recurrent apnea
10.   Neonatal asphyxia
11.   Transient persistent fetal circulation
12.   Symptomatic polycythemia
13.   Thrombocytopenia
14.   Developmental delay
15.   Seizure disorder
16.   Optic atrophy
17.   Spastic quadriparesis with athetoid features
18.   Possible kernicterus due to neonatal hyperbilirubinemia

---

[10] *Id.* (emphasis added).

This case review represents the necessity for very close inspection of the hospital records. The significance of the cerebral spinal fluid glucose alerts the viewer of the presence of untreated hypoglycemia. Oftentimes, it is necessary for the attorney to ask himself—What could have caused this problem? And, maybe more important—Could the physician have become aware of the problem? Should the physician have become aware of the situation? Obviously, if the physician should and could have identified the problem and yet failed to do so, the attorney has a viable cause of action.

CHAPTER 25

CASE REVIEW: PREECLAMPSIA

§ 25.1   Medical Issues

The medical issues in this case involve:

1. Hypertension
2. Preeclampsia

The first area of negligence relates to the doctors' failure to adequately define and treat Gail Morris's preeclampsia during the prenatal period. There was some degree of preexisting hypertension prior to the pregnancy in question. There was an increase in Gail Morris's blood pressure noted in November of 1979, prior to this pregnancy. At that time her pressure was 136/82, which is by definition within the upper range of normal and is known to present some degree of risk in case of pregnancy. Also, at the time of her first prenatal visit on June 11, 1980, Gail Morris's blood pressure was 132/80 which again shows a tendency to develop gestational hypertension.

Any evaluation of 30 mm or more in the systolic and 15 mm or more in the diastolic pressure is considered abnormal in pregnancy regardless of the absolute levels observed. Levels in excess of 140 systolic and/or 90 diastolic are considered hypertensive levels in pregnant women. It is recognized that such blood pressure levels in females of the reproductive age are much too high to constitute meaningful criteria for detecting significant diseases. Pressures in excess of 125/75 prior to 32 weeks of gestation are associated with significant increased fetal risk, as are levels over 125/85 at term.

The second area of negligence relates to the time when Gail Morris was hospitalized, by Dr.Nichols, at St. Michaels Hospital on February 11, 1981. The admitting diagnosis was severe preeclampsia. Dr. Nichols failed to provide fetal well-being studies and failed to meet the standard care for treating a patient with severe preeclampsia. By not terminating the pregnancy immediately upon hospital admission, Dr. Nichols permitted the pregnancy to continue, thus increasing the chances of fetal compromise due to the hazardous environment associated with severe preeclampsia.

§ 25.2 Prenatal Care

Mrs. Gail Morris was a 29 year old, five feet nine inches tall, 155½ pound, para 1-0-0-1 when first seen by Dr. Nichols on August 23, 1976. Dr. Norman, her family practitioner, had prescribed Diuril (a diuretic) for her on several occasions through 1974-1975, and her blood pressure on February 20, 1976, was 130/90. She was seen by Dr. Nichols on June 11, 1980, and reported that her last regular menstrual period had commenced on May 3rd. At that visit, the pelvic examination revealed the uterus to be four weeks in size. The pregnancy test was positive. Her weight was 173½ pounds, her blood pressure 132/80, and the calculated expected date of confinement was said to be February 10, 1981.

She was seen again on August 25, 1980, at which time her weight was 180½ pounds, and her blood pressure was 110/70. The fetal heart was heard with the Doptone instrument. She was seen again on September 30, 1980, at which time she weighed 188 pounds (representing a 7½ pound weight gain in approximately five weeks), and her blood pressure was 134/62 with the uterine fundus 19 cm. in height; there was no urine specimen at this visit. On October 13th, she weighed 191¾ pounds, but the blood pressure was not recorded. There were six subsequent antepartum visits, the last occuring on February 11, 1981. However, on January 9, the uterus was measured at 29 cm (it should have been at least 36 cm), and the vaginal examination revealed the cervix to be uneffaced and closed. She reportly refused an ultrasound examination, but the physician noted: "Patient informed that she may have an IUGR (Intrauterine Growth Retardation Syndrome)." Her last recorded weight was 221½ pounds (from the visit of February 6 until February 11, she had gained 12½ pounds in only five days). At the visit of February 6th, her blood pressure was 120/90 and her urine contained a trace of albumin. Her blood pressure on the visit of February 11th was 184/106 and 184/126 and, inexplicably, there was no urine specimen. The physician's note reads: "Will admit for preeclampsia." Thus, it is quite clear that as of February 11th, this patient was suffering from severe preeclampsia.

She was admitted to St. Michael Hospital at 11:45 p.m. on February 11, 1981. It appears that there was no complete physical examination done on admission to the hospital, but the admission blood pressure was 170/110. The admission orders included an order for Valium, 5 mg, four times daily. The nurse's notes for her admission state that her lower extremities were "somewhat edematous," and she was complaining of a "light headache." Her blood pressure, according to the nurses, was 180/110 and her weight was 220½ pounds, with the pulse of 80 and her urine 1+ for albumin. At 2 p.m., the blood pressure was said to be 150/70; and by 6 p.m. it was 170/96, with the fetal heart 144. At 8:30 p.m., she offered no complaints, however, her blood pressure was 166/100.

At 4:50 a.m. on February 12th, the day following admission, her blood pressure was said to be 160/90.

At 4:50 p.m. on February 13th, the blood pressure was 178/110 and the fetal heart 144. At 9 a.m., the blood pressure was 160/90 or 154/104, and the fetal heart 140. It appears that at 11 a.m., a consent was signed for cesarean section. There appears to have been no urinalysis carried out on February 13th. At 2 p.m., the blood pressure was 150/90, or 140/90 and the fetal heart 148. At 4:50 p.m., the blood pressure was 178/110 and 200/130, with the fetal heart 132. Despite the fact that the consent had been signed at 11 a.m. and the decision for caeserean section had been crystalized at 4:50 p.m., the patient was not taken to the operating room until 8:45 p.m.—representing a considerable and unnecessary delay in definitive treatment for this deteriorating, obstetrical situation. This constitutes a violation in the standard of care.

§ 25.3   Pathophysiology of Preeclampsia

Nearly one-half liter of blood per minute must be delivered to the placenta at term. It is clear that any mechanism which alters the utero-placental blood flow will drastically inhibit, or compromise, the amount of blood passing through the placenta per minute. Vasospasm (constriction) will definitely impede the blood flow.

The vascular phenomenon associated with the changes in the placenta in pregnancy complicated by hypertension and preeclampsia show a high incidence of placental infarcts due to thrombosis in the uteroplacental arteries; and thus, there is an increased incidence of abruptio placentas, and a signifi-

cant increase in the fetal morbidity and mortality associated with any hypertensive pregnancy (no matter what the cause).

Preeclampsia is a hypertensive disorder of pregnancy which is associated
with proteinuria, edema, and, at times, a coagulation abnormality. It usually
occurs primarily in women carrying their first pregnancy. Preeclampsia usually appears after the 20th week of gestation and, most commonly, near term.
Gail Morris was carrying her third pregnancy and had no problems with
preeclampsia during her first pregnancy. This is an indication that the
problems Gail experienced with her third pregnancy were probably a combination of a preexisting hypertensive state, which was then compounded by the
preeclampsia. Because preeclampsia can progress rapidly to a convulsive
phase (termed eclampsia), it is still a major cause of fetal and maternal death
today.

Choriodecidual (placenta) blood flow is reduced up to 60 percent when
pregnancy is complicated by maternal hypertension. The reduction in choriodecidual blood flow is related directly to the clinical severity of the maternal
hypertension. In other words, the higher the maternal blood pressure, the
greater the reduction in utero-placental blood flow. See **Chapter 14**.

There is a natural tendency toward placental inadequacy in the latter weeks
of pregnancy, and this placental inadequacy is aggravated by hypertension,
preeclampsia, and prolonged pregnancy. Therefore, the defendant doctors
were negligent in allowing this pregnancy to continue post-term, since the doctors were aware of Mrs. Morris's problems: (1) previous hypertension in the
nonpregnant state, (2) suspicion of intrauterine growth retardation, and
(3) clinical signs of preeclampsia.

One of the major avenues of criticism in this case is the doctors' failure to
take measures to prevent the onset of severe preeclampsia. The standard of
care dictates that when there is an early indication of possible mild preeclampsia (as evidenced by either a slight elevation of blood pressure, protein in the
urine, or preexisting hypertensive disease), the pregnant patient should be advised as early as possible in the pregnancy to adhere to a strict regiment of a
few hours of bed rest daily (lying on her side), and to increase the proportion
of protein in her diet.

Along with the bed rest and increase of protein in the diet, the patient (in
whom preeclampsia is suspected) should also be seen for frequent office visits.
It is well understood that preeclampsia is a progressive disease which, at
times, can become explosive. Initially, most patients with this disease have
very mild signs and symptoms. Therefore, it is of utmost importance to realize that once the disease is detected, even in its mildest form, the patient is to
be observed at very frequent intervals to detect even the slightest change in her
condition. Once the disease progresses from a mild preeclampsia to severe
preeclampsia, the mortality rate for the mother and the fetus increases at least
threefold.

§ 25.4 Pathophysiology of Fetal Hypoxia and Its Relation to Preeclampsia

Severe toxemia or preeclampsia is known to be a significant indicator of possible fetal asphyxia at birth. Severe preeclampsia has also been shown to cause hypoxic and/or ischemic episodes during the intrauterine environment.

Louis Gluck was one of the pioneering doctors doing research in developing antepartum testing to determine fetal lung maturity. Gluck was instrumental in developing the use of the L/S ration for determining fetal lung maturity. In his studies, Gluck has shown that fetal lung maturity is accelerated in cases of perinatal stress such as severe preeclampsia. Gluck has further concluded that fetal lung maturity is usually reached by 35 weeks gestation; however, in cases which are compromised by severe preeclampsia, fetal lung maturity has been found to be accelerated as early as 32 to 33 weeks.[1]

One might contend that since the doctors were uncertain about the expected date of confinement, they were hesitant to induce labor for fear of fetal lungs not being mature. However, the fetal lung is mature as early as 33 weeks' gestation in cases complicated by perinatal stress.

One main area of concern in this case would be to relate the central nervous system damage in the baby to the "relatively brief period of preeclampsia" in the mother. The literature overwhelmingly states that there is a significant reduction in placental blood flow for preeclampsia.

The brain of a *term* infant is well developed and has just undergone (as term approaches) an enormous increase in the relative volume of cortex and white matter. This volume increase is associated with the extension of neccessary brain connections. The increase in the volume of cortex and white matter causes an increased demand for cerebral blood flow to meet the increased metabolic activity of the cortex and white matter. This is the reason why reduced uteroplacental blood flow, as a result of the severe preeclampsia, may have caused serious injury to the infant, Anna Morris. The blood flow to Anna's cortex (her brain) and white matter may have been reduced, just as its needs were increasing.

The common denominator of hypoxic-ischemia injury is deprivation of the supply of oxygen to the central nervous system. Brain damage can occur by

---

[1] Intrauterine Asphyxia and the Developing Fetal Brain, edited by Louis Gluck, M.D., 293-307 (Year Book Medical Publishers, Inc., 1977).

either (1) *hypoxemia*—diminished amount of oxygen in the blood supply; or (2) *ischemia*—diminished amount of blood perfusing to the tissue.

Cerebral functions in the fetal brain fails when the brain is deprived of oxygen. This reduction in oxygen is detrimental due to the fetal brain having relatively low energy reserves and a relatively high metabolic rate.

The defendant doctors were negligent in failing to prevent the hazardous situation which developed when Gail's preeclampsia went both undetected and untreated in the last weeks of her pregnancy. Very careful observations must be made by the attending doctors in regard to the earliest possible signs and symptoms of preeclampsia. If preeclampsia can be detected at the earliest stages, the chances of preventing the hazards associated with severe preeclampsia often can be prevented.

> Whether or not one can prevent preeclampsia is a moot question. The incidence is declining, but no single factor or combination of factors can be shown to have been instrumental in this phenomenon. *Antepartum* care has been given most of the credit for alerting physicians to the earliest premonitory signs so that the disorder can be detected at its beginnings in the mild and more readily treatable forms. Thus, it can be credited with reducing the incidents of the severest forms of preeclampsia and eclampsia and thereby reducing the morbidity associated with them. . . .
>
> If one recalls that all the prodromal manifestations of preeclampsia are essentially silent insofar as the patient is concerned, one begins to appreciate how very important astute periodic observations by the physician are in detecting the disease process in its earliest phases. Regular examinations for the development of hypertension, proteinuria and weight gain and for the appearance of edema, are imperative.[2]

Therefore, when Gail Morris presented to Dr. Nichol's office on February 6th, 1981, she met all the criteria for preeclampsia, as evidenced by (1) elevated blood pressure of 120/90, (2) six pound weight gain, and (3) protein in the urine; immediate hospitalization was mandated.

On February 6, 1981, when Mrs. Morris had positive signs of preeclampsia, she was only four days before her expected due date of February 10, 1981. The closeness to the due date eliminated the risk of delivering a premature infant if the need to terminate this pregnancy arose due to an increase in the severity of the preeclampsia.

One must keep in mind that at this time (February 6, 1981), the defendant doctors were entertaining the possibility that the pregnancy was complicated by a possible intrauterine growth retardation. Thus, when Mrs. Morris

---

[2] J.P. Greenhill & E.A. Friedman, Biological Principles and Modern Practice of Obstetrics 406 (W.B. Saunders Co., 1974).

presented on February 6, 1981, with concrete signs of preeclampsia in addition to the intrauterine growth retardation, the *mandatory* course of action was immediate hospitalization with bedrest and immediate fetal well-being studies to evaluate the intrauterine growth retardation, and possible placental insufficiency as a result of preeclampsia. The accepted standard of care would dictate hospitalization, including:

Bedrest. Lowers blood pressure by increasing the perfusion of blood of the kidneys and relieves pressure on the vena cava. By lowering the maternal blood pressure, the utero-placental blood flow is improved due to the lessening of vasospasm

Fetal Well-Being Studies. Nonstress testing, oxytocin challenge testing, and fetal monitoring with earliest signs of labor.

Ultrasound and Amniocentesis. Ultrasound for placental localization, and amnioscentesis for L/S ratio to determine fetal lung maturity.

Observation of Mother and Fetus. Vital signs including blood pressure and fetal heart tones every four hours, frequent urinalysis for protein, 24-hour urine for total protein, frequent measurements of plasma creatinine, daily weight, and intake and output.

See **Chapter 14** for further discussion of care under these circumstances.

Medical textbooks assert that ambulatory treatment of preeclampsia has almost no place in modern obstetrics. It is axiomatic that any patient exhibiting symptoms of preeclampsia must be hospitalized and thoroughly evaluated, especially when the preeclampsia manifests itself close to term. It is, of course, universally accepted that the only cure for preeclampsia is termination of the pregnancy.

Ultrasound and amniocentesis for L/S ration (maturity of fetal lungs) become imperative when preeclampsia develops much earlier in the pregnancy—when there is a genuine risk of the fetus being so premature that it would not survive extrauterine life.

By the time Gail Morris was hospitalized on February 11, 1981, she was one day post-term. Based on Dr. Nichols's personal knowledge of this patient's past menstrual history, there was little question as to the accuracy of this patient's due date.

If Dr. Nichols had hospitalized Gail Morris earlier in the pregnancy when she first began to exhibit signs of preeclampsia, an ultrasound and amniocentesis could have been performed.

The severity of Gail's preeclampsia was such that termination of the pregnancy, as soon as possible, was the only choice. When preeclampsia becomes this severe, the risk of losing the mother and greatly interfering with the fetal blood supply is so great, that all obstetricians agree that the pregnancy must be terminated as quickly as possible. There is a direct relationship between the severity of the hypertension and the impairment of uteroplacental blood flow.

If, however, Gail had been hospitalized on February 6, 1981 and the aforementioned protocol carried out, there is every indication that Anna Morris would have avoided the hazards associated with intrauterine life, which was severely compromised by the subsequent severe preeclampsia.

The hospital records from St. Michael's Hospital indicate that Gail Morris was admitted on February 11, 1981, at approximately 12 noon. The admitting diagnosis was pregnancy with toxemia. The doctor's order sheet reveals that Dr. Nichols phoned-in the following orders:

1. Blood pressure and pulse every *six* hours (blood pressure, reflexes, and fetal heart tones should have been monitored every 30 minutes to one hour in a patient with such severe preeclampsia).

2. 1800 calorie diet (patient should have been kept NPO (nothing by mouth) or clear liquids only, due to the possibility of seizures developing and/or the necessity of a general anesthetic).

3. Valium 5 mgs qid (Phenobarbital is the drug of choice for preeclampsia; Valium is known to increase the incidence of hyperbilirubinemia in the newborn).

4. Heat-stable alkaline phosphatase daily (HSAP is one of the *least* effective ways to determine placental function, and most doctors feel it is *not useful at all*).

5. Urinalysis for albumin daily (urine should be checked for albumin frequently—a minimum of every four hours in order to detect a worsening of the condition: "[P]roteinuria varies greatly not only patient to patient, but in the same patient from hour to hour."[3] It should be noted that on February 13, 1981, from 1 a.m. until the cesarean section was performed at approximately 9 p.m., the nurse's notes reveal that the nurses failed to check the urine for protein at all on February 13, 1981. You will recall the doctor had ordered the urine tested for protein every day. However, it appears that the nurses failed to perform this test on February 13, 1981.)

6. BUN every second day (this seems to indicate that Dr. Nichols had no intention of an early termination of this pregnancy).

---

[3] J.A. Pritchard, M.D., & P.C. MacDonald, M.D., Williams Obstetrics, 16th ed., 680 (Appleton-Century-Crofts, 1980).

7. Bedrest with bathroom privileges (bedrest should have been ordered with the patient in the lateral position in order to improve the blood flow to the kidneys and lessen the pressure on the vena cava).

Gail Morris met the criteria for "severe preeclampsia" since she had repeated blood pressures of 170/110 and brisk reflexes. This severe preeclampsia was now imposed upon the defendant doctors' previous suspicion of intrauterine growth retardation, thus increasing the likelihood of fetal jeopardy. However, *no* tests were performed to ascertain the state of fetal well-being. It is well known that once a patient is diagnosed as preeclamptic, and *especially* when the preeclampsia becomes severe, that the intrauterine environment becomes very deleterious for the baby. Intrauterine demise in association with progressive placental insufficiency is a well known risk of severe preeclampsia. When severely elevated blood pressure is evident, the uteroplacental blood flow is severely impeded, thus causing hypoxic and/or ischemic injury in the fetus. It is well known that the fetus is particularly at risk close to term due to the brain's increased metabolic rate.

Dr. Nichols should have admitted Gail Morris directly to the labor and delivery area on February 11, 1981. Upon admission to the labor and delivery area, a fetal monitor should have been applied to establish fetal well-being. Also, if Mrs. Morris had been admitted to the labor and delivery area, the residents and nurses would have been more available to carefully monitor her (i.e., frequent blood pressure checks, frequent urinalysis for protein, and frequent observation of the fetal monitor pattern).

Usually, when a patient is admitted with severe preeclampsia the following regime is followed:

1. Admit to labor and delivery
2. Bedrest on left side
3. Frequent urinalysis for protein
4. Vital signs every 30 minutes
5. Intravenous fluids to establish correct hemodynamic balance
6. Administration of magnesium sulfate
7. Continuous fetal monitor
8. Intake and output—accurate measurement
9. Termination of pregnancy—either by a trial induction of labor or cesarean section
10. Baseline lab work to include clotting studies to ascertain whether or not any coagulopathy was developing
11. Insertion of a CVP line.

When Dr. Nichols hospitalized Mrs. Morris on February 11th, the admitting diagnosis was severe preeclampsia. It should be noted that Mrs. Morris was post-term. Therefore, every step should have been directed toward the immediate termination of the pregnancy. It is well known that any continuance of the pregnancy past this point only poses a greater threat upon the mother's life and fetal well-being.

In severe preeclampsia (as evidenced by the diastolic blood pressure of 110), the risk of cerebral hemorrhage or infarction in the mother is so great, that delivery of the baby must be carried out as soon as possible. Shortly after admission, the nurse's notes clearly state that Gail Morris's condition had somewhat stabilized and thus, she would have been a perfect candidate for either an immediate induction of labor or cesarean section.

In this case, tests to determine fetal lung maturity by means of an ultrasound for placental localization and an amniocentesis for L/S ratio were *not* warranted based on:

1. The severity of the mother's preeclampsia, as evidenced by the severe hypertension, necessitates the termination of the pregnancy no matter what the status of the fetal lung maturity. The risks of a cerebral infarction or hemorrhage in the mother is significant once the diastolic pressure reaches 115 to 120; and

2. When severe preeclampsia exists, the hypertension is known to interfere with the uteroplacental blood flow, thus creating an unfavorable intrauterine environment.

The only specific treatment of preeclampsia is termination of the pregnancy. Because the baby may be premature, however, the tendency is widespread to temporize in many of these cases in the hope that a few more weeks of intrauterine life will give the infant a better chance. Such a policy is justified in the milder cases. In severe preeclampsia, however, waiting may prove to be ill-advised, since the sequela of preeclampsia itself may kill the fetus and, even in the lower weight brackets, the likelihood of fetal survival may be better in a well operated neonatal intensive care unit than if left in the uterus.[4]

In addition to the above, bear in mind that at the time of admission on February 11, 1981, Dr. Nichols believed that the baby was possibly intrauterine retarded, which of course, further mandated fetal monitoring while preparations were made to deliver the patient as soon as possible (either by vaginal delivery or cesarean section). It is also known that hypertension and preec-

---

[4] *Id.* at 683.

lampsia cause the fetal lungs to mature early, so that even infants born at 34 to 35 weeks in a pregnancy complicated by hypertensive disease usually do not develop respiratory distress syndrome.

The next major area of deviation occurred when Dr. Nichols failed to prescribe magnesium sulfate (Mg SO_4), which is almost universally accepted as *the* drug of choice. It is used in *all* severe preeclamptics, especially, if not always, when brisk reflexes are present (usually thought to be a sign of central nervous system irritation in the mother).

The hospital record reveals that on February 13, 1981, the patient's condition and blood pressure were as follows:

Time per Record	Condition
12:20 a.m.	Complained of sinus congestion (in retrospect, this could have been a headache)
4:50 a.m.	Blood pressure—178/110 patient anxious

Comment.   Note the diastolic pressure of 110; yet it was five hours before the nurse checked her blood pressure again.

Time per Record	Condition
9 a.m.	Blood pressure—160/90, 154/104, no complaints
1:40 p.m.	Blood pressure + 150/90-140/90
4:50 p.m.	Dr. Williams in to do history and physical, blood pressure 178/110, 200/130, patient to have cesarean section at 1930 (7:30 p.m.) Dr. Nichols in

Time per Record	Condition
5:30 p.m.	Lying on left side quietly

Comment.   It is a violation of the standard of care for no blood pressure to have been taken after 4:50 p.m.. Anytime a blood pressure reaches this severe level (Gail's pressure was at 200/130), the patient deserves very careful observation and frequent, 15 minute to 30 minute, blood pressure checks.

Time per Record	Condition
7:50 p.m.	Blood pressure 150/110—198/124, pulse 96, fetal heart tones 148
8 p.m.	Foley inserted
8:45 p.m.	To labor and delivery per wheelchair

Comment. It appears that Gail was kept on the maternity floor (as evidenced by the transfer in a wheelchair) as opposed to being transferred to labor and delivery when the blood pressure recording of 200/130 was obtained. This is another gross deviation in the standard of care. Any patient with such severe preeclampsia must have constant monitoring of vital signs, including fetal heart tones, when a blood pressure reaches anywhere near 200/130. It is inconceivable that once the blood pressure of 200/130 was discovered, at 4:50 p.m. hours, that no one checked her blood pressure until three hours later, at which time it was severely elevated at 198/124. One of the common factors in fatal and nonfatal cerebral vascular accidents associated with pregnancy is hypertension. Physicians do not commonly use antihypertensive agents in patients with preeclampsia, but the clinician must be aware that when the diastolic pressure exceeds 110 mms, the patient is at an increased risk of a cerebral vascular accident and the pressure must be brought under control.[5]

Time per Record	Condition
8:50 p.m.	Received from floor postpartum per wheelchair
9:05 p.m.	To delivery per bed
9:10 p.m.	1000 cc's of IV solution started, left arm
9:25 p.m.	Spinal anesthesia
9:35 p.m.	Initial incision
9:38 p.m.	Viable female delivered

The delivery record states that no monitors were used. There is a discrepancy between the nurses' notes which state that the anesthesia was started at 9:25 p.m., while the delivery record states the anesthesia began at 9:05 p.m. This simply shows how inaccurate records can be.

The infant was delivered in a severely asphyxiated state with Apgars of 2 and 3. The baby's nursery records state that oxygen was given to the baby in the delivery room along with endotracheal intubation.

---

[5] E.J. Quilligan, M.D., & Norman Kretchmer, M.D., Ph.D., Fetal and Maternal Medicine 556 (John Wiley & Sons, Inc., 1980).

The nurses' newborn record discloses that upon admission to the nursery, the baby was cyanotic with some nasal flaring and rapid respirations. The infant went on to develop seizures approximately 12 hours after birth.

The infant has been diagnosed as having static hypoxia encephalopathy with seizure activity and profound mental retardation.

CASE REVIEW: PREMATURITY AND BREECH EXTRACTION

§ 26.1   Medical Issues

The medical issues in this case involve:

1. Prematurity
2. Total Breech Extraction
3. Entrapment of Fetal Head

Carol Zimmer was approximately 30 years of age at the time of the gestation under consideration. She had a previous pregnancy resulting in the birth of a 6 pound 4 ounce baby. Her last menstrual period occurred on March 12, 1975, and the expected date of confinement is variously stated in the records as December 19 or December 22, 1975. In actual fact, considering the intrinsic inaccuracies of Nagele's calculation of the expected date of confinement, a more appropriate estimation of the expected date of confinement would have been December 17, 1975. See § **9.7**.

The summary from United Hospital indicates that one week prior to her admission on October 6, 1975, leakage of amniotic fluid was noted and continued until the day of admission.

At the time of her admission at 8:45 a.m., on October 6, 1975, the patient had contractions five minutes apart. A vaginal examination was performed at 9 a.m. This revealed 3 cm cervical dilation with 80 percent effacement. The presenting breech was found at -3 station. The fetal heart rate was 140 beats per-minute and was found regular.

It was apparent that the breech presentation had been detected prior to admission. The in-patient records indicate clearly that at the time of the initial examination, there was an awareness of the breech presentation.

The discharge summary indicates that "labor progressed quite rapidly" following admission. Regretfully, there is no reference in the records to the time of complete cervical dilation. The patient was taken to the delivery room at 9:15 a.m. Thus, it is reasonable to assume that by that time, delivery was impending.

The records indicate that spinal anesthesia was administered at 9:25 a.m. Twenty-three minutes later, and only 33 minutes after the patient's transfer to the delivery room, a 2 pound 11 ounce baby was delivered by total breech extraction. The method of delivery (total breech extraction) is reiterated on at least three occasions in the obstetric records.

The baby was born with an Apgar score of 1 at one minute, and 5 at five minutes. It is stated in the summary that "difficulty was encountered in delivering the head as the cervix clamped down on it." This outcome is entirely predictable when the physician elects to deliver a premature fetus in breech presentation by total extraction.

The available records provided absolutely no explanation for the choice of the method of delivery. It has been established in the literature well before 1975 that the ideal method of breech delivery is what is usually called *assisted breech*. This approach allows spontaneous delivery of much of the body and calls for interference on the part of the obstetrician when the body is delivered up to the level of the umbilicus. In the absence of complications (such as fetal distress, prolapse of the cord, or arrest in the second stage of labor), there is absolutely no indication for total breech extraction procedure. In fact, generations of textbooks have emphasized the intrinsic dangers of this procedure, particularly severe in cases of premature birth, but contraindicated in cases of breech delivery under virtually all circumstances.[1]

A review of the hospital records provides no reference to any other complication with the exception of premature rupture of the membranes and premature labor. Since in the case of a multiparous woman a second stage of labor as long as 45 minutes is entirely within range of normal, there was no conceiv-

---

[1] J.C. Moir, Munro Kerr's Operative Obstetrics, 7th ed., 182 (Bailliere, Tindall & Cox Publishers, 1964); W.H. Pearse & D.N. Danforth, *Dystocia Due to Abnormal Fetal Pelvic Relations*, in Textbook of Obstetrics and Gynecology, edited by D.N. Danforth, 2d ed., 644 (Harper & Row Publishers, Inc., 1971); M.J. Eastman & L.M. Hellman, *Williams Obstetrics*, 12th ed., 423, 1162 (Appleton-Century-Croft Inc., 1961); J.P. Greenhill & E.A. Friedman, *Biological Principles and Modern Practice of Obstetrics*, 753 (W.B. Saunders Co., 1974).

able reason for terminating the labor by a "total breech extraction" only 33 minutes after what could possibly have been the earliest observation of full cervical dilatation. In fact, it has to be taken into account that even when examination indicates full cervical dilatation, the aftercoming head still may be captured by the contracting cervix. It is exactly for this reason that unwarranted interference is extremely dangerous in this clinical situation. It is largely for this reason that contemporary textbooks emphasized strongly that waiting patiently, until spontaneous delivery of most of the fetal body, is an extremely important aspect of the managment of premature breech presentation. See §§ **21.4** and **21.5**.

Following the delivery of a fetus with an Apgar score of 1, it could reasonably be anticipated that the process of labor and the technical details of delivery would be described in full detail. It was well understood in 1975 that a five minute Apgar score of 5, in the weight group of this baby carried an extremely high likelihood of cerebral palsy. Accordingly, full documentation of the case was warranted at the time of this birth, both for medical and possible legal reasons. It is entirely inexplicable, therefore, that even those details that are regularly recorded in virtually all hospitals of the United States, in cases of both normal and abnormal labors (lengths of first and second stages of labor, indications for operative intervention) remained unreported in the records of United Hospital.

Subsequent medical records note that eventually this child developed hypotonic cerebral palsy involving swallowing incoordination and mental retardation.

§ 26.2 Evaluation

The evaluation of this case has to take into account that the rate of permanent damage among babies delivered this much before term is relatively high. Based on a study that was conducted between 1958 and 1969 Lubchenco and her associates reported a neonatal mortality rate in the neighborhood of 50 percent for babies born with comparable gestation length and weight.[2] Studies conducted in the same center further indicated that the chances of survival much depended on the early Apgar scores; the overwhelming majority of those with a favorable Apgar score survived, whereas more than half of those with a low (less than 3) one-minute Apgar score perished. A comparable relationship emerged in the same study with regard to five-minute Apgar scores,

---

[2] Lubchenco, Searles, Brazie, et al., *Neonatal Mortality Rate: Relationship to Birth Weight and Gestational Age*, 81 J. of Pediatrics 814 (1972).

with scores of 6 or less carrying an unfavorable outlook. Based on studies conducted in the early 1970s, the same author concluded that among the babies born with a birth weight of less than 1500 grams, about two thirds survived with, or without, significant handicaps, and less than one third developed permanent handicaps.[3]

It appears, therefore, the Christian Zimmer, if delivered in optimum condition, would have had a favorable chance for reaching full mental and physical potential later in life. It has to be added that breech delivery of a premature baby is, and was in 1975, a significant complication; and difficulties in the process of delivery could have arisen even with the best obstetric management. However, under the conditions that prevailed before and during the labor of Ms. Zimmer, the probability of intrapartum complications was moderate. Insofar as the parturient had a favorable *breech score*, the election of total breech extraction under conditions that did not warrant such interference made the occurrence of severe intrapartum complications a near certainty.

Based on the above considerations, the following critical conclusions are applicable:

1. The records provide absolutely no explanation for the choice of total breech extraction in the course of the delivery of Christian Zimmer. The records indicate that the progress of labor was fast and provided a very favorable prognosis for spontaneous delivery of the body of the fetus. Whereas the length of the second stage was not stated, it is obvious that it was well-within the range of normal when extraction procedure was decided upon.

2. Whereas the reduction of the chances of healthy survival that the total breech extraction procedure entailed is difficult to quantitate, insofar as lasting fetal damage can occur as a result of gross prematurity itself, it is entirely fair to state that the chances of Christian Zimmer for a healthy life were reduced very substantially when, in the absence of acceptable indication, a difficult total breech extraction procedure was performed. Under these circumstances of his birth, Christian Zimmer had a less than equal chance to survive and, in case of survival, the likelihood of healthy development (both mental and physical) became slim.

---

[3] L.O. Lubchenco, G.A. McGuinness, A.L. Tomlinson, et al., *Aggressive Obstetric & Neonatal Management: Long Term Outcome*, in New Techniques and Concepts in Maternal and Fetal Medicine, edited by Leslie Iffy and Harold A Karninetzky, 123 (Van Nostrand Reinhold Co., 1979).

§ 26.3   Breech Delivery

There are several types of breech presentation. The Frank breech, or what is sometimes called the single breech, is when the infant's hips are flexed on the abdomen and the knees are extended so that the feet lie in front of the face or hand. This is present in approximately two-thirds of all deliveries of babies weighing more than 2500 grams. (Baby Zimmer was a Frank breech presentation). In a double or complete breech, the attitude is one of flexion. That is, both hips and knees are flexed with the feet present at the buttocks. This is similar to the attitude of sitting in an Indian position. Incomplete breech attitudes are of two types. One is a *single footing*, wherein one foot descends through the cervix ahead of the buttocks; or both feet, as in the *double footling position*. Footling breeches are more common in premature deliveries. See §§ 21.1 and 21.2.

Breech positions are common before the 32nd week, when the fetus can move freely within the uterus, because of the large volume of amniotic fluid. However, as pregnancy advances, fetal movement is restricted as relative space available is taken up more by the baby than by the amniotic fluid. Fetal motion plays an important part in decreasing the rate of breech presentation as the pregnancy advances.

Breech presentations are *nine* times more common at the 28th week of pregnancy than at term. Gross perinatal mortality is as high as 20-30 percent, but this can be reduced with good care. The most important cause of mortality associated with vaginal delivery of breeches include the following:

1. Anoxia resulting from delay in the delivery of the aftercoming head, and from prolapse cord, which occurs ten times more often than in normal vertex position (Baby Zimmer's head was caught by an incompletely dilated cervix).
2. Injuries, the most serious of which are those caused by intracranial hemorrhage and fractures of the spine with associated spinal cord injury. Also, there are problems with rupture of liver, spleen, and adrenal gland.
3. Complications of prematurity.
4. Developmental abnormalities.

The problem with breech deliveries is that the child's buttocks which are generally narrower than the fetal skull, descend first. Therefore, the cervix may dilate sufficiently for the buttocks and body to pass through the cervix, however, it is not sufficient for the aftercoming head. This results in additional time being necessary to allow for complete dilation of the cervix so that the fetal head can pass through the canal.

With a complete breech, or when both feet are flexed up towards the head (Frank breech), the legs provide an additional wedge in addition to the diameter to the body of the fetus to fully dilate the cervix and make room for the aftercoming head. However, this is not true with a single footling breech as the feet descent first and do not provide the additional wedge.

In managing a breech labor, the membranes should not be ruptured artificially because this may permit the cord to prolapse.

At delivery, the physician must be certain the cervix is completely dilated before attempting breech delivery. The buttocks, body, and even the shoulders can descend through a cervix that is not sufficiently dilated to permit the passage of the fetal head. This is particularly true with premature infants whose heads are larger than their shoulders.

There are three types of breech deliveries.

Spontaneous Breech Delivery. This is when the entire baby is allowed to deliver without manipulation by the attending physician. This most often occurs with very small premature infants with multipares with large pelvises and very rapid labor. This type of breech delivery is considered quite hazardous to the baby due to the precipitous type of delivery which causes increased pressures on the fetal head.

Partial Breech Extraction or Assisted Breech. This is the preferred type of delivery for any breech. The partial breech or assisted breech consists of a spontaneous controlled expulsion as far as the umbilicus, after which the doctor assists in the delivery of the shoulders and head. In this type of delivery, the physician watches until the buttocks descend toward the vaginal opening. When 8-10 cm of the presenting part is visible during a contraction, a large episiotomy is performed. Thereafter, the next few contractions will deliver the buttocks and abdomen through the vaginal opening, after which the rest of the body is supported by the physician and he then assists in the delivery of the shoulders and head. It is then that the application of the piper forceps should be used on the aftercoming fetal head in order to reduce the amount of pressure and traction exerted during the delivery. This is the preferred method of delivery.

It is important that the physician remember that downward traction is applied to the infant's pelvic girdle with the doctor's thumbs placed parallel over the sacrum. This affords the physician a bony prominence to hold onto as opposed to the risk of the physician exerting too much pressure on the soft tissue and organs of the abdomen. As the physician gradually pulls downward on the infant's body, he must be sure to keep the infant's back directly anterior until the axilla (armpit) comes into view and the scapula (the shoulder) emerges beneath the pubic arch. At this point, the physician assists with the delivery of the arm. After this, the body is then lifted upward and the posterior arm is delivered in the same manner. The head can then be delivered by manual manipulation alone. It can be brought through the inlet in a transverse or oblique diameter and then rotated to the anterior-posterior diameter of the lower pelvis and delivered over the perineum by flexion. As mentioned above, the use of piper forceps is thought to alleviate some of the trauma to the infant's head.

The head must be delivered within eight minutes after the umbilicus appears in order to prevent fetal anoxia. Maneuvers should be performed rapidly but deliberately avoiding undue haste as forceful traction at this stage may cause serious brain damage.

Complete or Total Breech Extraction.   Complete or total breech extraction is when the doctor manually extracts the entire infant from the birth canal. This is the most difficult and potentially traumatic of all obstetric operations, even when performed by experts, and often results in unacceptably high death and morbidity rates.

Complete or total breech extraction is divided into four maneuvers: (1) delivery of the breech and legs, (2) delivery to the shoulder, (3) engaging the shoulder girdle, and (4) delivery of the head.

The first step is effected by introducing the entire hand into the vagina and grasping both ankles and drawing them through the vaginal opening. Downward traction is then applied, and as the legs emerge, they are grasped higher and higher, and when the breech appears at the vulva, upward traction is made until delivery is effected.

One problem with breech deliveries, especially in the premature, is that the cervix may not be completely dilated at the time the rest of the body has descended through the cervical opening. Sometimes, an additional centimeter of dilatation is necessary to effectuate delivery of the head.

It is understood that once the umbilicus is delivered, the head must be extracted within eight minutes in order to prevent fetal anoxia. Therefore, an incompletely dilated cervix, or a cervix that is starting to clamp down on the baby's head because of contractions, may impede delivery of the head. If undue traction is then required to deliver the child, cerebral trauma may ensue from having to force the fetal head through too narrow an opening of the cervix.

The pediatric records show evidence that the "total breech extraction" was indeed traumatic to the infant, Christian Zimmer. The infant's arm was fractured in two locations, as well as both hands and feet being bruised and swollen. The nursery notes clearly describe these abnormalities, as well as x-ray evidence of the fractures. Clearly *only* a very experienced obstetrician should attempt to decompose (manually extract) a breech. Since there were two fractures of this baby's arm, as well as bruising of both hands and feet, there is evidence of excessive force.

Many hospitals require that two obstetricians be present to manage a vaginal breech delivery.

The brain damage suffered by Christian Zimmer is probably a result of a combination of hypoxia and trauma. In his book *Birth and Brain Damage*, Courville discusses both:

> We should recognize, in the first place, that true physical injuries of the brain are traumatic or mechanical effects of *exceptional* stress. The injuries that occur as a consequence of birth, however, differ from most traumatic lesions of the adult brain, which usually occur as a consequence of a sudden and severe violence. *Birth trauma*, on the other hand, results from an exaggeration of normal physiological stresses, which slowly increase to a degree so excessive as to result in brain damage. This damage may be due, of course, to certain structural abnormalities of the fetus, the uterus, or the birth passage, even though the force involved is normal. Traumatic effects may result also from traction on the fetus, such as excessive pull of the body against the head not yet delivered from the birth canal. [This appears to be the case of Christian Zimmer.] This traction often causes pressure on the medulla or damage to the spinal cord [from undue manipulation of the body of the infant while the head is in a fixed position], which results in itself in the production of an anoxic state.[4]

The child's birth history points out two distinct causes for brain damage:

1. The history of the baby's head trapped by the cervix, would account for the hypoxic brain damage due to compression of the umbilical cord by the cervix, and possibly premature separaton of the placenta (known to occur in breech deliveries).

2. Too much force used by the doctors in an attempt to hurry the delivery along and then, an undue amount of traction may possibly have been used in an attempt to free the entrapped head (This could account for the traumatic injury to Christian's brain).

The two fractures of this baby's left arm and subsequent ecchymosis of the hand, wrist, and feet point towards excessive force being used along with possible undue haste.

---

[4] Emphasis added. Cyril Courville, Birth and Brain Damage 23 (Margaret Farnsworth Courville, 1976).

When assisting in the delivery of an extended arm, *malrotation* may dislocate the shoulder or fracture the humerus. This seems to infer that the fracture of the humerus can be related to a malrotation or an incorrect maneuver being used by the physician.

Another area of concern with regard to the managment of this case from an obstetric point of view is in regard to the lack of close fetal monitoring at the time of labor and delivery. Fetal heart tones should be recorded regularly, preferably by an electronic fetal heart monitor, since occult or complete prolapse of the umbilical cord occur frequently in preterm breech deliveries. Also, if the fetal head is trapped by the cervix or lower uterine segment, the baby will suffer from anoxia due to cord compression between the fetal head and pelvic brim. Thus, continuous electronic fetal heart monitoring should take place right up until the time the baby is delivered. If no electronic fetal monitor was available at United Hospital in 1975, then the delivery room nurse should have used a doptone to continuously monitor the fetal heart tones for the 25 minutes the mother was on the delivery table.

The mismanagement of this preterm breech gestation seems to exemplify the problems commonly associated with the management of breech presentations.

CHAPTER 27

CASE REVIEW: HYPERTENSION, INTRAUTERINE GROWTH RETARDATION, AND DRUG ABUSE IN PREGNANCY

§ 27.1   Medical Issues

The medical issues in this case involve:

1. Hypertension
2. IUGR/SGA
3. Hypoglycemia
4. Hypothermia
5. Marijuana use in Pregnancy

Christina Sweet was born at Berman Hospital, on January 7, 1980 at 7:24 a.m. She was born to a gravida II, para 0, 25-year-old, white female after a full term pregnancy. The mother's last menstrual period was dated April 2, 1979, and the calculated estimated date of confinement (EDC) was January 9, 1980. Her height was 5 feet 5 inches, and her usual weight was 135-145 pounds. The prenatal records indicate that her past medical history was complicated by an episode of pelvic inflammatory disease, and that she had had an intrauterine

419

device present. It was further noted several places in the record that she smoked marijuana approximately three times-per-week, and that she took Bendectin for nausea. The prenatal records indicate that when she was seen on June 1, 1979, her blood pressure was 110/70 and the fundus was approximately a six-week size. On December 3, 1979, it was noted that her blood pressure had increased to 140/90 and that her weight was 147 lbs. A notation was made that the fetus was "small for EDC."

The admission note of January 7, 1980 reveals she was admitted to Berman Hospital. The history states that she complained of severe headaches for three months, and the she had had edema of the hands and face for three months. Her weight on January 7, 1980, was 170 lbs. There is no indication in the records that any stress testing was done to determine the integrity of the fetoplacental unit. The records state the Mrs. Sweet remarked that she had actually lost several pounds in the last month of pregnancy.

The obstetrical log book notes that on January 6, 1979 at 11:45 p.m., Mrs. Sweet was seen and examined. She was found to be fingertip dilated and to be having contractions every five minutes. The fetal heart tones were 140, the membranes were intact, the station was -3 and her blood pressure was 120/80. The log book notes that she was sent "home with instructions."

The records indicate that Linda Sweet was re-admitted at 2:15 a.m. on January 7, 1979. She was admitted in early spontaneous labor. Her initial examination showed her to be 1 cm dilated, 100 percent effaced, 0 station, membranes intact, and contractions every two minutes. After six hours of labor, she was found to be completely dilated. Her blood pressure was 140/90 at that time. The membranes were ruptured shortly before delivery, and thick meconium fluid was noted to be present. The fetal monitor was applied at 5:15 a.m. on January 7, 1979, when she was 2 cm dilated and at 0 station. There were several decelerations noted, as well as what appeared to be hypertonic uterine contractions on the terminal portion of the monitor tracing. Fetal heart rate decelerations and hypertonic uterine contractions are potentially detrimental to the fetus, especially a fetus that is marginally oxygenated and has experienced chronic intrauterine stress. See **Chapter 16**.

The labor record indicates that local anesthesia was used for delivery, and that Demerol had been given for analgesia during labor. It should be noted that Mrs. Sweet's blood pressure was 180/110 at 7:20 a.m.; 160/70 at 7:25 a.m.; and 150/80 at 7:40 a.m.

The records do not indicate whether a pediatrician was present at the delivery. The infant was somewhat depressed at birth with an Apgar score of 5 at one minute, and 7 at five minutes. The infant was noted to be meconium stained with a meconium stained cord. The placenta was also meconium stained on the fetal surfaces. The infant's weight was 4 pounds 11 ounces, her length was 18 inches, her head circumference was 13 inches, and her chest circumference was 10½ inches. She was described as being skinny, meconium stained, and she appeared intrauterine growth retarded. The records also note that after removing meconium stained mucus, the infant cried, and the color was fine. The records do not indicate that the vocal cords were visualized, or that deep tracheal suctioning was performed to free the airway of meconium. This represents a departure from the recommended approach and the standard care for infants with thick meconium at birth. In view of the subsequent diagnosis of meconium aspiration, pneumonia, and persistent fetal circulation, the failure to properly clear the airway is direct contributing factor to the infant's subsequent neurological damage.

The nursing records indicate that the infant was admitted to the special care nursery at 7:55 a.m., 31 minutes after birth. She was hypothermic at the time with a temperature of 94.3 F. At 7:55 a.m., Dr. Goodwin was paged, and at 8:15 a.m., he examined the infant. At 8:15 the infant had a dextrostick, which was 0 (indicating hypoglycemia). Attempts were made to start a scalp intravenous (IV) from 8:45-9:25 a.m. At 9:25 the IV was finally started. This represents a one hour and ten minute delay in delivering glucose to an infant whose dextrostick was 0. A blood glucose was obtained which was 10 (profound hypoglycemia). An intravenous with 10 percent dextrose was started, and 9 cc's of 25 percent dextrose in water was administered. In addition, Plasmanate was given. The infant's initial vital signs were pulse 120, respirations, 53, and blood pressure 36 (which is presumably a mean blood pressure, it is somewhat low). The nurse's notes indicate that the dextrostick was still 0 at 9:10 a.m., but that no tremors were present. The nurse's notes on admission mention that the baby was cold to touch and dusky. Her temperature was recorded at 94° F. She was placed under an oxyhood. She was noted to have irregular respirations on admission but no grunting or retracting. Her muscle tone was poor and her cry was only fair when stimulated. Initially, she was placed in 30 percent oxygen.

The prolonged attempts to start a peripheral IV for glucose administration in the face of a lethargic, limp, hypoglycemic infant, represents a departure from the acceptable standards of care. Hypoglycemia is an emergency situation in the newborn, and the easy access of the umbilical vessels make that the preferred route for the initial administration of glucose. This infant sustained hypothermia which compromised her already reduced glycogen stores and consumed an already diminished supply of glucose. The apparent absence of a pediatrician at the delivery of a known growth retarded infant with meconium staining, represents a departure from standard care and resulted in an additional insult to the infant. See §§ 16.1 through 16.3.

Following the initiation of intravenous glucose, her dextrosticks were fairly well-stabilized. The chest x-ray demonstrated marked pulmonary parenchymal changes consistent with aspiration pneumonia. Her physical examination revealed a liver that was 3 cm below the right costal margin. There was no murmur present. Despite several doses of Lasix, the infant had minimal urinary output. Although a diagnosis of congestive heart failure was made, this was apparently not due to a fluid overload situation, but rather to a combination of hypoxic myocardial injury and myocardial glycogen depletion secondary to hypoglycemia. Over the next several days as the hypoxia and hypoglycemia were corrected, the infant's heart returned to normal.

The nurse's notes at 9 a.m. on January 7, 1980, indicate that her blood pressure was 36/? (there's an arrow marked down which presumably means diastolic not registered). Her blood pressure had increased to 41/7 at 6 p.m. which is still somewhat borderline. Her hemoglobin was 16.6 gms on January 7th at Berman Hospital. She had several capillary blood gases done. Initially, the capillary blood gases indicated marked acidosis with a pH of 7.12, and a low capillary O_2 level.

The infant was then placed in 30 percent oxygen, and 4 milliequivalents of sodium bicarbonate were administered over several hours. These measures corrected the infant's pH level. However, the arterial blood gases were never done, notwithstanding the low oxygen level detected. Subsequently, blood gases were done at Charity Hospital which indicated that the infant was able to be normally oxygenated with 100 percent oxygen but was hypoxemic in 25 percent. It is likely that the infant sustained a prolonged period of relative hypoxia in the immediate neonatal period as a result of a inadequate assessment of her blood gases, and the inadequate delivery of the appropriate amount of oxygen.

The infant was seen in consulation by a pediatric cardiologist. The cardiologist felt that transfer to Charity Hospital was indicated. An EKG showed right ventricular hypertrophy and an echocardiogram showed the presence of all valves and chambers. There was no specific mention of any right or left systolic time intervals or shortening fraction. As mentioned previously, the chest x-ray initially showed a right pleural effusion and infiltrates consistent with aspiration pneumonia.

The infant was transferred to Charity Hospital in an oxyhood with 25 percent oxygen without apparent incident. Cardiac evaluation shortly after admission concluded that her low blood pressure was secondary to diminished cardiac output due to acidosis, hypoglycemia, and also hypoxic myocardial dysfunction. On the 9th of January, the chest x-ray showed that the heart size had decreased, and the right pleural effusion had reabsorbed. By discharge on January 14, 1980, the heart size was considerably smaller.

The remainder of the infant's course in the hospital was essentially unremarkable, and she was discharged at one week of age. Subsequently, she has been shown to have spastic diplegia and has delayed motor development. Her intelligence seems to be relatively preserved as is her skill level in social, language, and fine motor areas.

§ 27.2   Evaluation

Although the mother admitted to smoking marijuana two to three times-per-week, this did not have a substantial contributing role in the infant's current problems. Since marijuana use is frequently combined with poly drug abuse, the role of other substances of addiction is unknown. Specifically, the mother denies taking other drugs or agents during the pregnancy. Smoking, per se, can have a role in intrauterine growth retardation (IUGR), but the number of cigarettes per day usually must exceed one pack for there to be any measurable impact on the developing fetus. The placenta was examined in this case and found to contain multiple areas of fibrin deposition, and to be small and infarcted. This (along with the small size of the infant, the loss of subcutaneous tissue, and the relative head sparing of the intrauterine growth retardation) suggests that the etiology was placental dysfunction, particularly during the third trimester. A relative degree of pregnancy induced hypertension was also present and contributory. See **Chapter 14.**

As a noticeably small for gestational age (SGA) infant with thick meconium present, it could be readily ascertained that she was at risk for certain problems. An aggressive anticipatory approach was indicated. Since SGA infants frequently have loss of subcutaneous tissue due to loss of subcutaneous fat, these infants are especially vulnerable to hypothermia. See § **16.5.** This must be anticipated and the infant immediately wiped off, wrapped up, and placed in a warm area. It is uncertain why it took 31 minutes to get the infant to the special care nursery, and why her temperature was 94.3F degrees on arrival. Certainly, one must question the nursing care in the delivery room. As an infant born through thick meconium, she was at risk from meconium aspiration and was particularly at risk since she had evidence of intrauterine stress as well as acute intrapartum stress. The appropriate approach would have been to visualize the vocal cords, and to aspirate the airway to prevent meconium aspiration pneumonia. This was not done, and the infant subsequently developed meconium aspiration pneumonia. As a result of the pneumonia, persistent fetal circulation developed.

The SGA infant is known to be at risk for hypoglycemia (see § **16.3**). Early care should include the provision of adequate calories and the close following of the blood glucose. The general care of the infant should be such that factors known to increase the risk of hypoglycemia are avoided. Christina remained hypoglycemic for nearly an hour while multiple attempts were made to start a peripheral IV. In view of the emergency that neonatal hypoglycemia represents, it was entirely justifiable to begin an intravenous infusion through the umbilical vein, and then continue to search for a peripheral site. The diminished cardiac output due to hypoxic cardiomyopathy, the possible *hypoglycemia*, was a contributory factor to the infant's hypotension. This hypotension, in turn, lead to diminished perfusion of the central nervous system, and contributed to the subsequent seizure activity. The failure to assess arterial blood gases and to provide adequate oxygen, likewise contributed to hypoxic ischemic injury to perhaps multiple organ systems.

Prenatal identification of the slow growing fetus leaves the obstetrician with few therapeutic options since it is not known whether a growth retarded baby is better off in utero for as long as possible, or should be delivered prematurely before fetal distress ensues. This does not mean that the obstetrician is without the ability to assess the pregnancy and recommend measures that will optimize uterine blood flow such as bed rest in the left lateral recumbent position, and reduced activity. Such pregnancies should be regarded as high risk. A pediatrician should be present in the delivery room for the delivery of such an infant, and the obstetrician can evaluate the integrity of the fetal placental unit by performing estriol determinations and noninvasive stress testing. None of these were done during this pregnancy. See **Chapter 16**.

The presence of thick meconium at delivery should rapidly bring the presence of a pediatrician who is skilled at inspecting and suctioning the airway. Finally, all factors which are known to increase glucose consumption should be minimized or avoided in the small-for-date, growth-retarded infant. These would include (but not be limited to) hypothermia, hypoxia, and polycythemia. The stress to the fetus during labor cannot be overestimated when there is growth retardation present. Termination of attempts at a vaginal delivery should be considered when the fetal monitor tracing indicates fetal distress. Once hypoxia and/or hypoglycemia are identified, they should be promptly and sufficiently treated until the infant's own system can recover.

§ 27.3   Intrauterine Growth Retardation/Small for Gestational Age Syndrome

In gestational maternal hypertension, intrauterine fetal growth retardation (IUGR) is directly linked to the severity of the maternal blood pressure elevation. Thus, Christina may have suffered minimal intrauterine growth retardation. Intrauterine growth retardation/small for gestational age infants are prone to developing problems including hypoglycemia, hypothermia, and hyperviscosity. This condition is commonly referred to as the IUGR/SGA syndrome.

On December 3, 1979, there was strong evidence of intrauterine fetal growth retardation. Intrauterine growth retardation (IUGR) is characterized by:

1. Slow increase in fundus height
2. Decrease in normal 24-hour urinary estrogens
3. Lag and increase of fetal biparietal diameter on ultrasound

Intrauterine growth retardation can be caused by restricting the caloric intake of the mother. Intrauterine growth retarded neonates are highly predisposed to hypoglycemia due to lack of stored glycogen in the liver.

However, it should be noted that in IUGR, the fetal brain is saved from damage because of the fetus's ability to redistribute its blood flow to favor the brain. This was proven in experiments with monkeys, but there are no human parallels to these findings.[1]

The following is the most accurate way of assessing fetal welfare (in cases of possible intrauterine growth retardation):

1. Serial sonography to determine the growth rate of the fetal biparietal diameter
2. Weekly oxytocin challenge test
3. Twice weekly maternal 24-hour urinary estriol
4. Rate of uterine growth
5. Evaluation of fetal activity
6. Amniocentesis to determine the presence of meconium and measure the L/S ratio (L/S for fetal lung maturity).

To improve fetal growth (optimal):

1. The mother's diet is to be supplemented to achieve adequate weight gain;
2. Bedrest may be beneficial to fetal growth. Experiments show maternal exercise can lead to a reduction in total uterine blood flow. This is of little consequence in a normal situation; however, in intrauterine

---

[1] Intrauterine Asphyxia and the Developing Fetal Brain, 25, edited by Louis Gluck, (Year Book Medical Publishers, Inc., 1977).

growth retardation where there is little margin of safety, a reduction of uterine blood flow could adversely affect fetal growth.

Pregnancy can be allowed to go to term if you have:

1. Normal increase in fetal biparietal measurement
2. Normal uterine size
3. Normal oxytocin challenge test
4. Rising 24-hour urinary estrogen.

However, if fetal cephalometry shows a slower rate of growth with all other assessments normal, delivery is effected at 37 weeks or sooner if the LS ratio is indicative of fetal lung maturity.

Earlier delivery is indicated if the fetal biparietal diameter stops growing, or signs of distress develop.

Approximately one-third of intrauterine growth retardation fetuses will exhibit distress during labor. This high (one-third) incidence of possible fetal distress is why close and continuous monitoring of fetal well being is warranted throughout labor and delivery.

Intrauterine growth retardation fetuses are particularly susceptible to asphyxia, and labor is a particularly hazardous time.

It was known that the Sweet baby had evidence of intrauterine growth retardation (at 30 weeks gestation), which was compounded by:

1. Asphyxia—as evidence by the passage of meconium in utero;
2. Fetal metabolic acidosis (due to the hypoxia);
3. Severe fetal hypoglycemia;
4. Respiratory acidosis, secondary to meconium aspiration.

Generally speaking, intrauterine growth retardation neonates, without birth defects (the Sweet baby had none), *do not* (as a rule) fare badly *if* proper care is given (i.e., obstetrical, neonatal, and pediatric), whereas the remainder can suffer dire consequences.

The fetal monitoring done during Mrs. Sweet's labor was completely worthless, and thus, constitutes a deviation in the standard of care. The fetal monitor strips are of such a poor quality that they cannot be interpreted. Dr. Zate (the resident who ordered the external monitor) is negligent, as well as the obstetric nurses, for not adequately carrying out the order to monitor this patient.

Another serious violation in the standard of care exists on the part of the hospital obstetric nurses. When Mrs. Sweet was admitted to Berman Hospital on January 7, 1980 at 2:15 a.m., her blood pressure was 140/90, and she had a three-month history of edema of the hands and face. She also had a history of headaches.

Mrs. Sweet was a possible preeclamptic patient who consequently required careful observation. Yet the patient's blood pressure was checked only one additional time while in labor, and that was at 6:30 a.m. (elevated at 130/90). The next time her blood pressure was recorded was 7:20 a.m., when her blood pressure was 180/110. This was recorded in the delivery room, five minutes prior to the delivery. A blood pressure elevation of 180/110 is considered severe, and can reduce placental blood flow. Since Mrs. Sweet's blood pressure was not being monitored closely, we have no ideas to how long this elevated blood pressure existed. There were no blood pressures taken between 2:15 a.m. when she was admitted and 6:30 a.m., and none between 6:30 a.m. and 7:20 a.m.

One must constantly bear in mind that this pregnancy had already been diagnosed by Dr. Keyes as a possible intrauterine growth retardation, and thus, should be the goal to alleviate any unnecessary stress to an already compromised fetus. In his own words, the defendant doctor stated:

> A living female infant with a weight of four pounds, eleven ounces. The infant showed signs of intrauterine growth retardation. It had been noted that the infant was relatively small during her pregnancy, and on the flow sheet several times notes were made that the infant was small for the estimated date of confinement. However, there was no evidence of *any* hypertensive disorder. (Emphasis added).

Dr. Keyes further stated:

> After removing the meconium stained mucus from the airway, the infant cried very well and her color was fine. The infant was transferred to special care nursery in general good condition.

When Dr. Keyes took the baby to the special care nursery, 30 minutes after birth, the baby was described as dusky. The child was cold to the touch and the respirations were irregular with grunting and retractions; also, poor muscle tone was recorded. There was only a fair cry noted when stimulated. *This* description of the child on admission to the nursery hardly coincides with an Apgar score of 7 at five minutes.

It is difficult to understand how Dr. Keyes could possibly state that there was no evidence of *any* hypertensive disorder. You must remember that the mother had symptoms of:

1. Family history of hypertension;
2. On November 20, 1979 her blood pressure was elevated to 134/80 and edema (positive) noted. On December 3, 1979 her blood pressure was 140/90 and again we see (positive) edema; question small for dates.

On December 15, 1979, Mrs. Sweet told Dr. Keyes that the baby was not moving much at all any more. She stated that she felt a decrease of fetal movement. She states that Dr. Keyes said, "Don't worry about it, all babies are different." This is a deviation from the standard of care. It was widely accepted in 1980 that a decrease in fetal movement (especially in a suspected IUGR with hypertension) would warrant an oxytocin challenge test and careful monitoring.

The following is a summary of how Mrs. Sweet's prenatal care could have been improved to likely prevent fetal hypoxia:

1. On December 3, 1979, when blood pressure 140/90, positive edema, and small for gestational age were noted, the patient should have been henceforth considered a "high risk" and the continuation of her pregnancy monitored closely with hospitalization for optimum control of her increased blood pressure and edema. Patients are sometimes hospitalized so that careful serial blood pressure can be taken while the patient is being observed on total bedrest, with some time spent lying on the left side. (This increases the renal blood flow so the kidneys get better perfusion and work better).
2. While hospitalized, an oxytocin challenge test should have been carried out to evaluate placental function. This becomes especially important after Mrs. Sweet complained of decreased fetal movement. The oxytocin challenge test permits the physician to determine how well the placenta is functioning and how well it will tolerate the stress of contractions.
3. During the hospitalization, an amniocentesis should have been performed along with ultrasound to accurately evaluate fetal well being, fetal age, and lung maturity.

The amniocentesis should have been performed when the doctor had diagnosed possible intrauterine growth retardation. If this truly was an IUGR due to gestational hypertension, then the infant would be delivered as soon as its lungs are mature, but before any fetal hypoxia occurs due to placental insufficiency. The amniocentesis also affords an examination of the amniotic fluid to see whether any meconium has been passed.

The treating doctors failed to prescribe even the mildest froms of therapy for gestational hypertension, or possible preeclampsia, which would include:

1.   Maternal bedrest, lying on left side for several hours each a.m. and p.m.
2.   High protein diet with adequate calories
3.   Avoiding strenuous activity.

The above-mentioned amniocentesis with L/S ratio would also have helped prevent post-maturity. The doctors treating Christina at Berman Hospital believed she demonstrated signs of post-maturity.

Christina's neurodevelopmental abnormalities most likely were caused by perinata asphyxia, related to meconium aspiration, and poor air exchange. It must be remembered that this infant suffered some degree of hypoxia in utero (as evidence by the meconium), and thus was already in a state of metabolic acidosis at birth. It is well known that during a normal labor (without risk) there is a reduction of gaseous exchange across the placenta resulting in a relative degree of acidosis (asphyxia). Once a doctor sees evidences of meconium stained fluid, he must be alert to provide optimum newborn care, by anticipating the vulnerability of an already compromised infant. (In addition, Dr. Keyes was also aware of this mother's intrauterine growth retardation and gestational hypertension with blood pressure 180/110 five minutes before delivery).

The baby's APGAR scores were 5 and 7, which indicate a mild to moderately depressed baby; however, the validity of these scores must be questioned.

It should be noted that the anesthesia record is signed by M. Carole, CRNA. If, indeed, there was a nurse anesthetist present, this would be the ideal person to assess the Apgar score, not the obstetrician. It should be noted that the mortality rate in low scores (less then 6) is nearly 15 times that of high Apgar scores.[2]

The importance of suctioning meconium from the trachea and bronchi deserves special emphasis. Meconium is passed after an asphyxial episode in utero. If the asphyxial episode is accompanied by prolonged gasping, meconium will be drawn deeply into the lungs. This fetus *may* respond (recover) from this with regard to the acid-base balance, yet be born with lungs full of meconium. Such infants may initially be responsive and vigorously attempt to breath; however, if the amniotic fluid is heavily stained the doctor *must* suction the baby's mouth as soon as the head emerges from the vagina,

---

[2] Apgar & James, *Further Observations on the Newborn Scoring System*, 104 Am. J. Dis. Child 419 (2962); Drage, Kennedy, & Schwartz, *The Apgar Score as an Index of Neonatal Mortality*, 24 Obstet. Gynecol. 222 (1964).

before the baby is delivered. Then as soon as possible, after the infant is delivered, the doctor must observe the larnyx using a laryngoscope, irrespective of the initial responsiveness (even if the baby appears responsive and vigorous).

Under direct visualization of the vocal cords, endotracheal suction can be performed via an endoctracheal tube, in order to remove the aspirated meconium. Meconium should be cleared-out before administering any positive pressure or vigorous stimulation of the infant.[3]

If the amniotic fluid is only slightly stained with mecomium (as opposed to darker and somewhat thick), and *if* the infant is *actively responsive*, laryngoscopy and intubation are not necessary. This of course was *not* the case here. This infant was *not* actively responsive, it was just the opposite—depressed (i.e., Apgar 5, blue, hypotomic, hypothermic, and intrauterine growth retarded with its inherent hypoglycemia).

It should be emphasized that thick meconium cannot be removed from the lung using any type of nasal-pharynx suctioning (i.e., bulb syringe or DeLee catheter). These only clear the oral and nasal cavities. Deep endotracheal suctioning must be performed The meconium aspiration may have greatly contributed to this infant's hypoxia due to poor air exchange. The chest x-rays done at Berman Hospital and Charity Hospital demonstrate the presence of meconium aspiration pneumonia.

The next major problem to affect this baby occurred when there was a significant delay in treating her severe hypoglycemia. It is well known that hypoglycemia is usually present in intrauterine growth retardation fetuses. See § 16.3.

If the doctors in the special care nursery at Berman had started an umbilical catheter immediately after birth, and thereafter treated the severe hypoglycemia with a *constant*, low-dose glucose infusion, they could have avoided having to use a "large glucose push" known to *induce* hyperglycemia.

This baby's blood sugar was zero when admitted (31 minutes after delivery) to the special care nursery. This baby had a significant delay in treatment of the hypoglycemia due to the length of time the baby was kept in the delivery room. There was further delay in treating the hypoglycemia by the nursery personnel who attempted to find a peripheral vein to start an IV. This brought the time of treatment (for hypoglycemia) to 9:25 a.m., almost two hours after delivery, and over an hour after being admitted to the special care nursery. Since severe hypoglycemia is a known complication of intrauterine growth retardation, this should have been foreseen and an umbilical catheter should have been used initially in the delivery room. Hypoglycemia of this severity must be treated as soon as possible with systemic sugar. Unfortunately, in this case, they tried the nasogastric route first. Also, it appears that

---

[3] S.M. Shnider & G. Levinson, Anesthesia for Obstetrics 390 (Williams & Wilkins, 1979).

precious time was wasted attempting to start an IV in a peripheral vein since this baby was known to be "cold stress" (temperature on admission was 94.3F).

When you have a growth retarded infant that is asphyxiated (meconium fluid, low Apgar) and cold stress (decreased temperature), you will have a marked decrease in peripheral circulation due to the body's own defense mechanism of diverting the blood supply to its internal organs.

Since this baby was in a special care nursery an umbilical vessel catheter should have been used. Immediate therapy could have been started to treat the hypoglycemia and prevent severe metabolic alterations, which likely contributed to the overall neurological injury.

Untreated hypoglycemia can cause specific central nervous system damage. It commonly occurs in sick, small infants with other factors affecting outcome, such as anoxia, cerebral injury, or severe intrauterine malnutrition.

Symptoms of hypoglycemia in the neonate are:

1. Cyanosis
2. Tremors
3. Convulsions
4. Apnea (irregular respirations)
5. Apathy
6. High pitched or weak cry

The IUGR/SGA infant is *known* to be at risk for developing hypoglycemia, and early care should include the provision of adequate calories and the close following of dextrostick blood sugars. The general care of the infant should be such that factors known to increase the risk of hypoglycemia are avoided. This infant remained hypoglycemic for more than an hour while multiple attempts at starting a peripheral IV failed. The umbilical vein should have been used temporarily until a peripheral site could be found. The diminished cardiac output due to the hypoxic cardiomyopathy (persistent fetal circulation causing an open ductus with shunting from right to left) and possibly hypoglycemia were a contributory factor to the infant's hypotension, in turn, leading to diminished perfusion of the central nervous system and contributing to the subsequent seizure activity.

The hospital records indicate that this infant was delivered at 7:20 a.m. and was not admitted to the special care nursery until 7:55 a.m. Upon admission to the special care nursery, the infant's temperature had dropped to 94.3F. One hour after delivery, the infant's temperature was still very low at 95.8. This indicates that the infant was definitely allowed to cool excessively and be subjected to cold stress.

Very cold, freezing temperatures have obvious dramatic consequences. What is less obvious is that temperatures which feel hot to an adult may represent a dangerous cold stress to a baby, a stress that expresses itself in terms of morbidity and mortality. Even a moderately cool environment will inevitably require the baby to absorb more oxygen (threatening his life if he already has respiratory difficulty), and use more substrate as fuel (effectively creating artificial starvation). Thus, the effects of inadequate warmth has metabolic consequences, increasing metabolic acidosis, as well as purely physical effects. See § 16.5.

Immediately after birth, when a baby arrives naked, wet and practically asphyxiated, the body temperature falls abruptly unless special precautions are taken. If the delivery room temperature is about 25° C, even a lusty baby producing a maximum metabolic response to cold cannot match the rate of heat loss of about 200 K calories-KG-min (kilo calories per kilogram per minute). If he is small, ill, and asphxiated, the rate of fall of body temperature is dramatic. The period of time he is exposed to temperatures appropriate for adults must be minimized. Serious asphyxia may affect the baby's own homeothermy for many hours after birth. There is also risk in transporting an already cool baby down a hospital corridor.

The mother states that the baby's father was allowed to hold the infant in the delivery room. Since the father was fully clothed and gowned, there is no way any of his body heat could reach the infant. This caused the infant to cool even more. Also, the doctor stopped in the hospital corridor with the baby in a plastic bed (not an incubator) for the grandparents to look at the baby while the doctor spoke with the husband. The hospital corridors are usually very cool due to drafts from doors and windows opening and closing, and this atmosphere caused the baby to cool even more.

PART IV

NEGOTIATION AND ANALYSIS OF DAMAGES

CHAPTER 28

TAX-FREE STRUCTURED SETTLEMENTS

§ 28.1   Introduction

At least 90 percent of all settlements in birth trauma malpractice cases are structured settlements. The reasons for such settlements are exemplified when the plaintiff is young and severely retarded. If the negotiations and the agreement are handled properly, an injured child will be provided secure, tax-free, management-free, lifetime-guaranteed income.

Much has been said and written regarding the benefits and the management-free aspects of structured settlements. Few clients in any personal injury case have the sophistication to invest and protect large sums of money. We don't need studies to tell us that lump sum settlements are too often dissipated, squandered, or otherwise lost, long before the need for the money has disappeared. We, as attorneys, readily understand that transforming a lump sum payment into periodic payments will result in a tax benefit to our client which increase the overall payout by 20, to sometimes 50 percent. What we to understand is that the tax-free status does not come naturally as does the management-free status. The tax benefits accrue to plaintiff only if the attorney knows the law affecting structured settlements and incorporates those principles into the structured settlement agreement. It is this problem, the tax-free settlement agreement, and this problem only, to which the remainder of this chapter will be primarily devoted. There are many other concerns with structured settlements such as assignments and the liquidity of the company accepting the assignment, but those will not be dealt with here.

§ 28.2   Requirements to Exclude Periodic Payments from Gross Income

The parties to a structured settlement agreement generally include the following:

1. The plaintiff (alternatively referred to as claimant or annuitant)
2. A defendant
3. The defendant's liability insurer
4. An annuity provider

The agreement itself is an agreement between the plaintiff and the defendant, or sometimes both the defendant and the defendant's insurer. Often the obligation in the structured settlement agreement is satisfied by the purchase of an annuity which will necessitate a second agreement. The second agreement will be between the defendant, or sometimes the defendant and the liability insurer, on the one hand, and the annuity provider on the other. The second agreement is separate from the structured settlement agreement and should be considered merely as an investment by the party liable to the plaintiff used to fund the structured settlement obligation.

Internal Revenue Code § 104(a)(2) excludes personal injury settlement periodic payments from the annuitant's taxable income. Regarding a 1983 amendment[1] to this provision, the Senate reported:

> This provision is intended to codify, rather than change, present law. Thus, the periodic payments of personal injury damages are still excludable from income only if the recipient taxpayer is not in constructive receipt of or does not have

---

[1] Pub. L. No. 97-473, 96 Stat. 2605 (1983).

the current economic benefit of the sum required to produce the periodic payments.[2]

This amendment is codified a body of law established by a series of Revenue Rulings.[3] These rulings require the following conditions to be met in order to exclude payments from taxable income:

1. Plaintiff must not have *constructive receipt* of the sum required to produce the periodic payments.
2. Plaintiff cannot possess the *current economic benefit* or ownership rights of the annuity.
3. Plaintiff may not *control the investment* of the funding of the annuity.
4. Plaintiff may rely only on the *general credit* of the liability insurer and/or the defendant(s) for collection of the payments.

The precise nature of these restrictions is discussed in §§ **28.3** through **28.6**.

§ 28.3   —Constructive Receipt

Constructive receipt of income is a tax accounting concept that is applied to determine whether income that is earned but not physically or actually possessed by a taxpayer should be included in his taxable income for a given year. It is defined as follows:

> [income] is constructively received by him in the taxable year during which it is credited to [a taxpayer's account], *set apart* [for the taxpayer], or otherwise *made available* so that [the taxpayer] may draw upon it at any time. . . . However, income is not constructively received if the taxpayer's control of its receipt is subject to *substantial limitations*. . . . (Emphasis added)[4]

If the Plaintiff were to receive a lump sum payment, and thereafter, purchase an annuity, there would be no dispute that the monies generated from that principle would be taxable. Constructive receipt is a concept that prevents the plaintiff from doing indirectly what she could not do directly. If the plaintiff is given the choice between the lump sum payment or an annuity or structured

---

[2] S. Rep. No. 646, 97th Cong., 2d Sess. 4, *reprinted in* 1982 U.S. Code Cong. & Ad. News 4580, 4583.

[3] Rev. Rul. 65-29, 1965-1 C.B. 59; Rev. Rul. 77-230, 1977-2 C.B. 214; Rev. Rul. 79-220, 1979-2 C.B. 74; Rev. Rul. 79-313, 1979-2 C.B. 75.

[4] Treas. Reg. § 1.451-2(a), T.D. 6723, 1964-1 C.B. 74.

settlement that could be purchased with that same money, it would then be said that the monies were made available to the plaintiff-taxpayer, and therefore, taxable. For example, if during the settlement discussions, the defendant tells the plaintiff that the latter may either have a lump sum payment or a structured settlement which the same money could buy; and thereafter, the plaintiff indicates that she would take the lump sum, then changes her mind and asks the defendant to purchase an annuity, there is a high probability that the interest generated over and above the principle would be taxable. In that situation, the plaintiff had the money available. In essence, what she did was to invest that money in an annuity, but instead of purchasing it herself, she used the defendant as a conduit. One method of hopefully avoiding a situation where settlement negotiations could result in a taxable structured settlement is to take the position that the case can only be settled by way of a structured settlement and a lump sum settlement will not be acceptable.

The issue of constructive receipt is most often raised by the defendant. This issue is frequently raised by defendant in response to the plaintiff's inquiry about the cost of the annuity, as the negotiations get close to agreeable figures. The defendant argues that she cannot divulge the cost of the annuity since knowledge by the plaintiff would effectively make the periodic payments taxable. The revenue rulings discussed in § **28.2** do not indicate that knowledge alone constitutes constructive receipt. Although the IRS will not accept private letter rulings as precedent, the rulings certainly can be used to demonstrate the prior position and the logic that would be employed when the issue is raised. On May 16, 1983, the IRS issued a private letter ruling[5] dealing specifically with the question of whether disclosure by the defendant of the cost or present value of the annuity to fund the structured settlement results in constructive receipt to the plaintiff. This private revenue ruling citing Treasury Regulation § 1.451-2(a) concluded that knowledge is not determinative in deciding a question of constructive receipt, but unqualified availability is the decisive factor. Therefore, although knowledge coupled with a choice between the structured and lump sum settlement may make the subsequent agreement taxable, knowledge alone without the choice would appear not to. If the defendant persists in her position that this knowledge may make the agreement taxable, and that she, the defendant, has an obligation to the plaintiff (which she does not) that would be breached with the disclosure of this information, an interesting strategic move is to test the defendant's sincerity by agreeing to give the defendant a hold harmless agreement and release if disclosure affects the tax-free consequences of the agreement.

To ensure that the client's control of receipt of the funds is subject to substantial limitations so as to satisfy Treasury Regulation § 61.451-2, it is recom-

---

[5] Letter Rul. 83333035, May 16, 1983.

mended that language to that effect be incorporated directly into the structured settlement agreement. In the sample agreement in § **28.10**, an example of such language is contained in paragraph three. The language in this paragraph states that the plaintiff has no right to accelerate, increase or decrease the amount of the periodic payments. The effect of this language is to impose substantial limitations on the client's control of receipt of the funds.

§ 28.4   —Current Economic Benefit and Annuity Rights of Ownership

Although the revenue rulings, letter rulings, tax cases, and journal articles regarding the taxation of structured settlement benefits unanimously state as a condition of avoiding taxation that a plaintiff may not possess any current economic benefit or rights of ownership in the annuity or the sum invested to fund the annuity, specific guidance regarding the definitions of current economic benefit or annuity rights of ownership is very limited.

There are only two specific references and elaborations made regarding the kind of ownership rights that might jeopardize a plaintiff's tax-free benefits. In a landmark revenue ruling, the Commissioner of Internal Revenue emphasized the fact that the annuitant did not possess any of the rights of ownership, including the right to change the beneficiary.[6] In a letter ruling, the Commission found the structured settlement nontaxable for the following reasons: "The agreement provides that Taxpayer does not have the right to accelerate any payment or to increase or decrease the amount of the annual payments specified. Furthermore, the annual payments are not subject to assignment, transfer, commutation, or encumbrance."[7]

As will be noted below, the possession or nonpossession of the right to assign, transfer, commute, or encumber has been an important factor in determining the taxability of benefits in two analogous areas: in estate tax law cases regarding the taxation of life insurance policy proceeds, and in deferred compensation cases regarding the taxation of deferred annuity benefits. In estate tax law, the life insurance proceeds of a policy in which the decedent possessed no "incidents of ownership" are not included in the value of his taxable gross estate.[8] More specifically, if the policy was owned by the decedent in his name or if the decedent possessed any of the following five incidents of ownership, the proceeds of the policy were held to be taxable. To be

---

[6] Rev. Rul. 79-220, 1979-2 C.B. 74.

[7] Letter Rul. 7933078, May 21, 1979.

[8] IRC § 2042 (West 1979).

held not taxable according to Treasury Regulation § 20.2042-1, the decedent must not have possessed:

1. The right to change the beneficiary of the policy.
2. The right to surrender the policy for cash.
3. The right to borrow against the policy.
4. The right to pledge the policy as collateral.
5. The right to assign the policy or revoke an assignment of the proceeds of the policy.[9]

By way of further definition the regulation states,

> The term "incidents of ownership" is not limited in its meaning to ownership of the policy in the technical legal sense. Generally speaking, the term has reference to the right of the insured or his estate to the economic benefits of the policy. Thus, it includes the power to change the beneficiary, to surrender or cancel the policy, to assign the policy, to revoke an assignment, to pledge the policy for a loan, or to obtain from the insurer a loan against the surrender value of the policy.[10]

In addition, in *Chase National Bank v. United States*,[11] the Court held:

> A power in the decedent to surrender and cancel the policies, to pledge them as security for loans and the power to dispose of them and their proceeds for his own benefit during his life . . . is by no means the least substantial of the legal incidents of ownership. . . .

Rights of ownership are similarly defined for the purposes of determining the taxation of deferred compensation benefits. Deferred compensation is not taxable where an employee possesses no current economic benefit or ownership rights in the annuity that provides the periodic payment, i.e., the benefits cannot be subject to "anticipation, alienation, sale, transfer, assignment, pledge or encumbrance" by the taxpayer.[12]

To the extent that these analogies are appropriate, it appears that an annuitant of a structured settlement should not have the power to assign, alienate, or otherwise encumber the annuity and its benefits.

---

[9] Treas. Reg. § 20.2042-1(c)(2), T.D. 7312, 1974-1 C.B. 277.

[10] *Id.*

[11] 278 U.S. 327, 335 (1929).

[12] Rev. Rul. 72-25, 1972-1 C.B. 127.

To satisfy the above position, language similar to that found in Paragraph 7 of the Sample Structured Settlement in § 28.10 disclaiming all ownership rights can be used. This paragraph did not identify each of the different types of ownership interest, but simply disclaimed in general all ownership rights, actual or constructive, plus the right to change beneficiary.

§ 28.5   —Control of the Investment or Funding of the Annuity

Revenue Ruling 79-220 provides that a plaintiff who wishes to avoid being taxed cannot have the right to control the investment or the amount set aside to fund the annuity.[13] The precise meaning and implications of this condition unfortunately are not set forth in the cited revenue ruling or in any other revenue ruling, letter ruling, or tax court case. Accordingly, to determine the extent of control, if any, that a plaintiff may legitimately exercise without jeopardizing the tax benefits of the structured settlement, it is necessary to turn elsewhere for definitions and applications of the concept of "control."

Despite the tremendous variety in the cases and contexts in which control is defined (*i.e.*, to control the premises, to control the management of the corporation, to control the vehicle, to control the child, etc.), virtually every case cites one of two definitions: (1) "the power or authority to manage, direct, superintend, restrict, regulate, govern, administer or oversee. . . .";[14] or, (2) "to keep under check, . . . to restrain, . . . or to exercise a directing, restraining or governing influence over."[15]

The application of this common law definition of control to determine the degree of control allowed an annuitant or beneficiary of a structured settlement agreement implies a very constrained role for the annuitant plaintiff and his counsel, i.e., it appears that an annuitant would not be allowed to "direct, oversee or restrain" the liability insurer's (defendant's) selection of the annuity provider. Fortunately, however, precedent in an analogous deferred compensation agreement may offer room for increased participation by the plaintiff.

Goldsmith v. United States[16] was a case dealing with a deferred compensation annuity purchased by a hospital for an affiliated anesthesiologist. In that case the Internal Revenue Commissioner maintained that since Dr. Goldsmith had participated extensively in the selection of the annuity plan (i.e., despite

---

[13] 1979-2 C.B. 74.

[14] Black's Law Dictionary 298 (5th ed. 1979).

[15] 18 C.J.S. *Control* (1979).

[16] 78-2 U.S.T.C. ¶ 9804 *aff'd per curiam*, 586 F.2d 810 (Ct. Cl. 1978).

the fact that the agreement provided that the hospital "may fund or not fund" the annuity, the parties had agreed beforehand, at Dr. Goldsmith's insistence, that the annuity would be provided by Continental Assurance Co.), this participation constituted control and constructive receipt of the fund. The Court, however, held the deferred compensation agreement stood alone, and that direction and control exercised at the bargaining and negotiation stage did not jeopardize the tax advantages of the agreement.

> All the facts point to the conclusion that the determination of the amounts to be deducted, the choice of benefits and decision to fund, were decisions by the taxpayer, according to his desires. Even the hospital's bare legal right to discontinue funding could promptly be neutralized by the taxpayer's cancellation of the entire agreement (as provided for in the agreement). . . .
>
> These facts as to the origins and duration of the agreement have, however, little to do with constructive receipt, essentially a question of the product of the agreement when in force. Who brought the plan to the hospital's attention, whether the taxpayer persuaded the hospital to agree or vice versa, whose "personal requirements" are served by an agreement . . . are questions irrelevant to receipt, constructive or actual, under the binding agreement, in fact, reached. Objective matters such as the receipt of income from a bargain do not depend upon which party in the bargain dominated the other. If the employer's funding of the agreement does not work a constructive receipt to defeat a deferment of tax . . ., then it is no further ground for taxation that the funding was agreed by the parties at the suggestion or even the demand of the employee.[17]

The implications of this opinion for plaintiff annuitants in structured settlement cases suggest that a plaintiff may exercise directing or restraining control of the annuity investment at the negotiation stage. For example, she could require that the annuity provider have a Best AAA rating or that it possess reserves in excess of $12,500,000.00. She might negotiate that the annuity be provided by a third party insurer instead of a parent, subsidiary, or affiliate of the liability insurer to provide additional protection from insurance company insolvency. She might insist that the annuity company belong to an industry or government group that backs up the obligation of its members. However, as the opinion warns, the extent of the annuitant's control must be exercised only at the negotiation stage; the structured settlement agreement, standing alone, must not indicate any directing, restraining or overseeing influence by the plaintiff.

Just as it is often difficult for the plaintiff to find out the cost of the annuity because of the defendant's concerns about the tax-free status of the agreement, it is also difficult for the plaintiff to keep out of the agreement any reference to

---

[17] Goldsmith, 586 F.2d at 818.

the annuity company. Traditionally, when a defendant or defendant's liability carrier settled a personal injury claim, they would have no future responsibilities or contingent liability. Although they both now recognize that they must be "on the risk" to satisfy the fourth requirement of tax-free status as outlined in § 28.6, they have a penchant still for including a paragraph in the agreement to the effect they have satisfied their obligation to the plaintiff by purchasing an annuity from Insurance Company X. References to the annuity company should be excluded from any agreement. Since the defendant and his liability carrier must be "on the risk" of general creditors, the inclusion of such language in the agreement can only be construed against the plaintiff at a later date. Since the language in *Goldsmith* has already been approved, and since the court has said they would look to the four corners of the agreement, the exact language should be incorporated into an agreement as in the example in § 28.10 in Paragraph 7.

§ 28.6   —Collection of Periodic Payments as General Creditor

As a condition of nontaxation, Revenue Ruling 79-220[18] provides that the plaintiff must "rely on the general credit" of the liability insurer and/or the defendant for the collection of his monthly payments. The apparent rationale for this requirement is that such reliance signifies that the plaintiff has no ownership rights in the annuity and that the funding arrangement is a separate transaction that is "merely an investment" made at the obligor's convenience to provide a source of funds to satisfy its obligation to the plaintiff.[19]

The plaintiff then is a general creditor. Most commonly, a general creditor is an unsecured creditor who has no assets set aside to secure her debt. In Revenue Ruling 79-313,[20] dealing with a structured settlement agreement, the Commissioner held that the benefits were not taxable in that: "Under the agreement, M (the liability insurer) is not required to set aside specific assets to secure any part of its obligation to the taxpayer. The taxpayer's rights against M are no greater than those of M's general creditors."

Likewise, in a letter ruling, involving a personal injury structured settlement ruling, the Commissioner assured the plaintiff that his benefits were tax-free, noting that:

---

[18] 1979-2 C.B. 74.

[19] *See also* Rev. Rul. 72-25, 1972-2 C.B. 127 (deferred compensation).

[20] 197-2 C.B. 75.

You can only rely on the general credit of the school district's insurer for payment, as it will not be required to set aside sufficient assets or to secure its obligations in any manner. Your rights against the insurer are no greater than the rights of the insurer's general creditors.[21]

Although it seems to go without saying, in order to look to the general credit of the liability insurer and/or the defendant for the collection of monthly payments, it is absolutely essential that one, or both, of these parties sign the agreement along with the plaintiff. Although structured settlements have been used daily for almost a decade, some defendants and liability carriers still believe they do not have to sign structured settlement agreements. A structured settlement agreement is a contract, a contract that is entered into in consideration for the dismissal of the underlying action. If the defendant and/or defendant's liability carrier do not sign the agreement, the plaintiff has no recourse against either party. The plaintiff cannot look to the general credit of either of these parties unless they are signatories to the contract. Traditionally, when a case was settled, only the plaintiff signed the closing papers, the release and indemnification agreement, since the defendant and her carrier had no future responsibilities or liabilities. If you believe them, there are thousands of these alleged structured settlement agreements where plaintiff has dismissed a tort action in exchange for a contract action; if the plaintiff is the only signer of the agreement, she has no cause of action against anyone under contract law. The defendants do not like signing these agreements because they could result in long-term contingent liability. However, if the plaintiff must look to the general credit of the defendant and/or her liability carrier, one or both of these parties must sign the agreement.

A problem arises when the defendant wishes to include a paragraph in the agreement that states that in the event of a default, the plaintiff should sue the annuity company directly as opposed to suing the defendant. The defendant's logic is that since the annuity company is making the payments, why involve the defendant if the annuity company defaults. It may be logical to include a provision agreeing that the plaintiff can be assigned the general creditor's right against the annuity company. Although logical, it is contrary to the revenue ruling stating that the plaintiff can rely only on the general credit of the defendant or the defendant's insurer.[22] Therefore, although a defendant wishes to include such a paragraph in the agreement, plaintiff should be adamantly opposed. As can be seen in the Paragraph 7 of the example agreement in § **28.10**, language can be included to reaffirm that the plaintiff looks solely to the general credit of the defendant or the defendant's liability carrier.

---

[21] Letter Rul. 8042027, July 22, 1980.
[22] Rev. Rul. 79-220, 1979-2 C.B. 74.

By way of further definition, a general creditor is an unsecured creditor who has no lien or charge against the debtor's property to secure payment of his debt. Under Michigan common law, general creditors are "creditors who have no judgment or lien on the debtor's property."[23] Under the United States Bankruptcy Code, an unsecured creditor is a creditor whose claim is unsecured by a lien.[24] A lien is defined as a "charge against or interest in property to secure payment of a debt or performance of an obligation."[25] Interestingly, the code explicitly identifies judicial liens, that is, as "a lien obtained by judgment, levy, sequestration, or other legal or equitable process or proceeding,"[26] as liens establishing secured claims. The importance of this distinction between general creditors and judgment creditors becomes significant to the client and attorney when deciding whether or not the structured settlement should be incorporated into a consent judgment. In other words, if a structured settlement is incorporated into a consent judgment creating a judicial lien, it takes the plaintiff out of that category of a general creditor.

Given that a possessor of a judicial lien is not considered a general creditor, a question arises regarding the taxation of benefits flowing from a structured settlement agreement adopted or created by judgment. To the extent that judgments create a lien, and that general creditor status is forfeited, it would appear that tax benefits may be jeopardized in judgment arrangements. Again, unfortunately, no IRS ruling or tax case has addressed this issue. Some attorneys have suggested that to overcome the disadvantaged status of a general creditor, all settlement agreements should be adopted by a court and entered as a judgment. However, these writers seldom consider tax effects. Pragmatically speaking and considering the unequivocal revenue ruling condition that an annuitant have only the rights of a general creditor, the conservative attorney should thoroughly understand the situation creating a judicial lien and recognize that its creation may jeopardize the tax benefits of the settlement.

The United States Bankruptcy Court has held that the precise timing of the creation of judicial liens varies from state to state. For example, in *Matter of Smith*,[27] *In re Habeeb-Ullah*,[28] and *In re Washington*,[29] in Georgia, New York, and Virginia, a judgment creditor is considered a secured creditor from the date that the judgment is entered. In Michigan, a judicial lien on personal

---

[23] Dempsy v. Pforheimer, 86 Mich. 652, 658, 49 N.W. 465 (1891).

[24] 11 U.S.C. § 506 (1979).

[25] *Id.* at § 101(28).

[26] *Id.* at § 101(27).

[27] 17 Bankr. 541 (M.D. Ga. 1982).

[28] 16 Bankr. 831 (W.D.N.Y. 1982).

[29] 6 Bankr. 226 (E.D. Va. 1980).

property is not acquired until actual levy of an execution,[30] and a judicial lien on real estate is not created until the levy and notice of execution are registered with the county registrar.[31] Also, in *Schleowski v. Powlowski*,[32] a Michigan case, the court stated: "No lien is acquired on real estate in Michigan under a judgment until actual levy of an execution." There is, then, some authority in Michigan that even where structured benefits are adopted by judgment, a plaintiff may retain her general creditor status unless and until she levies execution for collection.

A way to avoid a judicial lien and some sort of preferred creditor status is to take the traditional consent judgment, and instead enter a consent judgment of dismissal with approval of the settlement. See § **28.8**. This type of order is obtained in the same manner as the traditional consent judgment would be obtained, but the form of the order is in effect a dismissal with prejudice. The consideration for the dismissal of this claim is that the defendant will sign the structured settlement agreement effectively exchanging the tort action and potential judgment on that action for the contract action.

§ 28.7   Payments for Lost Wages Are Taxable

Revenue Ruling 79-313[33] establishes that periodic payments for "personal injury, pain and suffering, disability, and loss of bodily function" are exempt from taxation. Although there is no structured settlement tax ruling, case or authority specifically on point, agreements should probably avoid statements or provisions that payments are made as compensation for "lost income." The general approach of the Internal Revenue Service on taxation of monies received as damages is set forth in *Hort v. Commissioner*.[34] This opinion provides that to determine whether and to what extent amounts received as damages, whether by compromise or as result of judgment, should be taxed as income, it is necessary to look to the nature of the item for which damages are a substitute. Applying this principle, the IRS has held that income received in settlement for claims of lost wages and for wages lost during periods of suspension is taxable.[35] Accordingly, it is advisable that structured settlements avoid references to compensation specifically for "lost wages."

---

[30] Mich. Comp. Laws § 600.6012 (1968).

[31] *Id.* at § 600.6051.

[32] 168 Mich. 664, 667, 134 N.W. 997 (1912).

[33] 1979-2 C.B. 75 (structured settlements).

[34] 313 U.S. 289 (1941).

[35] *See, e.g.,* Rev. Rul. 58-140, 1958-1 C.B. 15.

§ 28.8   Form—Order of Consent Judgment of Dismissal

STATE OF MICHIGAN
IN THE CIRCUIT COURT FOR THE COUNTY OF

ROSE DOE, Guardian of LISA DOE,
and ROSE DOE and HAROLD DOE,
Individually,

        Plaintiffs,

vs.

DETROIT HOSPITAL, a Michigan Corporation,

        Defendant.

_____

ORDER OF CONSENT JUDGMENT OF DISMISSAL

At a session of said Court held in the Courthouse, County of
_____, State of Michigan, on:
_____.

PRESENT: The Honorable _____
                    Circuit Court Judge

This matter having come on for hearing before the Court, the parties, after extensive negotiating, having achieved an amicable compromise of this matter; the Court having taken testimony at length on the record from ROSE DOE, the Mother of LISA DOE, and Guardian of her Estate, indicating that the settlement reached was in the best interest of the Plaintiff, LISA DOE, and the Court being otherwise fully advised in the premises;

NOW THEREFORE, it is hereby ordered that the settlement proposed by the parties, the terms of which are set forth on the record of this Court, dated _____, is hereby approved, the Court expressly finding that the settlement is in the best interest of Plaintiff, LISA DOE;

IT IS FURTHER ORDERED that ROSE DOE, in her capacity as Guardian of the Estate of LISA DOE is hereby authorized to execute a release and settlement agreement, made available for the Court's review and expressly approved, on behalf of LISA DOE, against Defendant, DETROIT HOSPITAL;

IT IS FURTHER ORDERED that this approval settlement between the parties is full and final; that Defendant DETROIT HOSPITAL, shall be and is hereby dismissed as a party with prejudice, thereby dismissing the entire cause of action and that no costs, interest or fees shall be taxed for or against any party to this action.

APPROVED AS TO FORM &
SUBSTANCE:

By: _____
    Attorney for Detroit Hospital

§ 28.9   Form—Satisfaction of Judgment

STATE OF MICHIGAN
IN THE CIRCUIT COURT FOR THE COUNTY OF

ROSE DOE, Guardian of LISA DOE,
and ROSE DOE and HAROLD DOE,
Individually,

            Plaintiffs,

vs.

DETROIT HOSPITAL, a Michigan Corporation,

            Defendant.

SATISFACTION OF JUDGMENT

NOW COME ROSE DOE, Guardian of LISA DOE, and ROSE DOE and HAROLD DOE, Individually, as well as LISA DOE, Individually, Plaintiffs by

and through their attorneys,_____,
and hereby acknowledge the terms of the attached Settlement and Release
Agreement, pages 1 through 7, executed by the aforementioned Plaintiffs
and _____ Insurance Company, in full satisfac-
tion of the Consent Judgment entered into by Plaintiffs and Defendant, DE-
TROIT HOSPITAL on _____   _____.

_____   _____
ROSE DOE, Guardian of Lisa Doe   HAROLD DOE

_____   _____
ROSE DOE   Attorney for Plaintiffs

§ 28.10 Form—Settlement and Release Agreement

Settlement,   Release   Agreement   made   this   ____   day   of
_____, 19 ____, by and among HAROLD DOE,
ROSE DOE and LISA DOE (hereinafter sometimes referred to as "Claimants"), and _____ INSURANCE COMPANY,
whose principal office is located in _____
(hereinafter sometimes referred to as "_____").

WITNESSETH:

Recital A: On or about _____, the
Claimants instituted a civil action in the Circuit Court for County of
_____, being Civil Action No.
_____, entitled, after amended Complaints, as follows:

ROSE DOE, Guardian of LISA
DOE,
and ROSE DOE and HAROLD
DOE, Individually,

        Plaintiffs,

vs.

DETROIT HOSPITAL, a Michigan
Corporation,
        Defendant.

Said civil action is hereinafter referred to as the "Civil Action". Since the inception of the Civil Action, Lisa Doe has reached the age of majority and the guardianship of her by Rose Doe terminated.

Recital B: The Claimants have fully resolved their disputes with all parties other than Detroit Hospital (hereinafter "Hospital"), which other parties have all been dismissed from the Civil Action.

Recital C: With respect to the claims and allegations set forth in the Civil Action against the Hospital, it is insured by Primary Insurer Insurance Company, Secondary Insurer Re-insurance Company and Excess Insurer (all of which are hereinafter referred to as the "Insurer").

Recital D: The Claimants and the Hospital, as well as the Insurers of the Insurer, have agreed to settle and enter a consent judgment of dismissal with respect to allegations in the Civil Action against the Hospital, without costs to any party except as hereinafter provided, in part under the terms and conditions set forth in this Settlement and Release Agreement.

Recital E: With respect to contribution to the payments to the Claimants under this Agreement, Primary Insurer will contribute Two Hundred Fifty Thousand ($250,000.00) Dollars, Secondary Insurer will contribute Five Hundred Thousand ($500,000.00) Dollars, and the balance of all payments to be made under the Settlement and Release Agreement are to be contributed by Excess Insurer. It is further understood that the said contribution of Primary and Secondary shall be made as a part of the lump sum payment called for in "Paragraph 2" hereinafter set forth.

NOW, THEREFORE, in consideration of the premises and the mutual covenants hereinafter contained, the parties hereto agree as follows:

1.   The Recitals A through E above are hereby incorporated into this Agreement by reference and made a part hereof as though set forth herein verbatim.

2.   The Defendant is to receive currently, in one lump sum, the total amount of Nine Hundred Thousand ($900,000.00) Dollars, which is to be allocated among the Claimants, and their attorneys as follows:

(a) $75,000.00 to Harold Doe;
(b) $75,000.00 to Rose Doe;
(c) $450,000.00 to Lisa Doe;
(d) $300,000.00 as attorneys fees and costs.

Insurer, in addition to the amounts referenced in Recital E above, agrees to pay to the Claimants, the amount of One Hundred Fifty Thousand ($150,000.00) Dollars, of the total amount set forth above in this Paragraph 2. The Claimants acknowledge receipt of the above payments, which have been made prior to the execution and delivery hereof.

3.   In addition to the current lump sum payments due pursuant to Paragraph 2 hereof, Insurer agrees to make the following payments to Lisa Doe:

(a)   Monthly payments of four Thousand ($4,000.00) Dollars, such payments to commence as of the 15th day of January, 1983, and to continue on the 15th day of each month thereafter until the later of (i) January 15, 2002, or (ii) the death of Lisa Doe, and said monthly payments to be increased annually on the anniversary date of the commencement of such payments, at the rate of three (3%) percent per annum, compounded annually, and

(b)   Should Lisa Doe survive to the following dates, the amount set forth after such date:
  (i)   January 15, 1992—$100,000.00
  (ii)   January 15, 2002—$200,000.00
  (iii) January 15, 2012—$300,000.00
  (iv)   January 15, 2022—$400,000.00

Under no circumstances shall the above payee have the right to accelerate or increase or decrease the amount of the monthly or lump sum payments specified in this Paragraph. Any payment due and payable after the death or incompetency of Lisa Doe shall be paid to her personal representative.

4.   For the consideration set forth in this Agreement, the Claimants, and each of them, individually and collectively, for themselves, their heirs, executors, administrators, successors and assigns do hereby forever release and discharge the Hospital, its employees, agents, successors, and assigns (Hospital and such additional persons are hereinafter referred to as "Releasees") from any and all claims, demands and actions in favor of Claimants, arising out of any and all acts, omissions, occurrence, defect, failure to warn or other event through the date hereof, and all of the consequences, damages, and injury resulting or alleged to result therefrom or which may result or be alleged to result in the future, and even though the same are not presently known, and even though there is no reason to believe that they may occur (excepting only the agreements of Releasees under this Agreement), and particularly all such claims, demands, causes of action and other rights (including costs, interest and attorney's fees) which may be based upon or arise out of medical care and attention provided for Lisa Doe from the beginning of time to the present, including but limited to any and all matters and things which are, or were, involved in the Civil Action.

5.   It is understood and agreed that the injuries and damages of the Claimants and the legal ability of the Hospital therefor are disputed and denied, that this Agreement and Release does not constitute an admission of liability of the Hospital, and that this Agreement is to compromise and terminate any and all claims of every kind and character as set forth in Paragraph 4 above. All agreements and understandings between the parties in reference to the subject matter herein are herein embodied.

6.   The Claimants hereby acknowledge that neither the Hospital, the Insurers, nor their counsel, have made any representations with respect to the Civil Action and the matters herein released, except only as contained in this Agreement.

7.   Insurer may, but need not, purchase an annuity or other contract providing for the payments due from it to Lisa Doe under Paragraph 3 hereof and any payment to Lisa Doe, or her successor, made pursuant to any such annuity or other contract

shall operate as a pro tanto discharge of Insurer's obligation for such payment due and payable under Paragraph 3 hereof. Any such annuity or other contract shall be and remain the sole property of Insurer and neither Lisa Doe or any other Claimant shall have any ownership rights whatsoever, either actual or constructive therein, any right to change the beneficiary or other control in the policy, or any rights of a secured party therein, and Lisa Doe, or her successor, shall remain solely a general judgment creditor of Insurer pursuant to this Agreement.

8. The parties hereto will, and do hereby, direct their respective attorneys to approve and file an Order of Dismissal of or a consent judgment with respect to the Civil Action, with prejudice, against the Hospital.

9. This Agreement is conditioned upon the approval hereof of the relevant courts of competent jurisdiction including the _____ County Circuit Court.

IN WITNESS WHEREOF, the Claimants and the Insurers, through its duly authorized representatives, have set their hands and seals on the day and year first above written.

_____
HAROLD DOE

_____
ROSE DOE

_____
LISA DOE

CLAIMANTS

_____
By: _____
   Its: _____

INSURER

CHAPTER 29

ANALYSIS OF DAMAGES AND LOSS OF EARNING CAPACITY*

---

* This chapter was prepared by the authors from research conducted by Thomas Czubiak, an economist, of Farmington Hills, Michigan.

§ 29.1   Summary of Costs for Recommended Health Care and Loss of Earning Capacities

Mary Smith is presently classified as having cerebral palsy and spastic quadriplegia requiring daily physical therapy. Notwithstanding the physical therapy, she has contractures of all four extremities with evidence of developing hip dislocations. The prognosis for even standing is very dim.

Mary is able to chew normal foods, but she cannot feed herself. Presently, she is totally dependent on others for all activities, including daily hygiene.

Mary is also diagnosed as microcephalic (small skull from lack of normal brain growth). Accordingly, her potential for learning is in a very limited range.

Notwithstanding the above problems, the prognosis for a normal life span is very good with proper medical care and treatment.

Cost of Health Care by Registered Nurse	$4,789,252
Cost of Service by Physical Therapists	418,503
Cost of Service by Occupational Therapists	158,782
Cost of Service by Speech-Language Pathologists	114,599
Loss of Earning Capacity - Mary Smith	138,392
Other Professional Care	50,000
Total:	$5,669,528

§ 29.2   Periods of Health Care Costs and Loss of Earning Capacities

Nursing Care.   The data available indicate a need for 24 hours, seven days per week care for Mary Smith for the balance of her expected life. At an assumed trial date of January 1, 1986, she will be 3.7 years of age. United States Bureau of the Census data show a life expectancy of 75.7 years at 3 years of age or an additional 72 years of life. This time period is used to project nursing health care.

Therapy.   Based on available data, Mary Smith will require physical, occupational, and speech-language therapy at least three times per week. Accordingly, the cost of such therapy is projected for a period of 72 years.

Loss of Earning Capacity—Mary Smith.   This study assumes that, normally, Mary Smith would begin work as a college graduate at the age of 22 years. The Division of Labor Force Studies of the Bureau of Labor Statistics shows that the women who begin work at age 22 are expected to have 39 years of additional employment throughout their lives. Loss of earnings is computed for the 39 year period.

Other Health Care Costs.   Apart from therapy and home care costs, additional service costs such as nutritional counselling, pediatric care, neurological treatment, and others cannot be projected with accuracy. A flat amount of $50,000 is used in this analysis.

§ 29.3   Billing Rates for Selected Health Care Occupations

Table 29-1 on the next page lists billing rates for selected health care occupations based on 1985 data.

§ 29.4   Methodology Used to Compute Present Values of Future Health Care Costs and Loss of Earning Capacities

The basic problem in establishing the future cost of health care and the loss of earning capacity is to relate those costs and losses to a present fund that would adequately compensate for those future amounts. Future amounts of costs and losses must be discounted to a present amount because a fund established at the present time can be invested to produce income to apply against future cost of services. Future increases in health care costs, which follow the increase in prices and cost of living must be considered in conjunction with the returns that can be realized on the investment of a fund at the present time.

Future increases in health care costs as well as future rates of investment opportunities cannot be forecast with any degree of accuracy. Therefore, the only available approach is to determine past relationships of these two variables and assume that the relationships will continue in the future.

For example, assume that the cost of occupational therapy is $3,000 at the present time. Further, assume that this cost will increase at a rate of 10 percent each year for the next five years and the present yield on corporate Aaa bonds is 10 percent. In this case, the increase in therapy costs will offset the investment discount rate as shown in **Table 29-2**.

Table 29-1
§ 29.3 Billing Rates for Selected Health Care Occupations

	Registered Nurse	Licensed Practical Nurse	Occupational Therapist	Physical Therapist	Speech/Language Pathologist
Upjohn Health Care Services-Bingham Farms	$16.75/hr* 18.50/hr**	$14.05/hr* 15.80/hr**			
Quality Care Nursing Troy	$17.95/hr* 18.95/hr**	$15.00/hr* 17.00/hr**			
Home Health Care, Inc., Southfield			$60.00/visit	$60.00/visit	$60.00/visit
Macomb Health Care, Inc., Warren			$59.00/visit	$58.00/visit	$59.00/visit
Visiting Nurse Association of Metro Detroit-Detroit			$56.00/visit	$56.00/visit	$60.00/visit
Medical Personnel Pool, Southfield			$56.00/visit	$56.00/visit	
Rates Used in This Analysis	$16.75/hr* 18.50/hr**	$14.05/hr* 15.80/hr**	$56.00/visit	$56.00/visit	$59.00/visit

* Weekdays
** Weekends
Rates based on the authors' information in 1985.

Table 29-2

Year	Cost of Occupational Therapy (Increasing at 10% per annum)	Investment/Discount Factor (10%)	Present Value of Therapy Costs
1	$3,000	-	$ 3,000
2	3,300	.9091	3,000
3	3,630	.8264	3,000
4	3,993	.7513	3,000
5	4,392	.6830	3,000
		Total Present Value:	$ 15,000

When both the rate of growth and the discount or interest rate are the same, the two offset each other and the present value can be determined by multiplying the base amount of $3,000 by five years or $15,000 as computed above. If the present investment rate exceeds the rate of growth in costs, assume 11 percent, future costs should be discounted by 1 percent. In this analysis, a growth in costs in excess of the present investment opportunity is considered to be an offset.

It should be noted in the above example, a 10 percent increase in therapy costs and a 10 percent fund investment, will exactly cover future therapy costs by depleting the interest income and principal of the fund as shown in **Table 29-3**.

Table 29-3

Year	Interest Income 10% per annum	Cost of Therapy (Shown above)	Increase/Decrease in Fund	Fund Balance
				$ 15,000
1	$-	$3,000	($3,000)	12,000
2	$1,200	3,300	(2,100)	9,900
3	990	3,630	(2,640)	7,260
4	726	3,993	(3,267)	3,993
5	399	4,392	(3,993)	—

§ 29.5   Cost of Health Care by Licensed Registered Nurses

Billing Rate and Time Period. The billing rates used for registered nurse home health care are $16.75/hr for weekdays and $18.50/hr. for weekends. See § 29.3. The period of required care is 72 years.

Cost Calculation

Weekdays -	24 hours at $14.05/hr. for 261 days	$ 88,009
Weekends -	24 hours at $15.80/hr. for 104 days	39,437
Total Cost Per Year		$ 127,446

Projected Health Care Cost.   As shown in **Table 29-4,** the salaries of professional registered nurses increased by 10.3 percent during the period 1980 through 1983. **Table 29-5** shows an average investment opportunity in corporate Aaa bonds at 13 percent during the same period.

Table 29-4

CALCULATION OF INCREASES IN BASIC MONTHLY SALARIES IN SELECTED OCCUPATIONS

Intermediate Salary Ranges

Occupation	1980	1981	1982	1983	Compounded Annual Increase
Nurse - Professional RN					
- Minimum	$1,214	$1,351	$1,472	$1,472	
- Maximum	1,352	1,810	1,972	1,972	
- Average	1,283	1,581	1,722	1,722	10.3%
Licensed Practical Nurse					
- Minimum	$ 926	$1,091	$1,195	$1,195	
- Maximum	1,091	1,386	1,611	1,611	
- Average	1,009	1,239	1,403	1,403	11.6%
Physical Therapist					
- Minimum	$1,247	$1,429	$1,567	$1,646	
- Maximum	1,498	1,914	2,078	2,189	
- Average	1,373	1,672	1,823	1,918	11.8%
Occupational Therapist					
- Minimum	$1,247	NA	$1,446	$1,526	
- Maximum	1,593	NA	1,923	2,022	
- Average	1,420	NA	1,685	1,774	7.7%
Speech-Language Therapist					
- Minimum	$1,247	$1,332	$1,368	$1,368	
- Maximum	1,498	1,764	1,810	1,810	
- Average	1,373	1,548	1,589	1,589	5%

Source: Michigan Occupational Wage Information
               Michigan Employment Security Commission

Table 29-5

MOODY'S CORPORATE Aaa BOND YIELD AVERAGES

	1980	1981	1982	1983
January	11.09%	12.81%	15.18%	11.79%
February	12.38	13.35	15.27	12.01
March	12.96	13.33	14.58	11.73
April	12.04	13.88	14.46	11.51
May	10.99	14.32	14.26	11.46
June	10.58	13.75	14.81	11.74
July	11.07	14.38	14.61	12.15
August	11.64	14.89	13.71	12.51
September	12.02	15.49	12.94	12.37
October	12.31	15.40	12.12	12.25
November	12.97	14.22	11.68	12.41
December	13.21	14.23	11.83	12.57
Annual Average	11.94%	14.17%	13.79%	12.04%
		Four Year Average		13%

Source: Moody's Bond Record, 1984

Accordingly, the future costs for health care by registered nurses are discounted by the difference of 2.7 percent as follows:

$151,098 times the present value interest factor for 72 years at a 2.7% rate or 31.696331 equals $4,789,252.

§ 29.6   Cost of Health Care by Licensed Practical Nurses

Billing Rate and Time Period.   The billing rates used for licensed practical nurse home health care are $14.05/hr. for weekdays and $15.80/hr. for weekends. The period of required care is 72 years.

Cost Calculation

Weekly Cost:	3 visits at $56.00/visit	$ 168
Cost Per Year:	$168 times 52 weeks	$ 8,736

Projected Health Care Cost.   As shown in **Table 29-4**, the salaries of licensed practical nurses increased by 11.6 percent during 1980 through 1985, as compared to a 13 percent average yield on corporate Aaa bonds for the same period, **Table 29-5**. Future health care costs by licensed practical nurses are discounted by the difference or 1.4 percent as follows:

$127,446 times the present value interest factor for 72 years at a 1.4% rate or 45.092901 equals $5,746,910.

§ 29.7   Cost of Physical Therapy Treatments

Billing Rate and Time Period.   The billing rate used for physical therapy treatment is $56.00 per visit. The period of treatment used is three treatments per week for a period of 72 years.

Cost Calculation

Weekly Cost:	3 visits at $56.00/visit	$ 168
Cost Per Year:	$168 times 52 weeks	$ 8,736

Projected Therapy Cost.   **Table 29-4** shows the basic salaries of physical therapists increasing at a rate of 11.8 percent per annum, compounded. This increase compares with average yields on corporate Aaa bonds of 13 percent for the same 1980-1983 period. Future costs for physical therapy, therefore, are discounted by the difference of 1.2 percent as follows:

$8,736 times the present value interest factor for 72 years at a 1.2% rate or 47.905507 equals $418,503.

§ 29.8   Cost of Occupational Therapy Treatments

Billing Rate and Time Period.   The billing rate used for occupational therapy treatments is $56.00 per visit. The period of treatment used is three visits per week for a period of 72 years.

Cost Calculation

Weekly Cost:	3 visits at $56.00/visit	$ 168
Cost Per Year:	$168 times 52 weeks	$ 8,736

Projected Therapy Cost.   As shown in **Table 29-4**, basic salaries of occupational therapists increased by 7.7 percent during the period 1980 through 1983. This increase compared to average yield on corporate Aaa bonds of 13 percent during the same period. Future costs for occupational therapy are discounted by the difference of 5.3 percent as follows:

$8,736 times the present value interest factor for 72 years at a 5.3% rate or 18.175594 equals $158,782.

§ 29.9   Cost of Speech-Language Therapy Treatments

Billing Rate and Time Period.   The billing rate used for speech-language therapy treatments is $59.00 per visit. The period of treatment used is three visits per week for a period of 72 years.

Cost Calculation

Weekly Cost: 3 visits at $59.00/visit	$ 177	
Cost Per Year: $177 times 52 weeks	$ 9,204	

Projected Therapy Cost.   **Table 29-4** shows an increase in basic salaries for speech-language therapists of 5 percent for the 1980-1983 period or 8 percent below the average of corporate Aaa bonds for the period, **Table 29-5**. Future costs for this therapy are discounted by 8 percent as follows:

$9,204 times the present value interest factor for 72 years at an 8% rate or 12.450977 equals $114,599.

§ 29.10   Loss of Earning Capacity

This report assumes that, based on her parents' economic status and education, Mary Smith would have completed a college program and would begin employment at the age of 22 in the year 2004. Her work life expectancy beyond that period would be 39 years.

Table 29-6 shows United States Census Bureau data which indicate a starting salary for a female college graduate in 1980 at $9,936 per year. The compounded rate of growth during the period 1975 through 1980 was 8.2 percent per year.

Table 29-6

MEDIAN MONEY INCOME OF WHITE FEMALE PERSONS BY
EDUCATIONAL ATTAINMENT - 1975 AND 1980

Educational Level	1975	1980	Compounded Growth Per Annum
Median Income-Total	$ 3,703	$ 5,819	95%
Elementary School:			
Less than 8 years	$ 2,342	$3,725	9.7%
8 years	2,621	4,256	10.2
High School:			
1-3 years	$ 2,997	$ 4,303	7.5%
4 years	4,143	6,048	7.9
College:			
1-3 years	$ 4,238	$ 6,872	10.2%
4 years	6,700	9.936	8.2
5 or more years	10.047	15,042	8.4

Source: U.S. Bureau of the Census, Current Population Reports, series P-60, Nos. 105 and 132

At an approximate 8 percent growth rate per year, the starting salary of $9,936 would increase in 18 years to $39,704 ($9,936 times an interest factor of 3.996019). Since the growth of 8 percent compares to a current investment rate of 11 percent, the future earnings are discounted at 3 percent as follows:

> Present value of an annuity of $39,704 per year for 39 years — $39,704 times an interest factor of 22.808215 equals $905,577.

In order to reach the amount of $905,577 in 18 years, $138,392 would need to be invested at the present time and earn the present available long-term investment rate of 11% for a period of 18 years as follows:

> $905,577 times a discount rate of 11% for 18 years or .152822 equals $138,392.

§ 29.11   Other Professional Care

As indicated previously, additional professional treatment costs such as nutritional counselling, pediatric care, neurological treatment, and others cannot be projected with accuracy. An estimated amount of $50,000 for these services is included in the analysis.

The $50,000 amount is not discounted since available data from the Michigan Employment Security Commission show that the increase per year for these services exceeds the present long-term investment rates of 11 percent to 11.5 percent.

§ 29.12   Health Care Professionals

A description of the qualifications, duties, and responsibilities of various health care professionals is presented in §§ **29.13** through **29.16**. This description for the professionals whose services are being recommended will often add credibility and support for the figures presented. With this description, there should be no question what these professionals will be doing on a daily basis. When the job description is compared with the physical condition of the plaintiff, there should be no question that the recommended services are essential.

§ 29.13   —Occupational Description for Registered Nurses

Duties.   Registered nurses provide care, treatment, counselling, and health education to the ill, injured, and infirm. Duties include:

1. Determining nursing and health needs of patients
2. Carrying out prescribed medical and nursing treatments
3. Teaching and counselling patients and their families
4. Observing and reporting the condition of patients and modifying the plan of care if needed
5. Directing and supervising less skilled health personnel.

Registered nurses may specialize in one of the nursing services such as obstetrics, surgery, psychiatry, cardiac care, or intensive care. They may also work with special types of patients such as children, the aging, the chronically ill, or the physically or mentally handicapped.

Registered nurses may belong to state nursing organizations such as the Michigan Nurses Association and the Michigan National League for Nursing.

Special Requirements.   Registered nurses must meet certain requirements set by each state to practice nursing in that state. All registered nurses in Michigan, for example, must be licensed by the Board of Nursing of the Michigan Department of Licensing and Regulation. Applicants must be at least 18, have completed an approved nursing program, and have passed a written exam.

Education and Training. The required education for entry into the nursing profession includes the following levels of education:

1. A certificate-program of up to one year of study beyond high school
2. An Associate Degree—two years of study beyond high school
3. A Bachelor's Degree—four years of study beyond high school
4. A Master's Degree—five to six years of study beyond high school.

§ 29.14 —Occupational Description for Physical Therapists

Duties. Physical therapy personnel conduct medically prescribed treatment programs for patients to restore function, relieve pain, and prevent disability following disease, injury, or the loss of a body part.

Physical therapists, also known as physiotherapists, plan and administer the treatment programs. Their duties may include:

1. Evaluating the physician's referral and the patient's medical records to determine the physical therapy treatment required
2. Performing patient tests, measurements, and evaluations, such as range-of-motion and manual-muscle tests, gait and functional analyses, and body-parts measurements
3. Conferring with the physician, other therapists, social workers, nurses, and psychologists regarding patient cases
4. Evaluating findings and planning a written treatment program based on available patient data
5. Administering manual therapeutic exercises to improve or maintain muscle function
6. Teaching and motivating patients in nonmanual exercises such as isometrics and practical activities such as walking
7. Administering treatments involving the application of such agents as light, heat, water, and electricity
8. Evaluating the effects of treatments, and durations and adjusting treatments to achieve maximum benefits
9. Administering deep and surface massage techniques

10. Administering traction to relieve neck and back pain
11. Recording patients' treatments, responses, and progress
12. Instructing patients and their families in physical therapy procedures to be continued at home
13. Training patients in the use of prosthetic and orthotic devices and recommending modifications
14. Directing the work of physical therapist assistants and aides.

Although there are no organized specialities, physical therapists may focus their efforts in the treatment of a specific group or disabillity in such areas as general practice, pediatrics, geriatrics, cardiopulmonary, or orthopedics. Physical therapists also may be actively engaged in such areas as research, teaching, consultation, administration, and community health.

Special Requirements.   All states and the District of Columbia require physical therapists to be licensed.   To practice in Michigan, a therapist must be licensed by the Board of Physical Therapy, Michigan Department of Licensing and Regulation.   The therapist must graduate from a board-approved physical therapy program and pass a one-day examination.

§ 29.15   — Occupational Description for Occupational Therapists

Duties.   Occupational therapy personnel conduct specialized therapeutic programs to help individuals with physical, psychological, or developmental problems to regain or improve physical or mental capacities or adjust to physical or mental handicaps.   The scope and objective of each treatment program varies according to individual patient needs and capabilities.   Occupational therapists plan, direct, and coordinate treatment programs.   Depending on the area of work, their general duties may include:

1. Testing and evaluating patients' physical and mental abilities
2. Selecting activities such as manual arts, crafts, homemaking, daily living skills and recreation to fit patients' needs, and capabilities
3. Planning individual therapy programs using selected activities
4. Counselling with other members of the treatment team to confirm that the programs are suitable
5. Teaching skills and techniques needed to do the activities
6. Designing special equipment to aid disabled patients

7. Evaluating patients' progress, attitudes, and behavior
8. Preparing patient progress reports
9. Instructing patients on how to adjust to home, work activities, and the social environment
10. Consulting with local, state, and federal governmental agencies and associations.

Although there are no recognized areas of specialization, occupational therapists usually work with certain types of disabilities and age groups. These therapists may work as staff therapists, senior therapists, supervisors, clinical directors, activity coordinators, administrators, consultants, researchers and educators.

Education and Training. Employers usually require an associate degree or a bachelor's degree for entering this occupation. After students complete the 6 to 9 month clinical practice period and graduate, they may take the examination to become registered occupational therapists.

§ 29.16 — Occupational Description for Speech-Language Pathologists

Duties. Speech-language pathologists are therapists who evaluate and treat speech, language, voice, and fluency disorders of children and adults. The duties of speech-language pathologists may include:

1. Identifying speech, language, voice, and fluency disorders and evaluating causative factors
2. Planning, directing, and conducting therapy for impairments such as aphasia, stuttering, and problems of articulation caused by organic and nonorganic factors
3. Providing guidance and counselling to patients and their families
4. Consulting with other professionals concerned with the patient's welfare, such as physicians, psychologists, physical therapists, social workers, and teachers
5. Referring patients to other specialists if the disorder is diagnosed as not being one of speech and language
6. Recording the method of treatment and the patient's progress
7. Acting as a consultant to educational, medical, and other professional groups

8. Conducting research related to the development of diagnostic and remedial procedures or the design of apparatus

9. Teaching their expertise in colleges and universities.

Speech-language pathologists work with patients who may have other conditions such as hearing impairment, brain injury, cleft palate, mental retardation, and emotional problems. They may specialize in therapy and research in
specific areas of interest.

Special Requirements. The American Speech-Language-Hearing Association offers a certificate of clinical competence in speech-language pathology
and/or audiology to qualified applicants. To qualify for the certificate of
clinical competence individuals must have a master's degree in speech pathology, or its equivalent, complete a nine-month clinical fellowship approved by
the association, and pass a national written examination.

Speech-language pathologists working in elementary or secondary schools
must meet certain state requirements. In Michigan, for example, they must
meet the standard for a teaching certificate and be qualified to work with
handicapped children.

PART V

CASE PREPARATION AND TRIAL EXAMINATION

CHAPTER 30

INITIAL CLIENT INTERVIEW

§ 30.1 Introduction

Often our most reliable source of facts and information, our client, is overlooked. Because of the vast amount of information that is available in the medical records; because of the multitude of depositions that we anticipate taking; and because we sometimes feel our clients are no match for the technical knowledge of the defendant, we often fail to discuss in detail the minute to minute events of labor and delivery from the person who often remembers the most. Pain has a way of engraving events into one's memory. There are few mothers who do not remember in detail the events surrounding the birth of their child.

The client may not have all of the following information at the initial interview. The gaps can be filled from the medical records when they become available. By using this chapter as a guide when evaluating the medical records, a comparison of the client's interview information and the recorded data can be made. When all of this information is extracted from the records, the case is ready for expert review.

The remaining sections in this chapter are suggested areas to cover with the client in the initial interview with a brief explanation, where needed, as to why the information may be helpful. For a more complete discussion of medical topics, consult the **Index** at the end of the book.

§ 30.2   Personal Data

Client Name: First, Middle, Last. The client's name at the time of birth may have been different and should be clarified.

> **Address:**   The client may be living with one parent or in a foster care facility making the address different from the parents.
>
> **Date of Birth:**
>
> **Social Security No.:**   Often medical records are filed under the client's social security number.
>
> **If Deceased, Date of Death:**

Mother's Name: First, Middle and Last. Clarification of the client's last name and the mother's last name can prevent delays when requesting medical records if there has been a name change.

> **Mother's Name as Stated on the Child's Birth Certificate:**   First, Middle and Last.
>
> **Address:**
>
> **Phone Number:**
>
> **Social Security No.:**
>
> **Birth Date:**
>
> **Occupation:**

Father's Name: First, Middle, and Last. If the parents are unmarried, did the father sign the paternity papers?

> **Address:**
>
> **Phone Number:**
>
> **Social Security No.:**

Birth Date:
Occupation:

Date malpractice was first discovered: Oftentimes parents of children with cerebral palsy, for example, will come to an attorney long after the statutory date for medical malpractice has run.   Inquiry should be made regarding the exceptions that often exist for this fixed statutory period.   There may be an exception for minors, as in Michigan, where the minor is given one year from reaching her 18th birthday within to file an action.   There may be a discovery rule for the parents' claim.

List all physicians/hospitals you believe were guilty of negligence/ malpractice:

Address:
Speciality: Are the physicians medical doctors or osteopaths?   Were they board certified specialists such as obstetricians or pediatricians?

Date of Last Treatment: When did the doctor you feel was negligent last care for the child or when was the child last discharged from the hospital that you feel was negligent?   This information is often essential in determining when the statute of limitation would run on the fixed statutory time period. For example, in Michigan the statute of limitation is two years from the last date of treatment.

§ 30.3   Medical Data

Number of pregnancies.   Gravida (G) is the term used on the obstetrical records to count the number of times a woman has been pregnant.   Some complications are more prone to occur in the first pregnancy such as toxemia. Numerous pregnancies ending in miscarriage may result from a preexisting medical condition such as diabetes.

Number of live births.   Para (P) is the term used on the obstetrical records to describe the number of live births.   Not all pregnancies result in the birth of a healthy child.   If the pregnancy results in the birth of a full term infant who is stillborn, the para does not increase.

Abortions.

> **Elective.** Frequent elective abortions can result in damage to the uterus and a tendency toward premature delivery in subsequent pregnancies.
>
> **Spontaneous.** Frequent spontaneous miscarriages may be a sign of maternal disease such as diabetes or uterine deficiencies. An incompetent cervix dilates easily resulting in premature deliveries.

Infertility. Mothers who have treated for infertility may have had an artificial insemination with the use of donor sperm or the husband's sperm. Infertile mothers often take medication to promote conception and maintain the pregnancy once fertilization occurs. The use of medication in the first trimester is always questionable.

Previous Pregnancies. If the patient has had complications in previous pregnancies, it would identify her as a high risk patient. If previous pregnancies have been normal, while the pregnancy in question exhibited numerous complications, the physician should be alerted to these problems.

> **Date/Year.** Frequent closely spaced pregnancies may result in infants of small size. Widely spaced pregnancies may indicate problems with fertility.
>
> **Sex.** Some congenital anomalies, such as hemophelia, are sex linked so it is important to have information regarding the brothers and sisters of the client.
>
> **Doctor/Hospital.** If siblings were delivered by the same doctor, then the doctor has personal knowledge of the mother's obstetrical history. If the siblings were delivered in the same hospital, then the mother's previous charts are available from Medical Records.
>
> **Vaginal/C-Section..** If a mother had delivered vaginally previously it indicates that her pelvis is large enough to accommodate delivery. If she had a previous cesarean section, subsequent deliveries are usually performed by repeat section.
>
> **Length of Labor.** With each successive labor, the length usually telescopes, meaning the classic first labor usually is approximately 12 hours, while the second is 6, and the third labor is nearer to 3 hours. These are approximate guidelines to alert the doctor how soon to anticipate delivery.
>
> **Birth Weight.** If siblings have all been large babies, there is a possibility that the mother exhibits a tendency toward diabetes. If previous pregnancies have resulted in small babies, there is a possibility she is prone to intrauterine growth retardation.

Pregnancy/Delivery Complication.   Some complications are prone to recur such as a difficult delivery from a narrow pelvis while other complications such as fetal distress may be an isolated incident.

Rubella Titer.   This titer is used to evaluate the mother's immunity to German Measles. Mothers who are not immune are in the greatest danger of exposure to the virus during the first three months of pregnancy. Her forming fetus may develop congenital anomalies such as heart defects or blindness.

Herpes.   The presence of genital herpes can be fatal to the newborn if the child is delivered vaginally in the presence of active lesions. Mothers with active herpes are usually delivered by cesarean section.

§ 30.4   First Trimester of Pregnancy

Last Menstrual Period (LMP).   If the date is accurately known, the due date can be easily calculated. Nagele's rule is: To the first day of the last normal menstruation, add seven days, subtract three months, and add one year to obtain expected date of delivery.

Estimated Date of Confinement (EDC).   The length of pregnancy is determined by this date and postmaturity is calculated from it. If the LMP is uncertain, then other obstetrical milestones are used to calculate an approximate date.

Initial Prenatal Visit.   If the patient does not see her physician until the second trimester, the fetus is fully formed and there is little the physician can do to detect or prevent anomalies. A baseline blood pressure is taken on the first visit. Other subsequent blood pressures are measured against this initial reading.

Dates and Results of Ultrasound.   Ultrasounds done early in pregnancy are more accurate than those done closer to term. Serial ultrasound, readings taken a week or month apart are valuable in detecting subtle growth changes.

Prepregnancy Weight.   When the mother is of small physical stature her fetus may suffer from intrauterine growth retardation.

Total Weight Gain.   The weight gain during pregnancy should be at least 15 pounds or more above the prepregnancy weight. A progressive weight gain of

½ to 1 pound per week is considered normal. Large weight gains are often indicative of complications.

Menstrual History. If the mother has a history of a regular menstrual cycle each month, then the obstetrical dates are more accurate. If the last period before conception was different from previous periods, it is possible conception actually occurred the previous month. Occasionally, mothers will have bleeding at the time the fetus implants in the uterus, 14 days following conception and this can be mistaken for a normal menstrual period.

Cycle. 28-30 days is the normal menstrual cycle. Variations in each woman's cycle are usually very slight.

Length. 3-7 days is the usual length of a menstrual period.

Flow. The rate of menstrual flow is a subjective evaluation made by each woman. An unusually heavy flow may actually be a miscarriage at 3 to 4 weeks with little disruption in the menstrual cycle.

Family/Mother's History. The presence of any health problem in the family background will necessitate additional testing during pregnancy. Congenital anomalies may occur which the physician is unable to control. These anomalies often are detectible in the first trimester, allowing the mother the option of elective abortion rather than delivering a defective child.

Diabetes. A family history of diabetes requires a glucose tolerance test during pregnancy to evaluate the possibility of gestational diabetes, which is latent diabetes precipitated by pregnancy with a return to normal following delivery.

Hypertension. The presence of a maternal blood pressure above 140/90 prior to pregnancy or before 20 weeks of gestation constitutes chronic hypertension.

Seizures. Studies suggest a higher incidents of perinatal mortality and congenital anomalies among infants of epileptic women. There is a possibility that anticonvulsive drugs and not the epilepsy may be responsible.

Congenital Anomalies. Certain congenital anomalies such as cleft lip and palate are transmitted genetically. The presence of any anomalies in the maternal or paternal family should be investigated for genetic transmission.

Rh Factor.   An Rh negative mother with an Rh positive child may develop Rh sensitivity as early as the 20th week of pregnancy. Rhogam may be given to counteract this effect. If the father is also Rh negative, there is little chance that a mother will conceive an Rh positive child. The Rh factor of both the mother and father should be obtained.

Nausea and Vomiting.   Morning sickness is an indication of high estrogen level, which is important for a healthy pregnancy. Mothers who experience morning sickness are less likely to abort in the first trimester.

Spotting.   Mothers who spot in the first trimester of pregnancy have a higher incidence of congenital anomalies.

Ultrasound for EDC.   The ultrasound done in the first trimester of pregnancy is accurate to within 10 days of estimating the gestational age of the fetus. This helps to establish an approximate EDC if the obstetrical dates are questionable.

Vitamins and Iron.   Prenatal vitamins and supplemental iron started in the first trimester can prevent maternal anemia and improve fetal formation by increasing the supply of oxygen and nutrients to the developing fetus.

Smoking.   Mothers who smoke an average of 10 cigarettes per day reduce the birth weight of their infant by about 6 ounces. If more than 15 cigarettes are consumed per day, birth weight is reduced by over 10 ounces.

Caffeine.   A high intake of caffeine is thought to contribute to congenital anomalies.

Alcohol.   Alcoholic mothers give birth to infants with a fetal alcohol syndrome, characterized by an abnormal physical appearance. Mothers who ingest an occasional social drink do not experience this problem.

Drugs.   Numerous prescription medications and street drugs result in congenital anomalies. This list of teratogenic drugs is very long. The potential benefits of any medication taken during pregnancy should be measured against the potential risk to the fetus.

Marijuana.   Mothers may continue to smoke marijuana when they are unaware conception has occurred. Marijuana used by both mother and father is thought to alter generic makeup and may increase the incidence of congenital anomalies.

Accident.   Injuries from automobile accidents and falls may be detected by x-rays. Radiation of the fetus in the first trimester of pregnancy can result in congenital anomalies.

Illness.   Maternal infections can attack the fetus and placenta and result in congenital malformations and spontaneous abortions. Bacterial infections may be treated by antibiotics. The TORCH viruses of Toxoplasmosis, Rubella, Cytomegalovirus, and Herpes are known to be destructive to the fetus and the placenta.

§ 30.5   Second Trimester of Pregnancy

Weight Gain.   Large weight gains may be indicative of gestational diabetes or preeclampsia. Lack of weight gain may indicate intrauterine growth retardation (IUGR).

Fetal Movement.   The date that fetal movement is first detected is an obstetrical milestone which confirms the EDC. Quickening usually occurs about the 19th or 20th week in the first pregnancy and a week or two earlier in subsequent pregnancies.

Fetal Heart Tone.   At 10 weeks of pregnancy, fetal heart tones are audible with various electronic listening devices, such as a Doptone. They are strong and regular and can be counted in the second trimester. The physician should record the total number of fetal heart tones counted in one minute on each prenatal visit.

Contractions.   An episode of premature contractions may be caused by some separation of the placenta from the uterine walls. Abruption of the placenta is the premature separation of the placenta before the delivery. A small abruption may subside spontaneously. A complete abruption will result in a fetal death.

Glucose Tolerance Test (GTT).   If there is a family history of diabetes, a glucose tolerance test will rule out the possibility of gestational diabetes. If the mother is obese, has a poor obstetrical history, or has given birth to previous large infants, a glucose tolerance test should be done during pregnancy.

Ultrasound.   In the second trimester an ultrasound may be done to identify the exact location of the placenta. Placenta previa occurs when the placenta is located partially or completely over the cervical opening. Ultrasounds also record fetal growth and rule out the possibility of multiple pregnancy.

Rhogam.   Rh negative mothers should be given Rhogam at 20 weeks of pregnancy to avoid intrauterine sensitization.

§ 30.6   Third Trimester of Pregnancy

Weight Gain.   A weight gain of more than two pounds per week or six pounds per month may indicate the early onset of toxemia.

Illnesses.   Maternal infection including upper respiratory tract infections or urinary tract infections may percipitate premature labor.

Hypertension.   An increase in the systolic pressure of at least 30 mm Hg or a rise in the diastolic pressure of at least 15 mm Hg, or the presence of a systolic presure of at least 140 mm Hg, or a diastolic pressure of at least 90 mm Hg is considered hypertension. These levels must be noted on two occasions at least six or more hours apart and should be evaluated against previously known blood pressure levels.

Swelling.   Edema of the feet may be normal during pregnancy. Edema of the hands or face may be an early sign of toxemia and results from fluid retention.

Spotting.   Spotting in the third trimester may be symptomatic of placenta previa and ultrasound in usually done to detect a low lying placenta. The premature separation of the placenta may also result in painless vagina bleeding.

Contraction.   Braxton-Hicks contractions are the painless contractions mothers experience throughout pregnancy. Painful contractions occurring at regular intervals, getting closer together, and lasting longer could be signs of premature labor. Tocolytic drugs may be used to arrest premature labor in the early stages.

Headache.   Increased blood pressure from toxemia may result in maternal headache and usually occurs in the advanced stages of preeclampsia.

Employment.   Mothers who work until their EDC often experience employment related stress such as dependent edema of the feet if their job requires long hours of sitting or standing. An early leave of absence may be necessary to reduce the detrimental effects of these stresses.

Classes.   Prenatal and Lamaze classes are often provided by the physician or the hospital. They provide physical and psychological conditioning for the parents as they approach labor.

Fetal Movement and Fetal Heart Tone.   Fetal movement usually decreases as labor approaches although fetal heart tone should remain strong and regular. The physician evaluates and records the fetal heart rate and the character of the fetal heart tones at every prenatal visit.

Instructions Regarding Signs and Symptoms of Labor. The physician should instruct the mother regarding what symptoms she should watch for if complications are developing. The physician should instruct the patient regarding the early signs of labor and at what point she wishes to be notified or when the mother should go to the hospital.

Spontaneous Rupture of Membranes/Leaking. Once the membranes rupture, the fetus is no longer in a sterile environment. The danger of infection entering the uterus through the birth canal and infecting the fetus or the placenta is very great. Delivery should take place in 12 to 24 hours.

Post-Maturity. A pregnancy is considered post term after 42 weeks and testing should be performed regularly to determine fetal well being. After 42 weeks of gestation the placenta begins to deteriorate and the amniotic fluid is decreased. The longer the pregnancy goes post-term, the greater are the dangers.

Stress Testing. A fetal activity such as a nonstress test (NST) should be performed at 42 weeks. The oxytocin challenge test (OCT) should be done if the NST is questionable.

§ 30.7 Labor

Time Labor Started. The incidence of fetal distress increases rapidly after 24 hours of labor. It should be recorded in the hospital records when labor began.

Contractions. In preliminary labor, the contractions are mild and infrequent and often, mothers do not know they are truly in labor.

> **Frequency.** Contractions are timed from the beginning of one contraction to the beginning of the next contraction to determine how frequently they are occurring.
>
> **Length.** The length of the contraction is timed from when the mother begins to feel the uterus tighten until it is completely relaxed. This records how long contractions are lasting.
>
> **Type.** Mild type of contractions occur in preliminary labor and increase to strong contractions during the transition period.

Time Physician was Notified. If the patient is unable to contact her physician, she may delay admission to the hospital. Once the mother is admitted to the hospital then the resident doctor or hospital personnel are responsible for notifying her physician of her arrival.

Instructions Received. When a mother notifies her doctor that she is in labor, the doctor may instruct her to remain at home for a period of time or to precede directly to the hospital. These instructions are often critical if the fetus is in distress on admission to the hospital.

Hospital Admission. Patients are often checked in an examining room by a resident physician before they are admitted to the labor and delivery area. The individual who accompanies the patient to the hospital may have a better memory of the events than the mother. If the mother is not in active labor, she may be discharged from the hospital with instructions to return when contractions are closer together or stronger.

> **Date.** The date of the first labor admission may be different from the birth date and should be recorded.
>
> **Time.** Hospital procedures may differ depending upon the time of day that the mother is admitted.
>
> **Attendant.** The name of the individual who accompanied the mother to the hospital and may have a better recollection of the events than she does.
>
> **Examined by Whom.** On admission to the hospital a mother may be examined by someone other than her own physician.
>
> **Examined Where.** Was the mother examined in the doctor's office before admission or was she examined in labor room on admission to the hospital.

Total Length of Labor. Prolonged labor results in fetal distress. When labor exceeds 24 hours, fetal morbidity and mortality is increased.

> **Preliminary Labor.** This phase of labor is marked by cervical dilation from 0 to 3 cm. A patient is not in active labor until she reaches 3 cm. of dilation and 100% effacement.
>
> **Mid-Labor.** This phase of labor is from 3 to 7 cm of cervical dilation. Arrest of labor can occur in the midlabor phase and is identified by a two-hour period in which no progress occurs. The effacement and cervical dilation remains the same, the fetal station does not change in an arrest of labor.

Transition.   This phase is from 7 to 10 cm of cervical dilation. The cervix is completely dilated at 10 cm. Delivery is imminent during transition and no medication should be given at this time, as the infant will be influenced after delivery.

Descent.   The infant leaves the uterus and moves down the birth canal during the period of descent. Two hours is the total time that a mother may push the infant to delivery before operative intervention is necessary. Operative intervention may include a forceps delivery or cesarean section.

Time Fetal Monitor was Applied.   The external monitor can be applied at any stage of labor, but the membranes must be ruptured and the cervix dilated to 3 cm for the internal scalp lead to be applied to the fetal head.

Time Membranes Ruptured.   Once the membranes rupture delivery should take place in 12 to 24 hours to prevent intrauterine infection. A large or small amount of amniotic fluid is abnormal. The presence of meconium in the amniotic fluid of an infant in a vertex presentation may be a sign of fetal distress. Infants in the breech position may excrete meconium from the pressure of uterine contractions.

Artificial Rupture of Membranes (AROM).   The progress of labor can be stimulated by artificially rupturing membrane to increase the pressure of the fetal head on the cervical opening. The physician should not rupture the membranes until she is certain the mother is in active labor to avoid having them ruptured for a prolonged period.

Appearance of Amniotic Fluid.   The fluid that surrounds the infant in the uterus is normally clear. If it is green tinged it may indicate the presence of meconium, a sign of fetal distress.

Amount of Amniotic Fluid.   A small amount of thick amniotic fluid may indicate that the infant is post mature.

Intravenous Medications.   Intravenous fluids prevent maternal dehydration during the course of a lengthy labor. Drugs administered intravenously pass through the fetal circulation within three minutes.

Induction.   Labor may be stimulated by the administration of Pitocin. A physician should be present in the labor and delivery area for a pitocin induction.

Monitor.   The fetal heart tone should be monitored for several minutes to establish a base line before any medication is given. Fetal monitoring should be continuous throughout the induction to detect fetal distress.

Infusion Pump.   An infusion pump is a monitoring device used to count intravenous fluid drops. It is used to monitor the dose of medication a mother receives. A pitocin induction is usually started with 2 to 3 drops-per-minute and increased every 15 minutes until contractions are occurring.

Physician's Presence.   The private physician may not be present until the late stages of labor. Preliminary and midlabor may be supervised by a resident. When no resident is available, the private physician should be present sooner.

Analgesic.   Pain medications given to a mother in labor are detectible in the fetal circulation within 3 minutes and may continue to depress the infant's respiration long after delivery. Narcotics may inhibit efforts to establish spontaneous respirations following birth.

Bleeding.   The pink tinged amniotic fluid is normal after membranes are ruptured. Scant bleeding from the pressure on small blood vessels in the cervix is responsible for this. Bright bleeding may be the result of an abruption or placenta previa.

Mother's Awareness of Vital Signs.   The patient has a right to be informed of the progress she is making during labor. The opening of the cervix (dilation and effacement) and the advancement of the fetus (position and station) will often have a strong influence on the fetal heart tones.

Dilation.   The opening of the external cervical os is expressed in centimeters. When the cervix is fully dilated it is at 10 cm.

Effacement.   The obliteration of the internal opening of the cervix is called effacement. The uneffaced cervix is 2 to 3 cm long. When it has shortened a ½ it is 50 percent effaced. When the internal opening is completely obliterated, effacement is 100 percent.

Position.   Infants usually deliver in the vertex or head first position. The infant is in a breech position when it is coming buttock or feet first. The head is the largest diameter to be delivered. It is dangerous for the head to be delivered last.

Station.   The level of the fetal head in the maternal pelvis is expressed as station. When the most dependent part of the head is at the level of the ischial spines, the station is referred to as zero. Levels of -1, -2, or -3 cm mean the head is not engaged in the maternal pelvis. Levels of +1, +2, or +3 cm indicate that the head has passed through the ischial spines in preparation for delivery. Each station is the approximate equivalent of one centimeter.

Fetal Heart Tones.   FHTs should be checked every 15 minutes in active labor if electronic fetal monitoring is not used.

Pushing.   The descent of the fetus through the birth canal is the most hazardous position of labor and is strongly influenced by the mother's ability to push. Mother should not begin pushing until cervical dilation is complete. Two hours is the longest a mother should push before operative intervention with forceps or cesarean section.

Crowning.   The appearance of fetal scalp at the vaginal opening indicates that delivery is imminent. If regional anesthesia, such as a spinal is to be used, it is to be given when the fetus is crowning so there is no interference with the mother's ability to push.

Time to Transfer to the Delivery Room.   A delay in the performance of the delivery following a transfer of the mother can result in fetal distress. Haste during the transfer may be indicative of emergency conditions.

Pelvimetry.   During arrest of labor, pelvimetry (x-ray of pelvis) may be performed to detect the presence of pelvic disproportion. Cephelopelvic disproportion (CPD) exists when the diameter of the infant's head is greater than any diameter of the maternal pelvis.

§ 30.8   Vaginal Delivery

Anesthesia.   Regional anesthesia such as a spinal may influence the mother's ability to deliver the infant by pushing. It should not be administered until the head is crowning. Local anesthesia is not necessary for the performance of an episiotomy.

Episiotomy.   The incision made to enlarge the vaginal opening is made in the skin between the vagina and the rectum. If a large episiotomy is needed to reduce trauma for a premature infant or a very large baby, the episiotomy can be extended to the right or left buttock to avoid extension of the incision into the rectum.

Physician who Delivers. If the patient's physician is not an obstetrician, it may be necessary for the physician to obtain a consultation with an obstetrician if problems are encountered during the labor or delivery. Most hospitals have a policy requiring the presence of an obstetrician for any type of operative delivery.

Forceps. The use of any type of instrument other than outlet forceps increases the risk of birth trauma. Mid or high forceps are considered operative delivery and should only be done by an obstetrician with considerable experience.

Presentation. The smooth, round crown of the infant's head passes through the birth canal with the least resistance and is usually delivered first. Infants who deliver in any other position other than the occiput anterior have a greater incident of arrest of labor and birth trauma.

Remark Made by Personnel. Often a chance remark made by someone in the delivery room is the first indication to the mother that something is wrong.

§ 30.9 Cesarean Section Delivery

Repeat C-Section. Mothers who have delivered previous infants by cesarean section are scheduled for repeat ones to avoid rupture of the uterine scar during labor. Some obstetricians are allowing cesarean section mothers to have a trial of labor if the previous C-section was done for fetal distress or breech presentation rather than cephalopelvic disproportion. If the mother's pelvis was too small to delivery vaginally the first time, she will always have this problem.

Emergency C-Section. If there is evidence of fetal distress or hemorrhage, an emergency cesarean section should be performed. Depending on the level of competency of the hospital, an emergency C-section can be performed in 15 to 30 minutes if emergency personnel are available. Cesarean section for breech presentation and cephelopelvic disproportion are not considered emergencies if there is no evidence of fetal distress.

Physicians who Performed Surgery.   If the patient's physician is a general practitioner, the physician may not be a surgeon and therefore will require that assistance of an obstetrician or a surgeon to perform the cesarean section.

Pediatrician in the Delivery Room.   For most C-sections, but particularly an emergency C-section, a pediatrician in the delivery room is essential to care for the infant after delivery.

Amount of Time Required for Surgery.   In an emergency C-section, the infant can be delivered within five minutes after the initial skin incision is made. Further delays are related to the preparation of the operating room and availability of personnel.

§ 30.10   The Newborn

Apgar Score.   The infant is given a score from 0 to 2 in the areas of heart beat, respirations, muscle tone, reflexes and color.   It is a good indication of the status of the infant at birth and within five minutes of birth.   The maximum score is 10,   Most infant receive a 9 as their hands and feet continue to remain somewhat cyanotic.

Birth Weight.   High birth weight may be an indication of gestational diabetes.   Low birth weight in the full term infant may be a sign of intrauterine growth retardation.   A premature infant has low birth weight as well as reduced gestational age.

Cry.   Failure of the infant to cry spontaneously after birth may be an indication of asphyxia or fetal depression.   Normally infants cry spontaneously once mucus is suctioned from the nose and mouth.

Cord Around the Neck.   The normal umbilical cord is two to three feet long and somewhat elastic.   If it is wrapped around the neck, it can be removed without difficulty after the head is delivered but before delivery of the body is complete.

Resuscitation.   Prolonged asphyxiation requiring extensive resuscitation both in the delivery room and in the nursery may result in central nervous system damage.

Resuscitator. If a pediatrician is available in the delivery room, the pediatrician assumes the responsibility for the resuscitation. In his absence, the anesthesiologist or nurse anesthetist might assume this responsibility. If the mother's condition is stable, the obstetrician could also offer assistance. If no one else is available, the resident or nurses might have to assume this responsibility.

How Long Did Resuscitation Take. If resuscitation is initiated quickly and performed effectively, it is possible that adequate profusion of the infant's tissues can prevent central nervous system damage.

Why Was it Required. Fetal distress in labor, meconium aspiration, or respiratory depression from narcotics are all reasons for delayed respirations at birth.

Infant's Appearance. The normal infant is pink faced with flexed arms and legs, spontaneous respirations and a lusty cry. A limp, cyanotic infant with a poor cry and gasping respirations strongly indicates fetal distress.

Medications Given. Narcan or similar medication to counteract the effects of narcotics may be given to the infant in the delivery room to combat respiratory distress. Sodium bicarbonate may also be given to counteract acidosis from anoxia.

Injuries Suffered by Infant. Manipulations in the birth canal may result in skin abrasions or broken bones. A fractured clavicle may occur while attempting to manipulate the shoulders of a large infant out of the birth canal.

§ 30.11 Nursery Admission

Newborn Nursery. Infants are transported to the nursery in an incubator for warmth. Usually they are assessed by the nursery nurse. An admission physical or an admission assessment form are usually part of the newborn records and provide an accurate evaluation of the infant following delivery.

Newborn Intensive Care Unit (NICU). Infants with low Apgar scores should be admitted directly to the NICU for specialized, critical care by experienced personnel. If the hospital does not have an NICU, arrangements are made for the infant to be transported to a hospital with those facilities.

Date Parents First Aware of Injury.   Infants with central nervous system damage may not exhibit symptoms for two or three days at which time tremors or seizures may occur.   Parents may be unaware of any damage until the child starts missing developmental milestones in infancy.

§ 30.12   Subsequent Care

Doctors Who Have Treated the Infant Since Delivery.   Records from speciality doctors such as pediatricians or neurologists may help to establish the cause of the client's injuries.

Hospital Admissions Since Delivery.   Children with cerebral palsy, for example, are prone to other medical problems and frequently have a long list of hospital admissions.   The records from these admissions provide an accurate picture of the child's subsequent development.

Clinic Care.   If the family is indigent, it is possible the child's medical care was provided by a clinic associated with the hospital or university.

School/Early Intervention Program.   Once a diagnosis of a birth injury is made, the family is usually referred to a social worker through the county or state.   The child is often enrolled in an early intervention program through the school district in an effort to develop his full potential.

> **Psychologist.**   Psychological testing will be performed on the child and evaluations of the parents will be made.   These reports are usually included with the school records.
>
> **Physical Therapy.**   A therapist may be provided through the school program or may visit the home through the Public Health Department.   Efforts are made to improve the child's mobility and prevent contractures.
>
> **Occupational Therapy.**   The therapist will assist in obtaining devices such as specialized wheelchairs which will facilitate the care of the infant.
>
> **Surgery Performed.**   Operative intervention may make it easier to care for the child by releasing muscles but it does not improve the cerebral palsy.
>
> **Genetic Counseling.**   Parents should have genetic counseling to determine if there is a possibility of a subsequent child suffering from the same injuries as the client.
>
> **TORCH Studies.**   Toxoplasmosis, Rubella, Cytomegalovirus, and Herpes are maternal diseases which can be detected in the newborn to determine if the birth injury resulted from them.

Chromosone Studies.   Chromosonal defects in the parents may be responsible for the abnormality the child suffers. Studies should be performed to rule out this possibility.

§ 30.13   Assessments of Damages

Mobility.   Spastic cerebral palsy and other birth injuries severely limits the amount of mobility a child will have. Often these children are unable to ambulate and are confined strictly to a specialized wheelchair.

Verbal.   Difficulty with muscle control in the face and mouth makes it difficult for the child to verbalize effectively.

Social.   Behavior problems can result from the frustration the child experiences. If the child is volatile it makes it difficult to provide therapy.

I.Q.   It is difficult to test intelligence due to the child's limited ability to communicate. Specialized testing must be utilized.

Prognosis.   Some limitations can be improved with surgery or various types of therapy so that the client's life span may be improved. The physical and mental potential may be severely limited.

Who is the Primary Care Giver.   Often the client requires so much physical care that the parents are unable to accomplish this alone, and the child is institutionalized or placed in a foster home.

How are Expenses Covered.   The client may be receiving state aid or expenses may be covered by a private insurance. The Crippled Children's Society often aids the parents with financial assistance.

CHAPTER 31

BIRTH TRAUMA INTERROGATORIES

§ 31.1   Introduction

§ 31.2   Questions and Comments

§ 31.1   Introduction

The philosophy of interrogatory use in a birth trauma case is not substantially different from any other medical malpractice action. One must always weigh the benefit of the efficiency obtained in the use of interrogatories against the spontaneous, less prepared answer obtained by way of deposition testimony. We will not reiterate here the standard questions that are often used in a medical malpractice action, but attempt to provide some of the more specific questions used in birth injury cases with a brief comment, where applicable, regarding the reason for the question.

§ 31.2   Questions and Comments

Q1. Please state the name(s), address and job title of the person answering these Interrogatories and all person(s) who assisted in gathering the substance information for same.

Comment: Oftentimes the administrator of a hospital will sign answers to interrogatories submitted to the defendant hospital, but there may be additional people who actually provided the information for the answers. These individuals may be in charge of the labor and delivery area, nursery, newborn intensive care unit, or simply a knowledgable head nurse. Whoever these individuals are, they are often potential deponents, especially when there is conflict between the answers to interrogatories and the deposition testimony.

Q2.   Please state the total number of inpatient beds at the Defendant Hospital at the time of the Plaintiff Minor's delivery.

Comment: The above question is of assistance if there is a community or locality standard of practice applicable such as the situation where a general practitioner performed the delivery. In such situations, it is often necessary to show that the plaintiff's independent expert practices in a similar locality. Establishing that plaintiff's expert practices at a hospital with a similar number of beds assists in laying this foundation.

Q3.   State the total number of labor beds available at the hospital at the time in question. With respect to said labor beds, state the number of patients occupying said beds during the time that Plaintiff was confined to the labor room during the admission in question.

Comment: The above information is usually available through a labor log that is kept in the labor area. This answer permits one to make a comparison, when coupled with subsequent answers to interrogatories and deposition testimony, of the ratio of hospital personnel to the number of patients in labor. This, of course, can be a value where there is understaffing of hospital personnel in the labor area.

Q4.   State the total number of delivery rooms available at the hospital at the time in question. With respect to said delivery rooms, state:
   (a)   The total number of deliveries accomplished in each room in the two hours preceeding the delivery in question;
   (b)   The time(s) for each delivery;
   (c)   Whether any of the above deliveries were by cesarean section, and if so, identify each.

Comment: The above information may have many functions. It may demonstrate that the delivery room was not available. If there were a cesarean section performed shortly before the time the plaintiff alleges the same should have been accomplished as to the plaintiff, it will demonstrate the availability of the personnel to perform such a procedure.

Q5.   Please state the total number of bassinets and isolettes available at the Defendant Hospital at the time of the Plaintiff Minor's delivery.

Comment: The above information will give the plaintiff's pediatric, neonatologist, or pediatric neurologist expert an idea of the facilities available at the defendant hospital in evaluating the appropriateness of the neonatal care.

Q6.   State the total number of births per year, at the Defendant Hospital for each of the five full years immediately preceding the Plaintiff Minor's birth. With respect to said birth, state:

   (a)   The total number of said births which were by way of elective cesarean section;

   (b)   The number of births that were by emergency cesarean section.

Comment: The above information is again an indication of the experience at the defendant hospital, and in particular, as to emergency cesarean sections.

Q7.   State the facility level classification for the Defendant Hospital with respect to deliveries and neonatal care (i.e., level I, II, or III) at the time of Plaintiff Minor's delivery, and state the facilities or services that the Defendant Hospital could not provide that would have entitled them to the next highest classification level in the event they were not a level III hospital.

Comment: The American College of Pediatricians has classified nurseries with Level I being the lowest and least equipped to handle high risk deliveries and Level III being those hospitals with the neonatal intensive care unit. This information is valuable if the delivery is expected to be high risk. In those instances, the defendant should anticipate the need for the neonatal intensive care unit, and if one is not available in the defendant hospital, the patient should be transferred to a hospital where those facilities are readily available so the anticipated depressed infant can be properly treated.

Q8.   State whether there were any "facilities," as used in Mich. Com. Laws Ann. § 600.2912a(b), which were not available to the Defendants, or reasonably available in the community, which would have been utilized in the care and treatment of the Plaintiff(s) had they been available. If so, state:

   (a)   The particular facility, equipment, instrument, device or other technology that was not available;

   (b)   How and when the Defendant would have utilized that as stated above;

   (c)   What information or results Defendant reasonably anticipates would have been obtained with the use of the above facilities, equipment, instrument, device or other technology.

Comment: This question has specific reference to a Michigan statute which in part provides that even with a specialist, the standard of practice must take into consideration the available facilities. That may well be the law in jurisdictions even without such a statute. The defendant can take the position that in an emergency that arose which was unexpected, and they acted appropriately in light of the equipment and facilities available to them. This question attempts to anticipate defenses and provides information that the plaintiff's expert must have before rendering an intelligent, informed opinion.

Q9. State whether an "apgar scoring" was performed on the Plaintiff Minor in the within matter. If so, state:
- **(a)** The position, title, or job description of each individual performing an "apgar scoring";
- **(b)** The specific time or period of time during which each of the above persons performed their individual "apgar scoring";
- **(c)** Whether each of the above "apgar scoring" was recorded, and if so, identify the time when each was recorded.

Comment: More frequently than anticipated, the apgar scoring is optimistic in favor of the defendants. Accordingly, the individual who performs the apgar scoring is almost always deposed. This question identifies an individual.

Q10. State whether there were any written rules, procedures or protocol, at the time in question, at the Defendant Hospital when the Plaintiff was admitted for labor and delivery with respect to *required consultation* on an obstetrical patient. If so, state:
- **(a)** The substance of this written rule, procedure or protocol;
- **(b)** All places where said document is located (i.e., Medical Staff By-Laws, Medical Staff Rules and Regulations, Nursing Manual, etc.).

Q11. State whether there were any written rules, procedures or protocol, at the time in question at the Defendant Hospital when the Plaintiff was admitted to labor and delivery with respect to *recommended consultation* on an obstetrical patient. If so, state:
- **(a)** The substance of this written rule, procedure or protocol;
- **(b)** All places where said document is located (i.e., Medical Staff By-Laws, Medical Staff Rules and Regulations, Nursing Manual, etc.)

Comment: Regarding the above two interrogatories, certain states have public health code regulations which require consultation, and that the necessity for consultation in certain situations be in writing. In addition, the American College of Obstetricians and Gynecologists has guidelines as to when consultation should be obtained. These interrogatories attempt to determine whether those regulations and recommendations have been incorporated by the hospital into their rules, regulations, and procedures.

Q12. State the name and last known address of each person in the labor room for the labor in question. With respect to each, state:
- **(a)** Their position, title, or job description;

(b) The duties and responsibilities that they in fact performed during the labor in question.

Q13. State the name and last known address of each person in the delivery room for the delivery in question. With respect to each, state:

(a) Their position, title, or job description;

(b) The duties and responsibilities that they in fact performed during the delivery in question.

Comment: Regarding the above two interrogatories, most, if not all, of the above individuals will ultimately be deposed. The answer to this interrogatory will usually establish the list of initial depositions that must be taken.

Q14. State whether it was the policy of the hospital at all times relevant hereto to comply with the standards as promulgated by the Joint Commission on Accreditation of Hospitals.

Q15. State whether the hospital herein requested certification from the Joint Commission on Accreditation of Hospitals within the last ten years, and if so, state each year that said certification request was made. With respect to the above request, state:

(a) Whether the hospital was certified by the Joint Commission on Accreditation of Hospitals for each of the above requests. If there were any deficiencies relating to the Obstetrical and Gynecological Department, Department of Surgery and/or Department of Pediatrics for each or any of the requested certifications, state:

  (i) The specific deficiency;

  (ii) The correction recommended by the Joint Commission on Accreditation of Hospitals;

  (iii) Whether said deficiency was corrected and when;

  (iv) The date the corrected deficiency obtained subsequent certification, if applicable.

Comment: The above two interrogatories attempt to identify deficiencies in the hospitals' policies and procedures in the Department of Obstetrics and Gynecology, Surgery and Pediatrics as established by the Joint Commission of Accreditation of Hospitals. If the hospital is an Osteopathic Institution, the interrogatory would relate to the American Osteopathic Hospital Associations' Committee on Hospital Accreditation.

Q16. State whether a fetal heart monitor was utilized during the labor and/or delivery in question. If so, state:

(a) The model and/or manufacturer's name of the monitor used;

(b)   Whether there was a formal written order to use the fetal heart monitor, and if so, the name of the person writing such an order and the date and time ordered;

(c)   Whether fetal heart monitor tapes were made at the time the fetal heart monitor was originally connected and started monitoring the fetal heart tones;

(d)   The time the fetal heart monitor originally started monitoring the fetal heart tones and the time it was disconnected, including therein the times when it was stopped and restarted, if applicable;

(e)   Whether fetal heart monitor tapes were produced by said monitor at all times during its use, and if not, the specific time the tapes were produced during its use;

(f)   Whether all the fetal heart monitor tapes were originally produced or maintained and are presently available, and if not, state:

   (i)   The times that are not available;

   (ii)   Specifically why the above times are not kept as a permanent record;

   (iii) If they were kept for a period of time, and discarded, when they were discarded and on whose order.

Comment: This question oftentimes provides a wealth of necessary information. Fetal heart monitors may vary from manufacturer to manufacturer, determining the particular manufacturer, and subsequently obtaining their publications should assist in obtaining a thorough understanding of the monitor and the tapes produced. Further, although most hospital personnel note on the fetal monitor tape the time the monitoring commences, on occasion this is omitted. Oftentimes there are stops and starts in the tape and the times are not recorded. This interrogatory hopefully will permit the attorney to correlate the specific information on the tapes with the clinical observations and other notations on the chart.

Q17. State whether there were any written rules, by-laws, procedures, guidelines or other documents which relate to when and how the fetal heart monitor should be used, at the time in question. If so, state:

(a)   The name and/or description of the place(s) where said document(s) is maintained;

(b)   The date the document was originally authored;

(c)   The author of the original document;

(d)   Whether said document has been amended since originally authored, and if so, state:

   (i)   The date(s) amended;

   (ii)   The author who made each amendment.

(e)   State verbatim, word for word, the content of each of the above documents, or in the alternative, attach copies.

Comment: Since electronic fetal heart monitoring is an innovation of the last decade, many obstetrical departments have internal guidelines and procedures for their use. The existence of these documents may be valuable in examining the people using the monitor. Their absence, when coupled with an absence of knowledge of the proper use of the monitor by hospital personnel may be of assistance in establishing hospital responsibility.

Q18. If a fetal heart monitor was utilized in the within labor, state the name and last known address of each person responsible for monitoring or watching the monitor and/or monitor strips to determine whether the fetal heart tracings and/or material tracings were within acceptable medical limits. With respect to each of the above individuals, state:

(a) Specifically the formal training each received in fetal heart monitoring and/or fetal heart monitoring tape interpretation;

(b) The title, place and date of each lecture, seminar, meeting or other conference attended with respect to fetal heart monitoring and fetal heart monitoring tape interpretation;

(c) The group, organization or individual(s) who organized and presented each of the above lectures, seminars, meetings or conferences;

(d) The number of hours and/or days each of the above lectures, seminars, meetings and/or conferences lasted, and the number of days and/or hours each of the above individuals attended each;

(e) Whether any written material was provided at any of the above lectures, seminars, meetings and/or conferences, and if so, state:

  (i) Describe all written material by title of subject matter and author;

  (ii) Whether the individuals still have copies of said materials, and if so, identify the individuals, and the materials they still retain.

Comment: Again, since the electronic monitor is an innovation in this country of the last decade, many people assigned the responsibility of monitoring the tapes lack the necessary education and training to appreciate the significance of the recordings. This question may assist in establishing that lack of experience or knowledge. The interrogatory is often more effective than asking the same question at the time of deposition where the response is vague and often equivocal.

Q19. State the name and last known address of every Board Certified obstetrician/gynecologist who had staff privileges at the Defendant Hospital at the time of the Plaintiff Minor's birth.

Q20. State the name and last known address of every Board Certified pediatrician who had staff privileges at the Defendant Hospital at the time of Plaintiff Minor's birth.

Q21. State the name and last known address of every Board Certified neonatologist who had privileges at the Defendant Hospital at the time of Plaintiff Minor's birth.

Q22. State the name and last known address of every Board Certified perinatologist and/or fetal medicine specialist who had privileges at the Defendant Hospital at the time of the Plaintiff Minor's birth.

Comment: The above four questions establish what specialists were available at the defendant hospital for consultation and assistance with a high risk pregnancy and distressed newborn.

Q23. State the specific time that the Plaintiff Minor was transferred from the delivery room, and the specific time (s)he arrived in the nursery. With respect to that time in the interim, state:

(a) Where the newborn infant was;

(b) The name and last known address of each individual who was caring for the newborn in this interim;

(c) The position, title or job description of each of the above referred to individuals;

(d) What care, treatment or other services were rendered to the newborn by each of the above referred to individuals in this interim time period.

Comment: In a depressed newborn, the transfer from the delivery room to the nursery or neonatal intensive care unit should be prompt and with sufficient staff and equipment to insure that the infant is properly cared for in transition. If the infant is described as being more depressed in the nursery than the description in the delivery room, it may be due to an unduly long transfer time and/or lack of appropriate medical attention during the transfer.

Q24. Please state the name and last known addresses of the Head Nurse, and Nursing Supervisors, of labor and delivery at the time the Plaintiff Mother was admitted to the Defendant Hospital.

Comment: These are additional people who may be deposed, depending upon the deposition testimony of the individuals actually involved in the care and treatment of the mother and infant.

Q25. State whether there was any written protocol at the Defendant Hospital at the time of the delivery in question with respect to resuscitation and subsequent care and treatment of a depressed newborn. If so, state:

(a) The date(s) that protocol was established and the date(s) amended thereafter if applicable;

(b) The author(s) of said protocol(s);

- (c) When, and/or how, this protocol was made available to the medical and nursing staff;
- (d) State verbatim, word for word, the contents of each protocol, or in the alternative, attach a copy.

Q26. State the name and/or description of each and every instrument, other piece of equipment, or material that was available *in the delivery room* at the time of Plaintiff Minor's birth to resuscitate newborns. With respect to each, state:
- (a) If it was used;
- (b) The time it was used;
- (c) The name of the person(s), and their job description or position, who utilized each of the above.

Q27. State the name and/or description of each and every instrument, other piece of equipment, or material that was available *in the nursery* at the time of the Plaintiff Minor's birth to resuscitate newborns. With respect to each, state:
- (a) If it was used;
- (b) The time it was used;
- (c) The name of the person(s), and their job description or position, who utilized each of the above.

Comment: The above three interrogatories provide background information to depose the individuals who cared for the depressed newborn in the delivery room and nursery.

Q28. State whether there were any written rules, by-laws, procedures, guidelines or other written instructions posted or otherwise displayed in the labor and delivery area with respect to the use of Pitocin at the time in question. If so, state:
- (a) The date said rule(s), procedure(s), guideline(s), protocol(s) or other written instruction(s) was originally posted;
- (b) Specify each and every location where posted;
- (c) Specifically how posted, and if by sign, the dimensions of same;
- (d) State verbatim, word for word, the information as contained on each sign or posting.

Comment: Some states have public health regulations with respect to posting in the labor and delivery area guidelines for Pitocin or Oxytocin use.

Q29. State whether there were any complications, abnormalities or other factors during the prenatal care which contributed to or was a direct cause of any of the Plaintiff Minor's subsequent problems. If so, state:
- (a) The specific complicating factor or abnormality;
- (b) The date when each of the above first manifested itself;
- (c) How it first manifested itself (i.e., physical exam, lab test, etc.);

    (d) What treatment if any, was rendered in an attempt to abate or eliminate said complication or abnormality.

Q30. State whether the Defendant has any information or opinion(s) that the cause of the Plaintiff Minor's injuries are due to some other factors other than alleged in the Plaintiff's Complaint. If so, state:

    (a) Each and every fact or opinion(s) which may relate Plaintiff Minor's condition to some factor(s) other than as contained in Plaintiff's Complaint;

    (b) The individual(s) who may testify or provide information with respect to each of the above.

Comment: The above two interrogatories are an attempt to ferret out potential defense positions as to the cause of the plaintiff's minor's injury.

Q31. State whether blood gas studies were performed on the newborn infant while at the Defendant Hospital. If so, state:

    (a) The date and time the blood was drawn for each test;

    (b) The time the results were reported for each test;

    (c) The results of each test, and the range of normal for each for the hospital lab.

Comment: The exact time blood was drawn from blood gas studies must be correlated with the clinical treatment. For example, the pH may appear artifically high if the blood for the gas studies was drawn after sodium bicarbonate was administered. The information may not be in the medical records, but should be recorded in the lab log books.

Q32. State whether there was telephone contact between the attending physician and those persons monitoring the Plaintiff Mother's labor after the latter was admitted to the hospital. If so, state:

    (a) The date and time of each telephone contact;

    (b) The person initiating the call;

    (c) All parties who took part in each call;

    (d) The length of time each telephone call lasted;

    (e) Any and all information conveyed by and between the parties, and identify which party conveyed what information.

Comment: Telephone calls between the nurses, interns, or residents and the attending physician are sometimes an indication of a change in the status of the labor. More importantly, these calls help establish who was taking responsibility for labor and who was making the final decisions.

Q33. State the name and last known address of each resident, intern, registered nurse, LPN or other individual, other than the attending physician, who examined the Plaintiff Mother while the latter was in labor at Defendant Hospital. With respect to each, state:

(a) The date and shift each of the above individuals would have had contact with the Plaintiff Mother.

Comment: Again, this question identifies people who may need to be deposed.

Q34. Please state the names of all members of the governing Board at the Defendant Hospital at the time of the Plaintiff Minor's birth, and today.

Comment: Depending upon the size of the community, this question often provides information utilized in voir dire.

Q35. State where cesarean sections could have been performed at the Defendant Hospital at the time of the delivery in this action (i.e., labor room, delivery room, and/or operative suite).

Q36. With respect to each and every location where cesarean sections could have been performed, state:

(a) The number of people and job identification or description necessary to perform the cesarean section;

(b) The specific act and/or acts needed to prepare each of the above locations for cesarean section;

(c) Assuming all personnel are available in the hospital, the average amount of time it would take to prepare each of the above referred to areas and have the people available to commence the cesarean section from the time the notice is given until the time the procedure commences.

Comment: These two questions provide information with respect to the speed within which the cesarean section could be performed. Smaller hospitals may not be able to perform cesarean sections anywhere other than the operating suite. Some physicians take the position that they will not perform a cesarean section unless they have a full operative team. The time within which a cesarean section can be performed may be important to the plaintiff's proximate cause of proofs.

CHAPTER 32

DIRECT EXAMINATION OF EXPERTS

§ 32.1 Direct Examination of an Obstetrical Expert Regarding Pitocin, Preeclampsia, Post-maturity, and Cesarean Section

Direct Examination by Mr. Stanley Schwartz:

Q: May I have your full name, please.

A: Tom Raymond.

Q: What is your profession or occupation?

A: I am a physician.

Q: Duly licensed to practice in the State of Michigan?

A: Yes, sir.

Q: And would you kindly tell us what states you are duly licensed to practice in other than the State of Michigan?

A: New York State and California.

Q: How long have you been licensed to practice medicine in the State of Michigan?

A: Since 1960.

Q: And have you practiced continuously from that date to the present?

A: Yes, sir.

Q: From what medical school did you graduate?

A: University of Michigan.

Q: And what year did you graduate from University of Michigan?

A: 1959.

Q: And where did you take your undergraduate work?

A: The University of Chicago.

Q: After completing medical school, did you take an internship?

A: Yes, sir.

Q: And where did you take that internship?

A: Ford Hospital.

Q: And what specifically is an internship?

A: Well, an internship in the days that I took my internship was a rotation, 12-month rotation, through a series of subspecialties in medicine, and it was a requirement in those days for licensure.

Q: Is that a one-year program?

A: One-year program, yes.

Q: So when you indicate a rotating internship, you are referring to being involved in disciplines other than obstetrics?

A: That is correct, yes.

Q: And do those disciplines include areas of specialty such as pathology?

A: Pathology, ophthalmology, surgery, emergency room, urology, neurology, psychiatry.

Q: And after completing your internship did you take a residency?

A: Yes, I did.

Q: And would that be immediately after completing your internship?

A: That is correct.

Q: And what is a residence program?

A: Well, a residency is a period of training preparing someone for a specialty practice.

Q: And by a specialty practice, are you referring to an area such as obstetrics and gynecology?

A: That is correct, yes.

Q: And where did you take your residency?

A: Also at Ford Hospital.

Q: In the course of your studies, did you learn about the anatomy of the brain?

A: Yes.

Q: Of the central nervous system of the fetus?

A: Yes.

Q: Did you study the female reproductive system?

A: Yes, sir.

Q: How long was the obstetrical program?

A: Three years.

Q: And that is a three-year concentrated course of study in obstetrics and gynecology?

A: Yes. Well, it was actually a four-year concentrated course, but since I had a year of pathology before I went, I did a three-year program.

Q: Could you tell us what the field of obstetrics deals with.

A: Well, it encompasses the care of pregnant females with a view toward guiding them through a pregnancy safely with a resultant healthy baby and mother.

Q: Is that one of the cardinal responsibilities of the obstetrician, to guide the mother and fetus through the prenatal period to ultimate delivery of a healthy child?

A: Well, that is the bedrock responsibility of the obstetrician, yes.

Q: Is it necessary for the obstetrician to know the fetal physiology and pathophysiology so as to be aware of problems that might occur during the prenatal period?

A: Well, I think it is consistent with one's training and the contract that one makes with the patient for care to be reasonably expert in those areas.

Q: Will you tell me whether or not it is true that in order for a baby to be born without brain damage, it is imperative that the obstetrician have knowledge of fetal physiology and pathophysiology?

A: Well, I think two things are important. One, they have to have the knowledge, and, two, they have to act consistent with the knowledge.

Q: And could you define for us what is meant by fetal physiology?

A: Well, fetal physiology is simply the mechanics and workings of the fetus, the body of the fetus with respect to its environment.

Q: And pathophysiology?

A: Pathophysiology deals with derangements of that mechanism.

Q: And what is meant by the term fetus?

A: Well, fetus is a passenger in the uterus waiting for delivery.

Q: That is, the fetus is nutured in the uterus and ultimately a child is born?

A: That is correct.

Q: What is meant by prenatal care?

A: Well, prenatal care is a discipline, really, in which we carry a pregnant woman through her pregnancy with the idea of: one, preventing problems; two, assuring she has good nutrition; three, taking care of problems that arise in the course of the pregnancy, with the idea that it would prevent problems following delivery of the child.

Q: After completing your residency program, did you join the staff of any hospitals?

A: Yes. I was on the staff of Sinai Hospital, and I was also on the staff of Beaumont Hospital.

Q: In 1979, were you on the staff of any hospitals?

A: Oh, yes. Sinai Hospital, Beaumont Hospital, and Providence Hospital.

Q: Are those hospitals members of the Joint Commission of Accreditation of Hospitals?

A: Oh, yes, I am certain they are.

Q: Are you board certified?

A: Yes, sir.

Q: What does it mean to be board certified?

A: Well, board certification means that, one, you have completed requirements set up by the American Board of Obstetrics and Gynecology, educational requirements, and, two, you have been examine both—well, the first time I took my boards—in a written and clinical exam. I was recertified in 1979. At that time it was simply a written examination.

Q: Was it necessary for you to become recertified?

A: No.

Q: Why did you?

A: Well, I thought it would be a good test of my own knowledge, and, second, I think that it is imperative for me and for most physicians to sharpen their skills and update their knowledge; and to have this test was a good indication of how I was doing.

Q: Is this a national test as distinguished from a local community test?

A: Oh, yes. It is given by the American Board of Obstetrics and Gynecology. It is voluntary, purely voluntary.

Q: This is a national board? In other words, it is a test that one may take in Michigan, and an obstetrician practicing in another state would take the same test.

A: The same test in every state, yes.

Q: If one passes the test, he is certified?

A: That is correct.

Q: In the field of obstetrics and gynecology?

A: That is correct.

Q: Are you a diplomate?

A: Yes.

Q: And what does it mean to be a diplomate?

A: Well, a diplomate means that you have passed the board, and they give you a certification. It is a diploma.

Q: Are you a fellow?

A: I am a fellow of the American College of Obstetrics and Gynecology.

Q: And how does one become a fellow of the American College of Obstetrics and Gynecology?

A: You apply for membership, are sponsored by two or three people, and fulfill the requirements of the college.

Q: May one practice medicine and specialize in obstetrics without becoming board certified?

A: Oh, yes.

Q: There are physicians who do do that?

A: That is correct.

Q: They do not take the test?

A: That is correct.

Q: Do you do any teaching?

A: Yes.

Q: And are you associated or affiliated with any medical schools?

A: Yes. I am a professor of obstetrics and gynecology at Wayne State.

Q: How long have you been a professor?

A: Well, I was made an assistant professor in 1965, so that is 18 years I have had professorial rank.

Q: So you are engaged in the academic field of medicine as well as private practice?

A: Oh, yes, private practice. I have always had a private practice.

Q: And you maintain a private practice at the present time?

A: Yes, sir.

Q: And where is that private practice located?

A: It is in the Medical Center in Detroit.

Q: Do you attend lectures?

A: Oh, yes.

Q: And the lectures which you attend, do they relate to prenatal care and how to treat patients suffering from, for example, preeclampsia?

A: Oh, yes. There are just lectures generaly to update my knowledge and skill. Our practice consists of fairly high risk group of patients. So, therefore, I attempt all the time to keep my skills up in that area and learn new techniques.

Q: So you have attended lectures where the subject or the topic of preeclampsia was discussed?

A: That is correct, yes.

Q: Have you also conducted lectures dealing with the subject of preeclampsia?

A: Yes.

Q: And you are familiar with what preeclampsia is and how to treat a patient suffering from preeclampsia?

A: I think so, yes sir.

Q: And are you familiar with what the standard of practice would dictate or require an obstetrician practicing in the State of Michigan to do in caring for a patient experiencing preeclampsia?

A: I believe I am qualified, yes.

Q: Have you had the opportunity of discussing the condition with fellow practitioners?

A: Oh, on a regular basis, certainly.

Q: Based upon your knowledge, your experience, the fact that you have attended lectures dealing with preeclampsia, as well as having conducted courses or lectures dealing with preeclampsia, do you believe that the care and treatment for women experiencing preeclampsia during their pregnancy is universally accepted in the United States?

A: With some minor exceptions, I think that the treatment of preeclampsia is pretty much standardized throughout the country, yes.

Q: Do you believe that you are qualified to testify here today with respect to the standard of care required of physicians in the State of Michigan as it relates to the manner in which patients experiencing preeclampsia should be treated?

A: Yes, sir.

Q: You have seen other fellow practitioners treat patients with preeclampsia?

A: Oh, yes.

Q: By the way, is one of the purposes of caring for a patient during the prenatal period to safeguard the fetus from brain damage?

A: I would say that is one of the purposes, yes.

Q: If preeclampsia is not treated commensurate with the standard of practice, in your opinion with a reasonable degree of medical certainty, could the fetus suffer brain damage?

A: The answer to that is yes.

Q: Have you conducted academic studies with respect to subjects dealing with prenatal care and treatment?

A: Well, I haven't done any, any research work, if that is what you mean by academic studies, but I certainly have done a lot of reading.

Q: And has your reading confirmed and corroborated your understanding as to what the standard of practice would dictate a physician do in caring for a patient suffering from preeclampsia?

A: Yes. Well, reading and experience both.

Q: Consequently, what you do as part of your everyday activities relating to treating patients and your knowledge of preeclampsia is also confirmed by your academic knowledge?

A: That is correct, yes.

Q: Do you believe you are qualified to render an opinion as to whether or not Dr. Gordon's care and treatment of Sally Armstrong measured up to the standard of care and skill required and called for in the treatment of women during the prenatal period as it existed in the year 1979?

A: I think so, yes.

Q: Doctor, we have been discussing and using the word "preeclampsia." Would you kindly define that term for us?

A: Well, I would like to define it, if I may under an umbrella of hypertensive disorders, because I think as seen against that background it is a little more intelligible. Is that okay?

Q: Yes.

A: Well, first of all, I think there are, by definition, several factors that obtain in hypertensive disorders of pregnancy. One is prior to 20 weeks or prior to pregnancy if a woman's blood pressure is above 140 over 90, then she is termed a hypertensive patient.

Now, at 20 weeks or later if a woman who has hypertension develops some significant edema and, proteinuria, that is, spillage of protein into the urine, then she has not preeclampsia superimposed upon hypertension. The vast majority of hypertensive patients exhibit the following: usually there is a rapid and sudden increase in weight and there is edema, that is, fluid.

Second, and I think the tricky part is that the patient conceivably could have normal blood pressure, that is, normal in the terms that we commonly think about it. But by definition preeclampsia occurs if the systolic blood pressure rises 30 points over what we have been observing, or if the disastolic rises 15 points or more. So, therefore, a woman, as I say, could have a blood pressure of 130 over 85 and that could still be an abnormal blood pressure for her. With that blood pressure she would fall into the category of having preeclampsia. Third, there is spillage of protein in the urine.

Now, the old thinking, and when I was a medical student we used to call it a triad, and since the late 1960s and the early 1970s that is an outdated concept. In other words, all three do not have to be present for it, to be preeclampsia.

Q: The triad that you are referring to that existed up until the late 1960s or early 1970s, relates to proteinuria, edema, and hypertension?

A: That is correct, yes.

Q: Based upon your knowledge and experience, would you say that the standard of practice as it existed in 1979 would compel an obstetrician to consider preeclampsia even if less than the three factors existed?

A: That is correct, yes.

Q: All right.

Q: You have discussed preeclampsia as encompassing a syndome characterized by those three factors.

A: Yes.

Q: Can you tell us something about the etiological factors or the pathology that manifests itself and brings about those conditions?

A: Well, I don't think anybody really knows what causes it. There are many theories, but I don't think there is anyone who really knows the cause. But some of the things that do happen in preeclampsia—one, there is the sudden weight gain; two, there are significant changes in blood pressure; three, there may be kidney damage; and four, there is poor placental profussion, that is, the blood doesn't flow through the placenta in normal limits.

There may be changes in the eye grounds, that is, in the examination of the eyes, there may be some bleeding or what we call retinopathy in the small blood vessels of the eye, and, of course, the same caliber blood vessels occur in the brain, and they occur in the kidney. So, the same changes, what we call angiospasm, that is, the vessels clamped down, and these changes occur throughout the body. We just happen to use the eye because it is a window. There may be convulsions which can be very, very serious, and attendant with a high incidence of maternal mortality and also about a five percent fetal wastage.

Q: Is the term preeclamptic toxemia the expression that is used?

A: Well, that is an old term. When Diekman and some of the early people were doing the work in toxemia back in the late 1940s and early 1950s, the theory was that a toxin was elaborated by the placenta to cause all of these symptoms. Well, the term toxemia stuck, but the rest of the beliefs have gone by the boards.

Q: What does toxemia mean?

A: Well, toxemia is a misnomer, but a term that is used to indicate these hypertensive disorders of pregnancy.

Q: You also indicated that with preeclampsia there may be some retinopathy changes.

A: That is correct.

Q: Is that an early change or a late change in the condition?

A: You do not see it in early preeclampsia. You see retinopathy changes in the eye grounds as the preeclampsia progresses and becomes aggravated.

Q: In other words, a late event?

A: Usually a late event, yes.

Q: You also used the term placenta profussion. What is the placenta?

A: Well, the placenta is an organ that does a number of things. One, it manufactures hormones which are important for the fetus and the mother. Two, it acts as a transfer organ between the mother and child. Basically, what it does is to help remove the waste products from the baby and shift them to the mother so she can safely remove the waste products the baby makes. Then in turn by a number of mechanisms the mother passes food, nutriments, protein, minerals, etc., and oxygen to the fetus.

Q: So it passes from the mother through the placenta to the fetus?

A: That is correct.

Q: So are we talking about three entities: the placenta, the mother, and the fetus?

A: That is correct.

Q: After the baby is born, by the way, what happens to the placenta?

A: The placenta is expelled.

Q: Are these three separate entities, the placenta, the fetus and the mother, existent with separate metabolic functions?

A: Well, they all have separate metabolic functions but they are very interdependent. Like my hand does different things than my ear, but I need my hand for my body to function well.

Q: Does the welfare of the fetus depend upon the health of placenta?

A: Very largely, yes.

Q: If the placenta is affected, in what way could or might that affect the fetus?

A: Well, if there is poor placental perfusion, you do damage to the placenta, malformation of the placenta or alteration of the caliber of the blood vessels; then the infant is going to get much less oxygen than it would ordinarily.

Q: Why is oxygen important for the fetus?

A: Well, it needs oxygen to survive. It needs oxygen to grow, and it needs oxygen for its development.

Q: Can the fetus suffer brain damage if there is a deprivation of oxygenation to the brain?

A: Well, I suspect that the commonest cause of brain damage is lack of oxygenation, yes.

Q: Is that called anoxia?

A: Anoxia or hypoxia. There is a wide variety of terms for that.

Q: And anoxia means a lack of oxygen?

A: Specifically, anoxia is a total lack of oxygen. Hypoxia means a diminished amount of oxygen. They can occur in a continuum.

Q: You made reference to angiospasms. Is that the primary pathophysiological change that occurs with preeclampsia?

A: Well, the angiospasm seems to be the one of the things that everybody agrees on that happens in preeclampsia, yes.

Q: And what is meant by angiospasms?

A: Angiospasm simply means there is a narrowing of the caliber of blood vessels, so, therefore, the heart has to push harder and pump harder to push through an adequate supply of blood.

Q: Does this cause an effect upon the placenta?

A: Oh, yes. It causes it to age, number one. Number two, therefore, the blood vessels suffer. Often there is not enough oxygen profusing through the placenta, so there is a literal rotting like damage to the blood vessels of the placenta. There is some hemorrhaging, and then there is an attempt to repair this hemorrhage by scar tissue.

Q: When the hemorrhage occurs, what effect, if any, does that have with respect to oxygenation of the fetus?

A: Well, it can reduce it, and it often does reduce it depending on the amount of damage and the length of time the infant and placenta are exposed to the insult.

Q: What do you mean by the term insult?

A: I am referring to the hemorrhaging and angiospasms.

Q: If there is diminished oxygenation to the fetus, can that destroy the brain cells?

A: Yes, sir, it can destroy the brain cells.

Q: Do brain cells regenerate?

A: No, they do not.

Q: Can a child, then, survive but be born with brain damage because of a diminution of oxygenation to the brain of the fetus by reason of placental insufficiency?

A: That is possible, yes, sir.

Q: And it does happen?

A: Oh, yes.

Q: And it does happen with preeclampsia?

A: It does happen with preeclampsia, that is correct.

Q: What correlation, if any at all, exists by and between weight gain of the mother and the triad—the proteinuria, the edema, and the hypertension?

A: Well, in regards to weight gain, I am talking now not of just a pound or two or three of weight gain, I am talking about sudden, excessive weight gain in the neighborhood of eight maybe ten pounds a month which is a really significant weight gain. The excessive weight gain is the red flag that hits most of us when we are treating pregnant women, that this person is a likely candidate for some kind of toxemia, if you will, whether it be preeclampsia or eclampsia.

Q: Does the weight gain cause the increase in blood pressure?

A: We really do not know what causes the increase in blood pressure except that there is an associated angiospasm frequently that will follow, and then this is apparently what causes the rise in blood pressure.

Q: I see.

A: Now, there is another theory about various mechanisms of a renninogen tensive system, and it has to do with the kidney. But whatever happens there is an elevation of blood pressure whether it is by the mechanisms of angiospasm or by the mechanism of the renninogen tensive, which, in turn, causes spasm; so the bottom line is there is an angiospasm, a spasm of the blood vessels.

Q: You previously used the term high risk pregnancy. Would a patient experiencing preeclampsia be classified as a high risk patient?

A: She becomes a high risk patient when preeclampsia is diagnosed or detected, yes.

Q: And with that characterization, what then is done for a patient who is a high risk patient?

A: Well, I think that, number one, she has to be carefully watched. Number two, one does a test to determine what is going on, and, three, I think that ideally you would like to develop some sort of plan to keep the risk to a minimum. I think the philosophy is much better to keep out of trouble than to get out of trouble.

Q: What is meant by post-maturity?

A: Well, by definition post-maturity is pregnancy that has gone beyond two weeks beyond the estimated date of confinement.

Q: Have you had the opportunity of reviewing documents submitted to you with respect to the care and treatment rendered to Sally Armstrong during her prenatal period as well as and including her hospitalizations, which would also encompass the hospitalization wherein the child, Susan Armstrong, was born?

A: Yes, sir.

Q: Have you reviewed Dr. Gordon's records?

A: Yes, sir.

Q: Have you reviewed Dr. Gordon's deposition?

A: I read it once, yes.

Q: Based upon your review of those documents, are you in a position to render an opinion with respect to whether or not in the care and treatment of Sally Armstrong, Dr. Gordon acted commensurate with the standard of practice for obstetricians in the State of Michigan in the year 1979?

A: Yes, sir.

Q: All right. Are you aware of the fact that this child was born 28 days past the expected date of confinement (EDC)?

A: Yes, sir.

Q: The baby weighed eight pounds eleven ounces at birth?

A: Yes, sir.

Q: Are you aware of the fact that the mother weighed between 120 to 125 pounds before she became pregnant?

A: Well, you did not inform me of that. In one of the nurse's records, the nurse took a history from the patient and the patient said she gained 69 pounds.

Q: Okay. That would bring it down to a weight of 120-125 pounds before pregnancy.

A: Roughly, yes.

Q: Based upon your review of the documents that we have just discussed, do you have an opinion as to whether or not the doctor departed or deviated from the standard of practice?

A: Yes, I do.

Q: And what is that opinion?

A: Well, I think that there were some significant deviations from standard of practice.

Q: All right. I am going to ask you to advise us, starting from the time that the doctor first treated this woman, how and under what circumstances the doctor deviated from the standard of practice?

A: Well, I think that in reviewing the patient's prenatal record, the patient had preeclampsia, if we use the definition that is commonly accepted in this country. By August 12th, the patient had significant elevations in her diastolic pressure well over the 15mm that is used as a guide. The patient spilled albumin on a fairly regular basis, and, and I think that at this point in time, by August 29th, especially on that day she had a 30mm increase in diastolic pressure and spilled a trace of albumin. At that point in time I think the patient obviously had preeclampsia.

Q: When did preeclampsia initially exist?

A: Well, I think that probably by the 1st of August, but by the 12th of August there was some evidence at that time that the patient was preeclamptic. And, of course, all along with the patient spilling traces of albumin, I think that that could have been investigated.

Q: In your opinion, could the symptoms have been recognized as developing preeclampsia?

A: Well, I think they would have certainly put the patient in the category, and also in the high risk category.

Q: And what would the ordinary, prudent physician specializing in the field of obstetrics in the year 1979 have done, commensurate with the standard of practice in August of 1979, when first cognizant of those factors that you have just alluded to?

A: Well, I think the patient would have been seen more frequently, perhaps on a weekly basis. Second, the patient would have been put to bed. And some dietary changes were certainly in order; that is, the high protein, low carbohydrates diet.

Q: Why are these important?

A: Well, because I think that the patient is losing protein through the kidneys, and we know that high protein diets sometimes ameliorate preeclampsia.

Q: What other things should the average, prudent physician have done in managing a patient with the condition that existed in Sally Armstrong in the month of August, 1979?

A: Well, I think those things were enough at that point—just a little closer observation and some definitive dietary things. Also somewhere along the line I think the patient was given a diuretic, and I am not really sure what month that was. But diuretics are really no-no's in the treatment of toxemia in pregnancy.

Q: Let us stay for the moment with the month of August.

A: Okay.

Q: Did you also notice weight gains that should have put the doctor on notice of potential preeclampsia?

A: Yes. In the month of August, the patient gained eight pounds, which is a pretty spectacular weight gain. I think that, in view of the fact she had gained nine pounds between May and June, and then again gained an additional nine pounds between June and July, in August to gain eight pounds is a pretty spectacular weight gain even for the most liberal physicians.

Q: Did the doctor, commensurate with the standard of practice, properly care for the patient?

A: I think not. I think that under the circumstances with the patient having this kind of weight gain, and this kind of elevation of blood pressure, and a trace of albumin, I think the patient should have been hospitalized at that time.

Q: Did the failure of Dr. Gordon to act, commensurate with the standard of practice, cause an acceleration or advancement of the preeclamptic condition?

A: Well, I think the failure to act certainly served to aggravate the condition, yes.

Q: In your opinion, with a reasonable degree of medical certainty, had he acted propitiously, as you outlined, in August of 1979, would the preeclamptic condition that this patient was experiencing have been abated and avoided?

A: I think so, yes.

Q: You indicated that Dr. Gordon gave the patient a diuretic. I believe it would have been on August 12th that he gave her a diuretic.

A: Yes, that is right, I think there is a "D" there. That means diuretic, yes.

Q: Why would that be violative of the standard of practice?

A: A diuretic does not do anything for preeclampsia. It is not good treatment. Not only that, there is some evidence it does more harm in terms of reducing blood volume, which further causes angiospasm, and causes the heart to work even harder to push the volume that is in the blood system along.

Q: Did the doctor, to your knowledge, continue to administer diuretics to this patient from the month of August up until the time of ultimate delivery?

A: I will have to look. I think there was another—I read somewhere here—I cannot really put my finger on it.

Q: All right.

A: The patient was given phenobarbital to take for some length of time. I think it was 100 mg.

Q: That is a barbiturate?

A: Yes, sir.

Q: All right. Staying with the—

A: Also a diuretic.

Q: —the diuretics. Accepting the fact for the moment that Dr. Gordon continued to give this patient diuretics from August 12th to the time the patient was confined to the hospital on or about October 30th, 1979, I ask you as to whether or not, with a reasonable degree of medical certainty, the administering of the diuretics caused or aggravated the preeclamptic condition?

A: Well, I think it does two things. One is I think it gives physicians a false sense of security. He may see some diminution of systolic blood pressure and maybe a little diminution in diastolic blood pressure, but you are not really treating the condition, and I think since that obtained, you may aggravate the condition. So to that extent I think that helped aggravate the condition, yes.

Q: By the way, systolic would be the top number on the blood pressure, and the diastolic the bottom number?

A: Yes, that is correct.

Q: And by aggravating the condition, I will now ask the tandem question, do you have an opinion with a reasonable medical certainty as to whether or not the aggravation of the preexisting condition was a causative factor in the brain damage to the child?

A: Well, taking the whole record, I think that is correct, yes.

Q: Now, moving to the month of September, did Dr. Gordon hospitalize the mother?

A: I don't see any hospitalization in September.

Q: What, if anything, do you see with respect to the care and treatment rendered to the patient by Dr. Gordon in the month of September?

A: Well, I see that she was given diuretics on the 16th, and on the 20th, and then there is a note on 9-20 that says "induce" in his record. So it leads me to think that, that he was thinking in terms that the pregnancy was not going well.

Q: Did the patient have preeclampsia in September?

A: Oh yes. Absolutely. No question about it.

Q: Did he treat the patient commensurate with the standard of practice for preeclampsia during the month of September?

A: I don't think so.

Q: What should he have done in the month of September that up to that time he had failed to do?

A: Hospitalize the patient again.

Q: Bed confinement?

A: That is correct.

Q: Should he have imposed strict dietary measures?

A: Oh, yes.

Q: Why?

A: Well, because I think that here again you see we have a condition that is very treacherous. It needs some very vigorous therapy in order to avoid problems for the mother and infant, and from what I can see in the record this was not done.

Q: Should he have taken blood pressure readings more often than he did in the month of September?

A: Yes, I think that there should have been certainly more readings, and certainly I would have loved to have seen some, some total albumins rather than just a random specimen. The 24-hour urine albumins, rather than just a random specimen.

Q: And by this failure to do that, would that also be violative of the standard of practice?

A: I think so, yes.

Q: Why should there have been additional albumin testing?

A: Well, because albumin varies from hour to hour in every patient, and random sampling is like playing the lottery: it is nice if you hit it, but you cannot count on it. It just does not give you the kind of information that one needs. You need something a little more thorough, and just one sample isn't worth it.

Q: The patient was confined to the hospital for the first time in October, early October of 1979, is that correct?

A: I think 10-8, I believe. Yes. Let me see the dates here. Well, she came in on 10-7. Yes.

Q: Okay. What if anything occurred during that hospital confinement?

A: Well, the patient was admitted on 10-7, and she was given bed rest. She was ordered to bed with just bathroom privileges and daily weights, which is fine, and then there are blood pressures three times a day; but then she was put on a low salt diet again, and here I think that something a little more vigorous than the diet could have been done.

   Also urinalysis every day, a morning specimen, I assume. Only one time a day is really not very helpful to tell us what is going on with this patient. A one shot sample does not do much.

   Again, Diuril was given; apparently it was a vocal order, and the patient was put to bed. I presume she was observed in bed and with the pressures taken. He then got an x-ray pelvimetry, and then after obtaining the x-ray pelvimetry he then attempted an induction of the patient.

Q: Now, what is a pelvimetry?

A: Well, a pelvimetry is an x-ray measurement of the bony pelvis of the mother. Sometimes it tells us some significant things about infants, and in this case it tells us that the infant was a reasonably mature infant. In other words, the distal femoral epiphyses were present in this infant, and so the infant had to be at least 36 weeks gestation. When you see the femoral epiphysis present, that means the baby is physically at term. It also told us the mother had a huge pelvis.

Q: The baby was a term baby at that time?

A: Yes, for all intents and purposes, it was a term baby.

Q: October 7th would have been—

A: That is October 10th. October 7th was her expected date of confinement (EDC). The x-ray was October 10.

Q: Okay.

A: Yes.

Q: So that when the x-ray was taken on October 10th, the mother would have been three days past her EDC.

A: Well, I think a better way of saying it was the baby was at term.

Q: All right.

A: Yes.

Q: You indicated that the mother was suffering from preeclampsia?

A: Yes.

Q: Do you have an opinion, with a reasonable degree of medical certainty, as to whether or not the preeclamptic condition that existed on October 7th caused any problems to the placenta?

A: Well, the preeclampsia is an ongoing problem, and I am sure that as long as there is an ongoing problem there is ongoing damage. Now, just what kind of damage there was to the placenta at that time, I couldn't say.

Q: Is it more likely than not that damage was being done to the placenta?

A: Yes.

Q: Was there any test performed during that confinement to determine as to whether or not fetal distress existed?

A: Well, she was in the hospital for, I think, four days. So you are asking me for that total time.

Q: Yes, for the total confinement of October 7th.

A: As I recall, the induction was done on the patient, and I believe she was monitored during this admission. Yes, a monitor was on.

Q: I would like to ask you to accept for the moment that a monitor was attached.

A: Yes.

Q: That would be commensurate with the standard of practice, to attach monitor?

A: Yes.

Q: When a patient is being induced with Pitocin in 1979, correct?

A: That is correct.

Q: And that was done in this case?

A: That is correct.

Q: You have not seen the tracings?

A: No, sir, I have not.

Q: You do not know what the tracing revealed?

A: No, sir, I do not.

Q: Assuming for the moment that the tracings are normal, is that classified as an OCT test?

A: It can be classified as an OCT test, yes.

Q: What is an OCT test?

A: The initials stand for Oxytocin Challenge Test.

Q: How is the test performed?

A: By administering intravenous pitocin in order to produce contractions so as to be able to interpret the fetal heart rate response.

Q: Is that accurate?

A: Well, it is a reasonably accurate test, but I don't think there is any single test that, that can answer all the questions.

Q: Let me ask it in this fashion. Would the standard of practice as it existed in October of 1979, have dictated that the obstetrician treating a patient such as

Sally Armstrong, perform any other test to determine fetal distress other than that which was performed during her confinement at the hospital?

A: Well, given the circumstances in this case, can I answer it that way?

Q: Sure.

A: Okay. Given the circumstances in this case, where the obstetrician began to induce the patient, there are tests that have to be made. You have to get a pelvimetry, especially if it is the woman's first child. A pelvimetry then tells us whether or not there is room for the baby to come through.

Second, the pelvimetry, the x-ray, also told us that this infant was at term.

Third, amniocentesis was available, which was done at another admission. Once you set your hand to induce the baby, the obstetrician commits himself to a course of action. I don't like to commit myself to a course of action unless I have all the facts in hand, and I think that an amniocentesis should have been done. Then at that point with all that information, the decision to do the induction could have been made.

Q: What about an estriol level test?

A: An estriol level test is a very valuable, probably the most valuable, placental profusion function test there is.

Q: Should that have been performed?

A: I think so in this case.

Q: Would it be commensurate with the standard of practice to have performed an estriol level test?

A: Given the fact that the induction was stopped, I think so, yes.

Q: Taking into consideration the fact that the child ultimately had brain damage, taking into consideration the child was term, taking into consideration that the mother had preeclampsia with all of the sequela that existed as you have indicated, do you have an opinion, with a reasonable degree of medical certainty, as to what the estriol test would have revealed had it been performed at that time?

A: Well, I suspect that the estriol levels here may have been low. They may have been normal, but they could have been low, and they may have been decreasing. In other words, serial estriols are needed; daily estriols in this kind of situation are needed in order for us to get a good test of placental profusion. At this point in time they may have been normal. They may have been low.

Q: Were estriol levels performed during the second confinement?

A: No, sir.

Q: If they had been performed, do you have an opinion, based upon a reasonable degree of medical certainty, as to what they would have revealed?

A: Well, I believe we would have seen some diminishing estriold

Q: Would that have been an indication of possible fetal distress?

A: I think so.

Q: And would it be violative of the standard of practice on that second admission not to administer an estriol level test?

A: I think so, yes.

Q: What is an estriol level test?

A: An estriol level test is a test that can be done either on blood or urine, or amniotic fluid for that matter, but it is more often done on blood or urine. It is a measure of the intactness of the fetal maternal placental unit. Certain compounds are made in the mother and transferred to the fetus; then the fetal adrenal and fetal liver do things to them and pass them back to the placenta. The placenta makes the estriol, sends it back to the maternal kidney, and the maternal kidney excretes it. Therefore, what happens in essence is that we are checking the baby and the placenta function with the estriol levels.

Q: Is it a more accurate test than the OCT test?

A: Infinitely more accurate.

Q: Infinitely more accurate in determining fetal distress?

A: That is correct.

Q: In your opinion, would the standard of practice as it existed in October of 1979 have required the doctor to deliver this child by C-section?

A: Well, given the fact that the doctor intervened to induce this patient and started the induction, then I think the standard of practice absolutely indicates that we should go ahead and complete the delivery. If the induction does not do it, then you do a C-section.

There is just no rationale to do an induction and then stop because the preeclampsia does not go away, it only gets worse. The only cure for preeclampsia is to get rid of the placenta?

Q: Evacuate the uterus?

A: That is right. The only way you get rid of the placenta is to deliver the baby. So if on day one there is an indication of doing an induction, well, it becomes even more imperative on day two and day three and day five and ten and fifteen, etc.

Q: Do you have an opinion, based upon a reasonable degree of medical certainty, as to whether brain damage would in all likelihood have been prevented had this child been delivered by C-section in early October of 1979?

A: I think, yes. My opinion is yes.

Q: The child would have been normal?

A: I suspect the child would have been normal, yes. I feel strongly it would have been normal, because it would have had two weeks outside of a hostile environment.

Q: It is more than two weeks. The child was born November 2nd.

A: Oh yes. That would be three weeks, is that right?

Q: About three, three and a half weeks.

A: Oh, yes. The baby just stayed in a hostile environment for three and a half weeks. There was no advantage to keep the baby in the uterus, not a single advantage from any way of reasoning, that this child benefitted from being in the uterus three extra weeks.

Q: When you say a hostile environment, tell us in your opinion, with a reasonable degree of medical certainty, as to what happened during those three and a half weeks?

A: Well, the baby got less oxygen and the placental profusion got worse. The nutriments were not very good. The baby was subjected to the loss of albumin of the mother, which, in turn, affects her ability to nourish the child.

The child was also affected by the swings in blood pressure, which I am sure this woman had. She went up to 170 over 110. That signifies considerable increase of angiospasm. We have only spot blood pressure; we have no idea what she did on a 24-hour basis. So keeping the baby in this environment just does not help in any way, shape, or form.

Q: Is it your opinion the baby was born brain damaged?

A: Yes.

Q: And is that opinion based upon a reasonable degree of medical certainty?

A: Yes.

Q: Doctor, considering the problems of preeclampsia, and you have informed us of the problems in the hostile environment, I now ask you whether or not you have an opinion, based upon a reasonable degree of medical certainty, as to whether or not when this child was ultimately born it was born post-maturely?

A: Oh, yes, I think so, very definitely.

Q: And why do you believe the child was born post-maturely?

A: Well, I think the baby had a fair amount of desquamation, according to the pediatrician, the baby had a fairly marked desquamation of the skin, and I think this is indicative of post-maturity.

Second, I think that the four weeks overdue by dates is another indication of post-maturity.

Q: When you say desquamation, how does that come about? What happens to the baby?

A: Well, the baby literally ages. They are wrinkled up, just like wrinked old men or women, and their skin peels off very easily.

Q: As a matter of fact, then, in tandem with that, what about the fact that the baby was born with breast buds?

A: Well, that is seen not uncommonly in post-mature babies, but that is simply a function of maternal hormonal influence, and—

Q: Is this seen often in postmature babies?

A: It is seen most often in postmature babies, in my experience.

Q: Why? What happens?

A: Well, just increased exposure to the maternal hormones. The fetal liver is very immature and it is not working very well, so it cannot neutralize the estrogens. So the estrogen will affect the baby's breasts.

Q: This baby weighed eight pounds eleven ounces upon birth.

A: Yes.

Q: We laypeople sometimes think of a post-mature baby as being big, 11-12 pounds. Is that true?

A: Oh no. Post-mature babies can be very small.

Q: Why is that?

A: Well, depending on a number of factors. It depends often on the degree of placental dysfunction.

Q: Is there usually dysfunction when you have post-maturity, an aging process of the placenta?

A: One of the causes, yes. There is placental dysfunction with post-maturity, but with some infants the problems of the placental problems start very early, and so you will get babies who are quite small with the placental dysfunction. It occurs for a number of reasons, and if the placental dysfunction starts early, these babies are very tiny.

Q: Is a post-mature baby high risk?

A: Oh, yes, very high risk.

Q: Why? Again, what happens when a woman passes her EDC and a determination is made the baby is post-date?

A: Well, when a woman passes her EDC and like other systems, the placenta begins to age and it is just not a very efficient organ, it does not clear away the waste product as efficiently. The baby does not get as much oxygen, does not get the nutrients.

Q: Can that cause brain damage?

A: Well, depending on the length and severity, yes, it can cause brain damage.

Q: In your opinion you indicated that this baby was born post-maturity?

A: That is correct.

Q: In your opinion, with a reasonable degree of medical certainty, did that cause and contribute to the brain damage of the child?

A: I think it contributed to it, yes.

Q: The primary factor was the preeclampsia?

A: I suspect it was a preeclampsia. In other words, there is a whole series of things that went on. The baby had a long period of insult in the uterus. The mother was treated with phenobarb for long periods of time. Also, she was given Azo Gantanol on a number of occasions, and there is a report from Ford Hospital, where I trained, written by Nash in 1956 or 1957 that indicated that gantanol did, in fact, could cause some brain damage in children. There were two cases reported by Nash which indicated there was some intracerebral hemorrhage which they thought was secondary to the Gantanol.

Q: Commensurate with the standard of practice in 1979, I ask you whether or not that should have been known by the physician?

A: Well, I think that Azo Gantanol should have been given with some care in pregnancy, yes. I don't think there is a proven cause and effect relationship between brain damage and gantanol, but I think that there are sufficient causes not to give drugs, and especially with the fact that culture was negative. I am hesitant, most of us are hesitant, to give pregnant women antibiotics when we do not have some culture to back it up.

Q: Was it violative of the standard of practice for the doctor to have given the Gantanol?

A: Well, I think so, with a negative culture, I think yes.

Q: And did he give the Gantanol?

A: I think he gave the Azo Gantanol, I think it was the first admission, if I am not mistaken. Azo Gantanol one tablet four times a day, and the urine showed only occasional bacteria, but that could be contamination, and when the culture was returned, I believe it showed no growth—yes, there is no growth in the culture. So I don't see, really, what benefit was obtained by giving the patient Azo Gantanol.

Q: The mother was also given phenobarbital, was she not?

A: Yes.

Q: And when was that given to her?

A: Well, phenobarbital apparently was given to her during the latter part of the pregnancy, and I think that phenobarbital is, is kind of a dangerous drug. I think most people agree, certainly agreed in 1979, phenobarbital did not have much use; it was an old drug that we used in the old days, 1956, 1957, 1958; it was used in the treatment of preeclampsia, but I don't know anybody, at least the colleagues, that was using phenobarbital.

Phenobarbital traverses the placenta very easily, so that when the baby is born, the effects of phenobarbital last for approximately two or three days.

Second, phenobarbital may lower blood pressure slightly, especially systolic blood pressure, and this can give you sort of a false sense of security in terms of the progress of the preeclampsia.

Third, it also is given to prevent convulsions, at least to guard against convulsions. In the old days we thought it was a pretty good anticonvulsant. Well, it is not a bad anticonvulsant; but we have a much safer one to use in pregnant women, which has been used for a long time, and that is magnesium sulfate, and it can be given much more safely and with much more specific effects.

Q: Was it violative of the standard of practice for Dr. Gordon to have administered the phenobarbital?

A: I guess I would have to say yes. I don't know what good it did, frankly. It is just not a drug that was used anymore in 1979.

Q: Is phenobarbital a barbituate?

A: Yes.

Q: And is this a central nervous system depressant?

A: Yes.

Q: In your opinion, with a reasonable degree of medical certainty, did the administering of pheonobarbital to the mother affect the fetus?

A: I think it does. I think it decreases oxygenation considerably in many babies, yes.

Q: And in this particular case, did it?

A: Well, I think what happened is there is a whole group of problems, and one is the preeclampsia. One is the lack of high protein diet. Another is the phenobarbital. Then there is the diuretic. So these are all cumulative effects that perhaps singly—well, preeclampsia singly certainly is enough—but added, it is like weighing someone down. If a person carries 50 pounds with minimum ability and then you add more pounds, then, they collapse, and I think this is what we are seeing here.

Q: Are you stating that the preeclampsia caused the brain damage?

A: I think that is probably the main causative affect, yes.

Q: And the phenobarbital would have aggravated the preexisting condition?

A: Yes. I think so. Well, let me rephrase that more accurately. The anoxia or hypoxia or, reduced oxygen, due to preeclampsia, was simply added to by the diuril and the phenobarbital and, and the procrastination, yes.

Q: What affect, if any, did the administering of phenobarbital, in your opinion, have upon the child when born?

A: Well, I think that the child suffered from bleeding in utero. That is number one. I think that the anoxia over a period of time caused some brain damage by, by virtue of bleeding at the small capillary level of the brain. That is number one.

Number two is I think that the, that the infant's vascular system, especially a cerebral vascular system, was very fragile, and once the infant was born and began to survive on its own and lead a much more sophisticated life outside the uterus, I think it was not able to do that and had a further bleed.

Number three, I think that the child may have demonstrated some seizures or certainly some gross neurological immaturities or deficiency or deficit, but this may have been masked by its phenobarbital level; that is, the phenobarbital may have tranquilized, if you will, the infant. So that on the surface the baby's neurological apparatus seemed intact, but actually what was happening was the deficits were being masked by the phenobarbital. When the bleed progressed and the phenobarbital wore off, then we began to see more neurological signs of the infant.

Q: Preeclampsia caused the anoxia?

A: Yes.

Q: The anoxia caused the cerebral bleeding?

A: Well, what happens is that it caused damage—the brain cells literally rot, you know. In other words, they just do not get enough nourishment and enough oxygen, and they have what we call necrosis, or they die, sort of a rotting process. This occurs at microscopic levels, and you do not see it unless you have got a microscopic section of tissue. Then what happens is that the lining of the small capillary vessels, these very fine linery vessels also rot, and there is this kind of bleed into the baby's head.

Q: So that when the baby was born it was experiencing a bleeding episode in the brain?

A: Either experiencing or had; I suspected it had experienced. You know, these hypoxic episodes were causing progressive brain damage to the child as it was growing.

Q: Now, between 48 and 72 hours, there was a seizure, is that correct?

A: Yes.

Q: Are you indicating that in your opinion, with a reasonable degree of medical certainty, the seizures did not manifest itself until that period of time by reason of the sedation?

A: I think there is a very strong possibility. I think there may have been a further bleed. The baby had a lot of peculiar neurological signs. At first it was on one side. Then it became diffuse, and so I think this was a continuing process. I don't think it's a one shot thing. In other words, I think it was just a continuum that got worse at one point, and I think the, that the phenobarbital may very well have masked a lot of neurological symptoms in the child.

Q: Is it your opinion that the baby experienced diffuse brain damage as distinguished from focal brain damage?

A: I think it had both. I think it was both focal and diffuse.

Q: Now, is your opinion predicated upon a reasonable degree of medical certainty?

A: Yes.

Q: What is the basis of your opinion that the baby had both focal and diffuse brain damage when born?

A: Well, I think that this child was suffering ongoing brain damage, and during the residency in the uterus, especially the last three weeks or so, I think that the child suffered significant brain damage at that point. I suspect that there was diffuse and focal damage as manifested by the kinds of signs the baby exhibited later on.

Q: Are you referring to the fact there were manifestations on one side?

A: One side and then the other side, and I think there was damage in the substrata of the baby's brain, and as the baby lived longer, these things just became more apparent.

Q: Reviewing the hospital record at the time of delivery, I ask you whether it makes reference to meconium?

A: Well, the only thing that I saw was that they aspirated the infant's stomach. There is a note by somebody here who aspirated the baby's stomach. It may have been the neonatologist, or the perinatologist, whatever, who said that he aspirated some yellowish fluid from the baby's stomach. There was a note in the record in which the doctor said that the infant's stomach was aspirated and there were three to five cc's of yellow fluid. So that led me to believe there may have been some meconium which indicated further distress, staining of the meconium fluid.

Q: What does meconium stained amniotic fluid mean?

A: Well, it simply means the infant is having some problems over a period of time as opposed to fresh meconium.

Q: Does that mean that the infant is having problems in utero?

A: That is correct, yes.

Q: What is meconium stain?

A: Well, meconium staining means the baby has moved its bowels in the uterus, and then after a period of time the amniotic fluid cleans out the system, but there is some staining that can be left behind as long as a week or 10 days.

Q: Is meconium staining of the amniotic fluid a sign of asphyxia in utero?

A: Well, per se, it may not be that. But when you reconstruct the whole case, the whole series of events, I think the baby was somewhat asphyxiated in utero. If you just take meconium staining by itself, it may not mean anything; but in terms of this particular situation, I think it is significant.

Q: Is it a reflex reaction of the sphincter muscle or nerves?

A: Yes.

Q: Now then, in your opinion, with a reasonable degree of medical certainty, did meconium staining exist in utero?

A: I suspect it did, yes.

Q: And in your opinion, with a reasonable degree of medical certainty, taking into consideration the facts of this case, do you have an opinion as to whether or not the meconium staining that existed in this case was indicative of fetal distress in utero?

A: I think so, yes.

Q: And is it your opinion, with a reasonable degree of medical certainty, that the fetal distress related to the preeclampsia condition?

A: Yes, sir.

Q: Now, Doctor, after the mother was discharged the first time from the hospital without a C-section having been performed, I ask you as to whether or not she reentered the hospital for a second admission?

A: Well, the second admission was around the 23rd of October, so it was almost two weeks later.

Q: During the two-week period of time, what treatment, if any, did Dr. Gordon administer to this patient?

A: Well, he simply saw her on the 16th, the 17th, and the 18th. He noted that blood pressure was 140 over 82 on the 16th. It was 130 over 97 on the 17th. He made a note there were no contractions. There were no albumin recordings on the 16th and on the 17th. On the 18th the blood pressure was 118 over 80, and the patient had one-plus albumin, and then on the 23rd he saw her again, the pressure at that time was 132 over 90. She came out of the hospital weighing 190 and on 10-23 she had gained six pounds when she was readmitted to the hospital.

Q: During that two week period of time what should the average, ordinary, prudent obstetrician have determined?

A: Well, again, I don't think that two week period of time should have happened. I think the baby should have been delivered.

Q: Was the patient still suffering from preeclampsia?

A: Yes, sir.

Q: Was this severe preeclampsia?

A: Well, by his definition it is severe preeclampsia.

Q: Do you consider it to be severe preeclampsia?

A: Yes, moderately severe preeclampsia.

Q: The patient was again admitted to the hospital, correct?

A: That is correct.

Q: What was done for the patient this second time?

A: Well the second time we have a number of albumins, that there is a three-plus albumin.

Q: What does that mean?

A: It means significant amount of proteins are being spilled in the urine. Second, it means there is a significant amount of insult to the kidney, and that this is indicative of severe preeclampsia.

Q: I might ask you what was her BUN (urea nitrogen) and serum creatinine during this period of time?

A: I don't see one in this chart.

Q: Do you recall what the BUN or serum creatinase as was prior to this admission?

A: I don't think I saw one of those, either. Yes. There was a BUN that was 18 on 10-8.

Q: That was while she was hospitalized?

A: That is correct.

Q: The first time?

A: Yes.

Q: What does that mean?

A: That is elevated. It means the kidneys are compromised somewhat.

Q: And would the kidneys be compromised by reason of the preeclamptic condition?

A: Obviously, yes.

Q: Is there any showing of a serum creatinase?

A: I did not see a serum creatinase at this admission.

Q: Okay. Going to that second admission, then.

A: Well, the patient had three-plus albumin, two-plus albumin which means the preeclampsia is probably more severe because of the increase in the amount of albumin. For years was one of the best indicators of whether the baby was going to be hurt or not was the amount of albumin spilled. At the medical center where I trained, we did, we used total albumins on a daily basis to, as a predictor of total outcome, and I still think it is a good test. We have more sophisticated tests now, obviously, but increasing albumin means that the baby is in trouble.

Also there was a type and cross match done when the patient was admitted, and so, again, I am prompted to think that the doctor is getting ready to deliver the baby and, in fact, he did start an induction on this patient on the 24th.

Q: Of October?

A: Of October, that is correct, yes.

Q: Were there any tests performed during that second admission other than the induction by Pitocin to determine if fetal distress existed?

A: Well, I suspected with the monitor on they used the oxytocin challenge test (OCT).

Q: Other than that test—?

A: What was the question?

Q: Were there any other tests?

A: No, other than just the urinalyses and that OCT.

Q: Were there any other tests to determine fetal distress that was performed other than the OCT test?

A: No.

Q: And would that be violative of the standard of practice?

A: I think so, yes.

Q: And should an estriol level test have been performed?

A: I think at least a serial estriol level test, yes.

Q: And you defined that before, and you testified in your opinion it would have revealed fetal distress?

A: I think at this time we would have seen fetal distress by estriol level, yes, serious placental difficulties.

Q: How is a patient induced?

A: In this case it was done the usual way, and using Pitocin, which is an oxytocin drug, which causes regular contractions in the uterus, and it was given by pump, I believe, which is the way is should be done. It was given by Hi-vac pump. It is a good pump. It measures accurately the amount of Pitocin that is given to the patient.

The monitor was also used. The Pitocin is put in intravenously in a diluted solution, and the patient is given gradually increasing amounts of this solution until we get a pattern that is commensurate with normal labor which is three contractions per ten minute period.

Q: In this case, there was not a successful vaginal delivery?

A: No.

Q: That permits you to conclude the oxytocin was not serving its purpose?

A: That is correct.

Q: How long was she administered the oxytocin?

A: It was just given during one day.

Q: The patient is lying down during that time?

A: Yes, usually.

Q: What effect, if any, does the administering of Pitocin for that long a period of time with the patient lying down have upon the fetus and the patient who is preeclamptic?

A: Well, with the patient lying on her back, aside from the Pitocin, for that length of time, unless she is moved from side to side, there can be some serious compromise of the oxygen and blood supply to the uterus. It is called a vena cava compression syndrome where the patient just lies on the vena cava, that is the main vein that takes all the blood back from the lower part of the body to the heart; and it could cause a decreased blood supply to the uterus.

Q: What about the Pitocin? Is that an antidiuretic?

A: Oh, yes, Pitocin has antidiuretic properties, yes.

Q: What effect, if any at all, does that have upon the preexisting preeclampsia?

A: Well, I think that unless there were severe degree of preeclampsia, it can be used. In this case the antidiuretic effect was probably not significant.

Q: What if anything should Dr. Gordon have done, during that second confinement that he did not do?

A: I think he should have delivered the baby.

Q: By C-section?

A: However. If induction did not take one day, do it again. Sometimes it takes two, three, four days to soften the cervix up, especially in a woman who has never had a baby. Obviously, he was worried or otherwise he would not have brought her in and would not have attempted induction. Again, when a decision is made to induce a patient, that means I commit myself to deliver this patient, so I think the patient should have been delivered.

Q: Was it violative of the standard of practice not to deliver the baby?

A: I think so, in this case, yes, in view of the fact that toxemia is a progressive disease and the baby gained nothing by being in the uterus for an additional two weeks.

Q: In your opinion, with a reasonable degree of medical certainty, was the failure of Dr. Gordon to act an omission that diminished the chances of a healthy baby being born?

A: I think so, in this case, yes.

Q: I assume that it is your opinion the damage was primarily done by failure to deliver the baby during the first confinement?

A: Well, I think that was the step in the wrong direction. There was an error, it was poor judgment at that point in time not to deliver the baby.

Q: Bad judgment?

A: Yes. It was incorrect judgment, yes.

Q: All right.

A: I think once that step was taken, then everything else just sort of spilled out of the bag. It is like holding a bag of potatoes. When you have a hole, they all fall through, and I think that is what happened in this case.

Q: The mother was again discharged a second time without a delivery?

A: Yes. she was in just two days.

Q: She was readmitted to the hospital a third and final time for delivery, is that correct?

A: That is correct.

Q: And that would be, when? October 30th or 29th?

A: October 30th.

Q: Doctor, when the patient was readmitted to the hospital for the third time, based upon your review of the hospital records, was the patient suffering from severe preeclampsia?

A: Yes, sir.

Q: Was the child delivered by C-section during that hospital confinement?

A: Yes, sir.

Q: Was the child born 28 days after the EDC?

A: Approximately 28 days, yes.

Q: Was an amniocentesis test performed?

A: Apparently it was, because there is a report here of amniocentesis.

Q: Were there any tests to determine whether or not fetal distress existed?

A: Other than the amniocentesis, no.

Q: Does the amniocentesis determine fetal distress?

A: It can in just a general way. For instance, if there is meconium after 32-34 weeks of pregnancy, it can indicate fetal distress, but mostly the amniotic fluid studies deal with, one, fetal maturity, and, two, malformations.

Q: What did this particular amniocentesis test deal with?

A: Well, there are two factors that were measured. One was the L/S ratio, and the other was creatinine level.

Q: There were no specific tests performed to determine the possible existence of fetal distress?

A: No. I guess not, no, there were none at all.

Q: The amniocentesis test was performed to determine L/S ratio?

A: That is right.

Q: What is the L/S ratio?

A: The L/S ratio is the ratio of two compounds formed by the fetal lung, and, and certain ratios indicate certain degrees of maturity of the fetal lung.

Q: Is that L/S ratio test for the lecithin to sphingomyelin ratio?

A: Yes.

Q: In this particular case there was a determination the ratio was 1.9 to 1.

A: Yes, the ratio was 1.9 to 1.

Q: To one?

A: Yes.

Q: This woman was preeclamptic, correct?

A: Yes.

Q: Of what significance, if any, is the L/S ratio when a woman is preeclamptic?

A: Well, the hooker in the L/S ratio comes in the following way. The two to one indicates, you know, lung maturity, and indicates probably a 38-week gestation.
Now, the hooker in preeclampsia comes that if there are small amounts of amniotic fluid, you can get erroneous readings. So the reading does not have that kind of validity. It is close, but—

Q: In your opinion, with a reasonable degree of medical certainty, taking into consideration the pelvimetry that was performed on October 10th and the desquamation of the child that existed after the child was born, do you have an opinion as to whether or not that L/S ratio was accurate?

A: Well, the L/S ratio, I suspect, was not all that accurate, but it really could not, did not make any difference. I mean, it is really not germane to the issue. This is not a test to do at this point in time when the patient is, you know, 30 days, or 22 days or 28 days overdue. That is a test you do way back when. That is a test, I suspect, he could have done early in September, or when he was thinking of inducing the child then. I don't think it is a test to be done at this point in time, so I think that the result may be spurious; number one, there is a high likelihood of it being spurious and, number two, I don't think it has any validity at this point in time. It is not a relevant test.

Q: When this mother was admitted to the hospital she had some ophthalmologic problems, did she not?

A: Well, she had some abnormal findings on funduscopic examination. She had, you know, the usual kinds of things you see with preeclampsia.

Q: Now, what were those problems—?

A: Well, it simply says here retinopathy, and he describes it as some blurring of the disc of the superior borders with an attenuation of arteries. He says there is no hemmorrhage or exudate, and I don't agree this is early hypertensive retinopathy, frankly. I think that some careful definitions again are in order here. I think that if there is some attenuation of the arteries, it is important to know what the L/S ratio is, but blurring of the borders of the discs indicates also some cerebral edema to me, and I think that takes it out of the category of just early changes.

Q: What does it mean?

A: Well, it means that the patient has had considerable swelling of her brain and she was in danger of having convulsion.

Q: That is severe preeclampsia?

A: That makes it very severe preeclampsia. This blurring is a serious sign to me, in my experience.

Q: The child was born with a nine Apgar?

A: Yes.

Q: What does that mean?

A: Well, the Apgar is kind of a rough test of the fetal condition. It is popular, and I think the shortcoming of the Apgar is that, that what it does is indicate primarily a very gross test of the infant, but it does not tell us anything about the infant's neurological problems at all. I mean, very minimal.

Q: Does the nine Apgar score cause you to change, alter or modify your opinions with respect to the fact that the child was born brain damaged?

A: Oh, no. No. Babies can have severe brain damage and still have good Apgar scores. You know, we have delivered mongoloids, children with Down's syn-drome—I did an anencephalic, that is, a baby with, with no cover over its head, and a monster—and the Apgar was eight, so that does not mean the baby has got good brain function or good neurological function.

Q: You are a qualified obstetrician, are you not?

A: That is correct.

Q: In the course of your studies, are you required to know the anatomy of the fetus and the brain of the fetus?

A: Yes.

Q: Are you required to know the anatomy, the pathology, and the physiology of the brain?

A: Yes.

Q: And of the central nervous system?

A: Yes.

Q: Taking into consideration the fact that the child demonstrated seizures between 48 and 72 hours after birth which manifested itself on the left side and later developed a right hemiparesis, what if anything does that permit you to con-clude with respect to the area of the brain that was damaged?

A: Well, if the baby had some problems on her left side, that means that there was damage on the right side of the brain. When there was damage, when there was the hemiparesis on the right side, there was damage also on the left side of the brain, and so right and left equal a whole, so there was diffuse brain damage.

§ 32.2   Direct Examination of an Expert in Vocational Rehabilitation on the Subject of Damages in a Birth Trauma Case

Direct Examination by Mr. Norman Tucker:

Q: Would you state your name, please?

A: Carl Smith.

Q: What is your occupation?

A: I am a vocational Rehabilitation Counselor in private practice.

Q: Are you associated with any particular business concern or any particular firm?

A: I am self-employed under the name of Carl Smith and Associates, Inc.

Q: What is Carl Smith and Associates, Inc.?

A: It is a vocational rehabilitation counseling firm that specializes in evaluating and providing services to individuals who have medical and/or psychological problems. We make determinations as to whether they can work and also arrange for and coordinate delivery of care they need in order to improve or maintain their employment and life situations.

Q: How many people do you employ?

A: Presently, there are four full-time employees in my organization.

Q: Are these people also vocational rehabilitation specialists?

A: Three are certified vocational rehabilitation counselors. I also have psychologists, nurses, and other medical professionals such as speech therapists and occupational therapists who consult with me on a regular basis in my work—who are not full-time employees, but work with me.

Q: What is your position with the firm?

A: I am the president and the primary clinician in terms of the work that is performed at Carl Smith and Associates, Inc.

Q: Do you hold any type of certification in your field of work?

A: Yes. I hold four certifications and my organization holds one. I am a certified rehabilitation counselor, which means that I have taken and passed an examination and maintained a minimum of 30 hours a year of continuing education units that are approved by the certifying agency. I am also a certified social worker under Michigan licensing regulations. I am a nationally certified counselor, in counseling within a broad sense, not just rehabilitation counseling. My organization is approved by the Department of Labor in Lansing, Michigan to provide rehabilitation services to people who are hurt in the State of Michigan and I am certified by the federal government to provide services to injured workers who are working for the federal government.

Q: For your certification as a vocational rehabilitation counselor, what qualifications are required?

A: Well, first of all there are educational requirements, usually a master's degree in either rehabilitation counseling or in a similar field such as psychology or counseling is required. And, then, a minimum number of years of experience depending on where you obtained your graduate degree from. If you have not graduated from a core-accredited school, you have to put in a minimum of one year practical experience before you can take the examination. If you graduate from a core accredited school, you can take the examination upon graduation.

Q: What is a "core-accredited" school?

A: It is a graduate school which is accredited by the Commission on Rehabilitation Education.

Q: So, you must have a master's degree?

A: Yes. In some cases a master's degree with an internship as part of your training is sufficient. In other cases, you have to have a master's degree and at least one year of practical experience before you can take the examination.

Q: And you have to pass an exam in addition to your educational requirement?

A: That is correct.

Q: Who certifies vocational rehabilitation counselors?

A: It is a national organization, the Commission on Rehabilitation Counselors Certification, which is in Chicago, Illinois. This organization is the one that has set up the testing and devised and validated the test and maintained the criteria for continuing education units. All of the units, 30 units per year, must be approved by their organization to apply toward an individual's recertification.

Q: Continuing education credits are required for certification?

A: Yes. An individual has to maintain at least 30 hours a year of education in order to maintain their certification. If they do not do that, then they have to retake the written examination to keep the certification.

Q: How often must you be recertified?

A: The recertification process is once every five years. If you do not demonstrate 150 hours of approved course work over a five-year period of time, then you have to retake the examination.

Q: Who approves the coursework?

A: It is approved by the Commission on Rehabilitation Counselor Certification. It has local representatives who look at the curriculum and its content and approve the course. You yourself can bring an existing course or class to the commission for approval, or the approval can be sought by and granted to the institution or individual that is setting up the class or course.

Q: How long have you been certified as a vocational rehabilitation counselor?

A: Certification process started in 1974. I have been certified since July, 1974. So approximately 10 years now.

Q: Prior to being certified, did you also work in the field of vocational rehabilitation counseling?

A: Yes. I started in this field in August, 1967, with the State of Michigan in the Wayne County area. My job at that time was to develop and run a program designed specifically to help those who had been hurt at work. Later on I helped develop a program for individuals who had been seriously hurt in automobile accidents. I rose through the ranks and was promoted to district supervisor before I left and went into private practice in January, 1976.

Q: Where did you receive your education prior to certification?

A: Well, my bachelor's degree was from Wayne State University with a major in psychology. My master's was from the University of Detroit with a major in counseling and a minor in industrial psychology in 1967.

Q: Did your academic course work focus on any special area?

A: The academic course work both at an undergraduate level and at a graduate level were primarily in the behavioral sciences. Also, my undergraduate training was in the exact sciences such as chemistry and biology, and I did my internship and my graduate program with the state vocational rehabilitation program. So, part of my education was, in fact, an internship as a vocational rehabilitation counselor.

Q: Was the internship required as part of your academic program?

A: Yes, it was.

Q: Where did you do your internship?

A: That was down at the Metropolitan Projects Office in Detroit, Michigan in 1967.

Q: Could you describe that internship?

A: Well, essentially, I was supervised by senior rehabilitation counselors and supervisors in the handling of cases that needed to be evaluated for rehabilitation services and also the provision of those services.

Q: Would you describe more specifically your tasks as an intern?

A: Evaluation, testing, determining vocational objectives, counseling, placement, and coordination of services.

Q: How many times have you been recertified?

A: I have just completed my second recertification process with somewhere in excess of 300 hours of educational credit over a five-year period.

Q: You have in fact taken twice the required number of hours of coursework?

A: Yes.

Q: In other words you met the coursework requirements as opposed to taking the exam?

A: Yes.

Q: Did your recertification coursework concentrate in any special areas?

A: Yes. The bulk of the work was done at medical institutions in seminars dealing with catastrophically disabled individuals. By catastrophically disabled, I mean individuals who have spinal cord injuries or brain damage in some form or another, or closed-head injuries or some other injury to the brain, or people who are severely burned, multiple amputees, and wheelchair dependent individuals.

Q: How long has Carl Smith and Associates, Inc. been in existence?

A: Since January, 1976, when I left the State of Michigan as a district supervisor and went into private practice.

Q: What does your work encompass?

A: The bulk of my work involves the provision of clinical services to individuals who are referred to my organization. By that I mean, people with many kinds of medical and psychological problems ranging from minor to very severe. It is my job first of all to evaluate them. I meet with them, take a history, review the medical records and the psychological testing records, and then do whatever diagnostic testing I deem appropriate in order to arrive at a conclusion as to whether they can work now and/or in the future; whether they are in need of any retraining or counseling services; whether they are in need of any medical referral or evaluative procedures. I also make recommendations for evaluative procedures when necessary. In addition, I am actively involved in the coordination of services for catastrophically disabled people. Usually, these are people hurt in auto accidents who fall into the category of spinal cord/closed-head injury and multiply disabled, but it also includes brain-damaged infants and children. I coordinate nursing care, physical therapy, occupational therapy, speech therapy, and purchase of equipment. I also counsel the family and the client to hopefully help them adjust to a very significant problem. In addition to that, I occasionally teach at the University and Medical School and I am a consultant to a number of medical facilities throughout the United States about rehabilitation counseling and services to these types of people. That's how I spend my time on a normal basis.

Q: Have you received any special recognition for your work in the field of vocational rehabilitation?

A: Yes, I have.

Q: What recognition have you received?

A: I have been awarded a Citation for Meritorous Service in Appreciation of Exceptional Contributions in Furthering the Employment of the Handicapped from the President of the United States for my work in dealing with severely disabled individuals. I have also been awarded certificates from a number of organizations, including the Department of Labor in Lansing for helping to develop guidelines for private rehabilitation professionals who practice rehabilitation counseling. I have also won awards for dedicated services in the field of mental health counseling of individuals who have significant psychological problems.

Q: Are there any professional organizations in your field?

A: Yes, there are.

Q: Do you belong to any of them?

A: Yes, I do.

Q: With which ones are you affiliated?

A: I am affiliated with the National Rehabilitation Association. I am also affiliated with the National Rehabilitation Counselor Association and am a past board member of the Michigan counterpart of that organization. I am a member of the American Personnel and Guidance Association and a member of the American Rehabilitation Counselors Association and past board member of that organization. I am the past president of the Metropolitan Detroit Rehabilitation Association, and I am also the past president of the Michigan Association of Rehabilitation Professionals in the private practice. I also belong to the National Association of Social Workers and the Michigan counterpart of that organization.

Q: How do your clients come to you?

A: From referrals primarily. I receive referrals from a number of sources. The vast majority of catastrophically injured clients I receive are referred by employers or their representatives. I receive a number of referrals from medical specialists who are the primary health providers for this population. I have also received referrals from representatives who provide the medical coverage for these individuals. In addition, lawyers representing a particular client or a particular company will refer clients to me. In addition, I get referrals from my former clients and my former employer, the State of Michigan.

Q: In your career as a vocational rehabilitation counselor, have you had occasion to evaluate and provide services for brain-damaged individuals?

A: Yes. A large number of brain-damaged individuals have been referred to me for evaluation and for provision of services.

Q: Are you personally involved in testing and interviewing the individuals that are referred to you?

A: Yes, I am.

Q: Are you able to estimate how many brain-damaged individuals, infants and adults, you have provided evaluation or treatment services to?

A: Clinical services to. I can't give you an exact number, but I would estimate that over the past 17 to 18 years I have dealt with an excess of 100 of these kinds of cases.

Q: How many children?

A: Forty to fifty.

Q: What is your goal in examining and evaluating brain-damaged children?

A: Well, the goal, first of all, is to determine whether there is any potential at all as it relates to future employment. If, after the evaluation has been completed and the records analyzed, future employment does not appear an appropriate alternative, based on present information, or it is felt that additional medical help might be needed in order to allow the individual to achieve employability, then I am critically interested in the subsequent medical treatment that the child will receive. If the individual is profoundly disabled as it relates to daily living activities, is unable to take care of herself, is unable to interact with the environment as a child, who cannot communicate, a child who is blind, a child who is severely paralyzed or mentally impaired, then we are really concerned with the quality of life issue. The goal is to give this child as much stimulation as possible to allow that child the opportunity to enjoy whatever limited abilities they have as they interact with the world. To repeat, I begin my job trying to come up with a job the child might be able to do in the future out of the Dictionary of Occupational Titles. Although somewhat difficult with a child, we can at least look functionally at these things. A finding of employability would be the best alternative. If I cannot do that based on the present knowledge, then obviously we wind up recommending that the child be bombarded with everything that is possible to hopefully reach the goal of maximizing the quality of life for her.

Q: How do you go about evaluating the future employability of these children?

A: When evaluating employability, in general, first you look at what skills are required to perform certain types of jobs. We get this information from the Dictionary of Occupational Titles which is the standard text published by the Department of Labor in the United States in Washington. Each job listed requires a certain level of physical demand, a certain level of educational demand and a certain aptitude. Then we test an individual and try to match an individual to those parameters, whether they are disabled or not. That's how career counseling works. When you talk about evaluating the employability of a brain-damaged child, it works somewhat differently. First, they are not ready for the world of work, they are too young. But there are certain kinds of developmental processes relating to employability that we can measure now, and from present measurements extrapolate into the future. For instance, the capacity to sit, stand, walk, and carry; the capacity to read, write, do math; intellect, visual acuity, and auditory acuity; the ability to interact with the environment—these are all factors that relate to what is required for employment, even at the lowest level of responsibility. So, my assessment includes observing and testing what I can test, depending upon the age of the child and looking at the activities of the daily living of this child. Obviously, the more normally they react to their everyday activities, the higher the probability is that they will be able to do normal work in the future—to do at least the simplest jobs that might exist—the unskilled work in the environment. The more disabled they are presently, the less that probability exists.

Q: How do you make a judgment about an infant as to what kind of work that infant will possibly be able to do 20-25 years down the road?

A: It is obvious you cannot pick out the precise job that they might or might not be able to do. The best that you can do under those kind of circumstances is to measure this child against a norm, and that norm would be other children who belong in the same age category as the child you are evaluating. So the closer they are to the norm, then the closer they would be to average type things, or norm type things if they were 18 and entered into the world of work. Obviously, if they are above the norm, then they would probably be above the average as it relates to jobs and occupations that exist in the dictionary. If, as we see with profoundly disabled children, they are way below the norm in terms of developmental milestones, in terms of intellectual capabilities and other factors, then with that kind of information, you can make a good estimate that they will be unemployable providing their condition remains the same.

Q: What has been your experience in this field as it relates to whether the present picture remains the same in the future?

A: In my 17 years of evaluating these kinds of clients, I have not seen miraculous recoveries after a period of recuperation of some significant time. My experience has been that the individual tends not to progress after a recovery period of a year or two years post-injury.

Q: Other than your own evaluation of the child, what else do you consider when you make that determination of employability for a child?

A: Other than observing the client (the child) and testing vocationally if I can—that is in reading, writing, spelling, math, and finger dexterity—those kinds of tests, I rely very heavily upon occupational therapy evaluation and treatments, physical therapy evaluation, and treatment, the results of neuropsychological testing, and the results of educational testing. Then I take all of that information and measure it against what is needed to perform the most minimally responsible job in the Dictionary of Occupational Titles. That's how I go about it.

Q: You test the child?

A: When I say I test the child, I test the child if the child is able to be tested from a vocational point of view.

Q: OK.

A: If the child is 1 year old, I can't test the child.

Q: If you cannot test the child what steps do you take?

A: If I can't test the child, then I look at the developmental milestones the child is making as compared to other children. I also look at what the diagnosis is from the medical people in terms of the functional limitations of this child. If those reports don't contain the kind of information that I need, then I use a standard set of questions that I ask the medical professionals and paramedical professionals in terms of the functioning of this child. Based on present functioning, I make a projection as to whether or not that child possesses the minimal functions to be able to perform work.

Q: What other things do you rely on?

A: Whether you are able to test them or not, you certainly want to see the child reacting in an environment such as an office situation and with you as a rehabilitation counselor. If it is possible, I personally interview them. The interview process, especially as it relates to infants and children, is done with the parents in attendance. And, if the child can communicate, certainly whatever interviewing and testing that can be done within the limits of their particular problems is accomplished. If they are unable to communicate or they are unable to respond, then the history and information is gathered from the parents along with information from the treating medical and paramedical professions. I may ask the child to draw a picture if she is capable of drawing. I take a very thorough history regarding the care needs of this particular child and compare those needs against those of a noninjured child of a similar age to see whether or not this child needs more or less care than children who are not injured. The history will note any special equipment that the parents need to use in care of this child and the therapy that is done at home other than that which is done by the professionals. I will take a look at the family structure and the interaction of this child and its parents in terms of that socialization process. This gives me, as a rehabilitation counselor, a much more objective look at this client than what I get by reading medical reports, which merely gives me diagnoses and functions.

Q: Are you acquainted with the plaintiff in this action?

A: Yes, I am.

Q: When did you first become acquainted with the plaintiff?

A: June 30, 1983.

Q: For what purpose did you see her at that time?

A: She was referred to me by her treating developmental medicine specialist for an evaluation relative to future needs that she may have as a result of severe brain damage.

Q: Did you do that evaluation?

A: Yes, I did.

Q: And how did you proceed?

A: I received from the medical doctor, medical records regarding this child and then I saw the child accompanied by her parents in my offices in Southfield. At that time I took a history of her regarding what had happened to her and the kinds of medical treatment that she has received in the past and her current ongoing treatment situation. I also took a history relative to her medication on an ongoing basis, and any other serious illnesses that she may have had experiencing that were unrelated to her brain-damage situation. We also talked at great length regarding a typical day's activities or daily living needs essential for taking care of Stacey. This included the equipment that she has to have at home, therapy that's done at home which augments the school therapy program, special transportational needs, special therapies that occur on a daily basis. Also, I had the opportunity to observe Stacey in the office and see her interact with her parents, and of course, interact with me. Then I generated a report to the physician regarding the current level of care and the present cost of future care based on his recommendation for future care along with recommendations of other professionals who evaluated her.

Q: In addition to your observations and interviews with the parents and the evaluation reports and records of the medical professional, did you do anything else during the time you spent with Stacey?

A: Well, part of the evaluation was to look at her potential employability into the future, and so part of the evaluation was to take that into consideration. Stacey was unable to perform many of the tests that measured the kinds of skills that are necessary for the world of work. But that was considered.

Q: So you were unable to do as much testing on her as you would have on an adult in the same situation.

A: Well, she was unable to perform the testing, but there are some adults that are also unable to perform the testing.

Q: Other than interviewing Stacey on June 19, 1983, and seeing her report, have you had any other contact with her?

A: Well, I've been to her home. I've seen her interact in her home situation, and I've also been in her school and talked with her teachers and her therapist and seen her interacting in the program plan there on a number of occasions. I believe I have seen Stacey, since the initial evaluation, probably two other times.

Q: Now, based on your personal observations, the tests, interviews, and records from her physicians have you been able to form an opinion as of Stacey's future employability?

A: Yes, I have.

Q: What is that opinion?

A: It is my opinion based on the results of my evaluation, observation, and review of all the material that I have seen in light of the requirements seen in the Dictionary of Occupational Titles that there are no jobs that exist that Stacey would be able to do, if she were to enter the work market place with the kinds of functioning that she currently demonstrates.

Q: What are the reasons for that opinion?

A: The reasons for that opinion are, first of all, that the jobs that I indicated earlier as described in the Dictionary of Occupational Titles require a minimum level of functioning as relates to a number of parameters. Stacey is profoundly disabled. She is unable to communicate, she is not able to take care of her everyday needs, she needs constant supervision. There are no competitive jobs, by that I mean jobs that pay $3.35 an hour where the individual works at least to a certain degree on their own, that she would be able to perform given this kind of current functioning. I arrived at the conclusion based on my observation of her which were confirmed by the medical diagnosis and the functional reports of the therapist, teacher, and other professionals working with her. Observing Stacey at home with her sister, brother, and parents further confirms the fact that Stacey is not the type of individual, based on her present level of functioning, who would be able to perform in the work world at the lowest level of competitive work that we know about.

Q: In the course of your work, is it necessary for you to be familiar with the compensation levels for the various types of employment available in the State of Michigan?

A: Yes, it is.

Q: And how do you familiarize yourself with these?

A: In a number of ways. First of all, a large portion of my practice includes dealing with individuals who have worked in the market place and been injured there and subsequently were referred to me for services. Second, as part of my job as a rehabilitation counselor, I have to be involved in placement in the work world, so I am out talking with employers on a regular basis weekly. Third, we rely on the United States Census Bureau and the Michigan Employment Security Commission for current data as it relates to average salaries and salaries in specific professions. That's how I keep abreast of all of the salaries for jobs in Michigan.

Q: When you evaluate the individual that has never worked, how do you determine the level of compensation that she would be able to earn?

A: Well, if they've never worked and are disabled and I want to determine what they would have been paid if they had not been injured, I'd have to take a look at the average level of compensation. Assuming that the individual would have been in the normal range to begin with, I can then look at the average salary that exists in the State of Michigan at any given point in time and conclude that an individual with the normal range of functions would be able to earn the average salary. They may have earned more than that and they might have earned less than that, but that's at least one way of looking at what the individual had she not been injured would be able to earn in the State of Michigan.

Q: Do you also make a determination of the level of skill at which they would have worked had they not been injured?

A: Well, we can look at the potential for that. Certainly, people who are in the average range can learn and do learn up to and including skilled work, and many people who are average do unskilled work. But, certainly compensation doesn't necessarily reflect the level of skill. As there are certain unskilled jobs that pay very good money, and of course skilled work usually pays excellent money.

Q: When you are making a determination of the employability of a person who has never worked who has never worked, how do you generally estimate the level of skill?

A: I take the average range. I indicate that if the individual would have been average, then an average salary and an average skill would apply, which would probably be in a semi-skilled ranged. At least they would have qualified for that. They might not be in the skilled category.

Q: Are you able then, based on your experience and on the evaluation of the individual in this case to give a reasonable estimate of what Stacey, had she not been injured, would have been able to earn?

A: If Stacey were to be able to enter the employment market place today in the State of Michigan at an average salary job—that average salary would be $27,000 a year. That is the average salary in Michigan.

Q: Based on her current level of function what would you expect her to be able to earn?

A: Presently? Given her present set of circumstances?

Q: Given her present set of circumstances.

A: Given her present set of circumstances, my opinion is that there would be no jobs that would exist that she would be able to do. So therefore, her earnings would be zero.

Q: Through your experience how long do people usually work?

A: That, of course, varies on the type of work that an individual is doing. Many people retire at age 62, some retire at age 65. Of course we know that under the law that individuals can work to age 70 if they can perform their work. So it really varies. My rule of thumb usually is that if an individual enters the work market place at the age 18, then she usually will retire somewhere in her early 60s, 62 to 65.

Q: In Stacey's case?

A: The same estimate, probably a total of about 45 years.

Q: As a vocational rehabilitation counselor, you say that you also arrange for and coordinate services, medical services, etc., and the acquisition of the equipment for disabled individuals?

A: Yes, I do, based on the physicians' recommendations and recommendations of the other consultants previously mentioned?

Q: Do you provide the service independent of a determination of employability?

A: Yes, it is independent of that evaluation.

Q: What special contribution does a rehabilitation counsel make regarding procurement of services or equipment?

A: The contribution is the knowledge of all of the available equipment, vendors, and service delivery people in the community, and an ability to make comparisons as it relates to a particular agencies or particular vendors of kinds of equipment that may be available from different sources. The family does not have experience in this situation. They really need to rely on someone who has had a lot of experience, in the sense of what's out there, in order to provide them with sufficient information so that they can make the best judgment regarding what they need to provide for the child, and, how much that is going to cost them over time.

Q: Have you arranged for and coordinated prescribed services and equipment for brain-damaged individuals, including children?

A: I have in the past and I continue to do so presently, yes.

Q: What types of services do you arrange for and coordinate?

A: I can give you a whole battery of services that need to be considered. They are not necessarily done in every case, but they are certainly things that we need to look at. As far as evaluations, I coordinate visual evaluations, hearing evaluations, speech, medical, orthopedic, neurological, psychiatric, psychological, educational, occupational therapy, and physical therapy evaluations. I also coordinate the treatment that may be recommended as the result of those particular evaluations.

Q: When you say coordinate, what exactly do you mean?

A: What I mean by coordinate is that, because of my relationship with the family, because I have gotten to know them and have evaluated them, I am relied upon to select or help select the providers of services for the family. So that I actually get involved with the family in terms of interviewing the professionals involved. I determine the costs that would be involved, coordinating delivery of those services for the family, and making sure that we have the right blend of professionals who can not only do a good job treating the child but also blend in with the family. We don't just treat a speech disorder or a learning disability, we really deal with the whole family as it relates to brain damaged children.

Q: Would the services you arrange for and coordinate include nursing care?

A: Yes, based on the recommendation and prescription of the physician, it is my responsibility to get involved with the hiring of nurses and the provision of prescribed nursing care for a child. The level of prescribed care varies. It may well be that a brain damaged child is on a ventilator, for instance. In this situation registered nurse care would be required for 8, 16, or 24 hours per day based on what the physician feels is needed. If certain medications or treatments need to be provided, the level may be licensed practical nurse care. Where there are no treatments of any significance to be provided, it may be care at a nurse's aide level. Whatever the level, it would be my job to work with the family and with the provider of services to get the blend that is most appropriate, that would help the patient the most. I would also get involved in the fees that are charged for these types of services.

Q: How do you determine the costs of these evaluations and treatments?

A: I talk to the providers of the service—the doctors, the therapists. Many times the client has already been billed for the services.

Q: What are the costs for the different levels of nursing care?

A: For R.N.'s about $22/hr; for LPN's about $14/hr and for nurse's aides about $8/hr.

Q: You also stated that you have arranged for purchase of equipment.

A: Yes, I do. If an individual needs a wheelchair. I get involved in the procurement of that wheelchair. In addition to wheelchairs, there is equipment that is attached to the wheelchair. There are trays, pockets, heel hoops. Whether it's an electric chair or whether it is an orthokenetic chair is determined by the medical or paramedical people, but to get the equipment and to get it to the family is part of the responsibility of a rehabilitation person.

Q: And, you are also familiar with the cost of this equipment?

A: Yes, since I am involved in coordinating the purchase of them, I become familiar with the cost and the periodic replacement needs of certain types of equipment. I also need to know costs to put together the list of equipment that a client may ultimately need in the future so that interested parties can take a look at what this child may need in the future.

Q: How do you determine the cost of the equipment?

A: I talk to the vendors and the clients.

Q: How do you determine the frequency of replacement?

A: I talk to the clients and the manufacturers.

Q: What is the cost of an electric wheelchair and how often does it need replaced?

A: An electric chair costs about $4,000, and it usually needs to be replaced every five to seven years.

Q: What have you calculated to be the cost of equipment over a life of a person like plaintiff?

A: Approximately $200,000.

Q: For what kinds of equipment?

A: Wheelchairs and accessories; transportation vehicle, repair and replacement parts.

Q: What else is of concern to you in the process of coordinating and arranging for services?

A: Other than the medical treatment and equipment, the major concern as the child grows up will be the environment in which she is living. If the child is going to remain with the parents and continue to grow, then, if the child is, for instance, wheelchair-dependent, one has to be concerned about designing the environment so that it will accommodate a wheelchair as far as doorways or access to the kitchen, access to the bathroom, rolling showers, light switches, floor coverings, the driveway. If the child needs therapy, a treatment area and often a recreation area will be necessary within the home structure. My concern as a vocational rehabilitation specialist is that the physicians and therapists prescribe the necessary structural changes and equipment that will be needed in the home and that an architect who has experience designing barrier-free living arrangements, would consult with the family in order to design this environment within the doctor's prescriptions.

Q: And you are involved in this process? You, as a vocational rehabilitation counselor?

A: Very much so because although we are dealing with a child now, this child will grow and the family has to be concerned with the kinds and costs of environments they will be purchasing in the future or present modifications of environments to accommodate the child.

Q: What would be a reasonable range of costs for these changes in plaintiff's case?

A: Eighty thousand dollars.

Q: Are there any other areas that you are concerned with regarding the provision of services?

A: Yes. I make the family aware of and discuss with them the need for potential alternatives to transportation. If the child is wheelchair-dependent and cannot be transported in the family car in a safe manner, certainly a need for a van with special lifts on it must be considered. Once the child grows up, if the child has the capacity to drive a motor vehicle, then the need for and costs of hand controls and lifts are costs that clients must consider.

Q: Have you had an opportunity to view the list of services and equipment prescribed or recommended by Dr. George for the plaintiff in this case?

A: Yes, I have.

Q: Based upon your experience in coordinating services and equipment and this list are you able to give a reasonable estimate of the cost of the recommended services to be performed?

A: Yes, I am.

Q: How did you arrive at your estimate?

A: I arrived at my figures by looking at, for example, the types of evaluations that are prescribed. I determined the cost of a single evaluation and the frequency of need and did a simple multiplication process to arrive at the cost per year. I did the same for the medical care, the therapies, the equipment, the medications, the cost of support care that Stacey needs on a daily basis and then added it up for one year and arrived at my figures.

Q: When you are calculating cost of future care, do you make adjustments to the present cost?

A: I don't make adjustments. I just calculate costs based on the present prevailing costs in the community. An economist would need to make any adjustments over time.

Q: I see you're reading from a document.

A: Yes, I am.

Q: Is that something that you generated?

A: Yes, this is a document that I personally worked out regarding Stacey. It covers all of the areas that we've been discussing relative to her care and needs into the future. I have made all of the calculations and placed them in this form and then added them up.

Q: So you have a list of specific items covered.

A: Yes, I have a list of each category and the items underneath as prescribed by the appropriate authorities. The cost of each of those for a year, the cost over a lifetime.

Q: Based on the frequency that these services would be provided?

A: Yes, based upon the frequency that they would be prescribed and needed. It included disposable items such as blow pads, alcohol rubs, and other things that Stacey needs because of her disability.

Q: You mentioned support care, what can you explain exactly by support care?

A: What I mean by support care is the care necessary to take care of Stacey's needs on a daily basis. Stacey has extraordinary needs because she has severe brain damage. Had she not had severe brain damage and been a normal child, then her parents would have to exert only normal parental supervision with Stacey. Unfortunately, Stacey is not a normal child and therefore, to take care of Stacey requires their constant attention. Extra attention that wouldn't normally have been required had she not been disabled. Since the family has other responsibilities to themselves and to their other children and cannot devote 100 percent of their time to the care of Stacey, they need according to the doctor the support care at a nurse's aid level for 24 hours a day, the cost of which is presently $8 per hour.

Q: So they would be using the support care to relieve themselves of some of the pressures of caring for Stacey in order to attend to their other children and their own needs?

A: Yes, to get some rest from taking care of the special needs of this child, to spend time with their other children and with themselves. The care they are providing Stacey is not normal parental care. It is special care because of their special problems and that is why the doctor has recommended that Stacey have nurse's aid support care 24 hours a day.

Q: Now, what is your total estimate of home care cost?

A: Based on her current needs, in terms of medical treatment, therapies, equipment, medications, she would need $84,293 per year to take care of her basic needs. If for any reason these needs would increase, then obviously she would need to spend more money on her current level of care.

Q: Assuming that Stacey is unable to remain at home for whatever the reason, what kinds of facilities would be appropriate for her?

A: Well, in order to provide Stacey with a quality of life that would be stimulating and give her the level of care that she currently is receiving at home, she should have to be put in a residential treatment facility. There are a number of these kinds of facilities throughout the United States that do provide 24-hour day, 7-day week care throughout adulthood.

Q: In your experience as a vocational rehabilitation specialist, have you had occasion to investigate these special treatment facilities?

A: I have had the opportunity to investigate them, to visit them and to refer individuals to them. I know individuals who currently reside in these facilities.

Q: Are you familiar with the availabilty of these facilities?

A: Yes, I am.

Q: Are there many of these facilities available for long-term residential treatment of a child?

A: In terms of long term treatment of the child, the answer to that is no, if you are talking about quality facilities that provide stimulation and provide quality of life rather than "warehousing." There are very few quality facilities that are available for life-time placement.

Q: What do you consider a quality facility?

A: I consider a quality facility a facility that is run and approved by the Joint Commission on Hospital Accreditation and provides occupational therapy, speech therapy, physical therapy, psychological counseling, recreational therapy, educational therapy, sensory stimulation, and supervision in an attempt to maximize the potential of the child. As opposed to a facility where they just essentially stay in their room all day, are fed three meals a day, and given therapy periodically.

Q: Would a quality facility provide essentially the same care that the child is receiving at home based on the prescription of the doctor?

A: Quality residential treatment facilities would have services comparable to what we are prescribed here. There may be an extra charge in addition to the daily room rate for some special services, but they certainly have available the same type of services that Stacey is currently receiving.

Q: And, you are familiar with the cost of these facilities?

A: Yes, I am.

Q: Based on your experience with the facilitites, are you able to give us estimate of the cost per day to plaintiff for residing in such a facility?

A: Yes.

Q: What is that estimate?

A: The level of care that Stacey currently needs would cost about $290 day, plus any cost for special medical services would be over and above the $290.

Q: Can you explain how you arrived at that figure?

A: I arrived at the figure based on my knowledge of the costs per day of these facilities. I also keep current on the costs of facilities throughout the United States by calling them and by visiting with them.

Q: As a vocational rehabilitation specialist, do you make recommendations beyond coordinating the prescribed services and determining the employability?

A: Yes.

Q: What other recommendations do you make?

A: Well, I provide counseling services as it relates to adjustment to disability not only to the client but to the client's family. For those clients who have some work potential, I get involved in making recommendations and prescribing prevocational training programs, vocational adjustment, retraining programs, job placement services, job modifications, job re-engineering, and on-the-job training to help that individual get back into the world of work. To get a job that would be consistent with their level of functioning, if they can perform competitive work. If they can't perform competitive work, many times I have been instrumental in attempting to get them placed in a sheltered workshop which is below competitive work and is paid on a piece rate. Unfortunately, there are not a lot of slots available for the number of people who could really use this type of service. It is not really employment. It is work activity which is good for the client, but it is not competitive employment.

Q: How about the individual that you determine to be unemployable?

A: If the individual is unemployable, it is very important that we maintain her present level of functioning and continue to reach for a higher level of function. It is very important that this child be provided with constant and intense stimulation.

My further recommendations will include the evaluation and the provision of services by individuals to provide sensory stimulation to the child through her environmental and through recreation just to maintain their life at a quality level.

Q: Then you make these kinds of recommendations in cases of brain damaged children.

A: Yes that's usually the area in which you make the recommendation.

Q: Based upon your experience and your evaluation of the plaintiff, do you have any recommendation beyond what has been described by the physician?

A: In order not to allow a deprivation to occur in her life situation and to prevent regression in terms of her functioning, it is important that she be continually evaluated for newer kinds of things that come on the market to help stimulate her to the highest level. We know from the literature and from experience that these individuals only get better through constant, intense stimulation, and these services need to be continued in order to maintain and maximize any potentials that might exists.

Q: Who would provide this continual evaluation?

A: A vocational rehabilitation specialist.

Q: What would be the fee for such services?

A: Fifty-four dollars per hour.

CHAPTER 33

CROSS EXAMINATION OF DEFENDANT PHYSICIAN AND EXPERT WITNESSES

§ 33.1   Cross Examination of Defendant's Neonatologist Expert Regarding Growth Retardation, Small for Gestational Age, and Hypoglycemia

Cross Examination by Mr. Stanley Schwartz:

Q: You have heard the term intrauterine growth retardation?

A: Yes.

Q: You have heard the term small for gestational age?

A: Yes.

Q: Are they synonymous?

A: Yes and no. I think they are, different causes, or one could be a cause of the other.

Q: An intrauterine growth retarded fetus would be small for gestational age when born?

A: Yes.

Q: How do you draw a distinction between the two?

A: I tend to think of the small for gestational age baby as the baby who is already born. I think intrauterine growth retardation can be diagnosed before delivery.

Q: So, with your definition they are and can be used in tandem with each other? By that I mean before birth and after birth definitions?

A: They could be, yes.

Q: What reasons, to your knowledge, exist for the necessity of a neonatologist being in attendance when an SGA baby is born?

A: An SGA baby, obviously, is small for gestational age and, therefore, can give problems related to birth, or because he is inherently small for gestational age, depending on the reason the baby is small for gestational age.

Q: Could a baby be small for gestational age by reason of infarctions of the placenta causing a diminution of oxygenation to the fetus during the in utero period?

A: Yes.

Q. And can, to your knowledge, a diminution of oxygenation to the fetus be caused by gestational hypertermian?

A. Yes.

Q: A baby born SGA as a result of an IUGR can suffer from hypoglycemia?

A: Yes.

Q: Hypothermia?

A: Yes.

Q: Hypoxia?

A: Yes.

Q: Polycythemia?

A: Yes.

Q: In essence, when an SGA baby is born, all factors or all events known to increase glucose consumption should be minimized or avoided, is that not correct?

A: Yes.

Q: Why?

A: Because you have hypoglycemia, and hypoglycemia can cause problems in the baby.

Q: Is it not true that a growth retarded neonate has poor nutritional recesses because of chronic starvation in utero?

A: Yes.

Q: And after delivery of that baby is it not true that any storage that the baby has with respect to glycogen, for example, is more or less rapidly depleted?

A: Yes.

Q: And factors that accelerate this depletion would include perinatal asphyxia?

A: Yes.

Q: Hypothermia?

A: Yes.

Q: Increased work requirements for breathing?

A: Yes.

Q: What is meant by hypothermia?

A: Hypothermia is a drop in temperature less than normal.

Q: If this baby had a temperature of 94.3 when first taken to the nursery, would that be classified as hypothermia?

A: Yes.

Q: If the baby on or after delivery had a temperature of 95.8, would that be hypothermia?

A: Yes.

Q: Hypothermia is compatible and consistent with small for gestational age?

A: It can occur with SGA babies, yes.

Q: Are not SGA babies more susceptible to experiencing hypothermia?

A: Yes.

Q: If the baby is suffering from hypothermia, will that require the baby to absorb more oxygen?

A: The requirement for more oxygen may be necessary, yes.

Q: And does the effect of inadequate warmth have any metabolic consequences?

A: It increases the metabolic rate.

Q: Does it increase metabolic acidosis?

A: It increases the need for oxygen. If there is lack of oxygen, then it will convert to an anaerobic metabolism and, therefore, produce acidosis.

Q: In a situation where a baby is born partially asphyxiated, is it necessary to insure the warmth of the baby?

A: Yes.

Q: Why?

A: A baby who is partially asphyxiated is already stressed and hypothermia would only add to the stress.

Q: If the baby is small, ill, and asphyxiated, the rate of the fall of body temperature can be dramatic?

A: Yes.

Q: With the awareness of the susceptibility that a small for gestational age baby may have concerning and including hypoglycemia and hypothermia, what if anything is accomplished under usual events, to keep the baby warm in the delivery room?

A: Usually there is a radiant warmer in the delivery room, and there are warm blankets in the delivery room. The baby is born wet, and that only causes more evaporation and more rapid cooling, so the first thing that is done is the baby is dried off, wrapped with warm blankets and placed under a warmer.

Q: Can you define what you mean by a radiant warmer?

A: A radiant warmer is a unit that gives off heat by transfer of heat from one solid object to another.

Q: Is it thermostatically controlled?

A: Yes.

Q: Where is it located?

A: The radiant warming unit is above the baby.

Q: How is the baby then transported to the nursery to be kept warm?

A: In an isolette.

Q: And what is an isolette?

A: An isolette is an enclosed box, an incubator, through which warm air is circulating.

Q: How is an SGA baby tested to determine if it is suffering from hypoglycemia?

A: A dextrose stick can be used on a peripheral blood, or a blood sugar can be drawn and sent to the lab.

Q: A dextrose stick would take only seconds to obtain the results?

A: Yes.

Q: And a blood sugar with a stat would take how long?

A: Possibly an hour.

Q: So that if I understand correctly, if a physician wishes to immediately determine if hypoglycemia exists, he would use a dextrose stick?

A: Yes, a dextrose stick is a screening procedure.

Q: And I would further assume that time is of the essence in treating and caring for a baby suffering from hypoglycemia?

A: Yes.

Q: And the earlier in time a baby is treated the better chance that baby has to abate the underlying condition?

A: Yes.

Q: And as hypoglycemia continues there is a great likelihood of brain damage occurring?

A: Possibly, yes.

Q: So that under usual procedure or protocol the physician, once he received the results of the dextrose stick, makes a determination as to whether or not the baby is suffering from hypoglycemia; and if so, he immediately treats the baby rather than wait for blood sugar results?

A: Yes.

Q: Did you make any determinations as to whether or not this baby was an intrauterine growth retarded fetus?

A: I saw the baby, and clinically the baby appeared to be small for gestational age.

Q: Then, it was not your function or desire to try to make a determination as to whether or not it could possibly or probably have been SGA prior to birth?

A: Well, it obviously was, but I did not make that determination before birth, only when I saw the baby.

Q: Did you make that determination after birth?

A: Yes.

Q: And what did you rely upon to make that determination?

A: First of all, the size of the baby, it was 2.1 kilos, and this was a term baby by clinical observation; therefore, that put it on the growth curve of 10 percentile, which is by definition small for gestational age.

Q: Is there more than one type of IUGR?

A: There is a breakdown into asymmetrical and symmetrical. If it occurs early, then the baby is small in all parameters: weight, head circumference and length, or symmetrical.

Q: What was this baby's head circumference?

A. Thirteen inches

Q. Is that normal?

A: The normal head size for a baby is 13 to 15, so I would assume it is at the lower end of normal.

Q: Did you make a determination in this particular case as to whether the IUGR that allegedly existed was symmetrical or asymmetrical?

A: It looked symmetrical.

Q: The baby was skinny?

A: It was small, yes.

Q: The skin was peeling?

A: The skin was peeling.

Q: And the baby was meconium stained?

A: Yes.

Q: What does it mean to be meconium stained?

A: It means that the baby passed meconium before birth, and it means if the skin and nails are stained, that the meconium had been in the amniotic fluid for 24 hours or greater.

Q: If the amniotic fluid, the bag of water, breaks and there is meconium, can that baby swallow that meconium?

A: Yes.

Q: When a baby is meconium stained, does that mean the baby is covered with meconium when born?

A: No.

Q: What does it mean?

A: When the baby is meconium stained, it means his skin, nails, and the umbilical cord are a yellowish color.

Q: If a baby is meconium stained, should any efforts be made to determine as to whether or not that meconium was down at the vocal cords or the larynx?

A: In what time period?

Q: At birth.

A: Yes, that could be done.

Q: Well, should it be done? You have a meconium stained baby. You have a situation where the Delee catheter is used, or a Delee trap is used. In your opinion should further investigation be accomplished by examining the vocal cords and the larynx?

A: You can examine the vocal cords, but if they are not covered with meconium, that does not rule out aspiration meconium, and if they are covered with meconium it does not rule in aspiration meconium.

Q: But should it be accomplished?

A: It could be.

Q: It could be. Should a laryngoscope be utilized to determine if there is any meconium down in the larynx?

A: If you want to determine there is meconium in the larynx, you should laryngoscope the baby.

Q: And if a baby is meconium stained, shouldn't one want to make that determination?

A: Yes.

Q: What is meant by the term brain sparing?

A: This is a term used in describing asymmetrical intrauterine growth retardation where, although the baby is small in length and weight, the head can have a normal size. The head appears to be larger than the rest of the baby, and this implies that the, what little nutrition there was went to developing the brain rather than to the weight of the baby or the length of the baby.

Q: So that means the organ that would be spared would be the brain?

A: Yes.

Q: And one way to determine as to whether or not the brain had been spared is to determine the size of the head circumference?

A: In relation to the weight and length.

Q: How does aspiration pneumonia occur?

A: The baby, because of hypoxia, makes an attempt to breathe intrauterinally and, therefore, aspirates amniotic fluid which contains the meconium, and this, therefore, gets into the lungs.

Q: Can an effort be made after the birth of the baby to aspirate meconium and avoid meconium aspiration pneumonia from developing?

A: Aspiration implies material in the lungs itself, and if it is already in the lung when the baby is born, nothing is going to get out that meconium. If meconium is in the nose or pharynx or trachea, that can be aspirated.

Q: What about the larynx?

A: The larynx, trachea.

Q: And there are different degrees of meconium aspiration pneumonia? Mild, moderate, and severe?

A: Yes.

Q: In this particular case, did you make any determination as to whether or not the child suffered from meconium aspiration pneumonia? And if so, whether it was mild or severe?

A: The baby had respiratory distress and aspiration was suspected. A chest x-ray was taken, and the first x-ray showed small, patchy infiltrates at the right base, and a small streaky infiltrate in the left medial base, which would indicate that some meconium was in the lungs.

Q: Was there any ventilation support for this child?

A: The baby was given oxygen.

Q: Other than oxygen, was the baby placed on a ventilator?

A: No.

Q: The baby was breathing on its own?

A: The baby was breathing on its own.

Q: Is that why you conclude it was mild as opposed to severe?

A: Yes.

Q: Was a dextrose stick employed in this case?

A: Yes.

Q: When in time?

A: There is a note on the chart at 8:15 that a dextrose stick was zero.

Q: And the baby was born at what time?

A: The baby was born at 7:24.

Q: What does it mean that the value was zero?

A: It means that the sugar in the baby was roughly less than 40.

Q: Would that mean the baby, in all likelihood, was suffering from hypoglycemia?

A: It meant the sugar is less than 40. It has to be at least 40 to register on the dextrose stick at the 40 level, so it means the sugar could be zero to 35-36.

Q: Which would mean the baby had, in all likelihood, hypoglycemia?

A: If you define hypoglycemia as less than 40.

Q: If one defines hypoglycemia as less than 40, the baby would be hypoglycemic?

A: Yes.

Q: If the baby was hypoglycemic at 8:15 with a value of zero, in all likelihood, the baby would have been hypoglycemic at the time of birth at 7:24?

A: Not necessarily.

Q: More likely than not?

A: I would say no, because right before birth the baby is still attached to the cord and placenta, and, therefore, the blood sugar should be whatever mother's blood sugar should be.

Q: Would the baby, in all likelihood, at approximately 7:50 have been hypoglycemic if at 8:15 it had a zero value?

A: Possibly, yes.

Q: Is it not true that hypoxia, especially when it is prolonged and associated with IUGR, it may cause neurological damage to the infant?

A: When it is associated with IUGR, it is difficult to differentiate what can cause damage because IUGR babies who do not have hypoglycemia are also most likely brain damaged.

Q: Are you saying that most IUGR babies are born brain damaged?

A: Most IUGR babies in developmental assessment later in life are not normal.

Q: You would not say that the hypoxia helps the condition?

A: No.

Q: It aggravates the condition?

A: Yes.

Q: And it can in and of itself cause brain damage?

A: Yes.

Q: And it is very difficult to determine, then, which factor caused what brain damage, is that not correct?

A: Yes.

Q: Hypoglycemia must be treated by the administration of sugar as soon as possible?

A: Yes.

Q: Would a peripheral vein be hard to find in a SGA baby suffering from hypothermia and stress?

A: Yes.

Q: Why?

A: If the baby is hypothermic and stressed, he probably has a somewhat shocky condition and in a shocky condition the peripheral veins are collapsed.

Q: If the peripheral veins are collapsed, could an umbilical vessel catheter be utilized in order to feed the baby sugar?

A: If someone was knowledgeable in using that, and all of the equipment is present to use it, yes.

Q: What type equipment is necessary to use or employ an umbilical vessel catheter?

A: You have to have a special catheter. You have to have sterile instruments to cut down on the vessel. It is an operative procedure.

Q: When in time was an intravenous procedure (IV) finally secured and dextrose administered?

A: Dextrose was administered at 8:20.

Q: How?

A: Orally by gavage.

Q: Do you know what reasons, if any, existed for the dextrose being administered?

A: Because the dextrose stick was zero at 8:15.

Q: And when it is administered orally, what effect does it have as compared to IV administration?

A: It is slower because it takes time to be absorbed.

Q: By the body?

A: Right.

Q: When do the records indicate that dextrose was administered either by gavage or intravenously?

A: Nine twenty-five.

Q: Was that by IV?

A: Yes.

Q: Is there any indication in the record that there were any efforts or attempts made to create a line for the IV?

A: Yes, Dr. Martin at 8:45 was attempting to start an IV.

Q: That was what the hospital record indicates?

A: Yes.

Q: And it was accomplished at 9:25?

A: Yes.

Q: Do the records make any reference to what efforts, if any, took place between 8:45 and 9:25?

A: Yes.

Q: To establish an IV line?

A: Yes. They say, Dr. Herman and Dr. Fox were attempting to start the IV line.

Q: Did you ever make inquiry of the two neonatologists as to what reason, if any, existed for their not attempting to utilize an umbilical vessel catheter?

A: No, I did not.

Q: Between 8:45 and 9:25, is it not true, that in all likelihood this baby was suffering from hypoglycemia and the brain was being subject to continuing metabolic alterations?

A: Yes.

Q: Did you state that all IUGR babies are born brain damaged?

A: No.

Q: Are you indicating that all SGA babies are born brain damaged?

A: No.

Q: One of the things one looks for in order to determine the possibility of brain damage in IUGRs would be congenital anomalies?

A: Yes.

Q: Isn't it true that another thing one looks for would be the circumference of the head?

A: Yes.

Q: If the brain is damaged, usually you will find the head circumference to be under normal limits?

A: Are you talking in regard to IUGR's now?

Q: Yes.

A: Because it depends on the relationship to the length and the weight.

Q: You would expect to find disproportion between the head length circumference and the rest of the baby?

A: In the asymmetrical type of IUGR.

Q: What about the symmetric type?

A: The symmetric type, they would all be 10 percentile or lower.

Q: There is a term, is there not, primary microcephaly and acquired microcephaly?

A: Yes.

Q: Acquired microcephaly is when the brain does not grow after birth by reason of brain damage, so the head is smaller?

A: Right.

Q: With IUGR babies, you have observed situations wherein the brain is not damaged, or smaller, because of the blood being directed to the brain for proper oxygenation, and as a result thereof there is a diminution or reduction of blood flow to other organs of the body?

A: Right, that usually occurs in the asymmetrical. It depends when the anoxia occurred.

Q: Isn't it true with an asymmetrical, as opposed to a symmetrical, the baby is usually very skinny and peeling of skin?

A: Peeling skin implies post-maturity.

Q: But isn't it true there is some peeling of skin or wrinkling with an asymmetrical?

A: Wrinkled skin indicates weight loss.

Q: Isn't it true with an asymmetrical you find the baby to be skinny?

A: Yes.

Q: Assume for the moment this baby suffered from hypoglycemia and that as a result of not being propitiously treated sustained brain damage—are you in a position now to tell us what brain damage was caused by the hypoglycemia as opposed to brain damage that might have been caused as a result of IUGR?

A: I don't think there is any way you can separate them.

§ 33.2   Cross Examination of Defendant Obstetrician Regarding Hypertension and Preeclampsia

Cross Examination by Mr. Stanley Schwartz:

Q: In the course of your practice, have you had occasion prior to 1981 to treat patients whom you classified as high risk pregancies?

A: I consider all patients high risk pregnancies.

Q: Do you consider some patients more high risk than others? In other words, is there a degree, or is it a relative term?

A: I assume you could feel that way.

Q: It is not true that some pregancies by reason of the condition of the mother cause you to consider the existence of a higher susceptibility for morbidity or mortality to the mother and/or the child?

A: Yes.

Q: Would you classify a mother suffering from preeclampsia to be a high risk?

A: Yes.

Q: The same thing holds true for gestational hypertension?

A: Yes.

Q: When a patient of yours is suffering from one of those conditions such as gestational hypertension and/or preeclampsia, do you treat the patient with more vigilance and diligence than you treat your other patients?

A: Yes.

Q: Do you ask to see the patient more often?

A: Yes.

Q: In normal pregnancies, how often do you see the patient?

A: Anywhere from 12 to 15 times, approximately.

Q: Do you see the mother more often in the third trimester?

A: Every week.

Q: Every week?

A: Yes.

Q: And if a mother is suffering from, let us say, preeclampsia or gestational hypertension in the third trimester, do you see the mother more often than every week?

A: We would admit her to the hospital.

Q: You admit the patient to the hospital when she is suffering from either one of those conditions?

A: That is correct.

Q: Is it important when a patient of yours is suffering from preeclampsia or hypertension, to admit that patient to the hospital in order to allow full bedrest and observation?

A: Full bedrest but they are allowed bathroom privileges? What do you mean by full bedrest?

Q: Is there a difference between full bedrest and bedrest with bathroom privileges?

A: Yes.

Q: When a patient suffers from preeclampsia or gestational hypertension that causes you to admit the patient to the hospital, do you admit the patient to the hospital with instructions for full bedrest or bedrest and bathroom privileges?

A: Usually bedrest with some bathroom privileges either for bowel movement or for bowel movement and for voiding.

Q: Are there any occasions wherein you would admit a patient suffering from gestational hypertension or preeclampsia and require full bedrest?

A: It all depends how severe her preeclampsia or toxemia is. If it is mild, the patient is allowed to ambulate to the hospital just to get her out of her environment at home and have her in the hospital. So it just depends, really, on the severity of the preeclampsia that this patient has.

Q: So you take into consideration the individualization of each patient's condition?

A: Yes.

Q: And you treat accordingly?

A: Yes.

Q: So, the degree of preeclampsia, be it mild or moderate or severe, would mandate what you do concerning bathroom privileges?

A: Yes.

Q: Is it not true that the committee for terminology of the American College of Obstetricians and Gynecologists has promulgated certain standards relating to the definition of hypertension?

A: There is a lot of controversy over that. Many men do not agree with their standards.

Q: Is it not true that hypertension is classified as a systolic of 140 or a diastolic of 90 or 30 mm of mercury systolis above normal blood pressure or 15 mm of mercury diastolic above normal pressure?

A: I think I would consider the patient, the anxiety of the patient I would consider a lot of patients coming into our office and having high blood pressure, and I have them taken at the hospital, they are normal tensive at the hospital, they are still frightened when they come into the office, and their blood pressure is taken and it is elevated in our office, and when they take it in the hospital or whereever they happen to work, it is always normal tensive, and this has occurred many times.

Q: Doctor, while you were giving your answer did you recall my question?

A: Yes.

Q: Let me add a postscript without repeating the question; assuming that the blood pressure is taken at six-hour intervals so that it is taken at least twice, both revealing the same elevated findings, would you classify the patient as being hypertensive?

A: Not on a real anxious patient.

Q: In other words, if a patient has anxiety, and even though you take it on two separate occasions with a six hour interval and it is elevated, you would not classify it as hypertension?

A: If I took it or hospital personnel took it, yes, I agree with your statement.

Q: When if at all do you classify a patient of yours as being hypertensive?

A: If I have seen her in the office on two separate occasions with an elevated blood pressure that has been taken several times by me, or by one of my aides in the office, and it is over 140/90, I would consider this most likely hypertension.

Q: Could you define for me what is meant by preeclampsia?

A: Preeclampsia is usually a combination of three things that comes, as you mentioned before, mild, moderate, severe, and it is, depends on the patient's blood pressure, loss of protein in the urine, and swelling or edema.

Q: Would weight gain be one of the signs of preeclampsia, abnormal weight gain? Excessive weight gain?

A: No.

Q: Are the signs that you made reference to, elevated blood pressure, proteinuria, and edema, classified as the cardinal or classic signs of preeclampsia?

A: Yes.

Q: A patient, if I understand correctly, can suffer from gestational hypertension without suffering from preeclampsia?

A: I believe in reading that preeclampsia, toxemia, gestational hypertension, pregnancy induced hypertension are all thrown together, and one man may decide to call it gestational hypertension, pregnancy induced hypertension. Another man may decide to call it preeclampsia. It depends on the article you read, and this is how he looks at it. So I feel that it depends on the article, and I would consider them all the same.

Q: Then if I understand correctly, by your definition a patient may suffer from elevated blood pressure classified by you as hypertensive without there being edema or proteinuria and you would classify it as preeclamptic?

A: I did not say that.

Q: Well, I thought that you said they are all the same.

A: I told you that in the readings they all feel that this can all be thrown in together.

Q: I am interested in you and what your thoughts are.

A: Would you please ask me that again.

Q: Yes, sir. The first question that I asked you, as a preamble to my other questions, was: Can a patient suffer from gestational hypertension and not be classified as preeclamptic?

A: If I understand your question, yes, she can be a hypertensive and not be preeclamptic.

Q: Whether a patient is preeclamptic or hypertensive, either one of those two conditions may cause a reduction of placental profusion?

A: You are asking me?

Q: I am asking.

A: Not necessarily.

Q: When you say not necessarily, are you indicating, then, that on occasion it can and on some occasions it will not?

A: That is correct.

Q: Are you, when you diagnose preeclampsia, or gestational hypertension, able to determine if the patient will suffer a reduction of placental profusion?

A: I would have a good idea.

Q: What information do you utilize to determine whether that particular patient will suffer a reduction of placental profusion?

A: The growth of the uterus over the past several visits in the office, doing an ultrasound on this patient and finding out what the placenta looks like, the amount of amniotic fluid, and the size of the fetus.

Q: Do you through the use of ultrasound determine diameters of the biparietal diameter, the size of it, the measurements?

A: Yes.

Q: That permits you to determine whether or not the fetus is small for gestational age or if there is intrauterine growth retardation?

A: Yes.

Q: You have a patient who is suffering from gestational hypertension or preeclampsia, you perform an ultrasound and you make a determination by ultrasound and other tests that you might perform that there is intrauterine growth retardation, are you then in a position to make a determination as to whether or not the patient who is suffering from preeclampsia or gestational hypertension is also experiencing a reduction of placental profusion?

A: I would assume so.

Q: You stated that one of the things you take into consideration in order to determine if there is a reduction of placental profusion is the amount of amniotic fluid?

A: Yes.

Q: If there is a larger than normal amount of amniotic fluid, does that assist you in negating the possibility of there being intrauterine growth retardation?

A: Yes.

Q: When you attempt to determine the gestational age, is it not true that it is best to perform the ultrasound in the second trimester rather than the third trimester?

A: It is best to do it in the first trimester.

Q: The first trimester. Okay. Is it as accurate in the third trimester as in the first trimester?

A: No.

Q: Is it as accurate in the third trimester as in the second trimester to determine gestational age?

A: No.

Q: It is less accurate?

A: Yes.

Q: In determining whether there is intrauterine growth retardation, does it make any difference which trimester the ultrasound is performed as far as accuracy is concerned?

A: Usually intrauterine growth retardation occurs in your third trimester. That is when you pick up, and that is when you do the ultrasound. You would have no reason to do it any other time.

Q: And when you do the ultrasound, what do you look for in determining as to whether or not there is intrauterine growth retardation?

A: The size of the fetus. The amount of amniotic fluid. The biparietal diameter versus the abdominal circumference of the fetus. That is all I can think of right now.

Q: Did you indicate that ultrasound can assist in determining whether or not the patient is preeclamptic—

A: I said that studies are showing that by looking at the placenta and grading the placenta it can determine whether that patient is going to develop preeclampsia on the average of 26 days before she develops preeclampsia.

Q: It puts you on notice of the possibility of the patient suffering preeclampsia?

A: Yes.

Q: The placenta is important for nutrition in carrying back waste, correct?

A: Yes.

Q: It assists in the transportation or transference of carbohydrates, amino acids, glycogen, and oxygen to the fetus?

A: Yes.

Q: And the fetus builds up a reserve that is necessary for protection against the stress that is imposed on the fetus during the labor period?

A: I am not aware of that. The fetus builds up a reserve?

Q: Is there a stress imposed upon the fetus during normal labor?

A: Yes.

Q: There is a reserve that exists, is there not, of the amino acids, carbohydrates, and glycogen in labor?

A: Yes.

Q: Would there be a deception of carbohydrates, glycogen, and amino acids during labor by reason of the stress imposed upon the fetus?

A: Usually a reduction, but I would not say a depletion.

Q: Is a fetus classified as small for gestational age or suffering from intrauterine growth retardation, more susceptible to suffering damage during the labor period than a baby who is not classified as small for gestational age or classified as suffering from intrauterine growth retardation?

A: Possibly, because of its lack of ability to sustain itself during stress.

Q: What is your definition of hypoxia?

A: A diminution of oxygen.

Q: To the tissues?

A: To the tissues.

Q: And anoxia would be a total cessation of oxygen to the tissues?

A: Yes.

Q: And would ischemia as opposed to anoxia and hypoxia be a diminution of the blood flow itself to the tissues?

A: Yes.

Q: Can a reduction of placental profusion cause a diminution of oxygenation to the fetus?

A: Possibly, but not probably.

Q: When?

A: Abuptio placenta, a heavily bleeding placenta previa, a mother going into shock and having no blood pressure, or very low blood pressure. Offhand, that is all I can think of.

Q: Even though there is a reduction of placental profusion, this reduction of placental profusion cannot cause a diminution of oxygenation to the fetus?

A: In extreme cases, yes. Not in preeclampsia.

Q: In extreme cases of what?

A: Placenta previa, abruptio placenta.

Q: It cannot cause, in your opinion, a reduction of oxygenation to the fetus if the patient is suffering from preeclampsia or gestational hypertension without an abruptio placenta or placenta previa existing?

A: That is correct.

Q: Why is it important to treat a patient suffering from gestational hypertension or preeclampsia?

A: So she does not develop eclampsia, so she does not go into coma and become anoxic and the baby would become anoxic. You are treating the mother. The elevated blood pressure is nature's way of giving that baby more oxygen, it is a way of giving that baby a better blood supply.

Q: Can hypertension in and of itself affect the placenta by causing infarctions of the placenta?

A: If it is severe enough, yes.

Q: What is severe, by your definition?

A: The placenta has a reserve of well over 50 percent. The blood supply of the placenta is anywhere from 500 to 600 cc's of blood per minute. The fetus only needs about 300 to 400 cc's per minute, so I would have to say approximately 50 percent infarction.

Q: Isn't it true that the fetus needs close to one-half liter of blood per minute from the placenta when the fetus is at term?

A: Three hundred to four hundred cc's per minute.

Q: Three hundred at term?

A: Yes, near term and at term.

Q: Are you, then, indicating that if there is a situation where there is an abruptio placenta of less than 50 percent, it cannot cause damage to the fetus?

A: I gave you figures of 500 and 600 cc's versus 300 and 400 cc's, and the baby has a 50 percent reserve. That would be a very critical point. I would say probably a third and the baby would be fine.

Q: An abruptio placenta of a third or less, the baby would be fine?

A: Right.

Q: Does the baby's need for blood increase and become greater at term as opposed to the seventh or eighth month of pregnancy?

A: Possibly.

Q: Prenatal care is a significant factor in determining or assessing the well-being of the patient?

A: Yes.

Q: It assists in identifying problems?

A: Yes.

Q: It allows you to determine how, if at all, to treat the patient?

A: Yes.

Q: And one of your prime objectives of prenatal care is to detect preeclampsia as early as possible if preeclampsia does in fact exist?

A: Yes.

Q: And to treat the patient accordingly?

A: Yes.

Q: Preeclampsia is a progressive disease, is it not?

A: Not necessarily.

Q: It can be?

A: It can be.

Q: And with the awareness it can be, your objective would be to attempt to diagnose the condition as early as possible and to treat it accordingly so as to abate the underlying condition and avoid it from progressing?

A: Yes.

Q: Preeclampsia at any given time can develop into eclampsia with developing convulsions?

A: Most patients on bedrest alone do fine, and they do not progress, so it is not a progressive disease because that means every patient that would come in would progress from stage one to two to three and on, and most of them do not.

Q: To avoid it from progressing, you treat the patient.

A: Yes.

Q: If a patient is not treated for preeclampsia, the disease can progress?

A: Yes.

§ 33.3 Cross Examination of Defendant Obstetrician Regarding Electronic Fetal Monitoring of Premature Infant during Labor

Cross Examination by Mr. Stanley Schwartz:

Q: Clinical fetal heart rate monitoring is an ongoing observation of fetal physiology?

A: It is an observation of what can be going on.

Q: It helps in determining the adequacy of the oxygenation?

A: That is right.

Q: The fetal heart rate pattern takes on certain characteristics under the influence of various hypoxic events?

A: That is correct.

Q: Consequently, would you not say it is important for the clinician to have a basic understanding of the physiology of fetal respiratory exchange and the consequences that might occur to the fetus by reason of hypoxia and/or anoxia?

A: All one needs to know are the results of what certain patterns might lead to based on one's own experience and the experience of others. But one may not necessarily understand what causes the problems related to oxygen deficiency.

Q: If I understand your answer correctly one might be put on notice of the possibility, if not probability of fetal distress, but not necessarily understand the underlying physiology or etiology giving rise to that manifestation?

A: That is right.

Q: Nevertheless, when time is of the essence it is imperative for the physician to take definitive action rather than to take time to understand the underlying causative factors giving rise to these distressful signs?

A: That is right.

Q: And if fetal distress exists, it is necessary to take the baby out of the unhealthy environment?

A: That is an important decision.

Q: And the earlier in time that decision is made, the better it is for the fetus?

A: Well, that may be qualified. That may be true in many cases, and not necessarily true.

Q: In other words, it is only after the birth of the baby that you can state whether it was wise or unwise to wait?

A: You are correct.

Q: There are certain signs and/or symptoms that exist during labor that allow the physician to determine whether these are warning signs, ominous signs or threatening signs, correct?

A: That is right.

Q: In dealing with fetal heart rate patterns and fetal heart monitors, is one of the things you look for a baseline?

A: That is correct.

Q: And the baseline will tell you the fetal heart rate?

A: Correct.

Q: You can see an increase or decrease of fetal heart rate in response to uterine contractions?

A: That is correct.

Q: There is a correlation between contractions and the fetal heart rate?

A: That is correct.

Q: If you cannot see the contractions, for example, or cannot find them depicted on the fetal heart monitor tape, it is difficult to determine whether or not you have variable decelerations or late decelerations or, per chance, even early decelerations?

A: You have to correlate them with the contraction.

Q: And the way that you best correlate them with the contraction is by an internal monitor as opposed to an external monitor?

A: It is a more efficient way of doing it.

Q: Both monitors show the contractions in tandem with the fetal heart rate, but the internal is better suited for that?

A: It is better suited because it is not altered by the patient's position or movement or stress of any sort.

Q: An internal monitor can tell you a little bit more about baseline variability and, most particularly, loss of baseline variability?

A: You are referring to beat-to-beat variability?

Q: Beat-to-beat, long-term, short-term, correct.

A: That will give you a better tracing.

Q: If an external fetal heart monitor shows evidence of loss of beat-to-beat variability, it is reasonably conclusive that by using an internal it would be greater?

A: That may be true in some cases, although sometimes you get a better tracing on the internal and your beat-to-beat actually looks better because it is a better tracing.

Q: If, in fact, the external shows some element of loss of beat-to-beat variability if an internal is applied, it would more readily reveal a loss of beat-to-beat variability and probably would show a greater loss of beat-to-beat variability?

A: If it had decreased beat-to-beat on an internal, you could rely on it pretty well that is really decreased beat-to-beat.

Q: The fetal heart monitor will pick up bradycardia?

A: Correct.

Q: It will pick up tachycardia?

A: Correct.

Q: Tachycardia would be a fetal heart rate above 160?

A: By definition, probably yes. We think in terms of 180 being a tachycardia.

Q: Would you, then, put characterizations on it: mild, moderate, severe tachycardia?

A: I would think 180 would be what we consider more severe.

Q: But anything over 160 would be tachycardia?

A: That is right.

Q: Tachycardia usually exists in the incipient stages of hypoxia, does it not?

A: It can.

Q: Is it not true that when hypoxia exists, quite often you will initially find tachycardia and the more severe the hypoxia becomes, the greater likelihood of the tachycardia changing to bradycardia?

A: I would agree that is probably correct.

Q: When you have bradycardia, you have a fetal heart rate below 120?

A: Assuming the normal is 120 to 160, anything below 120 would be a bradycardia.

Q: You would have mild, moderate, or severe?

A: Correct.

Q: And would severe be below 100?

A: Severe would be 100 and below, probably. We would not be alarmed by 110 or so as we would at 90 or 100.

Q: One of the most ominous signs of fetal distress would be a sinusoidal pattern?

A: That is correct.

Q: That clearly and unequivocally indicates fetal distress, correct?

A: Well, I have not seen it often enough to say that is true or not. I am not an expert in that.

Q: Notwithstanding the fact that you have not seen it often, are you, based upon your knowledge, able to state that when you do have sinusoidal patterns it alerts you to the fact that there is a strong probability of fetal distress?

A: That I would agree with.

Q: Would it also allow you to know that time is of the essence in the delivering of the baby and taking the baby out of an unhealthy environment?

A: That purely by itself without any decelerations or loss of beat-to-beat would alert you that probably you have to think about it, but not that you have to rush into it, as far as my interpretation.

Q: Are you indicating, then, that whenever you see, on a fetal heart monitor tape, ominous signs independent of bradycardia or loss of beat-to-beat variability, it does not compel or dictate that you deliver the baby as soon as possible but, rather, just watch the problem?

A: Observe the problem or other associated signs of danger.

Q: So, if I understand correctly, what you do is watch the pattern until it possibly turns to a loss of beat-to-beat variability or bradycardia?

A: Or improves.

Q: Once a loss of beat-to-beat variability exists, does that then call upon you to deliver the baby as propitiously as possible?

A: Only if you cannot correct it.

Q: Assuming you cannot correct it.

A: Yes.

Q: And the same thing would hold true for a bradycardia. Once you see that a bradycardia exists, that is, uncorrectable, you then make arrangements to deliver the baby?

A: I would.

Q: Isn't your responsibility to also watch those signs of fetal distress or the probability of fetal distress and attempt to deliver a healthy baby by preventing problems from occurring?

A: I would agree.

Q: Isn't it also true that when you see certain signs and/or symptoms during the labor period, putting you on notice of the possibility of fetal distress independent of bradycardia or loss of beat-to-beat variability, you are aware of the fact that if you are dealing with a premature baby there is a higher or greater possibility of damage than when dealing with a full term baby?

A: I would agree that is true, if the full term baby is healthy.

Q: Is it not true that as bradycardia becomes increasingly severe, it is associated with increasing fetal acidosis?

A: That would be true, if you had a fetal scalp pH to prove it. That is conjectural, otherwise, I guess.

Q: Well, when you say conjectural, at least, it is something that the physician considers as possibly taking place physiologically?

A: That is correct.

Q: And without a pH which did not exist in 1980, there is no way that the doctor can definitively know, correct?

A: That is right.

Q: But the doctor does undertake, at all times, to treat the patient in a way so as to avoid any deleterious consequences?

A: That is correct.

Q: You talked about loss of beat-to-beat variability being an indication of fetal distress.

A: Correct.

Q: As a matter of fact, it is of significance that time might well be of the essence?

A: Again, if it could not be corrected.

Q: So that what the doctor looks for is a loss of beat-to-beat variability, correct?

A: That is one thing.

Q: And as you indicated before, an internal monitor is better suited to make that interpretation?

A: I think so.

Q: Now, when you look at the tape, you are looking to see if the beats-per-minute vary?

A: Correct.

Q: In other words, if it is constant there would be no variation; it would be like a straight line, correct?

A: Correct.

Q: How much beat variation do you look for in order to determine that everything is normal?

A: I don't know that I have ever counted them. It is a matter of just looking and saying: Well, this looks like satisfactory beat-to-beat.

Q: If you see a straight line, that is definitely a loss of beat-to-beat variability, right?

A: I will agree.

Q: Is that the only thing you look for, then, a straight line, to determine if there is loss of beat-to-beat variability?

A: The straight line is the last, the end result of something that may have been decreased beat-to-beat before that.

Q: So a decreased or diminished beat-to-beat variability is also indicative of fetal distress?

A: It is a warning sign.

Q: So that even though the fetal heart monitor tape may demonstrate a line that is not straight, there, nevertheless, can be diminishment of beat-to-beat variability?

A: That is correct.

Q: Is a favorable fetal heart rate pattern one which fluctuates five beats per minute or more but does not fluctuate more than fifteen beats per minute with each uterine contraction?

A: I don't know that I have heard the definition, but I see what is meant by it now as far as the fluctuation of the short term fluctuation of five beats per minute.

Q: There are certain decelerations such as early deceleration, late deceleration, and variable deceleration, correct?

A: Correct.

Q: In essence, you will usually find depression of the fetal heart rate at a certain time during contractions?

A: That is correct.

Q: That would be usually classified as an early deceleration?

A: I would agree.

Q: A variable deceleration is a deceleration that has nothing basically to do with the contraction?

A: Well, it happens during the contraction in that sense.

Q: Can't a variable deceleration occur independent of the contraction?

A: It can. Then, I would guess, you might call it just a bradycardia or something of that nature. It is my impression that a variable deceleration occurs with the contraction, not before, not after.

Q: How do you define an early deceleration?

A: That is a deceleration that occurs actually before the contraction begins.

Q: Well, doesn't an early deceleration occur during the contraction and reach its peak of deceleration at the apex of the contraction?

A: It begins, actually, before the contraction begins, and then is over with by the time the contraction is over.

Q: And a variable deceleration need not necessarily be over at the end of the contraction?

A: It would not necessarily be over at the end of the contraction.

Q: Usually, if it is not over at the end of the contraction, there would be a late component to the contraction?

A: There would be a late component.

Q: And a variable contraction with a late component is a very ominous sign of fetal distress, is it not?

A: Is more worrisome than one that returns rapidly to baseline.

Q: A variable deceleration is most often associated with cord compression, correct?

A: Cord compression and head compression.

Q: When you have cord compression, there need not be total occlusion?

A: That is correct.

Q: And needless to say, when you are dealing with a premature baby, cord or head compression may cause damage or harm to the fetus?

A: If the monitor shows that type of a tracing, that would be worrisome.

Q: And when it becomes worrisome do you still, nevertheless, under the circumstances, wait for a loss of beat-to-beat variability or bradycardia that cannot be corrected to deliver the baby?

A: It depends upon the degree of problems that you have before. If you have a lot of decelerations, one deceleration in an hour is not going to alarm you. If you have one with every contraction, then you are not going to wait for any change in beat-to-beat, so it is a relative thing.

Q: If I understand your answer, you would want to act more rapidly with warning signs when you are dealing with a premature baby than with a full term, healthy baby, because of the susceptibility of the premature baby to damage?

A: Possibly.

Q: But you do accept the fact that premature babies are more susceptible to brain damage because their fetal reserves are less than a full term baby?

A: I would assume they are more susceptible to damage of any organ system.

Q: Isn't it true that if you have a number of late decelerations with a premature baby, those same numbers, let us say, three-four in one hour, can cause fetal distress more likely in a premature baby than in a term baby?

A: Well, the full term baby probably has more reserve if it is healthy.

Q: Isn't it true that distress occurs from stress when there is a depletion of fetal reserves?

A: That is probably true, but the termination of the pregnancy would not necessarily correct that.

Q: But there is no way of knowing until you deliver the baby, is that not correct?

A: That is correct.

Q: Can you now define late decelerations?

A: Late deceleration is a slowing of the fetal heart rate as the contraction ends.

Q: By your definition, then, at the end of the contraction the fetal heart rate does not go back to baseline?

A: Well, it may be at baseline all during the contraction. As the contraction stops suddenly, the heart slows.

Q: Have you ever heard it defined as a deceleration that takes place sometime during the contraction but at the end of the contraction it does not come back to baseline for at least 15 seconds?

A: It would start when?

Q: During the contraction.

A: If it started at the beginning of the contraction and did not come back for fifteen seconds, that would still be during the contraction.

Q: No. What I am saying is, it starts to decelerate sometime during the contraction but instead of coming back to baseline at the end of the contraction when the intensity or tonus of the contraction is lessened, it comes back more than fifteen seconds after the contraction.

A: Yes, that would be an element of late deceleration, but the pure late decelerations occur basically after the contraction is completed.

Q: Late decelerations are considered to be an ominous fetal heart rate pattern, correct?

A: That is correct.

Q: They are associated with fetal hypoxia and acidosis, are they not?

A: That is correct.

Q: Are these decelerations proportional to the duration and strength of the contraction?

A: They do not need to be.

Q: But they can be?

A: They can be.

Q: We talked about variable decelerations being attributable quite often to head compression or cord compression. Late decelerations are attributable, are they not, to uteroplacental insufficiency?

A: Correct.

Q: Such as abruptio placenta?

A: Correct.

Q: You can have variable decelerations change to late decelerations when there is considerable hypoxia existing by reason of cord compression?

A: That is correct.

Q: Also, late decelerations can be due to uterine hyperactivity?

A: By uterine hyperactivity, do you mean increased number of contractions per unit time?

Q: I mean, a limited resting period, or a short resting period.

A: Between contractions?

Q: Between contractions.

A: They might be seen in that situation. I am not sure.

Q: Doctor, if contractions occur every one or two minutes and last 45 seconds, or 60 seconds, it reduces the relaxation period between contractions?

A: That is correct.

Q: And when a contraction occurs, it is breath holding for the fetus. In other words, there is a reduction of oxygen?

A: Well, the contraction causes the uterus to contract. Whether it also compresses more blood into the fetus at that time rather than constricts it, I guess that is physiology that I would not say for sure about.

Q: You would accept the fact, however, that delivery of oxygen to the fetus is a critical function of uterine blood flow?

A: Correct.

Q: And that, in all likelihood, there is a reduction of uterine blood flow in the intervillous space at the time of contraction?

A: Well, I don't know if there is loss of blood flow in the intervillous space or where the blood goes with a contraction.

Q: Then, taking your understanding of the physiology, would there, in your opinion, be a greater prospect or opportunity for the fetus to receive oxygen during the relaxation period as opposed to contraction?

A: I would say probably during the relaxation period.

Q: So that relaxation period is important?

A: It is.

Q. If you have long contractions lasting several minutes, that can eliminate or reduce the relaxation period?

A. That is correct.

Q: And if you have hypertonic or tetanic contractions, one occurring, you know, more often than three minutes apart, that can reduce the relaxation period?

A: That can, although then you watch what happens to the fetal heart rate at the same time, and if it stays pretty stable, then, that is probably not affecting the fetus to any degree.

Q: When we talked about labor itself being stressful to the fetus, the contractions themselves are the stressful factors, are they not?

A: They are stressful, but that is part of the normal physiology of delivery, that the fetus can accommodate to in most cases.

Q: By reason of the fetal reserve?

A: Fetal reserve or just the process of nature, I guess, protects the newborn that way.

Q: And one of the ways nature protects the newborn relates to the capacity of the fetal reserve?

A: That is correct.

Q: When you are put on notice of stress existing in the fetus but not to the point where you see sustained bradycardia or continuous late decelerations or loss of beat-to-beat variability, you, nevertheless, know that attempts should be made to ameliorate stress to the fetus because as long as the stress continues the greater likelihood of fetal hypoxia and/or acidosis?

A: I will agree.

Q: The lower the Apgar score at birth, the more likely that the fetus during the labor suffered an acute bout of distress?

A: It possibly could occur just in delivery, if you considered the delivery period as part of the labor period, I would say that is true.

Q: It is true the longer the stress the more acidosis that develops and the more acidosis the greater the likelihood of low Apgar score?

A: That can be true, right.

Q: In this particular case, the Apgar score was 3, was it not?

A: It was 3 at one minute and 3 at five minutes.

Q: That is low?

A: Yes, that is low.

§ 33.4 Cross Examination of Defendant's Independent Obstetrical Expert Regarding Stimulation of Labor with Pitocin

Cross Examination by Mr. Stanley Schwartz:

Q: Is it not true that back in 1973 a fetal heart monitor was required to be attached when oxytocin was administered?

A: No, it was not true. It was encouraged but it was a matter of availability.

Q: Who encouraged it?

A: I cannot give you that answer.

Q: Do you recall posted in the hospital for review by active staff members a notice relating to oxytocin wherein it is stated, quote:

For induction or stimulation of labor, the use of Pitocin or prostaglandins is permitted by intravenous drip in a controlled fashion only. During such administration, a physician should be in constant attendance to monitor the patient in order to safeguard against adverse reactions. Electronic fetal monitoring should be done unless it is not feasible.

A: I cannot independently recall. I would not say it is unreasonable, but I cannot recall.

Q: Is it not true that when oxytocin is administered electronic fetal monitoring should be done unless not feasible was the accepted standard of practice in the Detroit metropolitan community in 1973?

A: I would say it is not the standard—that is my impression—I do not think it was the standard of practice in 1973 for hospitals in the metropolitan area to have such a rule.

Q: Your answer would be that it was not the standard of practice in 1973 for a physician to be required to use a fetal heart monitor each and every time he administered oxytocin to a patient prior to delivery?

A: I think it was not a requirement. It was not outside the standard of practice in 1973.

Q: As the chairman of the department, you promulgate certain rules and regulations that you expect to be followed by members of the hospital, correct?

A: I do.

Q: And if it is not followed by members of the hospital, you want to know why, is that not correct?

A: Yes.

Q: Would I be correct in stating that the standard of practice dictated back in 1973 that if a hospital such as United Hospital had a rule requiring that electronic fetal heart monitoring be utilized unless it was not feasible, it was mandated, commensurate, again, with the standard of practice, for the physician to dutifully follow that rule?

A: The key, of course, if "feasibility."

Q: Can you define what that rule means by "electronic fetal heart monitoring should be done unless it is not feasible?"

A: I would say, in my own mind's eye, that feasibility would include two things. One is the availability of equipment, and, I think, feasibility is probably a poor term in that it should say also indicated. There are certain times when it is more indicated than other times, and I think that is a judgment call.

Q: When is it more indicated than other times?

A: In a patient that has fetal distress, that is basically it. A patient with toxemia. High risk factors.

Q: High risk factors coming into the labor room?

A: Coming into the labor room. Known high risk patients. Patients with previous fetal demise.

Q: Is a fetal heart monitor more able to determine the subtle signs of fetal distress than a doptome or stethoscope of fetascope?

A: I would say it is more able than the other methods that you are saying, subject to proper interpretation.

Q: For the moment, going back to the alleged rule and regulation promulgated by the hospital wherein it states that the drip should be administered in a controlled fashion only, what is meant by controlled fashion?

A: It means to be delivered to the still pregnant patient in a way you can control the dosage of Pitocin.

Q: By an infusion pump?

A: By an infusion pump, Ivac, something that will deliver a measure of volume.

Q: Is that a Harvard infusion pump?

A: That is one of many.

Q: Why is it important to control the drip?

A: It is important to control the drip so you can control the dosage of the drug you are administering.

Q: To make sure there is not an overdosage?

A: Correct, and make sure that you have fairly constant dosage.

Q: The second sentence of the alleged rule states: During such administration, a physician should be in constant attendance to monitor. What is meant by constant attendance?

A: I am somewhat surprised it says a physician must be in constant attendance. That is not standard of practice either.

Q: Back in 1973—and, Doctor, I ask you for the moment again to accept the fact that there was such a rule and regulation—if a doctor does not believe that that rule and regulation, promulgated by the hospital, is in conformity with the standard of practice, does the physician have the right not to follow the rule?

A: I think rules in general can be bent as someone sees fit. He must be prepared to take the consequences of that bending of a rule. We are also open to somebody coming to us and saying: This rule is not proper. Will you change it, and, of course, we consider that, and there are, there is a method where people in the department would get together and say: Let us reconsider this rule.

Q: Back in 1973, to your knowledge, do you recall any meetings wherein this rule was questioned as it relates itself to the propriety of the rule?

A: I do not recall.

Q: When did you first become acquainted with the drug oxytocin?

A: Oh, it goes back to residency times.

Q: Did you every read any article by Caldyro-Barcia?

A: Yes.

Q: He was one of the leading authorities in the use and properties of oxytocin?

A: Probably one of the leading authorities in the mechanisms of labor and uterine physiology.

Q: In your reading, either in residency or thereafter, do you recall as to whether or not you have read any articles authored by Caldyro-Barcia relating to oxytocin?

A: I do not recall.

Q: The articles that you have read, or the books that you have read relating to oxytocin have assisted you in knowing when to use oxytocin, what the contra-indications are and what the adverse effects might be and how to safeguard against deleterious consequences?

A: I believe so.

Q: Any drug can be dangerous if imprudently used, is that correct?

A: I will have to agree with that.

Q: Are you familiar with what is known as the PDR, the *Physicians' Desk Reference?*

A: Yes.

Q: Is it a book that is sent to physicians all over the United States?

A: Yes.

Q: The manufacturer lists, among other things, what it knows to be the adverse effects and the contraindications to the drug?

A: Yes.

Q: And over the years you have received the PDR have you not?

A: Yes.

Q: And I assume that you have used the PDR?

A: I have used it.

Q: To your knowledge, in 1973 or prior thereto, did you ever look in the PDR to see what the manufacturers stated as it relates to the use of oxytocin and when it is contraindicated?

A: No, I am sure I did not.

Q: Based upon your familiarity with the drug, is it not true that your knowledge in 1973 assisted you in knowing that even with proper administration and ade-quate supervision, hypertonic contractions may occur?

A: That certainly could occur.

Q: Is it not true that you also knew, back in 1973 and prior thereto, that oxytocin was contraindicated when there was borderline cephalopelvic disproportion?

A: That is questionable because of the definition of borderline. I think you are getting into a judgment area that the physician says: Well, I think this pelvis is adequate. I think this one is not. The physician would have to use a judgment call.

Q: I am referring, not to the subjective aspects of the physician, but rather a situa-tion where the physician determines that it is borderline cephalopelvic disproportion.

A: I think, again, that is a judgment call.

Q: Assuming that a physician determines that there is borderline cephalopelvic dis-proportion, once that determination is made by the physician, is it not true that oxytocin is contraindicated?

A: If you are asking for a yes and no answer, I would have to say no, it is not true. There are circumstances where you might wish to use the drug.

Q: Did the PDR make reference to the fact that with borderline cephalopelvic disproportion oxytocin is contraindicated?

A: I am not familiar.

Q: Back in 1973, were you aware of the alleged fact that oxytocin could, under certain circumstances, cause tetanic contractions?

A: Yes, I was aware of that.

Q: Under what circumstances could oxytocin cause tetanic contractions?

A: It could cause it in two circumstances that I am familiar with. One would be a hypersensitivity to the drug, cause undetermined, and the other would be a situation where the drug is administered in too large a dose.

Q: Or not properly titrated?

A: That would be too large a dose.

Q: Back in 1973, oxytocin was manufactured by Parke-Davis?

A: Among others.

Q: To your knowledge, were there package inserts that are included in the bottling of oxytocin?

A: Yes, there are always package inserts in drugs.

Q: Is it not true that the official source for communicating drug information to the physicians would be the package insert?

A: I don't know what you mean by official. It is one way. A PDR is almost identical to what the drug insert says. The language in the PDR is the same as in the drug package.

Q: The oxytocic drug or agent is an artificial hormone?

A: Pitocin is a synthetic hormone at the present time, presumably identical to the pituitary hormone. It is manufactured naturally.

Q: It is to stimulate labor?

A: Yes.

Q: Does it increase myometrial and intrauterine pressure?

A: It increases intrauterine pressure and increases myometrial contraction.

Q: What does it do, if anything, with respect to the venous outflow?

A: The fact that the veins are traversing the myometrium, the contraction of the myometrium would decrease the venous outflow, perhaps.

Q: And would it also decrease the arterial inflow?

A: It could also decrease the arterial inflow depending on the strength of the contraction.

Q: And consequently would it not, then, interfere with circulation in the intervillous space?

A: Would it? Or could it?

Q: Would it?

A: There is a normal decrease of venous flow, and normally a decrease in arterial flow of the intervillous space during a contraction, whether it is an induced contraction or a stimulated contraction, or any kind of contraction. You are talking a matter of degree, and I would say by degree if one contraction is stronger than another contraction, the contraction will have less circulation to the fetus at that point. Less oxygenation to the fetus, I should say.

Q: If there is less oxygenation to the fetus, that can cause a late deceleration, can it not?

A: Yes, it can cause a late deceleration.

Q: How do you pick up a late deceleration by using a stethoscope, or a doptome, or a fetascope?

A: You could pick up late decelerations with a doptome with difficulty. If you are especially looking for them, you could pick them up. The big problem with that is, is the length of time that you are monitoring. But good nurses and good doctors pick up late decelerations with a doptome.

Q: The uterus at term is usually more sensitive to oxytocin than if administered in the sixth or seventh month?

A: Correct.

Q: Why is that?

A: I don't know the reason why.

Q: If there is an extreme sensitivity to the oxytocin, the patient can develop excessive activity, even tetany, which would be due to the oxytocin overdosage, is that not correct?

A: Yes, that is correct.

Q: So, therefore, this overdosage may occur at any rate of infusion?

A: That is correct.

Q: Okay.

A: It is unlikely to occur at a very slow rate of infusion, but it could.

Q: Are you familiar with Rule 9.22 of the Rules and Minimum Standards for Hospitals promulgated by the State of Michigan—

A: No.

Q: Which states, so there is no sophistry attached to my inquiry, which states:

The hospital shall require that there be staff policies concerning the use of Pitocin extraction and oxytocics during each of the three stages of labor, and the same shall be printed and posted in all delivery units?

A: I am not familiar with the rule. I am familiar with the idea we must post the oxytocin regulation.

Q: Are you a member of the Michigan State Medical Society?

A: Yes.

Q: Are you familiar with the committee of the Michigan State Medical Society that authored certain rules and standards for maternal health relating to the administering of oxytocin?

A: I am not familiar with the committee as it relates to oxytocin, no.

Q: Would not good nursing practice dictate that when oxytocin is administered, the blood pressure of the mother be checked?

A: Periodically.

Q: Every 10-15 minutes?

A: No. No. I think blood pressures in labor are probably checked every 15 to 30 minutes.

Q: What is meant by tumultuous uterine contractions?

A: I think basically it is a term that is used, and it is probably a poor one, but they are contractions that are probably of greater intensity and greater duration than expected for that stage of labor.

Q: Usually when there are tumultuous contractions, would there not be a shortened resting period between contractions?

A: You could have tumultuous contractions with a normal phase.

Q: When there are tumultuous contractions with negligible intervals present, what happens to the oxygenation of the fetal blood?

A: The oxygenation of the fetal blood could be decreased.

Q: Can that cause brain damage?

A: It could cause brain damage in an indefinite period of time. I think time is another factor that must be looked at.

Q: What if anything happens to the fetus when there is a rapid transit through the bony pelvis produced by tumultuous contractions with abbreviated or negligible resting periods?

A: The baby can be damaged in two ways. One, it could be damaged by the oxygen insufficiency which you referred to and, two, the baby could be damaged by possibility of intracranial hemorrhage, it could be damaged because the uterus ruptured and the placenta is extruded, etc. You could have all kinds of damage, but basically that would be the thing. The other thing that could happen is the pop-out effect. If the baby comes through very quickly and the pressure is suddenly relieved by a precipitious delivery, it seems to be detrimental to the child.

Q: Is it not true that rapid labor may therefore damage the fetus?

A: Possibly, yes.

Q: When cephalopelvic disproportion exists, not borderline, but actual cephalopelvic disproportion, or pelvic abnormalities, would that be a contraindication, back in 1972, to the use of oxytocin?

A: If you use the "absolute" as the adjective, I would say that with an absolute pelvic disproportion it is contraindicated.

Q: What is an absolute cephalopelvic disproportion?

A: When there is a bony protuberance that would obstruct labor completely, interspinous measurement of eight centimeters or less. There are certain absolutes which are just a matter of degree.

Q: Then within that confine, if they are not absolute, it is judgmental on the part of the physician?

A: If it is not absolutely, then it becomes judgmental.

Q: Some doctors would, some doctors might not use oxytocin?

A: Yes.

Q: What does a physician do in order to determine whether or not absolute cephalopelvic disproportion exists?

A: Basically he evaluates the size of the infant, as best he can, and he evaluates the size of the pelvis as best he can by pelvic examination, estimating the configuration of the bony pelvis, certain basic measurements that are limited as to what he can do, but that is the basic way of assessing a contracted pelvis.

Q: Does he do this clinically?

A: Clinically.

Q: Is he able to determine the diameter and size of the mid pelvis?

A: He can estimate the diameters of the mid pelvis clinically.

Q: Are there other portions of the pelvic cavity such as the inlet and the outlet that are more easily measured by clinical examination than the mid pelvis?

A: Yes, the outlet is more easily evaluated by clinical examination than the mid pelvis and the anterior-posterior dimension of the inlet is more easily demonstrated by clinical examination than is the mid pelvis.

Q: What about the transverse of the inlet?

A: The transverse of the inlet is very difficult to evaluate on a clinical basis. However, it is, of all the dimensions, it is the least likely to be contracted.

Q: Which portion of the pelvic cavity, inlet, mid pelvis, outlet, is the most narrow?

A: You are talking about a gynecoid pelvis, normal pelvis?

Q: A gynecoid pelvis and, for the moment, accepting that this was a gynecoid pelvis.

A: A gynecoid pelvis is a normal female-type pelvis. It refers to the relative dimensions and the bony architecture, outside of the dimensions, proper curvature of the sacrum, lightness of the bones.

Q: There are four basic types of female pelvis?

A: Yes.

Q: One if the gynecoid, which is the most common and normal, one is the platypeloid—

A: P-l-a-t-y-p-e-l-o-i-d.

Q: And what are the other two? Android?

A: Android, which is a male-type, and anthropoid, which is an ape-like pelvis.

Q: What is the average normal measurement of the ischial spines?

A: Nine centimeters, approximately. Eight centimeters.

Q: What is the average, normal AP (anterior-posterior) for the pelvic inlet?

A: Ten. I think it is 10.5.

Q: You think it is 10.5?

A: I think that is about it. That is a minimum, anyway. Yes, 10.5 is the minimum. It can go up to 11-12.

Q: What about the transverse of the mid pelvis? What is the average normal?

A: Average would be about 9.7 to over 10.

Q: Nine point seven?

A: Ten. About 9.5-10.5. About there. It is in the ballpark. The trouble is it is very difficult to measure clinically.

Q: It is difficult to measure?

A: Right; it is an estimation.

Q: What purpose, if any, does a pelvimetry serve?

A: In present day obstetrics?

Q: 1973 obstetrics.

A: In 1973, and present day obstetrics, very little, cephalic presentations.

Q: It serves no purpose, when you say very little.

A: Very little. It is useful in picking up certain anomalies of the fetus, in certain malpresentations it may be of use, in breech presentation it may be of use, but I think it has largely fallen into disuse, in obstetrics over the last 10 or 12 years.

Q: It determines the shape and inclination of the pelvis?

A: Yes.

Q: It determines the length of the diameters?

A: Subject to considerable error, yes.

Q: It is more accurate in determining the size of the diameters of the mid pelvis than a clinical examination?

A: I don't believe so.

Q: It determines the relationship and fit of the fetus to the pelvis?

A: Usually not any better than clinical examination will this determine the fit of the pelvis and the attitude of the fetus.

Q: What about the attitude of the fetus? Is it able to determine whether there is deflection of the head?

A: Yes, but so can clinical examination.

Q: Even when the baby is high up in the canal?

A: If the baby is out of the canal altogether, in other words, above the pelvic inlet, then the x-ray would be more useful than clinical, but if the baby has already come through the pelvic inlet, then the clinical will be every bit as good.

Q: Are you indicating, if I understand correctly, that the clinical examination is more accurate in determining the transverse diameter of the inlet and the distance between the ischial spines than a pelvimetry?

A: No, I did not say that.

Q: Is it less accurate?

A: I think that both of them make considerable error, and to say which is better or which is worse is very difficult. We have been grossly dissatisfied with the measurements by x-ray pelvimetry, and we find that many times a pelvimetry says the pelvis is adequate and it is not, and many times it is not adequate and the baby has come through without any difficulty.

Q: Do you use pelvimetry today? Or have you eliminated it in your practice?

A: Virtually eliminated.

Q: And in 1973 did you virtually eliminate it in your practice?

A: Virtually eliminated it in my practice.

Q: And your associates also virtually eliminated it?

A: Virtually eliminated it.

Q: And United Hospital has virtually eliminated it?

A: Virtually eliminated.

Q: Do you know of any other hospitals that have virtually eliminated it?

A: Almost all large obstetrical hospitals.

Q: In 1973?

A: I cannot tell you about all hospitals in 1973. I think that in current thought x-ray pelvimetry has fallen in great disuse except in circumstances of the breech.

Q: What views are taken with the pelvimetry? In other words, is it more than just an AP (anterior-posterior) view?

A: Yes. AP. Lateral.

Q: Standing lateral?

A: Depending on the technique and the ability of the patient to stand.

Q: To your knowledge, was there any portion of the pelvic structure that was more accurately depicted by pelvimetry in 1972 than clinical examination?

A: I would say if anything could be more accurately depicted than clinical examination and it would be the interspinous measurement.

Q: When Pitocin is administered, should the frequency, duration, and intensity of the contractions be checked?

A: Yes.

Q: Why?

A: To make sure that tetanic contractions do not occur; and if they occur, the Pitocin should be stopped.

Q: Are you familiar with what is meant by Montevideo units?

A: Vaguely.

Q: What is your definition of it? Or, can I help?

A: You may help.

Q: It is the product of the contractions arrived at by multiplying the intensity by the frequency?

A: I think that is appropriate, yes.

Q: The intensity is the rise in pressure produced by amniotic fluid and measured in millimeters of mercury?

A: Correct.

Q: And the frequency is the number of contractions on the Caldyro-Barcia plane of every 10 minutes?

A: Right.

Q: Is contraction defined as the shortening of a muscle in response to stimulation, or a stimulus, with return to its original length after the contraction has worn off?

A: Yes.

Q: What is meant by tonus?

A: All muscles, and especially smooth muscles, have a state where they are only partially contracted rather than fully contracted, and it is the partial contraction that we refer to as tonus.

Q: That would be the lowest intrauterine pressure?

A: That would be the lowest intrauterine pressure.

Q: The resting period?

A: Yes.

Q: And the intensity would be the amplitude and the rise of the pressure?

A: From the baseline or the tonus state.

Q: What would normal be? Thirty to fifty millimeter of mercury?

A: I believe so.

Q: What is meant by precipitous labor?

A: A precipitous labor would be one that is rapid.

Q: Usually with precipitous labor there is an amplitude of over 50 millimeters of mercury in the contraction?

A: I cannot give you that information.

Q: Are you familiar with the Friedman curve?

A: Yes.

Q: Do you use the Friedman labor curve in your own practice?

A: Yes.

Q: What is the Friedman labor curve?

A: Dr. Friedman drew a curve on the normal progress of labor, dilation, started with a flat, latent phase, then phase of acceleration, it slows down at the end as the patient is about to deliver, into a transitional phase, the pushing phase.

Q: Doctor, would that labor curve assist you in making a determination as to whether or not there is dysfunctional labor, or, contra to that, a precipitous labor?

A: Not necessarily. It depends on what, what stage you pick up the curve. In other words, if a patient comes in and she is already in accelerating phase, it would not assist you. If it is in a latent phase, yes, it might be well worthwhile.

Q: What is meant by tetanic contractions?

A: Tetanic contraction is a contraction that does not relax in a suitable interval of time. In other words, it persists to two or three minutes, something longer, without a relaxation phase. A permanent elevation of the baseline, I would say.

Q: When there are contractions, what if anything takes place with respect to the intervillous space and oxygenation of the fetus?

A: With contractions, the intervillous space, the circulation is slowed in the intervillous space, and there is decreased oxygenation of the fetus.

Q: And the oxygenation of the fetus takes place during the relaxation period?

A: Basically, yes.

Q: So that if the relaxation period is abbreviated to, let us say, five, ten, fifteen seconds, and then another contraction, that can cause hypoxia or anoxia to the brain of the fetus, can it not?

A: It can.

Q: Essentially, the blood flow to the placenta stops while the uterus is contracting, is that not correct?

A: It certainly slows down, anyway.

Q: What if anything takes place concerning increased pressure to the head of the fetus when tumultuous contractions occur?

A: I think that the fetus is basically subjected to pressures in all directions by the uterine contraction. The head does not receive any excess pressure until the cervix is fairly, almost completely dilated, and it is pressing against the pelvic floor, and there could be pressure on the fetal head, and it occurs in normal labors. We know the fetal heart tones drop due to head pressure.

Q: When there is almost complete dilatation of at least 8 centimeters there is also tumultuous contractions, is not true that the fetus is more susceptible to sustaining increased pressure on the head than in a situation where there are no tumultuous contractions?

A: There will be increased pressure on the fetal head if the contraction is very strong. However, if we compare this to where the head gets the most pressure and that is from the bearing down sensation, it will be fairly insignificant.

Q: Did you not mention that one cannot determine tumultous contractions unless the patient is monitored to determine the millimeter of mercury rise?

A: Yes.

Q: The contractions can also be.

A: By the hand on the uterus. It is a matter of observation.

Q: And that is why a nurse is called upon to check contractions when oxytocin is administered, correct?

A: Correct.

Q: And when she checks contractions, is she not called upon to determine the frequency and intensity and duration of those contractions?

A: That is correct.

Q: And if the doctor is not in attendance at the time the oxytocin is administered and the nurse is checking, is it not incumbent upon the nurse to record her findings with respect to intensity, duration, and frequency of contractions?

A: Record or notify or certainly observe.

Q: The effect of oxytocin on the uterus varies from patient to patient?

A: I will accept that fact.

Q: It depends on the stage of pregnancy?

A: Correct.

Q: And the activity of the uterus prior to the administering of the oxytocin?

A: Correct.

Q: The condition of the cervix?

A: Correct.

Q: And the metabolism of the uterine muscles?

A: I would expect so, yes.

Q: Is it not true that the uterus of patients with a soft, thinly effaced cervix over three centimeters dilated is easily stimulated by oxytocin, especially if the membranes are ruptured?

A: May and may not be.

Q: Have you ever read Bonica?

A: Yes.

Q: He is an authoritative writer in the field of anesthetics and obstetrics?

A: Right.

Q: I refer you to page 314 of his book, *Anesthetics and Obstetrics,*—do you accept or reject the statement:

> However, the uterus of patients with a soft, thinly effaced cervix that is over three centimeters dilated is easily stimulated by oxytocin, especially if the membranes are ruptured?

A: I don't recall the statement. I don't recall reading that statement.

Q: But do you agree with the statement?

A: I would say that in a patient who is in labor, yes. I would say it is probably easily stimulated with oxytocin, but—and it would be more easily stimulated with oxytocin than if you took the similar patient who had a closed cervix, or the membranes were intact.

§ 33.5 Cross Examination of Defendant's Independent Obstetrical Expert on the Causal Relationship between an Analgesic Administered during Labor and Narcotization to a Premature Infant

Cross Examination by Mr. Stanley Schwartz:

Q: Is it not true that Demerol crosses the placental barrier if given in significant concentrations?

A: Yes.

Q: Is it your belief that, in most instances, it does not produce fetal respiratory depression?

A: I don't think I can answer that question. It depends on what you mean by depression and it certainly depends on the dosage and when it's given.

I can certainly say that, in many cases, there does not appear to be respiratory depression and, indeed, I could say in most cases there does not appear to be respiratory depression.

Q: Would fetal respiratory depression be a more likely effect when large doses are given?

A: There would certainly be some sort of a relationship between dosage and depression, yes.

Q: When you write your articles, I assume you try not to be vague but be as specific as possible in talking about the dosage and timing with respect to, for example, Demerol?

A: I try to be precise.

Q: Let me refer you to an article that you authored in 1968 entitled _____ _____. Do you recall that article?

A: Yes, I do.

Q: I will show it to you if you wish.

A: If I need to, I will.

Q: I am reading from the first three sentences. And I would like you to explain to me what you meant by your statements back in 1968. And it reads:

Demerol (Meperidine) has been shown to cross the placental barrier in significant concentrations.

Now, that is the first sentence. What did you mean by crossing the placental barrier in significant concentrations?

A: A good deal of it gets across the fetal barrier, but a good percentage of it—

Q: But a good deal of it does get into the blood of the fetus?

A: That's correct.

Q: It goes from the placenta to the umbilical cord to the fetus?

A: That's correct.

Q: While in most instances it apparently does not produce fetal respiratory depression, Eastman called attention to the depressant effect of large doses. Do you recall presently, a number of years later, what you meant by large doses?

A: No.

Q: But you would state that the more the dosage or the greater concentration of dosage, the higher concentration in the blood stream of the fetus?

A: Yes.

Q: What is meant by respiratory depression?

A: It is an effect which is manifested by lack of or diminished respiratory effort.

Q: If there is respiratory depression, is there a diminution of oxygen intake?

A: In the newborn there is.

Q: Yes. I'm referring to the newborn.

A: Yes, in the newborn there could be. There is not necessarily. If you breathe adequately for the baby, then it doesn't really matter that there is respiratory depression.

Q: You mean by assisted respiration?

A: That's correct.

Q: All right?

A: If you breathe—

Q: By positive pressure, for example?

A: By positive pressure or intubation or in some other way see that a baby's oxygenated. Indeed, that is the treatment for respiratory depression.

Q: When the respiratory depression exists, there is a diminution of oxygen intake?

A: There is a potential for that.

Q: And I assume there is a retention of CO_2.

A: There is a potential for that.

Q: And I assume that, with a potential for the retention of CO_2, there can be respiratory acidosis?

A: There is a potential for that.

Q: Respiratory acidosis, if lasting for a period of time, can also be concomitant with metabolic acidosis?

A: I think it would take quite a bit of time, yes, several hours.

Q: I thank you for that qualification. I appreciate it. Respiratory acidosis and/or metabolic acidosis can cause brain damage?

A: I think only metabolic acidosis.

Q: What is respiratory acidosis?

A: Respiratory acidosis is an accumulation of carbon dioxide in the blood.

Q: What effect, if any, does that have at all upon the baby's brain, a newborn, if you know?

A: I think in the absence of metabolic acidosis, it probably has no ill effect.

Q: No ill effect?

A: Long-term ill effect, I probably should say.

Q: Is the brain prone—that is of the newborn—to damage from hypoxia?

A: Any brain is prone to damage from hypoxia. But it takes a good deal of hypoxia to produce brain damage.

Q: When there is a reduction in the oxygenation, would there then be a fall in the pH and a rise in the CO_2?

A: Usually, if it's severe enough, yes.

Q: The metabolic acidosis that you indicated occurs in a period of a few hours is due to a rapid depletion of the fetal glycogen?

A: No.

Q: What causes the metabolic acidosis?

A: The metabolic acidosis is caused by the excretion of certain ions which cause a base excess, the excretion of phosphate ions and others, in the kidney. And it takes some period of time for this to occur.

Q: Are you indicating then to my inquiry, with respect to glycogen, that glycogen has no effect itself upon the acidosis?

A: Glycogen relates here, but I wouldn't say it causes. When the cells do not have oxygen or adequate oxygen, they undergo anaerobic metabolism; and, in doing, they use glycogen which produces lactic acid. And that's what causes the acidosis.

Q: Can you define for me anaerobic metabolism?

A: It's simply metabolism without oxygen or with diminished oxygen available for the metabolism.

Q: Does the hypoxia then bring about, in a newborn, a condition known as anaerobic metabolism?

A: Yes. Potentially, yes.

Q: And what correlation, if any, is there between the release of lactic acids and anaerobic metabolism in a hypoxic newborn?

A: It's the anaerobic metabolism which entails the breakdown of glycogen that produces lactic acid.

Q: And is that breakdown itself the most common cause of metabolic acidosis?

A: I don't know. It's beyond my expertise.

Q: Is it not true that in a healthy newborn, with no deleterious consequences befalling the fetus during the labor period, a physician anticipates the newborn taking its first breath within 30 seconds of life?

A: I think that's usually true. It's a little less true of prematures, which are much more vulnerable, of course.

Q: And could you now define what is meant by the term premature?

A: There have been various definitions. Today, we try to define it in terms of gestational interval, sometimes also using birth weight 2500.

Q: The infant, here, weighed 1800 grams?

A: In that area, yes.

Q: So there is no doubt but that she was a premature baby?

A: That's correct.

Q: And if you took her weight or even her gestational history, it would be premature?

A: Yes.

Q: And I think the gestational period was 30 weeks?

A: That's what I recall.

Q: Would the most frequent cause of respiratory depression at birth be asphyxiation?

A: I don't know. I think so.

Q: You've heard of newborns being resuscitated?

A: Yes.

Q: What is meant by resuscitation of a newborn?

A: Resuscitation is trying to return a newborn, who is not in perfect metabolic balance, to a more perfect metabolic balance.

Q: Would the giving of oxygen to newborn be classified as resuscitation?

A: I believe so.

Q: Are most newborns given oxygen?

A: Certainly, virtually all prematures are given oxygen. I think probably most newborns are not given oxygen, but it's very frequently used.

Q: So, resuscitation in and of itself, by definition, is a broad encompassing term.

Q: It can include just the giving of oxygen, or it can include intubation or endoscopy, is that correct?

A: That's a very broad word, yes.

Q: When a newborn is oxygenated, is it important to clear the airway passages before the baby's oxygenated?

A: If there's obstruction, the giving of oxygen isn't going to get where it's supposed to get. And I would say, in most instances, we do suck out the baby's mouth secretions before we give it oxygen.

Q: Did you indicate that the records do not make reference to clearing of the passageways?

A: That's correct.

Q: Do all newborns suffering from respiratory depression also experience respiratory acidosis?

A: No, not if they're resuscitated quickly and if oxygen exchange is instituted quickly.

Q: So that the mode of treatment with respect to any baby suffering from respiratory depression is to attempt, as best one can, to quickly resuscitate the baby and allow the baby to breathe properly or receive sufficient amount of oxygen?

A: I would put it the latter way: to be sure that the baby receives adequate oxygen. Even a baby that doesn't breathe on its own can be well oxygenated.

Q: How long would you believe it takes for a baby suffering from respiratory depression to then experience respiratory acidosis?

A: With no exchange of oxygen, do you mean?

Q: With an attempt at exchange of oxygen, but, nevertheless, still suffering from respiratory depression?

A: Babies can get along on apparently relatively small amounts of oxygen for extended periods of time.

Q: All babies or some babies?

A: I don't know.

Q: Based upon your academic knowledge, your expertise, your personal experience, would you not say that babies respond differently to a lack of diminution of oxygenation?

A: I suppose there're also sometimes even unmeasurable peripheral factors that affect that. I really don't know. I suppose so.

Q: Would, for example, a healthy newborn be able to sustain itself, if there is for some reason a diminution of oxygenation for a period of time, better than an unhealthy newborn?

A: If a baby already is acidotic at birth, then clearly he would be less tolerant of more acidosis than one who is not acidotic at birth.

Q: When a baby is born acidotic at birth, does that necessarily mean that the baby, during the labor period, suffered respiratory depression?

A: I'm not sure that a fetus can suffer from respiratory depression. If a baby is born acidotic, then he probably suffered from a certain amount of asphyxia; but, I would not characterize it as respiratory asphyxia.

Q: A certain amount of distress?

A: Yes, that's correct.

Q: What is meant by anoxicencephalopathy?

A: It's a term used by pediatric neurologists to indicate a series of brain abnormalities that result from a lack of oxygen.

Q: It is correct to state that the longer a child suffers from acidotic conditions the greater the likelihood of brain damage?

A: No, I'm not sure that's true. I think perhaps the severity may be more important than the length of time.

Q: Severity of the acidotic condition?

A: That's correct.

Q: And going back to your definition, that would relate to metabolic acidosis as opposed to respiratory acidosis?

A: That's correct.

Q: In any event, as soon as the condition is reversed the better the prognosis?

A: Yes.

Q: One way to attempt to reverse acidosis is by oxygenation?

A: Yes.

Q: And decrease the CO_2?

A: Yes, by causing an exchange of gases across the lungs, yes.

Q: What is meant by blood gas?

A: It's a determination of the level of oxygen or carbon dioxide or, I suppose of any other gas in the blood sample, usually arterial sometimes venous.

Q: The Apgar score was originated by Virginia Apgar, I believe?

A: That's correct.

Q: The purpose was to basically determine, in a very simple way, the condition of the baby?

A: That was her purpose, to try to quantify the condition of the baby. And many think she didn't succeed very well and others think she did.

Q: The Apgar score basically determines whether or not the baby is asphyxiated?

A: Probably the one minute Apgar score doesn't.

Q: Doesn't.

A: Does not; because it can be low for several reason, one of them being drug depression. The five minute Apgar score comes closer to defining asphyxia.

Q: You've heard the term narcotization, have you not?

A: Yes.

Q: When you say drug depression, is there a difference, in your opinion, between the terms drug depression and narcotization?

A: I don't know. I don't use the term narcotization.

Q: By drug depression, are you indicating drugs the mother received may cross the placental barrier and cause a depression in the newborn?

A: I wouldn't like to say caused a depression in the newborn, rather caused a delay in spontaneous respirations. That's the primary effect, I think.

Q: If there is a delay in spontaneous respiration, concomitant with that, you may also find an effect upon the color and the heart rate?

A: At birth?

Q: At birth?

A: No, I don't think so.

Q: So that you could have depressed respiration but still have normal color and normal heart rate?

A: At the moment of birth, which is the time that you are talking about, describing the color and the heart rate, you don't know whether there is going to be depression of respirations or not.

Q: If there is respiratory depression, that can be due to drug depression?

A: It can be, but you don't know whether there is going to be respiratory depression at the moment of birth or not.

Q: When you see a newborn and you attempt to determine whether or not there is drug depression, what, if anything, do you do?

A: Look for respirations.

Q: And, if there is drug depression, what do you expect to find by way of sign and/or symptom concerning respiration?

A: Usually no respiration.

Q: Apnea?

A: Yes.

Q: Asphyxia?

A: Asphyxia may be present from something before birth, something unrelated to the drug, or it may begin to develop and, no you don't see asphyxia at the moment of birth.

Q: Have you ever heard the terms primary and secondary apnea?

A: Yes.

Q: Isn't primary apnea a situation where the baby, the newborn, breathes rapidly, gasps for breath, and then goes into the secondary apnea and turns blue and can't breathe?

A: Yes, that is correct.

Q: Are you stating that if you do not see a baby suffering from apnea immediately at birth, there can be no drug depression?

A: If the baby became apneic a few seconds later, after one gasp, then it still might be drug depression.

Q: So that baby could breathe spontaneously, gasp, and then go into drug depression and experience respiratory depression?

A: That's what I said, but I'm not sure.

Q: Is it your opinion that this baby was not narcotiud?

A: Yes, that's my opinion.

Q: Would you expect a baby who is suffering from drug depression not to cry spontaneously?

A: I think I would expect that; but, also, many babies that are perfectly normal don't cry immediately.

Q: If a baby is drug depressed, there are certain antagonists that may be given to the baby?

A: It is given or can be given?

Q: All right. Can be given?

A: Yes, there are certain antagonists that can be given.

Q: And is proper protocol, when a baby is suffering from drug depression, to administer Nalline?

A: That is not my practice, no. I have practically never given those. See, what you're concerned about is being sure that the baby has good respiratory exchange until it begins to breathe on its own. And if he can do that without giving an additional drug, I much prefer to do it that way. But I admit that some people use Nalline or one of the other drugs more frequently than I.

Q: If the baby is drug depressed, you take into consideration that the respiratory centers of the brain, the medulla oblongata, is effected.

A: That's correct.

Q: And if the baby is depressed by reason of drug intake during the labor period, your responsibility is to attempt, as best you possibly can, to oxygenate the baby; if necessary, artificially?

A: Until he can breathe on his own, yes.

Q: And there are terms such as tidal volume?

A: Yes.

Q: You say breathing on its own. You mean better than shallow breathing, do you not?

A: I mean breathing so that the heart rate is good and the color is improving. Those are the measurements that I go by because I see a baby only in the immediate delivery period.

Q: You expect, once the baby is breathing properly, for the baby to continue to breathe properly?

A: Usually; although prematures, as I'm sure you know, frequently have apneic episodes totally unrelated to anything other than their prematurity, as far as I know. That can occur for a day or two or three.

Q: Going back then to your evaluation as to whether and under what circumstances a baby may be drug depressed, you would consider the respiration at the time of birth, correct?

A: I think that's the primary determining factor.

Q: Would you consider the color?

A: No. That wouldn't really have anything to do with drug depression because turning cyanotic would follow the failure to oxygenate the baby after he's been born.

Q: Do I understand correctly that if a baby is suffering from respiratory depression, secondarily, will be the episodic event of cyanosis?

A: Yes, eventually.

Q: When you see a baby cyanotic, that necessarily means, does it not—I mean the entire body not just circumoral for example—that necessarily means the baby is not getting sufficient oxygen to its tissues?

A: Not getting sufficient oxygen. I'm not sure what you mean by sufficient oxygen to its tissues.

Q: Tissue nutrient is oxygen, is it not?

A: It means that it isn't getting as much oxygen as you like, but it doesn't imply any damage to the tissues.

Q: When the tissues of the body are cyanotic, it means that it's not getting sufficient oxygen?

A: That's correct.

Q: And by not getting sufficient oxygen, it allows you to conclude that the baby is not breathing properly?

A: That's correct. But this is something that can't be determined instantaneously.

Q: By instantaneously, you mean right at the time of birth?

A: Yes.

Q: Okay.

A: If a baby is not breathing, it takes a while for it to become cyanotic and, after it's breathing properly, it takes a while for the cyanosis to disappear.

Q: Assuming that the baby received oxygen almost from the immediate time of birth for a period of two minutes and then, at the end of two minutes, the baby was still cyanotic. Would that allow you to conclude that the baby was not receiving sufficient oxygen during that period of time?

A: I don't think I can tie these things up that precisely.

Q: It's outside your expertise?

A: Yes. And I think that you can't really tie those things up that precisely.

Q: If you see an Apgar score with a zero for color, isn't it true that more likely than not the baby would not receive a two for respiration?

A: I don't really know. I would think that that might be the case.

Q: Now, with respect to the heart rate, if you see a cyanotic baby, would you not expect that the heart rate would be below 100?

A: It depends on what's causing the depression. If it's been a severe asphyxia, yes. If it has been a less severe asphyxia, the baby can still be cyanotic and have a heart rate above 100.

Q: The longer the cyanosis exists, the greater the likelihood for the heart rate to go above 100?

A: The greater the length of time the acidosis and asphyxia has existed, that's absolutely true.

Q: And when you have acidosis and asphyxia, one of the signs or symptoms that you see would be cyanosis?

A: One of them might be, but you can have cyanosis without much asphyxia or certainly without much acidosis.

Q: Are there different degrees of cyanosis?

A: There probably are, but I would tend to think of them as deep and not so deep. I'm not sure I can quantify it very precisely.

Q: Can you have cyanosis of the extremities?

A: Yes, that's usual.

Q: And that's usually what you would find in a premature infant?

A: Yes. As a matter of fact, you see generalized cyanosis in premies. Premies are generally a very peculiar color.

Q: You would see cyanosis if the infant was suffering from hyaline membranes disease?

A: Hyaline membranes disease is not very often present at the moment of birth.

Q: It comes later on?

A: Yes, that's correct.

Q: Are you able to make a determination as to what underlying etiology exists to cause a baby to be cyanotic after two minutes of receiving oxygen by mask?

A: No, I am not.

Q: Would you expect a baby who is drug depressed to have poor or depressed muscle tone?

A: With Valium, yes. And I'm not sure with Demerol. I think not. But I'm not sure.

Q: If a premature baby does not suffer from hyaline membranes disease, it can nevertheless suffer from atelectacis and suffer respiratory difficulties, is that not correct?

A: That's correct.

Q: And could not drug depression, imposed on that preexisting condition in the premature baby, aggravate and worsen respiration?

A: Well, if you have a baby that is only using half of his lung, as you might have with atelectacis, two-thirds of his lung, and if you on top of that have him not breathe and not be oxygenated, then clearly that can make it worse.

Q: What effect, if anything, does hypothermia have upon the newborn?

A: You're beyond my expertise.

Q: Was this baby suffering from hypothermia?

A: The baby had some low temperatures.

Q: How low?

A: I recall a 96, I think.

Q: What about a 94? Do you recall that?

A: I don't recall it, no.

Q: 96 would be hypothermia?

A: I think you're beyond my expertise. I would think so but, since I don't take care of newborns, I'm not sure. It certainly sounds like it.

Q: If you state that 96 would be hypothermia, 94 would most assuredly be hypothermia?

A: If that is so, yes.

Q: Would babies suffering from respiratory depression be more susceptible to deleterious consequences from cold stress?

A: I don't know.

Q: Would cold stress, in an infant who is depressed at birth, have a tendency to increase the rate of metabolic acidosis?

A: I don't know.

Q: Is cyanosis compatible and consistent with low blood pressure in a newborn?

A: I would say that can exist separately. Many babies who are cyanotic, I'm sure, don't have low blood pressure.

Q: Do babies who have low blood pressure demonstrate cyanosis?

A: They may.

Q: Can muscle tone be affected by asphyxia?

A: Yes.

Q: If muscle tone is affected by asphyxia, is that the last category of observation in terms of Apgar scoring and neurological scoring to recover from asphyxia?

A: Possibly.

Q: Is it your opinion that drug depression can never cause brain damage?

A: Poorly treated drug depression has the potential of producing brain damage.

Q: In fact—

A: I think it's extremely unlikely.

Q: You wrote an article, did you not, indicating that resuscitation and the modes of resuscitation have less morbidity and more mortality in drug depressed babies?

A: I'm sure they have. I don't remember writing that, but I'm sure they have.

Q: Resuscitation is very important then in the caring of a drug depressed baby?

A: Yes.

Q: And, if proper resuscitation is administered to a newborn, in all likelihood that baby will recover?

A: Assuming there is not something else causing damage, yes.

Q: Cerebral palsy had been determined by many physicians as a waste paper basket definition, correct?

A: Waste paper basket diagnosis. They would like us to be more precise in telling what kind of cerebral palsy is present.

Q: A baby suffering from cerebral palsy is a baby who has had or experienced brain damage?

A: Yes. Brain damage is present in babies with cerebral palsy.

Q: And that brain damage is most often due to a diminution of oxygen to the brain of the fetus or the newborn?

A: I think so. But I reserve the right to change that opinion as we learn more about it.

Q: Medicine obviously is dynamic and not static?

A: That's correct.

Q: You, as an obstetrician, with respect to your caring for a newborn suffering from drug depression, would be obliged to make sure the baby receives adequate oxygenation?

A: That's correct.

Q: With respect to the care rendered to the baby, you would defer to a pediatrician or a neonatologist?

A: Yes.

Q: You would accept the fact, would you not, that any tendency toward respiratory depression of the infant may be increased by the use of Meperidine for maternal analgesia?

A: A qualified yes. If it's given several hours before, I don't suppose it does.

Q: Are you indicating that the timing of the drug influences the affect that it has upon the fetus?

A: It influences, yes.

Q: Are you indicating that if it's given several hours before the birth of the baby, it will have no affect upon the baby at birth?

A: I didn't say no effect, but minimal effect.

Q: When you say several hours, are you talking about two or more hours prior to birth?

A: It depends on its root of administration. If it's given intravenously, it reaches its peak effect in 30 to 60 minutes and thereafter—and before that, it has much less affect. If it's given intramuscularly, it takes a bit longer.

Q: Let's talk about intravenously. Its life span intravenously would be about six hours, would it not?

A: I believe so.

Q: The effect on the baby is dose related and time related, correct?

A: Well, level related, perhaps I should say that.

Q: Level related and what?

A: Which is, of course, dose and time related.

Q: Do you not also take into consideration the maturity of the fetus?

A: Yes. I tend to give less narcotics to premature fetuses than a mature fetus.

Q: Are you indicating inferentially if not expressly that you know that a premature baby is affected more significantly by reason of the immaturity of the liver to absorb and metabolize the drug than a mature fetus?

A: It's probably several factors. While the infant is in utero, the mother, of course, metabolizes the drug. Once it's born, of course, its liver, which is usually immature, has to metabolize the drug. Also, premature infants are more likely to have respiratory depression simply by virtue of their being premature.

Q: So that a premature baby is more likely to have respiratory depression than a full term infant, and drug depression can cause greater harm or injury to a premature baby?

A: Can cause greater depression, and if not properly treated, potentially cause harm, yes.

Q: Now, in your article you state:
Any tendency toward depression of the infant may be increased by the use of Meperidine for maternal analgesia?

A: Correct.

Q: When you take that into consideration, you also take into consideration the level relation?

A: Yes. That's, of course, an oversimplification.

Q: But the risk, nevertheless, is significant when the baby is premature?

A: I think it's greater that there will be respiratory depression with a premature than with a mature given the exactly the same set of circumstances.

Q: Respiratory depression due to drug intake?

A: That's correct.

Q: Could you tell me the parameters of time wherein it would have less affect than other times?

A: You're talking about intravenous?

Q: Intravenous.

A: Its maximum concentration in the baby appears to occur 30 to 60 minutes after use in the mother. So, before 30 minutes and after 60 minutes it has a lesser affect than it does between 30 and 60 minutes. Those are approximations, of course.

Q: Would you agree or disagree with this statement?
Maximum incidents of respiratory depression in infants occur when Meperidine is given to the mother one to two hours prior to delivery and no significant depression noted when the drug is administered one hour or less before delivery?

A: I think I'm referring to intramuscular and that is roughly true, yes. But I'm not sure. I would have to look at the paper if you want me to answer that.

Q: I would suggest you do look at it. It certainly does say "intravenously."

A: I recall now we did use intravenous Demerol, yes.

Q: Are you disagreeing with the statement now?

A: I think that is probably inaccurate. I think, with intravenous drugs, it's a shorter time.

Q: You are aware of the fact that this is your article?

A: I wasn't aware of it, but I'm now aware of it and it may be that we were inaccurate. It may be that that was what was believed at that time. I'm not sure.

Q: It is correct to state that the degree of fetal respiratory depression is dose related, correct?

A: Yes, I think so.

Q: And, therefore would you not state that it is desirable to restrict the dose to the smallest quantity that will keep the patient comfortable?

A: Yes.

Q: You're in a position to know what would be considered a more than average quantity of Demerol?

A: Yes. There was a fairly wide range of dosages.

Q: Do you know what the standard was in 1969 with respect to administering of Demerol?

A: I think there was a fairly wide dosage. I think from anywhere from 50 to 150 milligrams. And, again, I know what we used, but I think that the dosage range was at least that wide.

Q: 50 milligrams would be equivalent to 6 milligrams of morphine?

A: I don't know for sure.

Q: Demerol is a synthetic, is it not?

A: That's correct.

Q: Was the standard the same with respect to premature babies as to full term babies?

A: I have trouble with the word "standard" because I really am not sure exactly what the standard—

Q: Let's talk about what customarily, to your knowledge, was done.

A: If you would permit me to use that, then I believe certainly we, and I think in general, used less drugs in prematures than in matures.

Q: With the awareness that there is a high susceptibility of the premature to be drug depressed?

A: That's correct.

Q: Were you aware, back in 1969, as to the potentiating or synergistic effects of drugs upon one another?

A: Yes.

Q: Were you aware as to whether or not there was any potentiating or synergistic effect with respect to Demerol, Scopolamine, or Sparine?

A: Yes. We felt that the sedation was better when Scopolamine was given with the Demerol.

Q: Scopolamine crossed the placenta?

A: I think so.

Q: That's a depressant?

A: Maybe a very mild one. That's not its primary effect.

Q: Did you know what the effect, if any at all, Sparine had upon Demerol with respect to potentiating its potency?

A: I don't think I ever used Sparine. No.

Q: When brain damage does occur as a result of asphyxia, it results from decreased blood oxygen levels resulting in subcellular organelle damage; is that correct?

A: You're reading from my paper, and I don't remember at all saying that. That isn't the way I say it. I don't know anything about organelles or so forth.

Q: You have, on the back of the article, your references, correct?

A: Right.

Q: And most often, because you are such a prolific writer and you do, on occasion, take statements from others you necessarily make reference to the individual, correct?

A: That's correct.

Q: And, in this particular case, in your sentence:
Brain damage in asphyxiated fetus may result simply from decreased blood oxygen levels resulting in subcellular organelle damage.
You did not make reference to anyone, did you?

A: No.

Q: You will not argue with the fact that perinatal asphyxia is far from innocuous.

A: Innocuous, did you say?

Q: Innocuous?

A: It is not innocuous.

Q: It can kill and it can maim?

A: That's right.

Q: And, if a baby is suffering from drug depression and is not properly resuscitated, it can be maimed?

A: That's possible.

Q: Tell me first in this case as to whether or not, taking into consideration a 30-week gestation, you have an opinion concerning the propriety or impropriety of giving the dosage of Demerol, Scopolamine, and Sparine that was given in this case?

A: I think I could simply say that it was more than I would have given, more than I was in the habit of giving.

Q: Doctor, in your article published in 1968, you make reference to an article authored by Sol Shnider and Frank Moya, "Effects of Meperidine on the Newborn Infant," that was published in 1964?

A: Yes.

Q: I'm going to ask you if you agree or disagree with the statement contained in the article authored by Shnider and Moya:
To prevent neonatal depression, narcotics are usually avoided when delivery is imminent?

A: Yes.

Q: However, it has been suggested that Meperidine exerts its maximal effects on the infant when administered intramuscularly not one hour but two hours before delivery. You would agree with that, also?

A: I simply don't know what today's information is, whether it's changed from that or not.

Q: In this particular case, the mother received 100 milligrams of Demerol five and a-half hours before delivery?

A: Yes.

Q: What else did she receive at that time?

A: She received Scopolamine 100 units and Sparine, I guess it's 25 milligrams.

Q: If Sparine potentiates Demerol, affecting its potency to twice its affect, that would then be approximately 200 milligrams of Demerol, isn't that correct?

A: Scopolamine potentiates the analgesic effect, but I'm not sure it potentiates the respiratory depressive effect. And I simply don't know about Sparine.

Q: Are you indicating that Scopolamine potentiates Demerol?

A: We used to think that Scopolamine potentiated the analgesic effects. We didn't think that it increased the respiratory depression.

Q: But you don't know anything about Sparine, you indicated?

A: Not specifically Sparine.

Q: Now, two and a-half hours before birth, she received an additional 50 milligrams intravenous of Demerol, isn't that correct?

A: That's correct.

Q: So that obviously then, in a period of five and a-half hours before birth, she received 150 milligrams of Demerol, correct?

A: Correct.

Q: Forgetting for the moment about any alleged potentiating affects, would the entire amount of Demerol, that was given five and a-half hours before the birth of the baby, be out of the system when the 50 milligrams was given two and a-half hours before birth?

A: Probably not.

Q: When you evaluated the situation to make a determination as to whether or not, in your opinion, this baby was drug depressed, you most necessarily had to know and take into consideration the amount of Demerol, Sparine, and Scopolamine the mother received during the labor period, correct?

A: Not really because if the baby is not depressed he isn't depressed.

Q: So that in formulating your determinations that the baby was not drug depressed, you relied strictly upon the evidence that exhibited itself concerning the baby after the baby's birth and did not take into consideration the amount of drugs that the mother received during the labor period?

A: That's correct, not directly anyway.

Q: Would the amount of drugs the mother received during the labor period be consistent with drug depression?

A: In my experience, mild drug depression.

Q: Is it your opinion that the child's presently existing physical and mental handicaps are due to the fact that she was born prematurely?

A: I think that's the most likely explanation; yes, sir.

Q: Are you indicating that the prematurity caused brain damage?

A: That's an oversimplification probably. Prematurity is highly associated with cerebral palsy and brain damage. And so, in that sense, yes, I'm indicating, without at the moment specifying the mechanism, that relationship seems to exist here.

Q: Are you in a position to specify the mechanism?

A: Well, I think that most people think as do I, that in these cases, it is usually due to a bleed in the subependymal, which extends into the intraventricular areas and sometimes into the ventricles.

Q: An intracranial bleed?

A: Yes.

Q: Is that due to the friability of the vessels?

A: That's what is thought, yes.

Q: Can drug depression aggravate or activate or precipitate a preexisting condition with respect to friability of the blood vessels enhancing the prospects of a bleed?

A: There have been several studies that have attempted to determine what factors might be related to the subependymal bleed because not all premies have it, although a large numbers of them do.

§ 33.6   Cross Examination of Defendant Obstetrician Regarding Performance of Amniocentesis with Anterior Placenta and Oligohydramnios

Cross Examination by Mr. Stanley Schwartz:

Q: Is there a difference in the performance of an amniocentesis when there is an anterior placenta as opposed to a posterior placenta?

A: Well, we try to avoid the placenta if we can.

Q: Well, that was not my question.

A: Well, you asked me if there was a difference. Yes.

Q: It is more easily accomplished, that is, the performance of the amniocentesis without complication, when it is posterior? That is accepted, it is not?

A: There is less chance of hitting the placenta when it is posterior or fundal.

Q: One of the things I assume you instruct the resident to do in the performance of an amniocentesis is first to make a clear determination by reason of the ultrasound as to whether the placenta is posterior or anterior, correct?

A: I did. Yes.

Q: You did, because you knew it was important with respect to the procedure to know whether it is anterior or posterior?

A: Well, to be frank with you, the main reason we did them under the ultrasound was to localize the fluid and avoid hitting the baby.

Q: The ultrasound assists in doing the amniocentesis, so it is not done blind, isn't that correct?

A: Yes. But not just to avoid the placenta.

Q: Not just to avoid the placenta, but to do what?

A: To find where the fluid is.

Q: The pockets of fluid?

A: Pockets of fluid. And avoid hitting the baby.

Q: So the two things that the ultrasound assists in doing is to allow you to know where the pockets of fluid are located and to know where the placenta is situated to avoid it?

A: No, I didn't say that.

Q: All right. Does it assist in knowing where the placenta is located?

A: Yes.

Q: Is the object when an amniocentesis is performed to avoid the placenta?

A: If possible.

Q: In other words, if one can avoid the placenta, one does avoid the placenta?

A: I would say in 1984, yes.

Q: In 1982, no?

A: No.

Q: Are you indicating that even if one can avoid the placenta in 1982, it was not necessary to avoid the placenta? In essence, what scientific information came to you between 1982 and 1984 to cause you to now state that one should attempt to avoid the placenta if possible?

A: This case.

Q: What do you mean by "this case"?

A: I did not know what went on in this case would happen.

Q: What do you believe happened in this case that you did not know could happen?

A: A substantial amount of blood was transfused from the baby to the mother.

Q: Are you indicating that one of the placental vessels from the baby to the mother was ruptured or lacerated?

A: There are no vessels running from the baby to the mother.

Q: I am talking about the placenta.

A: There are no vessels running from the baby to the mother.

Q: Are there vessels in the placenta?

A: Exactly.

Q: What happens with those vessels? How does blood run from the mother to the baby, from the baby to the mother?

A: There is a pull in between, the way I understand it.

Q: Is blood transported to the baby?

A: From the mother, no.

Q: Is blood transported to the baby through the placenta?

A: Yes.

Q: Now, would it have been one of those vessels that lacerated?

A: I don't know.

Q: What do you mean, a substantial amount of blood was transfused from baby to mother?

A: A substantial amount of blood that was in the baby and the placenta got into the mother's system.

Q: Where did that blood come from?

A: The baby's blood.

Q: What caused it?

A: I don't know.

Q: Could it have been a rupture of one of the vessels of the placenta?

A: Possibly. I don't know.

Q: In other words, there was hemorrhaging?

A: I guess you could use the word.

Q: Now, I want you to come back with me to 1982. When you taught your residents, when you supervised your residents, did you instruct them as to whether or not they should attempt to avoid striking the placenta in the performance of an amniocentesis?

A: If possible. Yes.

Q: And why did you tell them, if possible, avoid the placenta?

A: To avoid a hematoma of the placenta, trauma to it.

Q: Isn't it also to avoid lacerating any of the vessels of the placenta?

A: Yes.

Q: And you know that if that occurred, namely, a laceration of any vessel of the placenta, it could cause deleterious consequences to the fetus?

A: No, I didn't.

Q: You did not know that it could cause morbidity and/or mortality?

A: You mean in the form of this transfer business?

Q: In the form of hemorrhaging to the baby.

A: I knew it could cause a placental hematoma.

Q: You did not know it could cause hemorrhaging in the baby?

A: Not like that. No.

Q: When you say not like that, no, did you know as to whether or not it could cause any hemorrhaging in the baby?

A: I did know that some cells may be transferred, which would cause a problem in the Rh immune system. In other words, Rh negative mother with a possible Rh positive baby could sensitize the mother to the baby. I did know that.

Q: Did you know as to whether or not a laceration of a vessel in the placenta could possibly cause hemorrhaging in the baby?

A: I knew it could cause a hematoma or an abruption of the placenta.

Q: Are you indicating, by your answer, that you did not know that it could cause hemorrhaging in the baby?

A: Not that type of transfer. No.

Q: Hemorrhaging and hematoma are two different things, are they not?

A: Hemorrhaging leads to a hematoma sometimes. Yes.

Q: Isn't a hematoma basically a blood clot?

A: Exactly. That would be a blood clot between the placenta and the uterus.

Q: Well, are you saying hemorrhaging can lead to a hematoma?

A: Yes.

Q: And in this particular case, that is in 1982, you indicated that you were aware of a hematoma occurring if there was a laceration of a blood vessel of the placenta?

A: I knew that was a rare occurrence with its sequela.

Q: Then are you indicating, in 1982, you were aware that a hemorrhaging can also occur, which could lead to a hematoma if there was a laceration of a vessel of the placenta?

A: Yes.

Q: But you knew that it was a rare occurrence?

A: Yes.

Q: And this rare occurrence, nevertheless, was one of the risks incidental to the procedure?

A: Yes.

Q: And that is why you told your residents to attempt, if they could, to avoid striking the placenta?

A: Yes.

Q: But if they can't do it,—

A: We went through placentas.

Q: You have no crystal ball? You have no way of knowing if you are going to hit a vessel in the placenta?

A: Exactly.

Q: So when you go through a placenta even today, you can go through a placenta without hitting a vessel, correct?

A: Yes.

Q: But you can also go through a placenta and hit a vessel, correct?

A: Yes.

Q: The ultrasound does not show the vessels, correct?

A: No.

Q: So back in 1982, you would teach your residents to avoid the placenta if they can, but if they can't, are you indicating that you told them that it would be safe to hit the placenta?

A: Yes.

Q: Did you indicate to them there might be greater risks in performing an amniocentesis when there is an anterior placenta as opposed to a posterior placenta?

A: Yes.

Q: If it is anterior, you can go through the placenta before you hit the pocket. Correct?

A: yes.

Q: And there can be injury because you might hit a vessel. Correct?

A: Yes.

Q: Did you teach them to rotate if they were not drawing out or extracting any fluid?

A: Yes.

Q: And can rotation of the needle or the bevel of the needle cause a greater risk of injury to a vessel as opposed to direct strike into the placenta and through the placenta without rotation?

A: I don't know.

Q: Is it not true that the thicker the placenta, the more likelihood there would be injury to a vessel of the placenta?

A: I would think so.

Q: Because there would be more vessels, correct? Doctor, could you answer that?

A: Yes.

Q: So that when one reviewed the inherent risks that might be incidental to the amniocentesis procedure, it is incumbent upon that individual to know the conditions, such as is it being anterior as opposed to posterior, correct?

A: Yes.

Q: Is it thick as opposed to thin, correct?

A: Yes.

Q: Does the amount of the amniotic fluid have any bearing with respect to the risk incidental to the procedure?

A: Yes.

Q: And if there is, oligohydramnios existing, that would be limitation or little amniotic fluid, correct?

A: Yes.

Q: So that would be an additional risk, correct?

A: Yes.

Q: Is it not true that the more times the needle is inserted, the greater likelihood of damage to the vessels of the placenta?

A: Yes.

Q: In this particular case, is it not true that it was an anterior placenta?

A: Yes.

Q: Is it not true that it was thick?

A: Yes.

Q: Is it not true that oligohydramnios existed?

A: Yes.

Q: Is it not true that there were two insertions of the needle?

A: Yes.

Q: Did you ever instruct your residents in 1982 and prior thereto with respect to when and under what circumstances they should abort the amniocentesis?

A: I never did more than two taps.

Q: That was not my question. When you instruct and taught your residents, did you ever say if such and such exists on the ultrasound or if such and such is determined to exist by you, I want you to abort the amniocentesis if there is no supervision?

A: They were with me when we aborted procedures.

Q: Wouldn't you, Doctor, if you were in attendance during this amniocentesis and determined it was an anterior placenta, thick placenta, oligohydramnios and you were unsuccessful in drawing fluid on the first insertion of the needle, abort the amniocentesis?

A: That is speculation.

Q: You are not able to give me an answer as to what you would have done?

A: No.

Q: So what you are saying is that you, as an active staff member of the hospital, having been in practice since 1973, in 1984 cannot tell me what you would have done in 1982 under the facts and circumstances I have just presented to you?

A: Right.

Q: Notwithstanding what you would have done, would you not say that it would have been incumbent upon a resident under the circumstances I just set forth for you to abort the amniocentesis if there was no attending physician supervising the procedure?

A: I can't tell you that, either.

Q: You don't know?

A: Right.

Q: And you never taught a resident when and under what circumstances to abort?

A: No.

Q: One of the things you teach your residents is never to do more than two taps?

A: Exactly.

Q: Would it be a violation of the standard of practice for a resident to pursue and not abort an amniocentesis when she knows that the placenta is thick, when she knows there is little amniotic fluid, when she knows it is an anterior placenta, and when she was unsuccessful in the first insertion to draw out fluid?

A: I would think if she could get out further away from the placenta, she would try it.

Q: As a practicing physician, what factors would you take into consideration and what would you do in inserting the needle the second time under the facts presented to you?

A: The first time when she was attempting to localize the fluid with the needle, I assume she would try it in the same place, but further away from the placenta?

Q: In the same place, but further away from the placenta?

A: Well, you keep saying this thickness. I wouldn't assume that she would go through a thicker part of the placenta.

Q: What about a suprapubic approach?

A: That is fine if you have a normal amount of fluid, but if there is no fluid there, it's impossible.

Q: You are saying it is fine if you have a normal amount of fluid? Is that what you are saying?

A: Exactly. You lift the baby's head.

Q: That is an easy procedure, it is not, just lift the baby's head?

A: Yes.

Q: So what you do with the ultrasound is to see where the pockets of fluid exist, correct?

A: Exactly.

Q: And this is what you teach your residents?

A: Yes.

Q: Well, if you have an anterior placenta and the only way you can get to the pocket would be through the placenta, are you indicating in 1982 that was permissible?

A: Yes.

Q: But not in '84?

A: I wouldn't do it.

Q: Because of what happened in this case?

A: Exactly.

Q: Well, you are a physician, you do a lot of reading and you use books for research?

A: Exactly.

Q: What books, if any at all, did you read to assist in making the determination that now you would not do it?

A: Just what happened here.

Q: Do any books corroborate your clinical evaluation of the situation not to do it?

A: No.

Q: Did you ever attempt to read any books or look at any research studies prior to 1982?

A: No.

Q: I am going to refer to David Danforth, *Obstetrics and Gynecology*, which you indicated is an authoritative treatise?

A: Yes.

Q: I am going to ask you if you agree or disagree with the statement that was stated in the 1982 edition:

> Since there is some danger of incurring a persistent high leak of amniotic fluid or even more serious of lacerating a large fetal vessel on the surface of the placenta, ultrasound should be used to locate the placenta before attempting amniocentesis.

A: Yes.

Q: Do you agree with it?

A: That's why I did do it under ultrasound.

Q: Correct. And one of the reasons to do it under ultrasound is to attempt to avoid the placenta?

A: Exactly.

Q: Do you also agree or perhaps disagree with the statement on the same page?

> The performance of a puncture should be in the lower part of the abdomen at the suprapubic site. By using this technique, you avoid piercing the placenta?

A: Sometimes you can, yes.

Q: So you agree with that statement.

A: If there is no fluid down there, sure.

Q: Are you indicating that even though you do an ultrasound, you can still go through the placenta to get to the pocket?

A: That is what I said.

Q: How do you know whether or not you are going to rupture or lacerate a vessel when going through the placenta?

A: You don't.

Q: And you taught your people accordingly?

A: I told them what I said before, to avoid the placenta, if possible.

Q: But if not possible, go through the placenta?

A: Through the edge of the placenta.

Q: Is injury to the fetus more common when the volume of amniotic fluid is small, compared to the size of the fetus?

A: If the amount of fluid is small, yes.

Q: Why is that?

A: If there is a lot of fluid that you can get into without going deeper into the cavity, the safer it is to the baby.

Q: If the baby is on the left side and the placenta is anterior, would you anticipate the placenta being more to the left than to the right?

A: No.

Q: It makes no difference. Is that what you are saying?

A: I don't know.

Q: You don't know the answer?

A: I don't think it necessarily would be true.

Q: If the baby is on the left side and the pockets are on the left side and it is anterior placenta, is it a violation of the standards of practice to insert the needle on the left side as opposed to the right side?

A: I depends on where the pockets of fluid are.

Q: So that where the pockets are, dictate where the insertion be made?

A: Yes.

Q: Notwithstanding the fact that it might have to be made on the left side with the awareness the baby is on the left side. Is that what you are saying?

A: Yes.

Q: So one follows and must observe the screen on the ultrasound, correct?

A: Yes.

Q: Does the hospital have both direct visualization and static?

A: Yes.

Q: What is the difference between the two?

A: Well, one is a freeze frame and one is showing what is going on at all times.

Q: You have personally carried out a suprapubic approach, have you not?

A: Yes.

Q: That is the safest way to avoid the placenta, is it not, after you lift the head, if it is necessary to lift the head?

A: Yes.

Q: Does it take more than one physician to do a suprapubic approach?

A: Yes.

Q: It takes two?

A: I would say yes.

Q: Why?

A: Well, we have one lifting, keeping the head out of the way, and one using the needle.

Q: Is it always necessary to lift the head?

A: Yes.

Q: Then you would expect the head to be engaged?

A: Not necessarily. If it is up against the cervix.

Q: If the head is unengaged, it is still necessary to lift it in a suprapubic approach?

A: I would say it would give you more of a chance to get fluid.

Q: So that no matter where the head is, basically, even if it is at a minus station, it is better to have two physicians in attendance when a suprapubic approach is performed?

A: Probably.

Q: Was there anyone in attendance with Dr. Jones so far as you know and the records reflect in the performance of the amniocentesis?

A: Not to my knowledge.

Q: Where would you have been?

A: I was in the delivery room.

Q: Was it necessary in this particular case for the amniocentesis to be performed at the time that it was performed, as opposed to several hours later or a day later? In other words, was it critical to do it on this designated date and time?

A: I wouldn't say critical. No.

Q: Were you informed of the withdrawing of blood on the second entry of the needle in the amniocentesis?

A: No.

Q: Are you saying that even up to this time you don't know that blood was withdrawn with the needle?

A: Well, I got the report there. Yes.

Q: What report are you referring to?

A: Well, the report the amniocentesis. There was blood in the fluid.

Q: Assuming that there was blood in the aspiration or withdrawing of the needle in the second insertion and there was the bleeding that you took note of after the birth of the baby, isn't it true that more likely than not there would have been a laceration of one of the vessels of the placenta?

A: I am not sure, to be honest with you.

Q: You are not sure whether it might have been fetal or maternal?

A: Right.

Q: But at least you would consider that as a possibility?

A: It's a possibility.

Q: What procedure, if any, is called upon if blood is withdrawn at the performance of an amniocentesis?

A: Placing the patient on the monitor is what we have done for all those years.

Q: This would be done, would it not, whether or not you did withdraw fetal blood after the performance of an amniocentesis?

A: In my patients, yes.

Q: Taking into consideration your own academics, taking into consideration the pragmatics of your clinical experience, do you have an opinion as to whether or not there can be a greater risk of damage or harm to the fetus when fetal blood is withdrawn as opposed to when it is not withdrawn during the performance of an amniocentesis?

A: Yes. Possibly, yes.

Q: And that greater risk can be incidental to a hemorrhaging that would be taking place?

A: Possibly.

Q: In this particular case, inasmuch as the patient was not in labor, you would not be able to utilize the fetal heart rate in tandem with the contractions to determine ominous decelerations, correct?

A: Right.

Q: Would you expect if damage befell the fetus as a result of withdrawing of fetal blood or injury to a vessel of the placenta for there to be a tachycardia or bradycardia?

A: I would think so.

Q: When you looked at the fetal heart monitor, did you just look at the seconds or minutes readout or did you look at the whole strip?

A: I looked at the whole strip.

Q: And looking at the whole strip, were you not able to determine that there was fetal stress and/or distress existing as far back as 10:03, 10:04?

A: It appeared that way.

Q: So that from the time the monitor was attached there was fetal distress, correct?

A: Yes.

§ 33.7   Cross Examination of Defendant Obstetrician Regarding Premature Breech Delivery Complicated by Hypotension from Spinal Anesthesia

Cross Examination by Mr. Stanley Schwartz:

Q: Isn't it true that at the time of the 28th week of gestation, most babies are in a breech presentation?

A: Yes.

Q: Isn't it also true that if the membranes ruptured at the 28th week, the doctor usually is put on notice of the probabilities of a breech presentation existing?

A: Yes.

Q: Do you know whether or not Bott Hospital had electronic fetal monitors in 1972?

A: I do not believe so.

Q: Did you employ any particular type procedure with respect to caring for your patient, and/or treating your patient, once you knew that the patient was a breech and there was a rupture of the membranes?

A: At that point in time probably I would examine to confirm rupture of the membranes, consider hospitalizing the patient to observe for any evidence of any infection, and just watchful expectancy.

Q: Would you do anything to determine as to whether or not the head is hyperextended or hyperflexed?

A: Well, if the patient started labor, as I say, I don't believe ultrasound was available, so we would possibly consider an x-ray.

Q: Abdomen? Flat plate?

A: Yes.

Q: Why, if at all, is it important to determine hyperextension and/or hyperflexion?

A: It would make the delivery of the aftercoming head much more difficult.

Q: Is it more common in a breech to have hyperextension as opposed to a vertex presentation?

A: I would say I believe so, yes.

Q: And a flat plate x-ray would, in all likelihood, allow you to make the determination, of the existence of a hyperextension?

A: It could, especially if you have got both views, lateral and posterior.

Q: And the hospital had the necessary facilities to perform that test?

A: At that time, yes.

Q: With respect to infection, is it not true that the longer the period of time exists between the rupture of the membranes and delivery, the greater the likelihood of infection developing?

A: Yes.

Q: Your usual procedure or protocol would be to check the mother to make sure infection was not developing?

A: Yes.

Q: To check the mother's temperature and vital signs?

A: Yes.

Q: What else?

A: Do serial blood counts.

Q: What information would you have had to allow you to make the determination that this was a 30 week gestation?

A: Well, history.

Q: From the mother?

A: From the mother, and, of course, examination would reveal a small infant, which would go along with that.

Q: And you would know that the membranes ruptured?

A: Again, by history; on examination you would not feel the membranes, yes.

Q: A frank breech, is that sometimes called a single breech?

A: Single breech? I am not familiar with that.

Q: Are the hips flexed in a frank breech?

A: Yes.

Q: The knees are extended?

A: Yes.

Q: So the feet would lie in front of the face?

A: Yes.

Q: Would you have known then that this was a frank breech as opposed to other type breeches when you examined Mrs. Zick in the delivery room?

A: Yes.

Q: It is not necessary, I assume, to perform a C-section on every woman who is carrying the baby in a breech presentation, am I correct?

A: Yes.

Q: How did you come to the conclusion that this should be and can be a vaginal delivery as opposed to arrangements for a C-section?

A: When I first saw the patient, she was ready to deliver.

Q: If you examined her at 9:05 then, you would have examined her in the labor room, would you not?

A: Right.

Q: Is there an indication as to the dilatation at 9:15?

A: No.

Q: Is there an indication in your records of your examination as to the dilatation at 9:05?

A: Yes.

Q: And what was the dilatation at 9:05?

A: Three centimeters.

Q: At 9:15 when she was taken to the delivery room, would that mean under usual procedures she had reached full dilatation?

A: Yes.

Q: So that in a period of ten minutes, she advanced seven centimeters?

A: Yes.

Q: Is that unusual?

A: Not in a premature, no.

Q: Because of the smallness of the baby?

A: Yes.

Q: The smallness of the body?

A: Because of the size of the baby.

Q: Are you able to, with the same degree of assurance determine full dilatation when a breech presentation exists as opposed to a vertex?

A: It is more difficult in a breech.

Q: Why?

A: Because with breech full dilatation of the cervix is a relative thing.

Q: So that in a breech presentation, it is not uncommon for a physician to believe there is full dilatation when, in fact, there may not be complete dilatation?

A: Yes, but for practical purposes it would be complete dilatation.

Q: When you say for practical purposes it would be complete in the sense that the buttocks were coming down?

A: Yes, the baby was going to be delivering.

Q: The head is larger that the buttocks, isn't it?

A: Yes.

Q: In a 29 or 30 week gestation, you would expect the head to be larger than the shoulders, wouldn't you?

A: Yes.

Q: So that would be the largest part of the body coming down the canal?

A: The head, yes.

Q: You can conceive of situations wherein the buttocks is able to travel down the canal but the head can get caught?

A: Yes.

Q: And the buttocks can come down the canal even though there may not be full dilatation?

A: Yes.

Q: In this particular case, the child's head was trapped?

A: Well, it appears that the cervix clamped down on the head.

Q: The cervix clamped down on the head?

A: Yes, after the rest of the baby was delivered.

Q: Would this assist you in making a determination as to whether, in all likelihood, this was an incomplete dilated cervix?

A: Not really, no.

Q: It could or need not be?

A: Right.

Q: The second stage of labor is after full dilatation?

A: Yes.

Q: Was she a multigravida or primigravida?

A: Multigravida.

Q: In a multigravida the second stage of labor is what? The average tie is about 55 minutes from full dilatation to delivery?

A: Yes, or less, depending on type of delivery.

Q: In this particular case, how long was the second stage of labor?

A: According to the records, it would be approximately 30 minutes.

Q: In a breech presentation, the cervix may be sufficiently dilated to allow the buttocks, and even the body, to pass through but not be sufficient for the aftercoming head?

A: Yes.

Q: There are basically three types of extractions in a breech? spontaneous, total, and partial, correct?

A: Essentially.

Q: In a spontaneous, it would mean the baby would deliver spontaneously without any assistance from the physician?

A: Yes.

Q: In a partial, the buttocks and the legs would be delivered spontaneously down to the umbilicus, and the doctor assists in delivering the head and the remaining portions of the body and the arms, is that correct?

A: Yes.

Q: And in a total extraction, the physician assists in completely delivering the baby by grabbing its legs and bringing it down by extraction and maneuver?

A: Yes.

Q: Isn't it true that the risk of injury to the fetus is greater in a premature infant, in a breech position as opposed to a mature baby in a breech position, because the diameter of the fetal head in a premature is considerably greater than that of the shoulders?

A: Yes.

Q: In a total breech extraction, is there any pressure placed upon the abdomen, or the suprapubic area, by the physician?

A: There can be.

Q: And suprapubic pressure can place pressure on the head of the fetus?

A: If that is the reason for doing it.

Q: In this particular case, with a total breech extraction, would there have been, to your knowledge, based upon your usual procedure, pressure placed upon the suprapubic area?

A: There probably was, yes.

Q: And you knew then in 1972, as you do know now, that you must take into consideration the amount of pressure to be applied? In essence, excessive pressure can cause injury to the fetus?

A: Yes, but it is unlikely when you are doing suprapubic pressure.

Q: When you do suprapubic pressure, can't you put excessive pressure on the head causing the medulla to protrude into the foramen magnum?

A: It is possible.

Q: So, in essence, if that is possible, you make sure that you use as gentle pressure as possible to avoid injury?

A: Yes. You use sufficient pressure to facilitate what you are doing, and that is, deliver the baby.

Q: Were you required, so far as you know, to have an assistant at the time of delivery?

A: Not required, but it was highly advisable to do.

Q: The anesthetic should not be administered until the buttocks is down at the perineum, and visible, correct?

A: True.

Q: The reason being because the anesthetic, assuming it is a spinal, for example, could slow down the natural forces of contraction?

A: True.

Q: I assume you are aware of the fact that a spinal in and of itself can cause a reduction of blood pressure in the mother?

A: Yes, I am.

Q: And you are aware of the fact that if there is a reduction of blood pressure in the mother, within a period of five minutes it can cause bradycardia to the fetus by reduction of blood in the intervillous space?

A: True.

Q: So that when the spinal is administered, there should be continuous review and examination of the mother to check the vital signs, and in particular the blood pressure, to determine that hypotension does not exist?

A: True.

Q: Even though, as you indicated, you wished to deliver the baby as rapidly as possible, again, you take into consideration the fact that the forceful traction should not be utilized because that in and of itself can cause injury to the fetus?

A: Yes.

Q: Do you introduce both hands into the vagina to grab the ankles?

A: Well, frank breech, you would have to first bring one of the, one or both of the legs down before you can grasp the ankles.

Q: But, then, they are grasped and pulled?

A: Yes.

Q: And that is a downward traction, I assume?

A: Yes.

Q: And, then, at the vulva is there an upward traction that takes place?

A: Not usually.

Q: There is a continuous downward traction?

A: Yes.

Q: And when is the pressure put on the suprapubic area?

A: After the shoulders are delivered.

Q: What, if anything, does the assistant do?

A: Well, depending on the types of maneuvers that you would use, the assistant could either hold the baby or apply—

Q: Pressure?

A: —pressure.

Q: If the cervix is incompletely dilated, as the traction is applied and the baby is being brought down the canal, there can be a clamping down on the baby's head by the cervix?

A: Yes.

Q: Also, more forceful traction must be applied in bringing the baby down the canal if the canal, itself, is narrow?

A: If the canal is narrow, yes.

Q: If the baby was born with fractures of the arm in two separate locations, would that allow you to conclude that in all likelihood there was excessive traction employed in the bringing down of the baby in the canal?

A: No.

Q: What would have caused that, in this particular case?

A: It could have been caused by, in the delivery of the opposite shoulder and arm, when you use the arm that was fractured, to rotate the shoulder to become anterior so it can come under the pubes.

Q: Isn't it more likely than not, when the arm is fractured, taking into consideration the maneuvers you made reference to, there is a malrotation of the arm that takes place causing a fracture?

A: It is quite possible, yes.

Q: Is it not also true that excessive force in employing the traction can cause fractures of the arm?

A: It is possible, yes.

Q: Isn't it true that usually in a premature breech it is unlikely to have fractures of the arm take place because the baby is so small, that the baby usually slides out of the canal and the cervix?

A: Usually, yes.

Q: Do you have any opinion as to why a total breech extraction took place as opposed to, as you call it, an assisted breech?

A: More than likely because she had received the spinal anesthetic.

Q: Do you have any opinion as to what caused the cervix to clamp down on the head?

A: In this particular case, no, but it is not unusual in a premature breech for it to happen, and I have seen it happen many times during my training and experience.

Q: Can that cause injury to the baby?

A: It could. The clamping down could cause cord compression; it could also delay delivery of the baby.

Q: And the greater the delay, the more likelihood that anoxia can develop?

A: Yes.

Q: And if there is a clamping down of the cord, it is more common when there is a nuchal cord around the neck?

A: True.

Q: In this particular case, there was a nuchal cord, wasn't there?

A: Yes, there was.

Q: And you did indicate it does happen, so you were aware of this situation occurring, or the possibilty of it occurring, correct?

A: Yes.

Q: I assume that medicine is such that you must take into consideration the inherent risks incidental to any type of procedure and take definitive action to attempt to abate it or avoid it from occurring, such as safeguards?

A: True.

Q: What safeguards, if any, did you employ, with the awareness that this could happen in this particular case?

A: Well, in this particular case, there really was no opportunity to, in 1972, to ascertain whether the cord was around the neck or whether the cervix was going to clamp down on the aftercoming head.

Q: I understand, Doctor. I did not mean that. But back in 1972 you were aware, as you indicated, that the, there can be a clamping down on the head by the cervix in a breech presentation, correct?

A: Yes.

Q: You could not tell, you are not clairvoyant, as to when it would occur, correct?

A: Correct.

Q: So you take into consideration in caring for your patient the more conservative approach that this can happen to this particular patient, correct?

A: Correct.

Q: And with the awareness that this could happen to any particular patient, what if anything do you do to attempt to avoid it from happening?

A: Well—

Q: Or is it by serendipity? In other words if it happens, it happens, and if it does not happen, thank God it does not happen.

A: How can I best put it? You know certain things can possibly happen, and if they do happen, you take care of them as they happen.

Q: Is that your complete answer?

A: Now, if to prevent the whole situation, of course, would be to use another mode of delivery.

Q: So that what you do is to take into consideration the fact that it can happen and be aware if it does actually happen, you take definitive action to attempt to avoid injury to the fetus, once the clamping down occurs?

A: Yes.

Q: What, if anything, did you have available to take immediate action to avoid injury to the fetus if there was a clamping down in this particular case?

A: Well, at that particular point would be to continue with steady traction and usually with the steady traction—and I am not saying it is hard, but it is steady, the cervix will gradually—

Q: Loosen?

A: Dilate, and the head will come out.

Q: Have you ever heard of giving a general anesthetic such as holathane to loosen up the uterus?

A: I have heard of it.

Q: Didn't that exist in 1972?

A: Yes, it did.

Q: It is not your responsibility to give the general anesthetic, is it?

A: It would be important for him to do that.

Q: So you rely upon the anesthesiologist to do that, don't you?

A: I would.

Q: You know when in time the cervix was clamping down on the head? You would be able to know that, wouldn't you?

A: When we went to deliver the head.

Q: And you would try, as best you possibly can, to deliver the baby as rapidly as possible, correct?

A: Correct.

Q: Utilizing traction, correct?

A: Yes.

Q: And you rely upon the anesthesiologist in doing his job and his responsibility to protect the mother and the fetus, correct?

A: Yes.

Q: What was the mother's blood pressure before the anesthetic was administered?

A: 100/70.

Q: A systolic of 100 would be probably the minimum number to allow sufficient blood flow into the intervillous space, correct?

A: No.

Q: How low can it go to allow sufficient circulation?

A: It could go to 90.

Q: And that is even more dangerous than 100, isn't it?

A: Yes.

Q: When was the blood pressure next taken as disclosed by the record?

A: I believe at 9:30.

Q: Five minutes after the anesthetic was administered?

A: That is what it says on the record.

Q: What was the reading then?

A: It looks like 100/70.

Q: And what was it after 9:30?

A: That looks like 90.

Q: Twenty minutes later, at 9:45?

A: I cannot make out the time.

Q: What was the reading? 90 over what? 68?

A: In that vicinity.

Q: That is hypotension, isn't it? 90 over, with a systolic of 68.

A: It is a relative hypotension.

Q: Was there any other reading after that?

A: Two more, and they are essentially the same.

Q: With the awareness that a spinal can cause hypotension, is there any prophylactic treatment that can be administered to the mother in an effort to attempt to avoid that from occurring, such as infusion?

A: Well, intravenous infusion.

Q: Another way to prophylactically prevent it from occurring would be vasopressors?

A: Yes, but I think prior to that, just elevation of the legs, putting them up in stirrups, usually would help that.

Q: Left uterine displacement would also help, wouldn't it?

A: Yes.

Q: By the way, when the cervix clamps down on the head, that is basically an entrapment of the head, is it not?

A. Yes.

Q: What, other than a completely undilated cervix, can cause that to occur?

A: It can happen whether the cervix is undilated or dilated.

Q: Physiologically or pathologically, how does it happen if the cervix is fully dilated, with a small baby, two, two and a half pounds?

A: Well, the cervix is part of the uterus, and it is muscular, and it can happen I don't really know the exact mechanism, but it does happen.

Q: It happens more often when it is not totally dilated as opposed to being dilated, doesn't it?

A: I would presume so.

Q: Once it does happen, entrapment of the head, time is of the essence in attempting to relieve the pressure on the head because it is relaxing the uterus?

A: Right.

Q: And to reduce the pressure that might be on the umbilical cord causing a diminution or cessation of oxygenation to the fetus?

A: Yes.

Q: When the blood pressure drops after the administering of a spinal, the administering of vasopressor agents can restore the maternal blood pressure?

A: Yes.

Q: Would that be the responsibility of the anesthesiologist to determine when and under what circumstances to give vasopressors as opposed to you, the obstetrician?

A: Yes.

Q: When the maternal blood pressure drops systolically from 100 to 90, isn't it true that the uterine blood flow is also reduced?

A: Somewhat.

Q: When there is entrapment of the head, it is important for the baby to receive as much oxygen as possible, correct?

A: Correct.

Q: The lower the uterine blood flow in the intervillous space, the lower the oxygen to the fetus?

A: Yes.

§ 33.8   Cross Examination of a Defendant Pediatrician Regarding Newborn Meningitis

Cross Examination by Mr. Stanley Schwartz:

Q: What is meningitis?

A: It's an infection or inflammatory process involving the central nervous system, particularly the meninges.

Q: What is the meninges?

A: The meninges are membranes covering brain and spinal cord.

Q: When a high index of suspicion of meningitis exists should not treatment be immediatley rendered?

A: I wouldn't unless I diagnosed it.

Q: Would you say that when there is a high suspicion of meningitis, one should attempt to perform the necessary tests to confirm or rule out meningitis?

A: Yes.

Q: Some of the cardinal signs and/or symptoms of meningitis which would permit the physician to formulate, at least a suspicion of meningitis would be lethargy, neurological deficits, and irritability in a newborn.

A: These could be symptoms of a number of diseases including meningitis.

Q: Now when you examined this child, Beth, what signs and/or symptoms existed which would be compatible and/or consistent with meningitis?

A: Poor feeding, lethargy, irritability and seizure-like activity.

Q: Would seizures be an indication of neurological deficits?

A: It could be.

Q: Was it not important to determine the etiology of the seizures?

A: Correct.

Q: Did you, in this case, determine the etiology of the seizures?

A: No. She was tremoring, as I recall, and central nervous system diseases are associated with tremors. But, also other conditions are associated with tremors.

Q: Tell me what you did to determine the cause of the seizures.

A: Initially, I ordered a blood sugar and a serum calcium.

Q: Would that tell you whether or not the newborn had meningitis?

A: No.

Q: Can't meningitis cause seizures?

A: Yes.

Q: A blood sugar would assist in determining if hypoglycemia existed.

A: Correct.

Q: And the serum calcium—hypocalcemia?

A: Correct.

Q: And the findings were negative—consequently these two conditions were ruled out.

A: When those studies were returned as normal, yes. Those are two common causes of seizures, tremoring in infants, but it apparently was not the case with Beth, yes.

Q: Were there any other tests you performed or called for in an effort to determine the origin of the seizures?

A: Skull x-rays.

Q: And what else, if anything.

A: A lumbar puncture.

Q: And the reason why you ordered a lumbar puncture was to determine if the seizures were caused as a result of meningitis?

A: Correct.

Q: The more serious the disease, the more necessary it is to rule it out?

A: You might say that.

Q: You are aware of the fact that time is of the essence in treating meningitis?

A: Correct.

Q: When in time was the lumbar puncture performed?

A: The day after performing blood studies.

Q: About 24 to 26 hours after you examined the baby?

A: The following day, I don't know in terms of hours when it was.

Q: Did you perform the lumbar puncture?

A: Yes, I did.

Q: Why did you wait till the next day to perform a lumbar puncture?

A: By far, a much more common cause of the tremoring, seizuring child in my experience would be hypoglycemia or hypocalcemia as opposed to meningitis.

Q: Are you indicating that you wished to first rule out hypocalcemia and/or hypoglycemia?

A: Correct.

Q: You placed down on the consultation sheet—lumbar puncture correct?

A: Correct.

Q: I assume there would have been no difficulty in performing a lumbar puncture once you determined by blood study that hypocalcemia and hypoglycemia did not exist.

A: Yes.

Q: If a baby suffers from meningitis and a period of 24 hours expires before antibiotics are administered, will not the condition worsen?

A: Yes.

Q: It is an infectious disease.

A: Correct.

Q: And it is a fulminating disease.

A: Yes.

Q: Could you not have put a stat (immediately) on blood study rather than wait for the results for approximately 24 hours?

A: Could I have? Yes.

Q: How long would it take for the lab to obtain results of the two tests?

A: If you put a stat order, I would think you would have a result within one hour.

Q: Is there any reason in this case as to why you did not put a stat on the blood study when, as you indicated, your desire to perform the blood study was to rule out hypoglycemia and hypocalcemia before you performed a lumbar puncture?

A: I don't recall why.

Q: Ultimately you performed a lumbar puncture?

A: Yes.

Q: You talked about an inflammation of the meninges. That is the covering of the brain?

A: Correct.

Q: And in between the layers would be the cerebral spinal fluid.

A: That's right.

Q: And when you do a lumbar puncture, do you test or study the cerebral spinal fluid?

A: That's right.

Q: Did bacteria exist in this case?

A: Yes.

Q: If you chose to do a lumbar puncture on the date you first examined the child it would have been you who performed the puncture?

A: Yes.

Q: When meningitis exists, the meninges become infected?

A: That's right.

Q: And the brain begins to swell and press against the skull?

A: Yes.

Q: In essence, there is intracranial pressure?

A: Increased intracranial pressure, yes.

Q: And that is due to the inflammation on the swelling?

A: Correct.

Q: When the brain swells I assume the brain has no place to go because the skull holds it?

A: To a certain extent, you are correct.

Q: And the nerve centers are all in the brain?

A: Correct.

Q: Are the brain and spinal cord control movements of the lower extremities?

A: Right.

Q: Control speech?

A: Yes.

Q: Movement of the eyes?

A: Correct.

Q: Hearing ability?

A: Right.

Q: You indicated that time is of the essence in treating an infectious disease such as meningitis?

A: Correct.

Q: Is the danger of irreparable brain damage more likely when one fails to immediately treat meningitis as opposed to hypoglycemia or hypocalcemia or are they all of equal and immediate danger to the newborn?

A: To a newborn infant's brain, they could be equally devastating.

Q: Are you stating that one is not more devastating than the others?

A: Any of those conditions, except hypocalcemia is not as likely to cause damage, but depriving the brain of glucose for any prolonged period of time, just like depriving the brain of oxygen, it can cause irreparable damage.

Q: For the moment then, eliminating hypocalcemia, you are stating that depriving the brain of glucose for a prolonged period of time will cause irreparable brain damage?

A: Yes, that is correct.

Q: Now isn't it true that if you fail to treat meningitis immediately, it will cause brain damage within an extremely short period of time?

A: Yes, it can.

Q: You are aware of the fact that the treating physician called for x-rays to be taken prior to your being called into the case as a consultant?

A: Yes, sir.

Q: When you examined the baby the x-ray interpretive report was not part of the hospital record?

A: Correct.

Q: You later became aware of the fact that the x-rays, as interpreted by the radiologist, demonstrated "early infiltration within the right lower lobe segment, probably aspiration pneumonia."

A: Yes.

Q: If you had seen the x-ray interpretive report on the date you first saw the baby, would not your thoughts of meningitis been high on your priority list?

A: Not necessarily.

Q: It could be?

A: Possibly.

Q: It would have heightened the index of suspicion would it not?

A: Of an infectious process.

Q: Isn't meningitis an infectious process?

A: Yes, it is.

Q: Would that in any of itself cause you to perform a lumbar puncture at or about the time the blood studies were performed?

A: It might have.

Q: But in any event, it was not in the chart when you first saw the baby?

A: That is correct.

§ 33.9   Cross Examination of Defendant's Independent Obstetrical Expert Regarding Cephalopelvic Disproportion, Arrest of Labor, Forceps Delivery, and Use of Pitocin

Cross Examination by Mr. Stanley Schwartz:

Q: I assume that your knowledge with respect to electronic fetal heart monitors, external and internal, is much greater today than it was back in 1980?

A: Well, I would hope so, yes.

Q: As everything, and particularly medicine being dynamic and not static, your knowledge, without question, has advanced?

A: Yes.

Q: Back in 1980, as well as today, I would believe that the individualization of each patient's problem would be vital to good medical care and attention?

A: I think that would be a correct statement.

Q: In November of 1980, during your fellowship, did you also do teaching?

A: Yes, I did.

Q: And this would be at the medical school?

A: That's correct.

Q: And it would be at the hospital?

A: That's correct.

Q: And I assume that in 1980 you would teach that the art of obstetrics was not only in the manipulative skills of a particular physician, but also totally evaluating the patient's condition and the risk of the patient in an attempt to avoid difficulties and problems from occurring?

A: That's correct.

Q: Would it be correct to state that the probability that a fetus will be injured while descending through the birth canal is directly or indirectly related to the difficulties encountered during labor and the methods used to resolve them?

A: Yes.

Q: And I assume that the physician, such as you, would be aware of the fact that you had two patients: one, the mother, and two, the fetus soon to be brought into life as a viable person?

A: That's correct.

Q: And the safety of these two patients would be important to you, not just one?

A: That is correct.

Q: Would it not be true that one of the things, therefore, that must be done in the matter of obligation to the patients would be for the doctor to take safeguards in connection with situations which he must or should anticipate during a labor period?

A: That is correct.

Q: It is imperative for the physician, that is the obstetrician, to always think ahead?

A: Yes.

Q: One of the things that the physician must do is be aware of all premonitory warnings that might exist to put them on notice of any possibility of deleterious consequences befalling the mother or the fetus?

A: Yes, sir, that's correct.

Q: And to take definitive action as best as possible to attempt to avoid the problem from occurring?

A: That's correct.

Q: The ultimate goal of the obstetrician is to deliver a viable baby to a healthy mother?

A: That is correct.

Q: There are necessary axioms that I am giving to you, and it would be unrealistic for me to think that you would not say anything other than what you are saying because this is common sense, but bear with me and we will reach our ultimate goal.

A: Fine.

Q: What is meant by a high risk pregnancy?

A: A high risk pregnancy would be defined as any pregnancy in which the outcome for either the mother or the infant is less than the perfect result or anticipated to be less than the perfect result.

Q: Would it encompass situations wherein the physician knows of a high susceptibility of morbidity and mortality to the mother and/or the fetus by reason of a condition that the mother or the fetus is experiencing?

A: Yes, that's correct.

Q: Would labor be classified as a stressful period for the fetus under normal circumstances?

A: I would have to answer that as under normal circumstances by definition labor would not be riskful to the fetus.

Q: If there is a diminution of uterine blood flow during the labor period, that can cause reduction of oxygenation to the fetus?

A: Under normal circumstances it does not.

Q: When you say "under normal circumstances," are you indicating that under normal circumstances when there is a diminution or reduction of uterine blood flow to the fetus, there will not be any lack of oxygen to the fetus concomitant with that?

A: That's correct, under usual circumstances.

Q: What are the circumstances wherein there would be a reduction of oxygenation when there is in tandem with that a reduction of uterine blood flow?

A: Well, the only way I can answer that would be with respect to animal studies. I don't know any direct studies in the human.

Q: Are you referring to sheep, goats, monkeys?

A: That's correct.

Q: Are you referring to any particular studies? Volpe studies, Myers studies?

A: There are a number of studies from which one can draw conclusions, if I can either cite them or summarize them.

Q: I have been referring to a diminution of oxygenation to the fetus. Would a common denominator of hypoxic ischemia be a deprivation of supply of oxygen to the central nervous system?

A: Yes. I think that would be a fair assumption, fair definition.

Q: Would hypoxia be a diminished amount of oxygen to the blood supply, hypoxemia?

A: Hypoxemia means only a decreased amount of oxygen in the blood. It does not necessarily equate with the level of oxygenation.

Q: There is a difference between hypoxemia and hypoxia?

A: Yes.

Q: Could you define hypoxia for me?

A: Hypoxia would be an inadequate environment of oxygen. Hypoxemia would be a decreased oxygen concentration in the blood.

Q: And for the trilogy, would ischemia be a diminished amount of blood profusing the tissues?

A: No, not necessarily. A decreased amount of adequate oxygenated blood profusing the tissues.

Q: If there is not adequate oxygenation to the tissues, can there be damage to the tissues?

A: Yes.

Q: If there is hypoxia to the fetus, can there be brain damage?

A: Yes.

Q: Are you able to determine based upon your own studies, pragmatic and/or academic, as to how long it would take for an hypoxic event to cause brain damage to the fetus?

A: Generally, but not precisely.

Q: In a general term—a parameter in time?

A: Somewhere between four and eight minutes.

Q: Would anoxia be a total cessation of oxygen as opposed to a diminution of oxygen?

A: By definition.

Q: Would anoxia take less time to cause brain damage to the fetus?

A: Yes.

Q: Again, in general terms, are you able to give me some determination as to that period of time?

A: It depends on the degree and extent of hypoxia. It would be more of a graded response.

Q: Reviewing the hospital records, independent of any information which you may have obtained from defense attorneys, are you able to determine who delivered the baby?

A: No.

Q: Do you recall seeing Dr. Barton's name in the records?

A: I would have to rescan the records.

Q: Looking at the records, are you able to determine how the baby was delivered?

A: Yes.

Q: And how was the baby delivered?

A: The records note that it was a spontaneous vaginal delivery.

Q: What is a spontaneous vaginal delivery?

A: Spontaneous vaginal delivery by definition is one in which the baby deliveries as a vertex or head first without any assistance with forceps.

Q: And that would be of an L.O.A. (left occiput anterior), L.O.P. (left occiput posterior), or R.O.A. (right occiput anterior)?

A: From anywhere.

Q: From anywhere. In this particular case would forceps delivery have been contraindicated?

A: I can't tell from the hospital record.

Q: What information would you need to assist yourself?

A: I would have to know the station of the presenting part and an examination of the bony pelvis, a clinical examination of the bony pelvis.

Q: The pelvimetry would not help you?

A: I don't use x-ray pelvimetries, so I don't know.

Q: Would you have to know the degree of caput or molding?

A: That would be helpful to some extent, yes.

Q: In essence, it's more difficult to determine the true station when there is molding and caput?

A: That's correct.

Q: And the longer the second stage of labor lasts, the greater the likelihood of caput and/or molding?

A: There is a linear relationship between the two, but it is not that tight.

Q: But there is some relationship?

A: Correct.

Q: Do you consider Emanuel Friedman's writings to be authoritative in the field of obstetrics?

A: Yes.

Q: Have you read his books?

A: In the past.

Q: Are you familiar with any of his philosophy and beliefs with respect to the use of forceps causing high susceptibility of damage or injury to the fetus when taking into consideration the extent of a second stage of labor?

A: I am aware of that.

Q: And what does he indicate with respect to that preface?

A: Dr. Friedman, to the best of my recollection, reports a progressive increase perimorbidity and mortality in labor disorders such as a protracted active phase or a secondary arrest of labor with an associated abnormal second stage with both spontaneous low and mid-forceps deliveries, and a graded relationship among those.

Q: And does he also indicate there is an even greater relationship with low and mid as opposed to spontaneous?

A: That's correct.

Q: So as we sit here today, you are relying upon the belief that this was a spontaneous delivery?

A: I'm relying on what I can glean from the hospital records, and that's the case.

Q: I'm going to ask you to look at the nurses' records.

A: Yes.

Q: Now, on the 7th—do you have the nurse's notes?

A: Yes.

Q: Look at the bottom of the page, on the 7th when the patient is taken to the delivery room.

A: Yes.

Q: Do you see that?

A: Yes.

Q: When would that be?

A: 10:25 p.m.

Q: Now, turn the page. When is the next notation?

A: 10:40.

Q: Read that into this record, please.

A: "Dr. Barton—gives spinal anesthesia, apply low forceps."

Q: Is that the first time you saw that?

A: That's correct.

Q: How long have you had those records, Doctor?

A: Well, I can't read them on my records.

Q: You just read them?

A: Well, these are not mine.

Q: I see. So your records that were sent to you were not legible with respect to that passage?

A: Not that place.

Q: Could I see your records?

A: Yes.

Q: Thank you, Doctor. I am looking at the records that were sent to you at the time you were asked to evaluate the file. And I state to you quite frankly that I too cannot read that notation. I can read the other notations, but I can't read that one. And are you indicating that you could not also read it?

A: I would say that I could not read that at the time. Having read this, I can read this.

Q: "Having read this," meaning the record handed to you by the defense attorney?

A: That's correct.

Q: Did you ever call to tell them that, "Gentlemen, this is an important matter for me, and I want to give you a candid, honest opinion, and I can't give you an opinion until I see the entire record and it's legible"?

A: No. I have not discussed that with them.

Q: When you couldn't read it, did you try to obtain a better copy?

A: No, I did not.

Q: So all your opinions have been predicated on the basis of the fact that this was allegedly a spontaneous delivery without the use of any forceps?

A: That is correct.

Q: What is hypothermia?

A: Decreased body temperature.

Q: Do you recall the temperature of this baby when born?

A: No, I don't.

Q: Were you requested to evaluate the baby's neonatal care?

A: The neonatal records have been sent to me.

Q: But your area of expertise would relate to the obstetrical care rendered to the mother as opposed to the care rendered to the child at birth.

A: I think that you could say generally so. I do have some knowledge about neonatal care as well.

Q: Would it have been important to you to determine whether this baby was well taken care of after birth to know as to whether or not hypothermia existed?

A: I would be helpful.

Q: Can hypothermia cause hypoglycemia?

A: It can.

Q: Hypoglycemia can cause brain damage if not properly treated?

A: That is correct.

Q: Did you at all, before I make any further inquiry along those lines, examine the neonatal records to see what care, if any at all, was rendered to the child?

A: I have.

Q: And are you indicating that at this moment you don't recall or do not recall having seen anything with respect to the body temperature of the baby?

A: Not that I can recall. May I review that?

Q: Please do, Doctor.

A: I have the neonatal record in front of me.

Q: Do you have any information with respect to the body temperature?

A: I don't see the body temperature recorded.

Q: Would a body temperature of 94 be classified as hypothermia?

A: Yes, it would.

Q: Do you have any information as to blood gas studies?

A: No, I do not.

Q: Do you have any information with respect to blood sugar studies?

A: No, I don't.

Q: Could you identify the records you received with respect to the neonatal care?

A: All right. I have records here, then, date November 8th and November 10th of 1980.

Q: And what do those records contain?

A: Yes. The first page is a newborn pediatric record, gives a brief description of the baby and a physical examination, an Apgar rating, progress note, and discharge summary. And then on the following page there are some comments regarding head circumference. Another one, which I can't read, and then physical examination within normal limits, full term female newborn. Oh, I'm sorry, excuse me. I have some additional records. I forgot about this.

Q: Why don't you also, as you are reviewing those records, see if there is any indication as to temperature.

A: All right. Yes. On the nursery record I note a temperature of 94 degrees.

Q: That would be a severe case of hypothermia, would it not?

A: It is certainly hypothermia. Whether it's severe or not, is hard to tell. It depends on the temperature in the delivery room and how well the baby was dried off and wrapped up shortly after delivery. But a normal baby can become significantly hypothermic at the time of delivery if convected heat loss occurs.

Q: Is a baby suffering from neonatorum asphyxia more susceptible to experiencing hypothermia?

A: Yes.

Q: Hypothermia would be below what?

A: 96 degrees.

Q: Does the thermometer go below 94 degree?

A: I don't know. It's been so long since I've personally taken a temperature, I can't tell you.

Q: You indicated that a baby suffering from hypothermia is more susceptible to experiencing hypoglycemia than one who is not correct?

A: Correct.

Q: Was dextrostik used in 1980?

A: Yes.

Q: Did you see indication of the use of a dextrostik?

A: No, I don't.

Q: Are you able to determine, based on the information that you have, and without speculation or conjecture, whether this child might possibly have had hypoglycemia?

A: I'm not able to determine.

Q: A dextrostik or blood sugar would have been of assistance in making that determination, would it not?

A: That is correct.

Q: Fetal acidosis would be a pH of what?

A: Oh, certainly below 7.2.

Q: This baby had an Apgar of four at one minute, and six at five; correct?

A: That's correct.

Q: Would that allow you to conclude that the baby was distressed at the time of birth with an Apgar of four?

A: Well, I'd have to say that the Apgar score is very nonspecific. There can be a number of reasons for low Apgar scores.

Q: Seeing an Apgar of four, would allow you to conclude that there was a high probability of the baby being born distressed?

A: Only possibility.

Q: You would have had to be there to make that determination for yourself?

A: That's correct.

Q: So what you are indicating, if I understand correctly, without trying to invoke my interpretation to what you are saying, is that seeing a writing of four and six does not allow you to make any determination as to this baby's condition at birth?

A: In my experiencing of seeing Apgar scores over the years, the accuracy of the Apgar score is dependent upon who is scoring the baby and the institution in which it's occurred and the condition of the baby. All factors would be important.

Q: I would be correct in stating, however, that if you rated a baby as four, you would consider that baby to be distressed?

A: I would consider that baby to have some decrease in scoring of the five parameters that go into making up an Apgar score, and it may be due to several factors.

Q: Would the determinations of Apgar and its significance, if any at all, rest within the discipline of pediatricians and neonatologists as opposed to obstetricians?

A: It depends on the center in which it's occurring. By and large, it's more appropriate to have an individual who did not do the delivery give the Apgar score.

Q: Would a pediatrician, more than an obstetrician, be the one who would be required to determine the effects, consequentially, of a distressed baby?

A: In most circumstances I would say, yes.

Q: Still looking at the neonatal records, there is an indication of molding a caput, is that correct?

A: Yes. On the initial physical examination.

Q: And, I believe, if you will look at the nurse's entry, you'll see molding of head.

A: Female infant admitted to newborn nursery. No. 1, general condition appears satisfactory. Note: molding of head.

Q: What does it mean to have molding of head?

A: Molding of the head is the collection of edema fluid between the scalp and the skull as well as the shaping of the skull as it descends through the birth canal.

Q: And there is a linear correlation, as you mentioned, with respect to the time of the second stage of labor and molding?

A: A very rough linear correlation.

Q: The same would hold for caput?

A: That's correct.

Q: And the definition, of caput is?

A: Well, molding would be a combination of the bone changes and the collection of edema. Caput is primarily the collection of edema fluids between the scalp and the bone.

Q: How does the molding come about?

A: As the baby's head conforms to the configuration of the birth canal.

Q: Is there any correlation between the degree of molding and the narrowness of the canal as compared to the size of the baby?

A: In its broadest terms, I would say, yes.

Q: Would the same thing hold true for caput? By that I mean, a correlation between the degree of caput and the tightness of the canal itself.

A: Not necessarily.

Q: When you say "not necessarily," can you elucidate for me as to what you mean by "not necessarily"?

A: I could try. If a bony pelvis was more than adequate to accept the specific dimensions of the head, but the head was in a deflexed position at the time of the onset of labor, considerable caput may occur until adequate flexion takes place; and given that observation, substantial caput may form even if there is adequacy of the pelvis.

Q: By the way, did you indicate that you do not use pelvimetries?

A: Not in vertex presentations, that's correct.

Q: You rely upon clinical evaluation of the patient's condition?

A: That's correct.

Q: You rely upon clinical evaluation to determine the possible existence of cephalopelvic disproportion?

A: Well, I'd have to say that most obstetricians no longer use that term.

Q: Back in 1980 was the term used?

A: Yes.

Q: What other equivalent terms were used?

A: Poor progress in labor.

Q: Acknowledging that in 1980 the phrase cephalopelvic disproportion still was used, could we state that cephalopelvic disproportion, if it existed, might cause poor progress of labor?

A: Correct.

Q: Back in 1980, were you using pelvimetries to evaluate the pelvic structure?

A: Only in breech presentations.

Q: In 1980 and prior thereto, you had the opportunity of looking at pelvimetries?

A: That's correct.

Q: Would a pelvimetry also be of assistance in showing the degree of molding?

A: To some extent.

Q: Would it be important in a poor progress of labor for a doctor, if he could determine how much molding existed?

A: Only with respect to determining whether or not the presenting part was engaged in the pelvis; and, second, in terms of assessing the descent of the presenting part in the pelvis.

Q: Well, in line with what you are indicating, would the degree of molding be of assistance in evaluating as to whether or not the pelvic structure was of sufficient dimension to allow descent of a fetus without injury when there was poor progress of labor?

A: I don't believe that the degree of molding would be helpful.

Q: But you indicated that there is some correlation between the degree of molding and the tightness of the pelvic structure.

A: A loose correlation, but I think that the only true effect the observation of molding on the management of labor would be in the difficulty in assessing the accurate station of the presenting part.

Q: And one must necessarily know the accurate station of the presenting part when one uses forceps?

A: One must know the implications of molding and have an idea to what extent molding may interfere with accurate diagnosis of station.

Q: And the more experience one has, the more one is able to determine that?

A: If one equates experience with expertise, that would be true.

Q: By the way, going back to the notation we talked about, "applied low forceps," looking at that notation itself where Dr. Barton's name was mentioned, does that assist you in concluding who delivered the baby?

A: Well, this comment at 10:40 reads: "Dr. Barton gave spinal anesthesia. Applied low forceps." From the nurse's note, I would have to conclude that the same physician did both.

Q: Back in 1980, Doctor, if you recall the standard of practice, did it permit and allow a first-year resident to utilize forceps without the attendance of an active staff member when taking into consideration a second stage of labor going beyond two hours?

A: That would depend on the past experience of that individual and the degree of trust that the attending had for his experiences and expertise.

Q: So he would have had to receive permission, then, before doing it on his own?

A: In most cases I would say, yes.

Q: Because of the inherent risk incidental to that type procedure?

A: Yes. I would expand on that, if I may, though. Not having seen the comment about low forceps before, and with respect to the impact of spontaneous low forceps and mid forceps in protraction or abnormal labor disorders, as Dr. Friedman has written, I think it is important to add that the material and outcome was derived on material collected prior to major advances in the neonatal and obstetrical care. I think that most obstetricians would conclude that a low forceps delivery would not be of much significant increase in risk to a baby over a spontaneous delivery.

Q: Much of an increase?

A: That's correct. And I don't know that I could put a number on that, but I would have to say that a usual low forceps delivery would not subject the baby to a substantially increased risk over a spontaneous delivery.

Q: But the greater the stress that's imposed upon the fetus prior to the use of forceps, the greater the likelihood that the forceps will cause injury to the fetus?

A: I'm not sure how one equates those two. I would certainly agree that the imposition of a difficult mid-forceps delivery can certainly produce birth trauma which superimposed on birth hypoxia would synergistically increase the risk. I'm not sure that in an easy low forceps delivery one could make the same conclusion.

Q: Back in 1980, based upon the standard of care, was it permissible for a first-year resident to infuse the patient with Pitocin without first obtaining permission from the active staff member?

A: In most teaching institutions that would be correct.

Q: It would be a violation of the standard?

Q: If the institution required permission from the active staff member, then it would be a violation of the standard of practice?

A: It would certainly be a violation of the hospital policy. Whether or not that would violate standard of care would depend on the teaching institutions and the local community involved.

Q: Pitocin, when contraindicated, can cause damage and/or injury to the fetus and/or the mother?

A: Under certain circumstances it can, that is correct.

Q: In 1980, the term poor progress of labor was replacing the phrase cephalopelvic disproportion?

A: Yes.

Q: Can poor progress of labor be caused by a contracted pelvis?

A: Yes, it can.

Q: Can poor progress in labor cause stress to the fetus?

A: Yes, it can.

Q: Can poor progress in labor ultimately cause distress to the fetus?

A: Yes, it can.

Q: Is there a difference between stress and distress?

A: Yes. Fetal distress by current definition requires the presence of an abnormal fetal heart rate tracing and/or some abnormality of fetal blood gases and the evidence of acidosis. Fetal stress conceptually is anything up to that point but not including.

Q: Fetal stress can lead to fetal distress?

A: In common terminology, yes.

Q: There is a capacity for the fetus to withstand stress and not lead to distress?

A: Yes.

Q: But that capacity is diminished as stress continues?

A: That's correct.

Q: So that at any moment in time stress can lead to distress?

A: That's correct.

Q: And it is impossible, notwithstanding the electronic fetal heart monitor, for the physician to know exactly when in time stress has turned to distress?

A: That's correct.

Q: So when stress exists and it's demonstrable, the physician attempts to abate the stress?

A: Correct.

Q: To look ahead and avoid distress from occurring?

A: That's correct.

Q: Have you had the opportunity of reading Friedman's 1974 article, "Dysfunctional Labor"?

A: I have read it at one time, but not recently.

Q: Would you consider *Williams Obstetrics*, edited by Hellman, to be an authoritative treatise?

A: Which edition?

Q: The 15th edition?

A: The 15th edition would be authoritative at that point in time.

Q: Is it not true that in 1980 the medical dogma, as discussed in *Williams Obstetrics*, declared that perinatal injury was increased markedly in labor when the second stage of labor lasted longer than two hours?

A: I believe so.

Q: Notwithstanding the fact that you did not use pelvimetries in 1980, you knew the purposes of pelvimetries, correct?

A: That's correct.

Q: You knew that a pelvimetry also was used by some in 1972 to attempt to determine the pelvic structure measurements?

A: That's correct.

Q: Is it not true that it is difficult to determine the measurements of the transverse diameter clinically?

A: That's correct.

Q: Is it not true that it is easier to determine the measurements of the transverse diameter by pelvimetry?

A: If one wishes to know the transverse diameter, that is correct.

Q: Is it not true that there is and has been an awareness of margin of error with pelvimetry from zero point five to one centimeter in measurements?

A: There is a significant error in pelvimetry, and it's dependent upon the relationship of the patient's pelvis to the x-ray source from the film and the rotation of the pelvis at the time it's done. There is a great deal of error in pelvimetry.

Q: But the error in pelvimetry that you are referring to would relate to the positioning of the patient and of the fact that it is external rather than the manner in which the radiologist takes the measurements?

A: Well, the bony pelvic measurements are not going to change.

Q: You have had the opportunity of looking at the pelvimetry interpretation of this particular case?

A: That's correct.

Q: What is the normal measurement or the average normal of the transverse of the inlet?

A: Twelve centimeters.

Q: And looking at the interpretative report in this particular case, what is the transverse?

A: It says 11 point something here, and on this is written 11.3.

Q: Would that be a contracted transverse?

A: By pure definition, it would be a measurement that falls below two standard deviations from the mean which by definition would be abnormal.

Q: Now in this case, there was a transverse arrest, correct?

A: That is recorded in the hospital notes.

Q: There was a manual rotation?

A: That's correct.

Q: Manual rotation went from a transverse to what?

A: I presume an occiput anterior.

Q: Why do you presume an occiput anterior?

A: Because one would not generally rotate to a posterior.

Q: Why not?

A: If it rotated more easily, one could rotate to a posterior, but I'm assuming that it rotates to an occiput anterior because that would be by convention the usual attempt.

Q: Why would one want to attempt a rotation anterior rather than posterior?

A: Because delivering as an occiput anterior is the easiest way for the head to come under the pubic synthesis and delivered by extension.

Q: By spontaneous delivery without forceps?

A: That's correct.

Q: And is it easier to use forceps on an anterior than a posterior?

A: Yes, but it can be done on either

Q: But it is easier on an anterior than a posterior?

A: Yes.

Q: Please examine the records and see if it was a posterior or an anterior.

A: "After a manual rotation to the left occiput posterior, the patient was transferred to the delivery room, and under spinal anesthetic and episiotoma spontaneous assisted vaginal delivery, full term infant with molding."

Q: This was a posterior as opposed to an anterior?

A: That's correct.

Q: Isn't it true that whenever the pelvic inlet is less than 10 cm in its shortest A-P diameter or 12 cm transverse diameter, dystocia increases in frequency?

A: Correct, in the term fetus.

Q: What is the normal average A-P inlet?

A: The normal average A-P of the inlet exceeds 10 centimeters.

Q: Would the average normal be 12.5?

A: I can't recall the specific normal. But the lower limit of normal would be 10.

Q: What is the average normal of the interspinous?

A: The average normal would be approximately 10.5.

Q: Would there be a greater likelihood of a failure of rotation from a transverse position at the interspinous when it is less than 10.5?

A: It would, but the lower limit of normal would be 9.5, and it would increase below that.

Q: What was the interspinous in this case?

A: The interspinous was read as being 9.8.

Q: If in this particular case, subject to my ability to connect, the transverse was 11.3 of the inlet, and the interspinous was 9.8, would that allow you to conclude that this was in all likelihood a contracted pelvis?

A: I don't think that I can agree with that statement.

Q: Would it be a normal pelvis?

A: No, not if one compares it to thousands of radiologically determined measurements.

Q: It would be an abnormal pelvis?

A: It would be a smaller than average pelvis.

Q: Would it be a borderline pelvis structure?

A: That depends on its relationship to the head of the fetus; and if one doesn't know the size of that, it may be more than an adequate pelvis, it may be exceedingly generous.

Q: If you don't have ultrasound, you will only know that after the birth of the baby?

A: I think that ultrasound doesn't help with that either. And I would have to say that that would be majority obstetrical opinion with the exception of Dr. Friedman that pelvic adequacy in a given labor is measured by functional process and progress.

Q: Well, going back to my question: Would I be correct in stating that there is no way, then, that a physician could know the size of the head until the baby is born?

A: He may be able to determine some dimensions of the head, but can't be absolutely certain at any point in time what dimensions of the head are posed to the specific dimensions of the pelvis. Therefore, it would not be prognostically accurate information.

Q: So you'd have to know the size of the head and also the position of the head?

A: Size, position, and degree of flexion.

Q: I was referring to the position encompassing the flexion, but it would be a different factor, position and flexion?

A: Position and flexion are different phenomenon.

Q: You would expect, under normal circumstances, that the head is at the vertex and that it's flexed?

A: Correct.

Q: Is there a difference between extended and hyperextended?

A: Yes.

Q: If the head is extended, is that the military attitude?

A: It depends on the degree of extension and what is presenting. In the so-called sinciput presentation, that would be military presentation, that would be, yes, extended.

Q: In this particular case was the head extended or flexed?

A: May I see that x-ray?

Q: Yes.

A: Well, within my capability to read these films, I would say I don't know.

Q: Then, in following your statements, what does a physician do if labor goes three hours, four hours in the second stage, he knows there is a transverse arrest, he takes measurements that are less than average normal, he concludes that there is no way of knowing whether or not this is a contracted pelvis unless he knows not only the measurements of the size of the baby's head, but also whether or not there is flexion and/or extension, and he can't determine whether there is flexion or extension, and he can't tell the size of the baby's head until the baby is born?

A: I think what the obstetrician has to do at that point is to—and I believe that this would be appropriate management at the time of this case in 1980—the obstetrician would be required to demonstrate that there is adequate progress in terms of the descent of the presenting part, and if convinced that the bony pelvis was adequate by clinical examination and was not absolutely contracted.

Q: Am I correct in interpreting what you previously stated; namely, that taking into consideration the measurements that existed in this particular case, you would have to know the size of the head and the flexion and/or extention to determine whether or not contraction existed?

A: I would agree with that, yes.

Q: What is adequate progress of descent?

A: Well, the standards that are given, and the ranges are quite wide.

Q: Back in 1980?

A: Well, they are still the same. Labor hasn't changed. The stage of labor would be approximately 1 cm descent per hour.

Q: In this particular case, what was the station at 6:00 p.m.?

A: Station at 6:00 p.m. was recorded as plus one.

Q: And at 7:00 p.m.?

A: 7:00—I don't see a recording at 7:00 p.m.

Q: What is the next recording that you do see after 7:00?

A: Is this 7:05 or 8:05? I think that's 8:05 p.m.

Q: And what would that be?

A: Plus one station.

Q: And what would it be at the next recording?

A: Plus one station.

Q: What time would that be?

A: It looks like 9:05 p.m.

Q: Is there any recording between 9:05 p.m. and the birth of the baby?

A: No.

Q: Would that be adequate progress of descent?

A: Not by definition of normal standards, no, it's not.

Q: Do you know what, if anything, Dr. Barton did to determine the bony pelvis measurements in this particular case?

A: I assume that an x-ray pelvimetry was ordered.

Q: Do you know that reveals that he didn't have those results until after the birth of the baby?

A: I know nothing of that.

Q: Are you able to tell the station of the baby at the time the pelvimetry was taken?

A: Not for certain, no.

Q: Why "not for certain"?

A: On the A-P film I would have to say that the head appears to be at somewhere between a zero and plus one station on the lateral film, the same.

Q: Are you allowing for molding?

A: No. I think the molding has some affect on the clinical examination, but I think that one can by looking at those films make an estimate of where the biparietal bones are with reference to the mother's pelvis.

Q: And the biparietal bones would be four centimeters above the most presented part?

A: In the average term fetal head without molding.

Q: So in this case you have molding?

A: That's right. That's why I'm directing my inspection to where the parietal bones would be.

Q: Would that be also why you were giving yourself a one centimeter margin of error?

A: That is correct.

Q: A baby usually comes into the inlet in a transverse position before rotation?

A: That's correct.

Q: And where does it usually rotate?

A: As it goes through the level of the mid pelvis.

Q: Would that be at the ischial spine?

A: Correct, at or above.

Q: And the interspinous?

A: It's the same thing.

Q: In this particular case do you have an opinion as to why there was a transverse arrest?

A: No. I don't.

Q: Is it not true that there is a high existence of extension and hyperextension in the transverse position as opposed to an O-A position?

A: That's true.

Q: One of the reasons as to why there could well have been a transverse arrest in this case is the extension of the head?

A: Correct.

Q: Isn't it also true that extension of the head is more common in a posterior position than an anterior position?

A: Correct.

Q: If there is an extension of the head after rotation, manually, is it more difficult to utilize forceps than when there is no extension of the head?

A: Correct.

Q: What, if anything, does the doctor do, if extension of the head exists at the time of manual rotation, to insure that the baby is posterior and there is no further extension?

A: I don't know that there is much one can do.

Q: So that rotation, in and of itself, does not abate the condition of extension if extension does, in fact, exist?

A: That's correct.

Q: Most fetuses that begin labor in the L-O-T (left occiput transverse) position, for example, rotate the head 90 degrees L-O-T to L-O-A (left occiput anterior) to O-A (occiput anterior)?

A: Correct.

Q: And that would bring the occiput under the pubic synthesis?

A: That's correct.

Q: And then you have, usually, spontaneous delivery?

A: Correct.

Q: And if the head is arrested with the site of the sutures in the transverse diameter of the pelvis, that's a transverse arrest?

A: Correct.

Q: Looking at the hospital record in this case, from the time of the x-ray at or about 9:38, I believe, to the time of delivery, is there any indication of fetal condition?

A: Not that I can find from the hospital record.

Q: Are you able to state that fetal distress did not exist for the 75-minute period of time?

A: I am not.

Q: You know the difference between acute and chronic distress?

A: I think so.

Q: More likely than not a distressed baby, at birth, is due to acute distress as opposed to chronic distress?

A: Not necessarily.

Q: Is it more common for a baby who is acutely distressed during labor to be distressed at the time of birth as opposed to one chronically distressed taking into consideration the compensation period?

A: I don't know that anybody can answer that question accurately.

Q: Would you accept the fact that a neonatologist and/or pediatrician would be better suited to testify or explain those areas than an obstetrician?

A: Not necessarily.

Q: What is a neonatologist?

A: A neonatologist is one who specializes in the care of newborns.

Q: And that would be from the moment of birth?

A: Correct, but there is a great deal of overlap. A specialist in perinatal medicine is expected to have a solid understanding of neonatal life and its complications, and the converse is true with a neonatologist.

Q: There have been occasions, I assume, in your career where you were aware of the fact that a baby by reason of some underlying event, in all likelihood, was going to be born distressed and the child would require the assistance of a neonatologist and/or a pediatrician in the delivery room?

A: Absolutely.

Q: You would want assistance in the caring for the baby?

A: Correct.

Q: Did you have the opportunity of reviewing any fetal heart monitor tapes depicting events between the taking of the pelvimetry and the birth of the baby?

A: The only assumption that I can make is that from the hospital notes, as I have seen them, with respect of when the fetal heart rate monitor was applied, and calculating the total length of time that the heart rate monitor was applied, and assuming that these are the only heart rate tracings available, then beyond that time the answer is I did not.

Q: Is it mechanically possible for a patient to be transported to the x-ray department from the labor room and still have a fetal heart monitor attached?

A: It is possible.

Q: You've done that?

A: On occasion.

Q: It is also possible to detach the fetal heart monitor and reattach it at the time the patient reaches her destination, in this case, the x-ray department?

A: That is correct.

Q: In this particular case, approximately 75 minutes expired from the time the patient was transferred to the radiology department and the birth of the baby?

A: That seems to be a correct approximation.

Q: And there is no recording of any fetal heart rate by auscultation or otherwise during the period of time in the hospital record, is there?

A: None that I can find.

Q: I mentioned the name Volpe. Are you familiar with that name?

A: I am.

Q: Are you aware of the fact that he allegedly authored a book *Neurology of the Newborn*?

A: I am.

Q: Have you had the opportunity to read that book?

A: No, I have not.

Q: Notwithstanding the fact that you have not had the opportunity to read this book, you are, nevertheless, familiar with Volpe, and know that he has authored other books and articles; consequently, I ask you if you are in a position to advise me as to whether or not you find his enlightening writings to be authoritative?

A: I have read several of Dr. Volpe's articles. I cannot at this point in time cite the specific references. I would agree that Dr. Volpe is an authority in neonatal asphyxia and outcome.

Q: Would you not accept the fact that there is an increase of incidences of hemorrhaging with prolonged second stage labor?

A: What type of hemorrhaging?

Q: Subarachnoid?

A: A very modest increase and more related to the difficulty of the actual delivery.

Q: By use of forceps?

A: Correct.

Q: What about a prolonged second stage of labor and the use of oxytocin and the rapid acceleration or descent of the fetus and the relationship of subarachnoid hemorrhaging?

A: I don't know that there is any clear-cut data that demonstrates a relationship.

Q: When you say "any clear-cut data," are you familiar with Volpe's data concerning the relationship between oxytocin and precipitous deliveries?

A: I can't recall the specific details.

Q: Are you familiar with any studies and/or statistics relating to a direct or indirect correlation between subarachnoid hemorrhages and precipitous when oxytocin is administered?

A: Not specifically.

Q: Is there a term precipitous delivery?

A: There is.

Q: The mother was transferred to the delivery room at what time?

A: 10:25.

Q: The last recording of the station is at 9:05. As plus one?

A: That's correct.

Q: Is there any indication on the fetal heart monitor tape as to the station at the time the mother was transported to the x-ray department?

A: No.

Q: If the head was at the perineum when forceps were used at 10:54, how many centimeters, approximately, would the head have to descend between 9:05 to 10:54?

A: Approximately three.

Q: Would you consider a descent of four centimeters within a period of approximately 60 minutes to be a precipitous delivery?

A: No.

Q: Did you indicate that there was a definition of a precipitous delivery?

A: There are varying definitions.

Q: What is your definition?

A: A precipitous labor is one which, rather than precipitous delivery, is one which occurs in less than four hours.

Q: So you do not use the term precipitous delivery but rather precipitous labor and define it as such?

A: Correct.

Q: Does the uterine blood flow vary inversely with the intensity and frequency and duration of the uterine contractions?

A: In what species?

Q: Human.

A: Nobody knows.

Q: Are you indicating that the study relates only to animals?

A: That's correct.

Q: Again, whose studies?

A: Again, there are a variety of studies in which uterine blood flow has been measured with uterine contractility. They include Myers. There are a number of investigators who have studied that.

Q: When you treat your patients do you take into consideration the correlation that might exist between uterine blood flow and the intensity of the contraction?

A: Yes, because I think that data is applicable to humans.

Q: Is it not true that the steady delivery of oxygen to the fetus cannot be interrupted for even a short period of time without serious consequences befalling the fetus?

A: You would have to define "a short period of time."

Q: A minute, two minutes.

A: I would have to say that with an interruption of oxygenation for one to two minutes and then a reversal of those circumstances to return the rate of oxygen delivery to normal, that would not produce a problem with the fetus.

Q: What time parameter would you believe could or might cause a problem?

A: Probably, at least with acute cessation of flow, somewhere between six to eight minutes, and that would depend on the maturity of the fetus.

Q: Are you referring to a single period of time?

A: Correct.

Q: So that damage to the fetus may occur, if not during one period of time, over an extensive period of time?

A: It might.

Q: Is there a reduction of oxygenation to the fetus during a contraction?

A: There is a reduction of blood flow into the intervillous space. Whether or not there is a reduction in oxygenation depends on the circumstances.

Q: What is meant by hypertonic contractions?

A: Hypertonic contractions by definition imply an elevation of the base line intrauterine pressure above approximately 20 mm of mercury as a common denominator.

Q: Are you able to, by looking at the fetal heart monitor tape, with your comment that this might not have been an internal lead, ascertain the intensity of millimeters of mercury during a contraction?

A: I can't interpret that because I don't know what the numbers are on the graph.

Q: If you did know that, you would then be able to interpret it?

A: If I knew that the base line was zero and the top line, where the number four is recorded, represented 100 millimeters of mercury, I would be able to make more accurate statements, assuming that this was an intrauterine catheter.

Q: What is meant by a tetanic contraction?

A: A tetanic contraction is a contraction that does not return to the base line within the normal period of time. It's one that lasts. It is prolonged.

Q: Can tetanic contractions cause a reduction of blood flow into the intervillous space?

A: Yes.

Q: And can that possibly cause a reduction of oxygenation to the fetus?

A: Yes.

Q: And what is a normal contraction period of time?

A: Well, a normal contraction is approximately one minute from the beginning to the end.

Q: And a tetanic would be longer than a minute?

A: Yes, but it's generally defined as even longer. I guess the best way to express that is: If the contraction lasted a minute and 15 seconds, it would not necessarily be tetanic. If it lasted for over two minutes, it would be considered tetanic, but I don't recall a specific definition of what time element this required to call it a tetanic contraction.

Q: In a normal labor, active stage, accelerated stage, do you expect to find approximately three contractions every ten minutes?

A: On the average.

Q: And how long is the resting period?

A: Oh, at least one minute between contractions.

Q: If the resting period is less than a minute, does that have any affect upon the fetus?

A: Well, by deductive reasoning, that would decrease the amount of time, the amount of blood profusing the intervillous space and might produce hypoxia. The only way one could tell is to record the fetal heart rate.

Q: Can you tell me whether or not uterine contractions that are tetanic or contractions occurring with resting periods between them of less than a minute, can cause damage to the fetus when fetal reserves are low?

A: They may.

Q: How?

A: Depending on that point in time and the degree of fetal oxygenation and acid base status, it is entirely possible that decreased oxygen could be provided for fetal utilization so that it would result in anaerobic metabolism and metabolic acidosis. However, I don't know that anyone can tell clinically at what point one is starting in order to make that determination.

Q: Is there a term, arrest of dilatation?

A: Yes, there is.

Q: And what is meant by arrest of dilatation?

A: That means that dilatation of the cervix is not proceeding at the normal rate as established by previous standards.

Q: Is there a term secondary arrest of dilatation?

A: There is.

Q: What does that mean?

A: Secondary arrest is characterized by adequate progress during the active phase of labor up to a point at which arrest of subsequent dilatation occurs.

Q: What is the normal dilatation per hour?

A: In a primigravid patient or multiparous patient?

Q: Primigravid?

A: Primigravid would be approximately 1 and 1.2 cm per hour.

Q: Would you define a secondary arrest of dilatation when that does not take place?

A: Yes, that is correct, in the active phase of labor.

Q: In the active phase of labor, how many contractions usually occur during a ten-minute period?

A: Well, basically you need to have a cervix that is dilated somewhere three to four centimeters or beyond.

Q: Would that be the signal you would utilize—the degree of dilatation of the cervix as opposed to frequency of the contractions?

A: The frequency of contractions may be a cause of secondary arrest. I'm not sure whether one could define a secondary arrest as rare uterine contractility in terms of uterine activity, per se, inasmuch as patients may make adequate progress with minimal uterine activity.

Q: In this particular case what was the dilatation at 2:30, 3:00 p.m. in the afternoon?

A: At 2:10 p.m., five centimeters is recorded.

Q: At 2:10 would the patient, by your definition, be in the active stage of labor?

A: Yes.

Q: And what was the dilatation at 5:20?

A: 5:20 is seven centimeters.

Q: So there were two centimeters in a period of approximately three hours?

A: That's correct.

Q: Would that be classified as secondary arrest of dilatation?

A: That would not be a secondary arrest. That might be a very minimally protracted active phase arrest. I should say protracted active phase.

Q: Would that be a poor progress of labor?

A: That would be poor progress in labor, to a very minor degree.

Q: This is before there was full dilatation at 6:00 o'clock?

A: That's correct.

Q: And we discussed the descent from 6:00 o'clock on?

A: Yes.

Q: What is meant by gestational hypertension?

A: The presence of hypertension during pregnancy.

Q: Do you have a formula that you utilize?

A: There are certain standards, yes.

Q: And have these standards remained constant from 1980 to the present?

A: Yes, they have.

Q: And would this be the definition of the American College of Obstetricians and Gynecologists?

A: Yes, it is.

Q: Would the standard nomenclature back in 1980, define gestational hypertension as a systolic of 140 or a diastolic of 90 or 30 millimeters of mercury in excess of normal systolic or 15 millimeters of mercury in excess of normal diastolic?

A: That would be correct if one added to that that they were measurements that were persistent over time.

Q: Do you know whether or not this woman was suffering from gestational hypertension during her prenatal period?

A: I have not seen the prenatal records, but from the hospital records I would say, yes, she was.

Q: Are you in a position to determine, by looking at the hospital records, the extent of the gestational hypertension?

A: The diastolic pressure ranged, as best I can tell, somewhere between 90 and 100 mm of mercury.

Q: Would that be moderate, severe or mild?

A: Well, that would be mild.

Q: What would severe hypertension be?

A: It would be characterized by a persistent diastolic rate of 110 and systolic rate of 160 as a specific blood pressure criteria. There are other criteria for distinguishing between severe and mild.

Q: This patient, I believe at the time of admission to the hospital, had a diagnosis of mild preeclampsia, did she not?

A: I believe so.

Q: Is there a difference between gestational or pregnancy-induced hypertension and mild preeclampsia?

A: There is no difference between pregnancy-induced hypertension and preeclampsia. They are synonomous.

Q: A patient can have pregnancy-induced hypertension without edema proteinuria?

A: She may.

Q: Is it important to diagnose a patient who is suffering from pregnancy-induced hypertension or preeclampsia?

A: Yes.

Q: Why?

A: Because the development of pregnancy-induced hypertension carries some risk to the mother and to the fetus.

Q: That risk would involve the placenta?

A: In longstanding cases of severe preeclampsia there may be damage to the placenta.

Q: Without damage to the placenta, what injury, if any at all, can fetus suffer when a mother has pregnancy-induced hypertension?

A: Aberation of growth.

Q: Intrauterine growth retardation?

A: Correct.

Q: Intrauterine growth retardation did not exist in this particular case, is that correct?

A: By definition, since this baby weighed seven pounds, that would not let it fall below the ten percentile of birth rate for gestational age. Therefore, it did not meet the criteria for intrauterine growth retardation.

Q: Also, there is an amniocentesis, correct?

A: That is correct.

Q: And that amniocentesis was performed between 10:00 and 11:00, on the morning of the 7th?

A: That's consistent with my recollection.

Q: So again at that time of morning there was no indication of any fetal distress by reason of the amniocentesis?

A: Well, inasmuch as the amnionic fluid was recorded as being cleared or having absent of meconium staining, that would be correct.

Q: Would that be before the mother was in active labor?

A: She appeared to be in either early labor or in false labor at that time.

Q: It was many hours before full dilatation?

A: That's correct.

Q: Would I be correct in stating, therefore, that at the time of the amniocentesis was performed, there was no indication of a fetal problem?

A: That's correct.

Q: And further, there was no injury to the fetus as a result of any maternal hypertension that might have existed?

A: I would have to say that only by the absence of having meconium staining amnionic fluid, can I make the statement that there was no injury, ischemic injury to the brain at that time. It's possible that injury could have occurred in an earlier time, meconium passed or not passed, and then if it had passsed, been cleared from the amnionic fluid.

Q: That would be speculative?

A: Purely speculative.

Q: Is it not true that molding obscured the suture lines of the fetal skull, and these suture lines assist in correctly applying forceps?

A: Correct.

Q: Can intracranial hemorrhaging result not only from anoxia but also from direct trauma to the brain?

A: It can.

Q: Is there a term "mechanical injury" to the brain?

A: I'm not familiar with that term.

Q: Can intracranial hemorrhage occur as a result of the baby coming down a small birth canal and striking the pelvic structure as it descends?

A: The best way that I could answer that is that it has been proposed that that may occur. Whether it does or not, I'm not certain.

Q: And it can also occur as a result of a traumatic delivery?

A: That may occur.

Q: Improper application of forceps may cause a traumatic delivery?

A: It can.

Q: An enlarged caput may create the impression that the head is descending when in reality the advancement of the head is delayed or arrested?

A: Correct.

Q: Is it not true that the immediate effect of maternal hypertension is vasospasms and substantial reduction of uterine blood flow?

A: Well, there is certainly the evidence in that disease that vasospasm occurs. There is only one study that I'm aware of in which indirect measures of uterine blood flow occurred, and that study is over 20 years old and probably not reliable.

Q: You are familiar with the drug Pitocin or oxytocin?

A: Yes.

Q: You are familiar with the effects of oxytocin?

A: I am.

Q: And you knew the effect of oxytocin back in 1980?

A: To the best of my knowledge, they haven't changed.

Q: And the contraindications as to its use, have not changed?

A: Assuming that there are some.

Q: Are there some?

A: There are some.

Q: The drug can cause harm if imprudently used?

A: Correct.

Q: It's a synthetic hormone?

A: It is a synthetic hormone.

Q: Stimulates labor?

A: True.

Q: It increases intrauterine pressure?

A: Yes.

Q: It increases myometrial contractions?

A: True.

Q: It can interfere with circulation in the intervillous space?

A: If used injudiciously.

Q: Does it affect the blood pressure of the mother?

A: No, not unless given in huge bolus amounts.

Q: It basically stimulates the uterus to contract?

A: Correct.

Q: And it's important for intensity, frequency, quality, and duration of contractions to be continuously observed?

A: Correct.

Q: Back in 1972, was there any requirement on the part of the physician ordering the Pitocin to be in attendance during the administering of the Pitocin?

A: It depended on the hospital policy.

Q: Are you indicating there was no uniform policy that you were aware of, but rather it would rest within the determinations of the particular institution?

A: That's correct. Either a doctor or a nurse would be in attendance.

Q: But one or the other had to be in attendance?

A: Correct.

Q: Would a contraindication to Pitocin be fetal distress?

A: Correct.

Q: Would a contraindication to Pitocin be cephalopelvic disproportion?

A: That is a very gray area.

Q: And in 1980 was it a gray area as opposed to an accepted fact?

A: I would say that that would be a gray area in 1980.

Q: Let's go back, then, to 1980. The PDR was published in 1980, was it not?

A: Yes.

Q: There were pharmacological books available to physicians with respect to the properties of Pitocin and its effect?

A: Correct.

Q: Was the PDR an authoritative work with respect to drugs and its contraindications and use?

A: In an exceedingly conservative format.

Q: In essence, if I understand correctly, without paraphrasing your testimony, but in attempting to understand it, the safeguards or the comments made in PDR would be published by the manufacturer, and it would be quite conservative and therefore not necessarily followed by physicians?

A: Correct.

Q: Therefore, it would not be utilized for the purpose of setting standards?

A: That is correct.

Q: But it was followed, at least, as a reference?

A: Correct.

Q: Let's go to the gray area, then. Can you expand upon that term by telling me what you mean by it being a "gray area"?

A: Yes. Since physicians by and large nowadays, and certainly in 1980 began to direct their attention to the functional progress in labor rather than to the strict definition of cephalopelvic disproportion, they began to utilize normal labor curves such as Dr. Friedman's to assess the course of labor. If there was a protracted active phase or a secondary arrest of labor, then physicians would evaluate the situation clinically and perhaps augment uterine contractions with oxytocin and determine a finite length of time for progress to occur following the administration of oxytocin. As such, cephalopelvic disproportion would be a term that would not be used clinically, and therefore would put this entire issue into a gray area rather than black and white contraindication and indication.

Q: Are you stating that it was not a violation of the standard of practice to administer Pitocin when the physician knew that cephalopelvic disproportion (CPD) existed?

A: Well, I would say that the only way I could answer that is to contend that the physician never knows when absolute cephalopelvic disproportion exists.

Q: Then, contra to that, are you indicating that if by way of some divine determination you would know that it exists, it would be contraindicated?

A: Under those circumstances, if I would consider any circumstance in which the physician would be able to define that, the answer would be correct.

Q: And you are stating that under no circumstance could a pelvimetry determine the existence of CPD?

A: I don't believe I said that. There are certain circumstances where pelvic fractures have occurred where a developmental abnormality due to metabolic bone disease in which absolute cephalopelvic disproportion might be assumed.

Q: With those exceptions?

A: Correct.

Q: One of the pitfalls of oxytocin stimulation would be the existence of CPD and the head becoming fixed or wedged into the pelvis?

A: That is correct. And that is the determination that the obstetrician has to make based on clinical evaluation at the time.

Q: Is transverse arrest usually caused by cephalopelvic disproportion?

A: Yes.

Q: It is true, is it not, that the oxytocin would only correct the forces of labor and in no way alters the inadequate pelvis or abnormalities in the fetal size or malposition?

A: Correct.

Q: Would malposition be a contraindication to oxytocin?

A: No.

Q: By the way, least I forget, in this particular case there was an artificial rupture of the membranes, was there not?

A: Yes, at 2:10 p.m.

Q: And what was the station at that time?

A: Minus one.

Q: Looking at the record, do you have any opinion, without conjecture or speculation as to why the membranes were artificially ruptured?

A: I can't speculate.

Q: You don't know?

A: That's correct.

Q: Is there an increased risk of prolapsed cord when the membranes are artificially ruptured and the head is unengaged?

A: It depends on the degree of lack of engagement, and there is varying opinion as to that risk. My opinion is that rupturing membranes at a minus one station raises the risk of a prolapsed umbilical cord minimally, and those risks are outweighed by the benefit of perhaps accelerating the process of labor.

Q: What you are saying is that there are certain risks inherent to the procedure when the head is unengaged, be it minimal or substantial, but if the risks are minimal, they are probably outweighed by the benefits of rupturing the membranes?

A: Correct.

Q: What were the benefits in this case?

A: The benefit would be to accelerate the process of labor in someone who has been having contractions for many hours and may indeed have had a long, if not prolonged, latent phase of labor.

Q: So, it was an effort to expedite labor?

A: Correct.

Q: To move it along?

A: Correct.

Q: Because there is a correlation between the extent of labor and fetal distress?

A: There is a rough correlation between the extension of labor and fetal distress.

Q: Under certain circumstances, the earlier in time the baby is delivered, the better it would be?

A: Correct.

Q: The membranes were ruptured at 2:10 in the afternoon, and after about another eight and a half hours of labor the baby was delivered?

A: Correct.

Q: When oxytocin is administered, I assume it has to be adjusted according to the responses of the uterus?

A: Correct.

Q: What are some of the other contraindications to the use of oxytocin other than fetal distress?

A: The placental praevia, a previous vertical uterine scar; certainly in 1972 any previous uterine incision; a transverse lie of the fetus. Those would be the major contraindications.

Q: There is a difference between absolute and relative disproportion?

A: That's correct.

Q: You would agree that an attempt to overcome a CPD would not be to administer oxytocin if CPD, in fact, did exist?

A: In the presence of 1972 definition of absolute cephalopelvic disproportion, that would be correct.

Q: If relative disproportion exists, it may cause problems to the fetus when Pitocin is administered?

A: If one were not carefully following the progress of labor, that's correct.

Q: Is there a correlation between the extent of the second stage of labor and damage or injury to the fetus?

A: There is a correlation.

Q: The longer the time, the greater the likelihood of damage to the fetus?

A: That's correct.

Q: The average normal time would be two hours?

A: That's the upper limit of normal.

Q: What would be the average normal time?

A: Oh, an hour plus or minus, and then no primigravid mode.

Q: There seems to be two entries in the hospital record with respect to the period of time of the second stage of labor, but considering full dilatation at 6:00 o'clock and delivery at 10:54, it would be four hours and 54 minutes?

* * *

Q: If there is an arrest of labor, what effect, if any, is there upon the fetus when hypertonic or tetanic contractions occur in tandem with the arrest of labor?

A: Fetal distress, as we've previously defined it, may occur.

Q: And how did we previously define it?

A: As an abnormality of the fetal heart rate and/or evidence of acidosis by the scalp pH sampling.

Q: And with respect to fetal heart rate, again, we don't know what it was during the last 75 minutes?

A: Correct.

Q: With respect to fetal heart rate, back in 1980, were there signs such as ominous signs, threatening signs, suspicious signs of fetal distress?

A: Without using a fetal heart rate monitor?

Q: No, with a fetal heart rate monitor.

A: Yes. One could define certain abnormalities, yes.

Q: Were you able to determine the ischial spine as to whether they were prominent and posterior?

A: No.

Q: Were you able to determine whether or not the sacrum was long and straight or short and concave?

A: No.

Q: Were you able to determine as to whether the side walls were parallel or convergent?

A: No.

Q: Were you able to tell as to whether or not the sacral sciatic notch was wide or narrow?

A: No.

Q: Would I be correct in stating that there are five components of cephalopelvic disproportion, one of which would be size and shape of the bony pelvis? I'll go through the other four in a minute.

A: Size and shape of the bony pelvis may contribute to a disproportion of the fetal head and the pelvis.

Q: So the size of the fetal head would also be important?

A: Correct.

Q: And would the widest diameter of the head be the biparietal diameter?

A: In the presence of flexion.

Q: And in the presence of extension, what would it be?

A: It could be the occipitomental or the occipitobregmatic.

Q: Whether there is extension or flexion, there is no way of knowing if it is a large, normal, or small head?

A: Correct.

Q: The baby weighed what, seven pounds?

A: Correct.

Q: That's a full-sized baby?

A: That's a slightly smaller than average term size.

Q: The more normal the pelvis or the larger the pelvis, the more the head would have to be extended in order to cause a problem during descent, is that not correct?

A: I think that would be a fair assumption.

Q: There are certain things that put a fetus at risk at the time of labor, is that not correct?

A: Correct.

Q: One would be eclampsia?

A: Oh, yes.

Q: One would be hypertension without proteinuria or edema?

A: Very minimally so.

Q: One would be malpresentation?

A: Yes.

Q: Do the records indicate the last time the blood pressure was taken?

A: Prior to deliver?

Q: Yes, sir.

A: The last blood pressure recording that I see in the nurse's record is at 6:00 p.m. on November 7th.

Q: And what was the reading?

A: 150 over 90.

Q: Taking into consideration the hypertension that existed in this particular case, would good nursing practice dictate that each and every time the nurse checks the blood pressure it is to be recorded?

A: That may be over requesting what might go on in a busy service. It would be ideal. I'm not sure if it would be necessary.

Q: In any event, be it ideal or otherwise, good nursing practice would dictate, taking into consideration the facts in this case, that the blood pressure be checked more than just once in the last four hours of labor?

A: Correct.

Q: How often should they have been taken?

A: Oh, perhaps every 15 minutes, every 30 minutes.

Q: When the blood pressure is checked and not recorded, can you tell me how and under what circumstances, without speculation, the doctor is informed of the blood pressure?

A: Verbally.

Q: So that they would have to go to them and tell them each and every time, every 15 minutes, what the blood pressure reading was?

A: Correct.

Q: If I recall, the second stage of labor, as indicated in the hospital record started at 6:00 p.m. and this would have been, as you indicated, the last time the blood pressure was recorded, correct?

A: Correct.

Q: Would it be important for the physician to know the blood pressure reading during the last four hours and 54 minutes?

A: Correct.

Q: Why?

A: Because if the blood pressure increased sharply, the obstetrician may wish to consider treatment with specific drugs.

Q: Such as magnesium sulphate to avoid seizures?

A: Yes, and/or anti-hypertensive medication.

Q: Also, it would assist the physician in evaluating as to whether or not the baby should be delivered by C-section?

A: No, I'm not sure that would enter into the management or decision-making process as to the route of delivery.

Q: At least it would be another source of information for him to digest and make his evaluation of the patient's condition?

A: Correct.

Q: And to determine what care and treatment should be rendered to the patient?

A: Right.

Q: What is meant by fetal well-being studies?

A: Fetal well-being studies include those laboratory evaluations that insure the obstetrician that the fetus is in reasonably good health within the limits of the ability of those studies to provide that information.

Q: Would a patient suffering from preeclampsia be a good candidate for fetal well-being studies in 1980?

A: I think that that would best be answered by saying that fetal well-being studies were frequently utilized.

Q: Were any fetal well-being studies performed in this case?

A: No.

Q: If performed in this case, you do not know what the results would have been.

A: No, I do not.

Q: The delivery of a baby is a very critical period of time?

A: That's correct.

Q: As well as the hour and a half that precedes that time, correct?

A: Correct.

Q: And we do not have fetal heart monitor tapes for that period of time?

A: Correct.

Q: Is a 99.6 temperature considered to be normal during labor?

A: It is reaching the upper limits of normal.

Q: Could exhaustion of the mother, due to the extent and time of labor, be compatible and consistent with an elevated temperature?

A: It would depend upon the degree of hydration the mother had received during labor.

Q: Would you expect to find a certain degree of dehydration, taking into consideration the extent of time of the second stage of labor?

A: It would depend on how much intravenous fluid had been replaced.

Q: In this particular case, are you able to determine how much has been replaced?

A: No, I can't. I would add, though, that it's very common for a patient in labor to have a temperature of 99.6.

Q: But that can also be due to some element of dehydration?

A: It may.

Q: And also this was a 16-year-old girl; you're aware of that fact?

A: I am.

Q: The pelvic structure of a 16-year-old is usually smaller than that of a mature woman?

A: Well, there is clearly an increase in the growth of the pelvis around the time of puberty. However, there is a great deal of controversy as to exactly when and at what age that translates into clinical problems with the progress of labor.

Q: When you say "what age," are you saying, below that particular age, whatever it may be, there might be a problem?

A: That's correct.

Q: Under 14, do you know that it would cause a problem?

A: In most cases it will not necessarily cause a problem, but it might increase one's concern.

Q: And would 16 be a gray area?

A: It would be a gray area depending on the time of puberty.

Q: Do you know what an oxytocin infusion sheet is?

A: Yes, I do.

Q: Did you see an oxytocin infusion sheet in this particular case?

A: No.

Q: What is an oxytocin infusion sheet?

A: An oxytocin infusion sheet is a record which documents the time and quantity of and augmentation or reduction in the administration of oxytocin.

Q: Is uterine hyperstimulation a contraindication to the continued use of oxytocin?

A: Yes.

Q: Again, could you define uterine hyperstimulation?

A: Yes. Uterine hyperstimulation would be the use of oxytocin to the point that uterine contractions are spaced too closely and/or associated with an elevation of the base line intrauterine pressure.

Q: In this particular case, do you know why the pelvimetry was ordered?

A: I can only speculate.

Q: Could you give me your speculative thoughts?

A: Yes. I would guess that x-ray pelvimetry was obtained because the physicians caring for the patient wanted to know what the bony pelvic measurements were. And I would add to that that they wanted to know what those measurements were because they were concerned about the lack of progress.

Q: When did they order the pelvimetry?

A: 8:00 p.m.

Q: When was it performed?

A: At 9:45 p.m.

Q: Under normal procedure, would that be a reasonable and expected period of time between ordering of a pelvimetry and taking of one?

A: That would depend on whether an x-ray technician was present.

Q: And if an x-ray technician was not present, one would have to be called?

A: That's correct.

Q: And are you indicating that if one has to be called, an hour and 45 minutes would not be a protracted period of time?

A: Yes. It depends on how far a technician lives from the hospital.

Q: I'm just talking about what good practice would dictate. If a pelvimetry was called for by reason of the concern a physician might have, would you not say that good medical practice would dictate that there be at least one technician available to take the x-ray within, let's say, a 20-minute period of time?

A: That would be reasonable.

Q: The apparent indication for Pitocin in this case was transverse arrest, correct?

A: Correct.

Q: The Pitocin was administered at what time?

A: It appears to be approximately 7:00 p.m.

Q: 7:00 what?

A: 7:30 p.m.

Q: 7:30 p.m. on 11-6 the fetal heart tones, by auscultation, were 160 at 10:00 p.m. Normal is 120 to 160?

A: That's correct.

Q: Would 160 by auscultation be a high normal?

A: It would be normal.

Q: Are there any inherent built-in errors when it comes to auscultation?

A: Yes.

Q: And what would they be?

A: The fact that the fetal heart rate may vary, frequently around a mean, and so that if one has a heart rate of 140 beats-per-minute that is a real heart rate, and one counts for 15 seconds when it happens to be a little bit more rapid, multiplies by four, that may calculate out to a rate of 160, and the converse may be true as well.

Q: If there is a transverse arrest and the contractions are coming normally within a 10-minute period of time, and they are strong and the duration is normal, what purpose does the Pitocin serve?

A: It serves no purpose.

Q: In other words, isn't it true that one of the contraindications for Pitocin is when there is no purpose for its use?

A: That's correct.

Q: Looking at this record, do you see a purpose for its use? Look at the nurses' records wherein they indicate how often the contractions were coming and the fact that they were strong. Look at 3:35, for example, on 11-7.

A: I see that.

Q: It states, "Every three to five minutes"?

A: "Every three to five minutes."

Q: Look above that at 3:00 o'clock.

A: "Strong every three to five-minute contractions. I.V. infusing slowly." The clinical evaluation of the adequacy of labor can be very variable.

Q: I understand that, but the records do not indicate any?

A: That is correct.

Q: The records do not indicate any reason for the use of the Pitocin?

A: That's correct.

Q: The contractions appear to be coming at a normal rate and intensity?

A: Correct.

Q: Back in 1980, electronic fetal monitoring did not always provide unequivocal information?

A: That's correct.

Q: What is tachycardia?

A: It's rapid heart rate.

Q: Would that be a heart rate above 160?

A: If it's sustained over time, yes.

Q: Back in 1980, was that the definition of tachycardia?

A: A persistent and sustained fetal heart rate of 160.

Q: You have testified that Dr. Hon is an authority in the field of fetal heart monitor?

A: That is right.

Q: Isn't it true that Dr. Hon believes that tachycardia is strictly associated with fetal hypoxia?

A: He has.

Q: You've read Roger Freeman's book, *Fetal Heart Monitoring*?

A: I have.

Q: Isn't it true that Roger Freeman stated that it is difficult at times to determine fetal heart rate patterns?

A: Yes.

Q: Roger Friedman defines fetal tachycardia as a heart rate in excess of 160 beats-per-minute, correct?

A: Correct.

Q: Is it not true that with an external fetal heart monitor tape, what is depicted with respect to baseline variability, is usually greater than what actually exists?

A: That would be a fair statement that the equipment utilized in 1972. Although I would add that one can usually distinguish between what is truely beat-to-beat variability on that equipment and what is extraneous and what isn't.

Q: But if you determine variability to be five beats-per-minute, you must consider the fact that it could be less?

A: That's correct.

Q: Back in 1980, isn't it true that obstetricians practicing in the United States relied upon clinical evaluation and prolongation of the second stage of labor in deciding when to perform a C-section?

A: That's correct.

Q: Isn't it true that in 1980, it was believed that when tachycardia existed, it could be due to acidosis in the cord blood?

A: It was believed that hypoxia may be a cause of the tachycardia, and that may or may not be associated with acidosis of the cord blood.

Q: Was the initial response to hypoxia, tachycardia as opposed to bradycardia?

A: It varies from one fetus to the other. What is ordinarily seen is initially a lengthy acceleration of the fetal heart rate followed by lengthy accelerations in fetal tachycardia.

Q: The last stage would be the loss of beat-to-beat variability?

A: Yes. That doesn't always have to occur in that pattern, but that's frequently observed.

Q: Wasn't it true that by 1980, Dr. Hon had already come out with his writings indicating that tachycardia was a sign of hypoxia?

A: That's correct, but I think that most physicians relied upon the observations of a late uniform fetal heart rate deceleration as being more pathognomonic of hypoxia than tachycardia.

Q: That is when they relied upon the fetal heart monitor as opposed to relying upon clinical evaluations and a prolongation of the second stage, as you mentioned?

A: Correct.

GLOSSARY OF MEDICAL TERMINOLOGY

This glossary defines commonly used medical terms in the field of obstetrics; however, if further assistance is necessary, we recommend *Dorland's Illustrated Medical Dictionary*, 26th edition (W.B. Saunders Company, 1981), and *Taber's Cyclopedic Medical Dictionary)*, 14th edition (F.A. Davis Company, 1981).

Aberrant: wandering or deviating from the usual or normal course.

Abruptio Placenta: premature detachment of a normally implanted placenta; it is a life-threatening condition that is often accompanied by profuse hemorrhage, shock, and a decreased urine output.

Accelerations: a quickening, as of the pulse rate or respiration.

Acetone: liquid found in blood and urine in diabetes, other metabolic disorders, and after lengthy fasting, produced when the fats are not properly oxidized, due to inability to oxidize glucose in the blood.

Achondroplasia: defect in the formation of cartilage at the epiphyses of long bones, producing a form of dwarfism; sometimes seen in rickets.

Acidemia: excessive acidity of the blood, due to an uncompensated reduction in circulating alkaline substances or uncompensated increase in circulating acid substances.

Acidosis: a pathologic condition resulting from accumulation of acid or depletion of the alkaline reserve (bicarbonate content) in the blood and body tissues, and characterized by an increase in hydrogenation concentration (decrease in pH).

Adipose Tissue: connective or areolar tissue containing masses of fat cells.

Albumin: a simple protein normally found in blood, milk and muscle tissues; its presence in the urine is indicative of an abnormal condition somewhere in the body.

Alpha-fetoprotein: a protein found in the amniotic fluid. When this protein is elevated (determined by amniocentesis) early in a gestation, a diagnosis of a neural tube defect (anencephaly, spina bifida, etc.) can be made.

Amenorrhea: absence or suppression of menstruation.

Amniocentesis: procedure to remove amniotic fluid to detect genetic disorders or maternal-fetal blood incompatibility.

Amniography: roentgenography of amniotic sac after injection of a radiopaque substance into the amniotic fluid to diagnose fetal abnormalities.

Amnioscope: optical device for looking inside the amniotic cavity.

Amniotic Fluid: intrauterine fluid in which the fetus is immersed throughout pregnancy; it protects fetus from injury, maintains even temperature, prevents formation of adhesions between the amnion and the skin of the fetus, and prevents conformity of the sac to the fetus.

Amniotic Sac: the "bag of membranes" containing the fetus before delivery.

Amniotomy: surgical rupture of the fetal membranes; done to induce or expedite labor.

Anaerobic: (1) lacking molecular oxygen; (2) growing in the absence of molecular oxygen.

Analgesia: absence of normal sense of pain.

Android: resembling a male, manlike.

Anencephaly: condition in which the fetus has a congenital absence of brain and spinal cord.

Anesthesia: partial or complete loss of sensation with or without loss of consciousness as result of administration of an anesthetic agent, usually by injection or inhalation.

Anoxia: lack of oxygen supply to a tissue despite adequate blood flow to the area; often used interchangeably with the term hypoxia.

Antenatal: occurring before birth.

Antepartum: before onset of labor.

Anteroposterior Diameter: from front to back of the body.

Anthropoid: resembling man; an ape.

Anticholerigic: (1) blocking the passage of impulses through the parasympathetic nerves; (2) an agent that blocks the parasympathetic nerves.

Antimicrobial: (1) killing microorganisms, or suppressing their multiplication or growth; (2) an agent that kills microorganisms or suppresses their multiplication or growth.

Apgar Score: a numerical evaluation of 0-10 given to all infants 1 minute and 5 minutes after birth; the 1-minute score indicates whether the newborn is in need of immediate resuscitation and the 5-minute score correlates with its neurologic status and expected outcome.

Aphasia: absence or impairment of the ability to communicate through speech, writing, or signs, due to dysfunction of brain centers.

Apnea: temporary cessation of breathing.

Arteriography: roentgenography of arteries after injection of a radiopaque dye.

Artificial Insemination: mechanical injection of viable semen into the vagina.

Asphyxia: condition caused by insufficient intake of oxygen.

Aspiration: act of inhaling or sucking fluid or foreign substances into the air passages, as in the condition called aspiration vomitus; removal of abnormal accumulations of foreign substances from a body cavity by suction.

Asymptomatic: without symptoms.

Asphyxia Neonatorum: respiratory failure in the newborn.

Ataxia: failure of muscular coordination; irregularity of muscular action.

Atelectasis: condition in which lungs of a fetus remain unexpanded at birth; may be partial or total.

Athetoid: resembling or affected with athetosis (a condition wherein there are slow, irregular, twisting, snakelike movements seen in the upper extremities, especially in the hands and fingers, and performed involuntarily).

Athetosis: a condition wherein there are slow, irregular, twisting, snakelike movements seen in the upper extremeties, especially in the hands and fingers and performed involuntarily.

Atony: lack of physiologic tone, especially in an organ that contracts.

Atrophy: (1) a wasting away, a diminution in the size of a cell, tissue, organ, or part; (2) to undergo or cause atrophy.

Attitude: a posture or position of the body; the relation of the fetal members to each other in the uterus; the position of the fetus in the uterus.

Axilla: a small pyramidal space between the upper lateral part of the chest and the medial side of the arm, and including, in addition to the armpit, axillary vessels, the brachial plexus of nerves, a large number of lymph nodes, and fat and loose areolar tissue; called also armpit, fossa axillaris, and axillary space.

Axillae: plural of axilla.

Baroreceptors: a sensory nerve ending that is stimulated by changes in pressure, as those in the walls of blood vessels.

Basal Ganglia: ganglion is a general term for a group of nerve cell bodies located outside the central nervous system; occasionally applied to certain nuclear groups within the brain or spinal cord, e.g. basal ganglia.

Bicornate: having two horns or having horn-shaped branches, as the uterus of most mammals.

Bolus: a concentrated amount of medication or fluids given intravenously.

Brachial Plexus: network of lower cervical and upper dorsal spinal nerves supplying the arm, forearm, and hand.

Bracht's Manuever: for breech presentation, the breech is allowed to spontaneously deliver up to the umbilicus. The body and extended legs are held together with both hands maintaining the upward and anterior rotation of the fetal body. When the anterior rotation is nearly complete, the fetal body is held against the mother's sumphysis. Maintenance of this position leads to spontaneous completion of delivery.

Bradycardia: slowness of the heart beat, in the fetus, it means a rate of less than 120 beats-per-minute.

Braxton Hicks Contractions: painless uterine contractions occurring periodically throughout pregnancy, thereby enlarging the uterus to accommodate the growing fetus.

Breech: the nates, or buttocks.

BUN: blood urea nitrogen. A blood test to evaluate kidney function.

Caput Succedaneum: swelling produced on the presenting part of the fetal head during labor.

Carcinoma: a new growth or malignant tumor which occurs in epithelial tissue.

Cardiomegaly: hypertrophy of the heart.

Catheter: flexible, tubular instrument used for withdrawing fluids from or introducing fluids into a cavity of the body; frequently threaded into a patient's bladder in order to remove urine.

Caul: a portion of the amniotic sac which occassionally envelops the child's head at birth.

Central Venous Pressure: the pressure within the superior vena cava; it reflects the pressure under which the blood is returned to the right atrium.

Cephalic: cranial; pertaining to the head.

Cephalopelvic: pertaining to the relationship of the fetal head to the maternal pelvis.

Cerebral Palsy: a persisting qualitative motor disorder appearing before the age of three years due to a nonprogressive damage to the brain.

Cervix: any necklike structure; in obstetrics, it refers to the lower, constricted end ("the neck") of the uterus; it is the connection between the vagina and the uterus.

Cesarean Section: delivery of the fetus by an incision through the abdominal wall and the wall of the uterus.

Chorion: the outermost of the fetal membranes.

Chorionic Plate: in the placenta, that portion of the chorion attached to the uterus.

Clonus: alternating contractions and partial relaxations of a muscle occurring in rapid succession.

Coagulation: the process of clotting.

Coagulopathy: any disorder of blood coagulation.

Computerized Axial Tomography (Cat Scan): tomography where transverse planes of tissue are swept by a pinpoint radiographic beam and a computerized analysis of the variance in absorption produce a precise reconstructed image of that area.

Convulsion: a violent, involuntary contraction or series of contractions of the muscles.

Cor Pulmonale: heart disease due to pulmonary hypertension secondary to disease of the lung, or its blood vessels, with hypertrophy of the right ventricle.

Corticosteroid: any of a number of hormonal steroid substances obtained from the cortex of the adrenal gland.

Couvelaire Uterus: term for a severe uterine condition seen in some cases of separation of the placenta, in which the uterine musculature is disrupted and infiltrated with blood; also called uteroplacental apoplexy.

Cricoid Cartilage: the lowermost cartilage of the larynx.

Crown: when the largest diameter of the head is visibly encircled by the external vaginal opening.

Cyanosis: bluish or purplish discoloration of the skin due to deficient oxygenation of the blood.

Cystocele: hernial protrusion of the urinary bladder through the vaginal wall.

Cytomegalic Inclusion Disease: a disease, especially of the neonatal period, characterized by hepatospenomegaly (see below) microcephaly and mental or motor retardation. (Enlargement of both liver and spleen).

dl: deciliter one tenth of a liter, equal to 6.1028 cubic inches.

Defibrillation: stopping fibrillation of the heart through the use of drugs or by physical means.

Dextrose: a form of the common sugar, glucose; typically administered by intravenous infusion in order to replenish the patient's system with the necessary fluids and nutrients.

Dextrostick: trademark for a reagent strip designed for determination of blood-glucose levels with the use of fingertip venous blood.

Diethylstibestrol (DES):   a synthetic preparation possessing estrogenic properties. It is several times more effective than natural estrogens and may be given orally. It is used therapeutically in the treatment of menopausal disturbances and other disorders due to estrogen deficiencies.

Dilatation: dilation; enlargement of a cavity, canal, or blood vessel.

Diplegia: paralysis affecting like parts on both sides of the body; bilateral paralysis.

Doptone: an electronic device designed to monitor the fetal heart rate.

Down's Syndrome: the preferred term for mongolism; a variety of congenital moderate-to-severe mental retardation.

Dührssen's Incision: incisions made in the cervix uteri to facilitate delivery.

Dystocia: difficult labor.

Eclampsia: onset of convulsions and coma in a patient with preeclampsia, either during pregnancy or immediately after delivery.

Ectopic Pregnancy: development of the fertilized ovum outside of the uterine cavity.

Edema: an abnormal accumulation of serous fluid in tissues or body cavities that may cause visible swelling.

Effacement: the thinning and shortening of the cervix.

Embryo: an organism in the early stages of its development; in humans, this term refers to the stage from conception until the end of the seventh or eighth week of gestation; often called the fetus even at this early stage of development.

Emesis: vomiting; an act of vomiting.

Encephalomalacia: cerebral softening; softening of the brain.

Encephalopathy: any degenerative disease of the brain.

Endogenous: (1) growing from within; (2) developing or originating within the organism, or arising from causes within the organism.

Engagement: entrance of the fetal presenting part into the pelvis, the first stage of its descent through the birth (pelvic) canal.

Episiotomy: surgical incision of the patient's perineum; performed so that the fetus can pass through the vagina without injuring itself or its mother's tissues.

Erb's Palsy: a paralysis of group of muscles of shoulder and upper arm involving cervical roots of 5th and 6th spinal nerves. The arm hangs limp, the hand rotates inward, and normal movements are lost.

Erythroblastosis Fetalis: a hemolytic disease of the newborn characterized by anemia, jaundice, enlargement of the liver and spleen, and generalized edema (hydrops fetalis).

Erthrocyte: a mature red blood cell or corpuscle.

Erthropoietin: a glycoprotein hormone secreted chiefly by the kidney in the adult and by the liver in the fetus, which acts on stem cells of the bone marrow to stimulate red blood cell production.

Estriol: estrogenic hormone considered to be the metabolic product of estrone and estradiol. It is found in the urine of the female.

Estrogen: a hormone secreted by the ovary and the placenta.

Exudate: accumulation of a fluid in a cavity, or matter that penetrates through vessel walls into adjoining tissue, or the passing out as pus or serum.

Falx Cerebri: a fold of the dura mater which lies in the longitudinal fissure and separates the two cerebral hemispheres.

Fetal Hydrops: accumulation of fluid in the entire body of a baby with hemolytic (Rh) disease.

Fetography: roentgenography of the fetus in utero.

Fetoscope: a specially designed stethoscope for listening to the fetal heart beat.

Fibrinogen: a protein present in the blood plasma which through the action of thrombin in the presence of calcium ions is converted into fibrin; this is essential for clotting of blood.

Fibrosis: abnormal formation of fibrous tissue.

Fontanel: the diamond-shaped space between the frontal and two parietal bones in very young infants. This is called the anterior fontanel and is the familiar "soft spot" just above a baby's forehead. A small, triangular one (posterior fontanel) is between the occipital and parietal bones.

Foramen Magnum: opening of the occipital bone through which passes the spinal cord from the brain.

Forceps (Obstetrical): an instrument designed to extract the fetus by the head from the maternal passages without injury to it or to the mother.

Fundus: the upper rounded portion of the uterus between the points of insertion of the fallopian tubes.

Gait: manner or style of walking.

Genitofemoral: genitocrural, or pertaining to the genitalia and the leg.

Gestation: the length of time from conception to birth; synonymous with pregnancy.

Gestational Diabetes: that in which onset or recognition of impaired glucose tolerance occurs during pregnancy.

Glucose: the sugar which is the body's principal source of energy.

gm/dl: gram per deciliter.

Gravida: a woman who is or has been pregnant.

Gynecoid: woman-like, resembling a woman. Gynecoid type of pelvis is the type normally present in females.

Hematocrit: ratio of the volume of just the red blood cells to the volume of whole blood (expressed as a percentage); used to determine the presence of anemia, blood loss, etc.

Hematoma: massive accumulation of blood within a tissue or an organ.

Hemolysis: destruction of red blood cells.

Hemolytic: pertaining to, characterized by, or producing hemolysis.

Hemorrhage: bleeding, especially a profuse blood flow.

Hepatic: pertaining to the liver.

High Forceps: forceps delivery in which the forceps is applied to the head before engagement has taken place.

Homeotherm (or Homoiotherm): an animal which exhibits homoiothermy; a so-called warm-blooded animal.

Hyaline Membrane Disease: a respiratory disease of the newborn infant. It is characterized by dyspnea, expiratory grunt, cyanosis, limpness, and rapid respiration.

Hydatidiform Mole: an abnormal pregnancy resulting from a pathologic ovum (egg cell).

Hydramnios: polyhydramnios; excessive amount of amniotic fluid.

Hydrocephalus: abnormal increase in the amount of cerebrospinal fluid within the cranial cavity, causing enlargement of the skull (especially the forehead) and atophy of the brain.

Hydrops Fetalis: gross edema of the entire body, associated with severe anemia, occurring in erythroblastosis fetalis.

Hyperactivity: abnormally increased activity.

Hyperbilirubinemia: excessive concentrations of bilirubin in the blood, which may lead to jaundice.

Hypercapnia: excess of carbon dioxide in the blood.

Hyperosmolarity: abnormally increased osmolar concentration.

Hypertension: high blood pressure.

Hypertonus: increased tension, as muscular tension in spasm.

Hypertrophy: increase in size of an organ or structure which does not involve tumor formation.

Hypocalcemia: reduction of the blood calcium below normal.

Hypogastric: pertaining to lower middle of the abdomen or hypogastrium, which is the region below the umbilicus or navel, between the right and left inguinal regions.

Hypoglycemia: abnormal decrease in the sugar (glucose) concentration of the blood.

Hypopharynx: region of the pharynx that lies below the upper edge of the epiglottis and opens into the larynx and esophagus.

Hypotension: low blood pressure.

Hypothermia: a low body temperature, as that due to exposure in cold weather or a state of low temperature of the body induced as a means of decreasing metabolism of tissues and thereby the need for oxygen, as used in various surgical procedures.

Hypoventilation: reduced rate and depth of breathing.

Hypoxemia: insufficient oxygenation of the blood.

Hypoxia: reduced oxygen supply to the tissues despite adequate blood flow to the region; one of the components of asphyxia.

Hysterectomy: surgical removal of the uterus.

Icteric: pertaining to or affected with jaundice.

Indwelling Catheter: any catheter which is allowed to remain in place in the bladder.

Interspinous: interspinal; between two spinous processes.

Intrapartum: occurring during childbirth, or during delivery.

Introitus: general term for an entrance into a cavity, canal, or hollow organ.

Intubation: the insertion of a tube into a body canal or hollow organ, as into the trachea or stomach.

Ischemia: deficiency of blood in a part, due to functional constriction or actual obstruction of a blood vessel.

Jaundice: a condition characterized by yellowness of skin and whites of eyes, mucous membranes, and body fluids due to deposition of bile pigment resulting from excess bilirubin in the blood.

Kernicterus: a condition with severe neural symptoms, associated with high levels of bilirubin in the blood. Develops during the second to eighth day of life; prognosis is quite poor if untreated.

Ketoacidosis: acidosis accompanied by the accumulation of ketone bodies (ketosis) in the body tissues and fluids, as in diabetic acidosis.

Kielland's Forceps: obstetrical forceps having no pelvic curve, a marked cephalic curve, and an articulation permitting a gliding movement of one blade over the other, thus allowing the blades to adapt to the sides of the fetal head when the head lies with its long diameter in the transverse diameter of the pelvis.

Klumpke's Paralysis: the lower-arm type of brachial paralysis: atrophic paralysis of the muscles of the arm and hand, from lesion of the eighth cervical and first dorsal nerves. It often occurs in infants delivered by breech extraction.

Labor: process during which the fetus is expelled from the uterus through the vagina to the outside world; also called childbirth, confinement, delivery, and parturition.

Larynx: organ of voice production; located between the pharynx and trachea.

Lasix: trademark for preparations of furosemide (a diuretic in the treatment of disorders in which edema is a symptom and in hypertension).

Lecithin/Sphingomyelin (L/S) Ratio: test of fetal maturity; done to assess the development of the lungs.

Leopold Maneuvers: four maneuvers in palpating the abdomen for ascertaining the position and presentation of the fetus.

Lethargy: a condition of drowsiness or indifference.

Lie: the situation of the long axis of the fetus with respect to that of the mother.

Lightening: the sensation of decreased abdominal distention produced by the descent of the uterus into the pelvic cavity, which occurs from 2 to 3 weeks before the onset of labor.

Lumbosacral: pertaining to the lumbar vertebrae and the sacrum.

Macrosomia: abnormally large body.

Mauriceau Maneuver: a method of delivering the after-coming head in cases of breech presentation.

Meconium: the dark-green or black substance found in the large intestine of the fetus or newly born infant.

Membranes: amniotic membranes; the thin layer enclosing the fetus and the amniotic fluid within the amniotic sac.

Meningocele: hernial protrusion of the meninges through a defect in the skull or vertebral column.

Mentum: the chin.

mg/dl: milligram per deciliter.

mg/kg: milligram per kilogram.

mEq/l: milliequivalents per liter.

Mid-forceps Delivery: the application of forceps when the fetal head is engaged, but the conditions for outlet (low) forceps delivery have not been met; any forceps delivery requiring artificial rotation.

mmHg: millimeters of mercury.

Molding: the shaping of the baby's head so as to adjust itself to the size and shape of the birth canal.

Moro's Reflex: flexion of an infant's thighs and knees, fanning and then clenching of the fingers, with the arms first thrown outward then brought together in an embrace attitude, produced by a sudden stimulus, such as striking the table on either side of the child. It is seen normally in infants up to 3 to 4 months of age.

Morphology: the science of the forms and structure of organisms; the form and structure of a particular organism, organ, or part.

Multigravida: a woman who has been pregnant two or more times.

Multipara: a woman who has borne more than one viable infant or many children.

mU/min: milliunits per minute.

Myocardial: pertaining to the muscular tissue of the heart.

Myomectomy: surgical removal of a myoma (a tumor made up of muscular elements).

Nagele's Rule: a system to estimate the day in the year labor will begin, by counting back exactly 90 days from the day the last menstrual period began and add seven days to that date.

Necrosis: death of areas of tissue or bone surrounded by healthy parts; death in mass as distinguished from necrobiosis, which is a gradual degeneration.

Neonatal: pertaining to the newborn, usually considered the first four weeks of life.

Neonatologist: a physician whose primary concern is in the specialty of neonatology.

Nephrotic Syndrome: a condition characterized by massive edema, heavy proteinuria, hypoalbuminemia, and peculiar susceptibility to intercurrent infections.

Neuron: a nerve cell, the structural and functional unit of the nervous system.

Nonstress Test: measurement of the frequency of fetal movement and the response of the fetal heart rate.

Normotensive: normal blood pressure; a person with normal blood pressure.

Nulligravida: a woman who is not now and has never been pregnant.

Nullipara: a woman who has not yet delivered a viable infant.

Nystagmus: an involuntary rapid movement of the eyeball, which may be horizontal, vertical, rotatory, or mixed, i.e., of two varieties.

Occiput: the back part of the head or skull.

Oligohydramnios: abnormally small amount of amniotic fluid.

Oligomenorrhea: scanty or infrequent menstrual flow.

Oliguria: diminished urine output relative to fluid intake.

Optic Atrophy: atrophy of the optic disk resulting from degeneration of the second cranial (optic) nerve.

Oropharynx: central portion of the pharynx lying between the soft palate and upper portion of the epiglottis (a thin leaf-shaped structure located immediately posterior to the root of the tongue which covers the entrance of the larynx when the individual swallows, thus preventing food or liquids from entering the airway).

Oscilloscope: an instrument for making visible the presence, nature, and form of oscillations or irregularities of an electric current.

Osmolarity: the concentration of osmotically active particles in solution.

Osteogenesis Imperfecta: an inherited condition, usually transmitted as an autosomal dominant trait, in which the bones are abnormally brittle and subject to fractures.

Otoscope: an instrument for inspecting or for auscultating the ear.

Oxytocin: the hormone that stimulates the pregnant uterus to contract at the end of gestation; may be synthetically prepared; such preparations are sometimes given to induce labor or to strengthen ineffective uterine contractions during the intrapartum and/or postpartum periods.

Papanicolaou Smear: a test or study for early detection of cancer cells, especially the cervix and vagina; also called pap smear.

Para: reflects the total number of pregnancies that continued beyond the 20th week of gestation.

Parametrium: loose connective tissue around the uterus.

Parenchyma: the essential parts of an organ which are concerned with its function in contradistinction to its framework.

Parity: the ability of a woman to carry a pregnancy to a point of viability (500 grams birth weight or 20 weeks gestation) regardless of the outcome.

Parturient: a woman in labor.

Perinatal: occurring in the six-week period preceding, during, or after birth.

Perineotomy: surgical incision through the perineum.

Perineum: the area between the vagina and the rectum.

Peritoneal Cavity: region bordered by parietal layer of the peritoneum containing all the abdominal organs exclusive of the kidney.

Periventricular: around a ventricle.

Pharynx: the throat; its lower portion consists of the oropharynx and hypopharynx.

Phonocardiography: mechanical or electronic registration of heart sounds.

Phototherapy: the treatment of disease, e.g., bilirubinemia, by exposure to light, especially by variously concentrated light rays.

Piper Forceps: a special obstetrical forceps for an aftercoming head.

Pitocin: trademark for preparations of oxytocin. See oxytocin.

Placenta: the organ that joins the mother and fetus during pregnancy; its numerous blood vessels supply the fetus with oxygen and essential nutrients and remove its carbon dioxide and nitrogenous waste products; after delivery of the fetus, the expelled placenta (and the umbilical cord attached to it) is called the afterbirth.

Placenta Previa: condition in which the placenta is abnormally implanted in the lower segment of the uterus instead of the upper segment; painless hemorrhage in the third trimester is the most common sign.

Platypellic: having a wide pelvis.

Platypelloid: platypellic; having a wide pelvis, i.e., a pelvis index below 90.

Pleural Effusion: the presence of liquid in the pleural space.

Pneumothorax: an accumulation of air or gas in the pleural space, which may occur spontaneously or as a result of trauma or a pathological process, or be introduced deliberately.

Pneumonitis: inflammation of the lung.

Polycythemia: an excess of red blood cells.

Polycythemia/Hyperviscosity Syndrome: Increased viscosity due to large numbers of red cells, and marked by retarded blood flow, organ congestion, reduced capillary perfusion, and increased cardiac effort.

Polyhydramnios: excess of amniotic fluid.

Position: refers to where the fetus is situated in its mother's pelvis.

Postpartum: occurring after childbirth.

Postprandial: following a meal.

Preeclampsia: a condition characterized by high blood pressure, protein in the urine, edema and sudden, excessive weight gain. If this condition is neglected or not treated properly, the patient may develop true eclampsia.

Prenatal: before birth.

Presenting Part: the first portion of the fetal body to descend through the birth canal.

Primigravida: a woman who is pregnant for the first time.

Primipara: a woman who has carried one pregnancy beyond the 20th week, regardless of fetal outcome.

Progesterone: the pure hormone contained in the corpora lutea whose function is to prepare the endometrium for the reception and development of the fertilized ovum.

Prolapse: the falling down or slipping of a part of the body from its usual position. Prolapse of the umbilical cord—movement of the umbilical cord so that it lies ahead of the presenting part of the fetus instead of behind or alongside it. Prolapse of the uterus—downward displacement of the uterus into the vagina.

Prophylaxis: observance of rules necessary to prevent disease.

Pudendal: relating to the external genitals, especially those of the female.

Puerpera: a woman after labor; one who has just given birth.

Puerperium: the period following delivery until the reproductive organs return to normal prepregnancy size and shape.

Pyelogram: a roentgenogram of the kidney and ureter, especially showing the pelvis of the kidney.

Rectocele: hernial protrusion of part of the rectum into the vagina.

Rh Disease: Rh is chemical symbol for rhodium; a blood incompatibility with all Rh factors lacking.

Rickets: childhood disease resulting from a vitamin D or calcium deficiency; characterized by softening of the bones, with associated skeletal deformities, muscle pain, profuse sweating, enlargement of the liver and spleen, and general tenderness of the body.

Ringer's Solution: a solution resembling the blood in its salt constituents.

Roentgenography: the making of a record (roentgenogram) of internal structures of the body by passage of x-rays through the body to act on specially sensitized film.

Sacrum: the region of the vertebral column that is directly connected with, or forms a part of, the pelvis.

Sagittal: shaped like or resembling an arrow; straight.

Seizure: a sudden attack, usually in reference to convulsions.

Show (Bloody Show): popularly, the blood-tinged mucus discharged from the vagina before or during labor.

Sickle-Cell Trait: a single gene for sickle cell anemia affecting one out of twelve American Blacks.

Speculum: instrument for examination of canals. A vaginal speculum usually has two opposing portions which, after being inserted can be pushed apart, for examining the vagina and cervix.

Spina Bifida: congenital defect in walls of the spinal canal caused by lack of union between the laminae of the vertebrae. Lumbar portion is section chiefly affected.

Station: location of the fetal presenting part in the pelvis; evaluated from +5 to −5 or from +3 to −3.

Sternocleidomastoid Muscle: one of two muscles arising from the sternum and inner part of the clavicle.

Subarachnoid: between the arachnoid membrane and the pia matter.

Subdural: situated between the dura mater and the arachnoid.

Supine: lying with the face upward.

Suprapubic: above the pubic arch.

Symphysis Pubis: the junction of the pubic bones on midline in front; the bony eminence under the pubic hair.

Syntocinon: trademark for a solution of synthetic oxytocin.

Swaddling: restraining an infant by wrapping with strips of cloth to prevent hypothermia.

Tachycardia: abnormal rapidity of heart action, usually defined as a heart rate over 100 beats-per-minute.

Tachypnea: abnormal rapidity of respiration.

Teratogenesis: the development of abnormal structures in an embryo resulting in a severely deformed fetus.

Teratogenic Agent: a drug, chemical, virus, physical agent such as x-rays.

Term: a definite period or specified time of duration, such as the culmination of pregnancy at the end of 9 months.

Tetanic: (1) pertaining to or producing tetanus; (2) any agent producing tetanic spasms.

Thorax: the chest.

Thrombin: an enzyme formed in shed blood from prothrombin which reacts with soluble fibrinogen converting it to fibrin which forms the basis of a blood clot.

Thrombocytopenia: decrease in the number of blood platelets.

Thrombosis: the formation, development or existence of a blood clot or thrombus (blood clot that obstructs a blood vessel or a cavity of the heart) within the vascular system.

Tocodynamometer: an instrument for measuring the expulsive force of the uterine contractions in labor.

Toxemia: (1) the condition resulting from the spread of bacterial products (toxins) by the bloodstream; (2) a condition resulting from metabolic disturbances, e.g., toxemia of pregnancy.

Trachea: windpipe; the air tube that descends from the larynx and branches into the right and left bronchi, which directly feed the lungs.

Transplacental: through the placenta.

Trendelenburg's Position: one in which the patient is supine on the table or bed, the head of which is tilted downward 30 to 40 degrees, and the table or bed angulated beneath the knees.

Trimester: a period of three months.

Ultrasound: the use of high-frequency waves to "visualize" the morphology and physiology of the uterus, placenta, or fetus.

Umbilical Cord: a soft, easily compressible vascular structure that connects the fetus to the placenta.

Uremia: the retention of excessive by-products of protein metabolism in the blood, and the toxic condition produced thereby.

Uteroplacental Insufficiency: pertaining to the uterus and the placenta.

Uterus: the womb; a hollow muscular organ in which the fertilized ovum is normally embedded and developed into the fetus.

Vagal: pertaining to the vagus nerve.

Vagina: the canal in the female, extending from the vulva to the cervix of the uterus.

Vagus Nerve: the pneumogastric or 10th cranial nerve. It is a mixed nerve, having motor and sensory functions and a wider distribution than any of the other cranial nerves.

Vasa Previa: presentation in front of the fetal head during labor, of the blood vessels of the umbilical cord where they enter the placenta.

Venous: of or pertaining to the veins.

Ventilation: oxygenation of blood; can be by mask over mouth and nose or through endotracheal tube.

Vertex: the summit or top of anything. In anatomy, the top or crown of the head.

Viable: a term in medical jurisprudence signifying "able or likely to live"; applied to the condition of the child at birth.

Villous (Villose):   pertaining to or furnished with villi or with fine hairlike extensions.

Viscera: the internal organs of the body.

Vulva: the external part of the vagina.

Womb: the uterus.

TABLE OF CASES

INDEX

HANDLING BIRTH TRAUMA CASES
VOLUME 1

1991 Cumulative Supplement
Current through December 1, 1990

SCOTT M. LEWIS

Member of the Bars
of the States of Ohio
and Texas

and

MARK S. RHODES

Member of the Bars
of the States of Illinois
and New York

*Insert in the pocket
in the back inside cover
of the bound book.
Discard supplement
dated 1990.*

Wiley Law Publications
JOHN WILEY & SONS
New York · Chichester · Brisbane · Toronto · Singapore

ISBN 0-471-54059-5

PREFACE

The 1990 cumulative supplement to **Volume 1** provides greatly expanded discussions of recent case authority. There are significant developments in a variety of areas, including the following:

Wrongful pregnancy–wrongful birth–wrongful life. Discussion of the differences in these torts and their applicability, including relevant statutory authority.

Damages. Statutory authority dealing with caps and limitations on damages recoverable in birth malpractice cases is included, as are provisions relating to the periodic payment of damages. The applicable measure of damages for particular birth-related torts is detailed.

Products liability. Recent developments involving birth injuries sustained due to the use of particular drugs, including DES and Bendectin.

Standard of care. Increased discussion on the standard of care and problems of causation. There is also a discussion of jury instructions on these issues.

Rochester, N.Y.   MARK S. RHODES
February 1991

NEW IN THIS SUPPLEMENT

Note to the Reader: Materials that appear only in this supplement and not in the main volume are listed below. Materials new to *this* supplement are indicated by an asterisk (*) in the left margin in the list and throughout the supplement.

THE MEDICO-LEGAL LIBRARY FROM WILEY LAW PUBLICATIONS

AIDS AND THE LAW
  William H.L. Dornette

EMERGENCY MEDICINE MALPRACTICE
  Scott M. Lewis

HANDLING BIRTH TRAUMA CASES (TWO VOLUMES)
  Stanley S. Schwartz and Norman D. Tucker

OB/GYN MALPRACTICE
  Scott M. Lewis

PLASTIC SURGERY MALPRACTICE AND DAMAGES
  Jeffrey D. Robertson and William T. Keavy

PSYCHIATRIC MALPRACTICE
  Jeffrey D. Robertson

THE RIGHT TO DIE
  Alan Meisel

CHAPTER 2

IDENTIFYING THE DEFENDANTS

§ 2.1 The Complexity of Modern Medical Practice

Page 7, add at the end of the section:

A question may be presented as to the liability of the mother for actions taken prior to the child's birth when the child seeks to sue the mother for her negligence. Such a problem was raised outside the birth trauma situation in the case of *Stallman v. Youngquist,* 125 Ill. 2d 267, 126 Ill. Dec. 60, 531 N.E.2d 355 (1988). The child was injured in an auto accident while in utero. The child sued her mother and the other motorist involved in the accident. The trial court granted summary judgment for the mother. The appellate court reversed. The Illinois Supreme Court held that there is no viable cause of action against a mother for a claim of negligent infliction of prenatal injuries. The court looked to the status of parental immunity in Illinois.

The court cited *Grodin v. Grodin,* 102 Mich. App. 396, 301 N.W.2d 869 (1981), wherein it was held that a child's mother could be held liable for prenatal injuries just as anyone else. The Illinois Supreme Court criticized *Grodin* as missing the issue of family immunity. The *Stallman* court stated (531 N.E.2d at 359):

> A legal right of a fetus to begin life with a sound mind and body assertable against a mother would make a pregnant woman the guarantor of the mind and body of her child at birth. A legal duty to guarantee the mental and physical health of another has never been recognized in the law. Any action which negatively impacted on fetal development would be a breach of the pregnant woman's duty to her developing fetus. Mother and child would be legal adversaries from the moment of conception until birth.

Clearly, this deals with unintentional conduct resulting in injury. The court continued (*id.* at 360):

> It should be a legal fiction to treat the fetus as a separate legal person with rights hostile and assertable against its mother. The relationship between a pregnant woman and her fetus is unlike the relationship between any other plaintiff and defendant. No other plaintiff depends exclusively on any other defendant for everything necessary for life itself. No other defendant must go through the biological changes of the most profound type, possibly at the risk of her own life, in order to bring forth an adversary into the world. It is, after all, the whole life of

1

the pregnant woman which impacts on the development of the fetus. As opposed to the third-party defendant, it is the mother's every waking and sleeping moment which, for better or worse, shapes the prenatal environment which forms the world for the developing fetus. That this is so is not a pregnant woman's fault: it is a fact of life.

§ 2.4 Liability of a Physician for the Acts of an Agent, Employee, or Assistant

Page 13, add at the end of the section:

An interesting situation was presented in *Kavanaugh v. Nussbaum,* 71 N.Y.2d 535, 523 N.E.2d 284, 528 N.Y.S.2d 8 (1988). The trial court denied a motion to set aside a verdict on liability and entered judgment on some damage counts of the complaint. The appellate division modified the judgment and affirmed. The court of appeals affirmed and remitted the action, holding that the defendant obstetrician was not vicariously liable for the negligence of a physician who covered for him on the day prior to the birth. The evidence supported a finding of negligence and causation on the part of both the obstetrician and the emergency room physician. The plaintiff was awarded $1.5 million for pain and suffering and $740,000 for impaired earning capacity, which damages were apportioned between the defendants.

The mother was 44 years old. When she started bleeding, she went to the emergency room. There was a question as to whether the child was injured due to placenta previa which should have been detected at that time. The next day, an internal exam of the mother was performed and, upon the loss of the fetal heartbeat, a cesarean section was performed. The child was in distress, at only 31 weeks' gestation, and weighed only 3 pounds at birth. The Apgar scores of the newborn were 1 at 1 minute, 5 at 5 minutes, and 4 at 10 minutes. The baby was transferred to another hospital with better neonatal facilities, where a tracheotomy was performed, but the child suffered permanent debilitating injuries.

§ 2.5 Liability of Physician for Acts of Employees of a Hospital

Page 16, add at the end of the section:

Often there are numerous professionals working in the delivery room. The question is always presented as to vicarious liability in such situations. The case of *Boyd v. Bulala,* 877 F.2d 1191 (4th Cir. 1989), applying Virginia law, involved a claim for birth defects arising out of the failure to provide adequate medical care during labor and delivery. The trial court entered judgment for the plaintiff. The circuit court affirmed in part and reversed in part, holding that the statutory cap on recoverable damages in malpractice actions (Va. Code Ann. § 8.01-581.15 (1984)) was constitutional. A verdict was entered for the child in the amount of $1.85 million compensatory damages and $1 million punitive damages, for the mother in the amount of $1.575 million compensatory and $1 million punitive, and for the father in the amount of $1.175 million in compensatories. However, the Virginia statutory cap of $750,000 applied per claim exclusive of any punitive damage award. In support of its decision, the court cited *Etheridge v. Medical Center Hospital,* 237 Va. 87, 376 S.E.2d 525 (1989). In *Boyd,* a jury question was presented as to the physician's liability for the negligence of nurses. There was evidence of the physician's control over the delivery room, and the nurses could have been found to have been agents of the physician. Therefore, this was another ground for the liability imposed on the physician. Punitive damages were appropriate because supported by evidence of willful and wanton conduct, in that the physician diagnosed the plaintiff's condition over the telephone. The physician also failed to get the nurse's assessment of the stage of labor. The nurse was ordered not to call him until crowning occurred, which posed risks to the health of the mother and child. There was expert testimony that this violated the applicable standard of care. The physician lowered his standard of care at night so that he could get his rest.

§ 2.6 Partnership Liability

Page 18, add at the end of the section:

Practice Note. Counsel for the physician should make certain his client understands that one of the members of a partnership can bind the other members by his negligent acts. Despite the perfectly valid reasons for forming a business partnership, the vicarious liability of the partners outweighs the financial and other benefits of the partnership structure. The professional corporation is far more prevalent today among obstetricians and gynecologists, pediatricians, and other specialists, because of the insulation from liability provided members of the corporation for the negligence of the other members. Counsel for the plaintiff should fully explore, in interrogatories and depositions, the precise nature of the business organizations of which the defendant physician is a part. If the suit is against only one member of the partnership, the partnership itself may have its own insurance policy, thus increasing the settlement value of the case.

§ 2.7 Professional Corporations

Page 18, add after first full paragraph of section:

The liability of physician shareholders in professional corporations, including situations wherein multiple physicians treat the mother, was discussed in *Footit v. Monsees,* 26 Mass. App. Ct. 173, 525 N.E.2d 423 (1988), a wrongful death action for the death of the mother and the unborn child. The trial court entered judgment on the verdict for the defendant, which judgment was affirmed on appeal. The jury answers, to the effect that neither physician was negligent in the treatment of the mother or unborn child, were dispositive as to the physicians' liability and rendered immaterial confusing answers to other special questions.

The defendants were two board-certified obstetrician-gynecologists who practiced as a professional corporation. The suit claimed that they failed to diagnose the mother's medical condition and failed to perform appropriate tests or refer the patient, who suffered from coronary artery disease, to an internist or cardiologist for treatment.

The mother had regular prenatal examinations. The child was due in April 1983. In late December 1982, the mother had severe nausea and vomiting, but otherwise the pregnancy was normal. In early April, she had difficulty in breathing, severe nausea, and diarrhea. Three days later, she had further difficulty breathing and was examined by the defendant, who listened to the baby's heart and the mother's lungs and performed a pelvic exam, but never listened to the mother's heart. The defendant said that she had flu-like symptoms. Four days later, an exam showed that labor was imminent, but the defendant did not consider performing a cesarean, because the pelvic exam showed favorable for a vaginal delivery. Two days later, the mother was taken to the hospital with severe breathing problems. The fetus died and was removed by cesarean section. The wife encountered severe heart problems and died.

Such facts presented issues for the jury to consider with regard to liability. The jury questions were straightforward and dealt with the liability of each physician. With respect to each physician, the questions were:

Was the defendant Dr. _____, negligent with respect to his duty to [Mrs. Footit]?

Was the negligence, if any, of Dr. _____ the proximate cause of the illness and death of [Mrs. Footit]?

Was the defendant, Dr. _____, negligent with respect to the unborn child of [Mrs. Footit]?

Was the negligence, if any, of Dr. _____ the proximate cause of the death of the unborn child of [Mrs. Footit]?

The jury answered "no" to all questions and judgment was entered on the verdict for the defendants. The court ignored the answers to allegedly confusing special questions.

* *Page 19, add at the end of the section:*

In many cases in which a patient goes to an HMO or to a clinic or practice group, the patient does not necessarily see the same physician on each visit to the clinic. In one such case, the plaintiff brought suit against the physicians arising out of injuries sustained in a debilitating stroke that occurred during a therapeutic abortion required by the administration of Depo-Testadiol. A defendant physician recommended the injection of the hormone after examining the plaintiff and hearing her problems. One month after the injection, the plaintiff went to the same obstetrics group and saw a second doctor, who determined that the plaintiff was pregnant and had conceived about the time of the injection. This, coupled with the fact that the plaintiff had contracted a mild case of chicken pox, posed a risk of birth defects to the unborn fetus. The physician advised the plaintiff to undergo a therapeutic abortion. A third physician performed the abortion and prescribed birth control pills. The last physician failed to notify the plaintiff that the laboratory analysis indicated that the abortion procedure had been unsuccessful. She was again referred to the second physician. By this time she had visited the emergency room and was diagnosed as having a pelvic inflammation. The second physician performed a second abortion procedure on the plaintiff, and that evening she suffered a serious stroke which left her permanently impaired. The trial court entered judgment against the second physician, but granted judgment n.o.v. for the original physician who administered the hormone. The appellate court in *Coleman v. Atlanta Obstetrics & Gynecology Group, P.A.,* 194 Ga. App. 508, 390 S.E.2d 856 (1990), reversed in part and affirmed in part. The court held that the original physician could be held liable for any treatment by the other physicians which was foreseeable from the original negligent act of injecting the hormone without properly testing the plaintiff for pregnancy. The original physician was therefore liable for all resulting damages, including the unskillful performance of the first abortion and the second procedure that led to the stroke.

§ 2.9 Traditional Limitations of Hospital Liability

Page 22, add at the end of the section:

Hospital liability can arise in situations not involving the hospital-patient relationship. In *Jarvis v. Providence Hospital,* 178 Mich. App. 586, 444

N.W.2d 236 (1989), an unusual form of liability was sought to be imposed on the hospital. The father brought suit for the death of his daughter, who died in utero when the mother contracted hepatitis while working in the hospital's laboratory. The trial court entered judgment for the plaintiff. This was affirmed by the appellate court, which held that a wrongful death claim could be maintained even though the fetus was not viable at the time the hospital was negligent, since the fetus was viable at the time it was injured by the hepatitis virus. The cause of action could be brought even though there was no special relationship between the hospital and the fetus. The hospital was aware of the pregnancy and therefore it was under a duty to avoid any unreasonable risk of harm to the fetus. The negligence of the employee mother in delaying the completion and filing of an accident report for two days was not the cause of the injury (the mother cut her finger on a vial containing bilirubin from a hepatitis patient, but immediately cleansed the wound). She was 3-ü months pregnant when she was negligently informed that gamma globulin injections were not necessary. The fetus was not actually injured until it was eight months old. The court discussed viability at 28 weeks and stated that there can be a wrongful death action once the fetus has reached that age.

§ 2.10   Charitable and Sovereign Immunity

Page 23, add at the end of the section:

The doctrine of governmental immunity generally insulates city, county, and state hospitals from liability for negligent injury to a patient. Nevertheless, some states have enacted legislation designed to abrogate in part the broad granting of immunity enjoyed by governmental units. A Texas statute provides an illustration of governmental immunity and the waiver thereof. In 1969 the Texas state legislature enacted the Texas Tort Claims Act, pursuant to which liability was imposed on governmental entities for personal injury or death to patients "caused from some condition or some use of tangible property, real or personal, under circumstances where such unit of government, if a private person, would be held liable to the claimant." Tex. Rev. Civ. Stat. Ann. art. 6252-19, § 2 (Vernon Supp. 1985).

Under the Texas legislation, as interpreted by the Texas Supreme Court, if the plaintiff's injury arises from "some use" of hospital tangible property, the plaintiff does not have to prove that the property was defective or inadequate for the governmental immunity to be waived under the Texas Tort Claims Act. *Salcedo v. El Paso Hospital District,* 659 S.W.2d 30 (Tex. 1983). This interpretation broadens the rights of the patient to bring suit against a government hospital, because most acts of medical negligence involve "some use" or failure to use tangible property, (e.g., fetal heart monitor, Pitocin, X-rays) in the course of treatment or diagnosis.

*   In *Armendarez v. Tarrant County Hospital District*, 781 S.W.2d 301 (Tex. Ct. App. 1989), the plaintiffs sued for injuries sustained by the son during delivery. They alleged that the hospital and the physicians were negligent in using vacuum extraction equipment and proceeding with a vaginal delivery rather than performing a cesarean. The central issue was the application of governmental and official immunity. The trial court granted summary judgment for the defendants. The appellate court reversed, holding that there were questions of material fact which precluded the grant of summary judgment. With respect to the issue of official immunity, the court held that physicians working at government hospitals are not immune to tort liability when their duties are the same as those performed by private physicians in private hospitals. However, there was a factual question as to whether hospital residents were in a special position and were engaged in governmental functions such as might require the extension of immunity to them. With respect to the claims against the hospital district, the court held that Tex. Civ. Prac. & Rem. Code § 101.021 would not serve to extend immunity to claims arising from the negligent use of tangible property. This raised a factual issue as to whether the injuries were sustained due to the negligent use of the vacuum extractor or through other causes.

*   In *Surratt v. Prince George's County*, 320 Md. 439, 578 A.2d 745 (1990), the parents brought wrongful death and survival actions arising out of the death of their child 14 days after his birth. The parents claimed that the child died due to negligent prenatal treatment provided at the county hospital where the child was ultimately born. A health claims arbitration panel rejected the parents' claim. In determining the extent of governmental immunity, the court was required to look to the county's actions. The courts effectively limited the county's liability to $250,000 for each individual per occurrence, but greater recovery could be had to the limit of insurance coverage if in excess of $250,000. The court held that this effectively limited the county's liability to $250,000 or the limit of liability insurance for this claim.

When the patient suffers an injury at a hospital owned and operated by the federal government, the Federal Tort Claims Act governs the rights of the plaintiff to secure relief. 28 U.S.C. § 2674 (1976). Under the act, a patient may recover only if the action giving rise to the injury was the exercise of or failure to exercise a discretionary function or duty. *Id.* § 2680(a). A *discretionary duty* refers to a general or planning kind of function or activity as opposed to an operational activity. *See Wildwood Mink Ranch v. United States*, 218 F. Supp. 67 (D. Minn. 1963). Whether the hospital's actions causing the patient's injury are deemed discretionary or nondiscretionary depends upon whether the injury occurred prior to or subsequent to the patient's admission to the hospital. The admission of a patient is generally viewed as a discretionary function. *See, e.g., Denny v. United States*, 1971 F.2d 365 (5th Cir. 1948), *cert. denied* 337 U.S. 919 (1949). Once the patient has been admitted, however, the discretionary limitations evaporate, and the hospital must treat the patient without negligence. *See* J. Perdue, *The Law of Texas Medical Malpractice* 161 (1985); *Rise v. United States*, 630 F.2d 1068 (5th Cir. 1980); *Hicks v. United States*, 368 F.2d 626 (4th Cir. 1966).

§ 2.11 Modern View of Hospital Liability

Page 24, add before last sentence of section:

In *Parker v. Southwest Louisiana Hospital Association*, 540 So. 2d 1270 (La. Ct. App. 1989), a child was severely brain damaged when one day old due to a cardiac arrest or apneic episode while the child was in the hospital nursery. The trial court entered a verdict for the defendant. The appellate court affirmed, finding that the hospital complied with the requisite standard of care in observing a well baby at 10- to 15-minute intervals when the infant's condition did not require constant supervision. The court also found that the claimed failure of the staff to intubate the baby properly when they attempted resuscitation was not established by the evidence.

The complaint alleged a variety of failures to train and supervise the nursing staff. The complaint specifically alleged that the defendants failed to call for a "Code Blue" immediately when the child was found to be in distress and that the distress would have been discovered earlier had there been sufficient staff monitoring the children. The hospital had a separate nursery intensive care unit for the children whose conditions required constant supervision, but this baby was normal and required no such extraordinary measures.

The case discusses the incidence of sudden infant death syndrome (SIDS), which is 2 in 1,000 babies from 3 weeks to 6 months old. This baby went into arrest within 24 hours of birth; SIDS incidence is approximately 1.5 per 100,000 at that age. Therefore, the occurrence of apnea is very very rare in such a child. The court also recognized that a baby can turn blue within 60 to 90 seconds of when it stops breathing and that the amount of brain damage sustained by such a child is not indicative of the amount of time that the baby was left unobserved.

§ 2.15 Corporate Liability: Staff Privileges

Page 33, add at the end of the section:

In *Purcell v. Zimbelman*, 18 Ariz. App. 75, 520 P.2d 335 (1972), the patient was admitted to the hospital after an osteopathic surgeon found an intestinal obstruction. Dr. Purcell, a general surgeon, was asked to consult on the case. Dr. Purcell's initial diagnosis was either cancer or diverticulitis of the lower intestine. Dr. Purcell performed a sigmoidoscopic examination of the patient and then performed a surgical procedure known as a "pull-through" operation. In this procedure, the surgeon opened the patient's abdomen, removed a piece of bowel, and then took the end of the remaining bowel and pulled it through the peritoneal reflection into the rectum, where he attached it to the anus. All of the bowel and rectum below the proximal end of the resection were thus discarded. As a result of the procedure, the patient sustained a loss of sexual function, loss of a kidney, urinary problems, and a permanent colostomy.

The patient, Zimbelman, filed suit against Dr. Purcell and the hospital, and at trial, the patient's experts testified that the choice of the pull-through operation was below the standard of care of the average surgeon. The pull-through operation, the experts testified, should be performed only when the patient's disease is located below peritoneal reflection and not, as in Zimbelman's case, when the disease is shown to be located above the peritoneal reflection.

Zimbelman's theory was that the hospital had a duty to the public to allow the use of its facilities only by professionally competent physicians and that it breached that duty when it failed to take any action against Dr. Purcell, when it knew or should have known that he lacked the skill to perform bowel surgery. The hospital defended on the basis that Dr. Purcell was an independent contractor and there was no reason to believe he would commit a specific act of malpractice.

At the conclusion of the evidence, the jury returned a verdict on behalf of Zimbelman. The court of appeals affirmed the judgment and held that the patient has established at trial that the standard of care among hospitals was actually to monitor and review the performance of staff doctors and "to restrict or suspend their privileges or require supervision when such doctors have demonstrated an inability to handle a certain type of problem." 520 P.2d at 341.

Practice Note. An evidentiary issue raised on appeal concerned the admission at trial of evidence of four other cases in which Dr. Purcell's patient had filed malpractice suits against him arising out of the same kind of operative procedure (anterior resection) as that performed on Zimbelman. The hospital argued that evidence of these prior acts was inadmissible because the alleged negligent acts in the other cases were not precisely the same as those alleged in Zimbelman's case. The hospital's contention would be meritorious only if the evidence of the prior acts of the physician was admitted for the inference that the doctor was negligent on the date in question. Character evidence of this sort is inadmissible when offered to prove conduct in conformity with character. See Fed. R. Evid. 404(a). However, evidence of specific prior acts is admissible if relevant for some other purpose, for example, to prove plan, intent, or motive. In *Purcell* the evidence was relevant against the hospital on the issue of notice – that is, to show that the hospital knew of past complaints against Dr. Purcell and therefore should have taken action against him. One of the patient's experts testified that a negligence suit is ground for a competent hospital to review the doctor's records and that, when a hospital is joined in a lawsuit, review of the doctor's records is even more of a requirement. The court concluded that "evidence of the filing of the [other] lawsuits was admissible on the question of notice, not only as to the particular type of operation and ailment that was involved but as to the general competency of Dr. Purcell to continue to be a member of the medical staff." *Id.* at 340.

A hospital may be held liable under the theory of corporate responsibility even though it has no actual notice of the physician's incompetence if it fails to act reasonably to acquire existing evidence of the physician's incompetence. In *Gonzales v. Nork,* 20 Cal. 3d 500, 573 P.2d 458, 143 Cal. Rptr. 240 (1978), the hospital had no actual notice that the physician was deficient until some three years after he had operated on the plaintiff. The defendant-physician had performed a number of laminectomies prior to operating on the plaintiff, 38 of which were alleged to have been improperly performed. The court found the hospital liable because it had failed to learn of the defendant physician's background and lack of skill and also because it had failed to implement a system which would have permitted the hospital to learn of the allegations of incompetence and to monitor the information in the records of the doctor's patients.

The court applauded, in dicta, the action of the hospital in promptly restricting the defendant-physician's privileges upon learning of the past complaints against him. The restriction of privileges resulted in the resignation of the doctor from the hospital medical staff. At the same time, however, the court found that the hospital acted too late.

* A plaintiff mother was injured in the course of delivery and sued a hospital and private diagnostic clinic for damages. Two months prior to the delivery, she consulted with the physician at the clinic and received assurances that if in the course of the delivery she required epidural anesthesia, it would be administered by the particular physician or by an anesthesiologist who would insert the catheter. She was admitted to the hospital as a private patient of the clinic and its physicians. She was given an epidural anesthetic block to the epidural space of the spinal cord. The anesthesia was administered by a resident of the hospital. The first attempt to insert the catheter failed and punctured the layers covering the spinal cord, releasing spinal fluid. The second attempt struck a blood vessel. The third attempt was successful. Following the delivery, the plaintiff suffered various problems attributable to the puncture of the spinal cord covering and the loss of fluid. The trial court entered summary judgment for the defendants. That judgment was affirmed by the court in *Labarre v. Duke University,* 99 N.C. App. 563, 393 S.E.2d 321 (1990). The plaintiff's breach of contract claim failed because there was no consideration supporting the promise that the physician or an anesthesiologist would administer the anesthetic. The tort claim of the plaintiff was also rejected because she failed to allege that the resident who administered the anesthetic was negligent in administering the anesthesia. Such being the case, liability for those acts could not be imputed to the hospital.

*   In another case, the plaintiffs sued the hospital for the death of their child two months after birth by cesarean section. They sued the physicians and the hospital. The trial court granted the defendants' motions for summary judgment. The appellate court reversed the summary judgment for the hospital. In *Albain v. Flower Hospital*, 50 Ohio St. 3d 251, 553 N.E.2d 1038 (1990), the Ohio Supreme Court reversed the appellate court's judgment. The plaintiff mother was visiting friends when she started bleeding and was rushed to the hospital. Because her obstetrician did not have staff privileges at that particular hospital, he agreed to have the on-call obstetrician handle the situation. The mother was examined and the on-staff obstetrician was called. The on-staff physician was seeing patients in her office and gave care orders. She told the nurse that she would be at the hospital at 5:30. She went home and was called there and told that she had been expected. She arrived at the hospital at 8:00. She consulted with the plaintiff's obstetrician and transferred the plaintiff to another hospital which had a neonatologist. At 9:30, the plaintiff was examined by her regular obstetrician and the staff obstetrician, who determined that there was a possible abruptio placentae. The baby was delivered by cesarean section two hours later. The infant had suffered from neonatal asphyxia and died two months later. The court held that the hospital could not be held liable under the plaintiff's claims of negligence for the granting of staff privileges. The granting of staff privileges does not impart the necessary level of control over a physician so as to impose liability in respondeat superior. As for the claim that the hospital had a nondelegable duty to assure that physicians with staff privileges performed in a nonnegligent manner, the court rejected such a claim. The court found that hospitals only have a duty to assure that those with staff privileges are competent, and even a competent physician can be negligent in any given case. The hospital did not violate any duty owed to the plaintiff by failing constantly to supervise the actions of those physicians with staff privileges. The court also rejected an attempt to impose liability on theories of agency by estoppel or ostensible agency.

CHAPTER 3

PARTIES PLAINTIFF

§ 3.1 Birth Trauma Plaintiffs

Page 39, add after first full paragraph of section:

Problems arise as to the proper party plaintiff and whether the person can prosecute the claim individually or on behalf of another. In *St. Francis Medical Center v. Superior Court (Patterson)*, 194 Cal. App. 3d 668, 239 Cal. Rptr. 765 (1987), a mother sued for the death of her daughter and for her own economic damages sustained when she was required to take care of her daughter's children (her grandchildren). The daughter died allegedly due to the negligence of the hospital and physicians in connection with the daughter's giving birth. The trial court denied the defendant's demurrer, but the appellate court held that the mother individually could not recover the damages sought. She clearly lacked standing to bring a wrongful death action under the statute, although the daughter's children did have standing to sue the defendants. The plaintiff could not recover, as she could not establish that the defendants breached any duties owed to her. The mother's claim did not fall within any recognized exception which would impose liability for damage suffered by a third party. The court could, therefore, determine that, as a matter of law, no duty was owed to the mother and therefore there could be no recovery. The court also recognized that this type of damage might otherwise be recoverable by the children in a wrongful death action.

* *Page 39, add to footnote 1:*

Hatter v. Landsberg, 259 Pa. Super. 438, 563 A.2d 146 (1989), was a wrongful conception case. The plaintiffs brought suit arising out of a failed tubal ligation procedure. The trial court granted summary judgment for the physician. On appeal, the court affirmed in part and reversed in part. The court was required to consider the following statute (42 Pa. Cons. Stat. § 8305):

(A) Wrongful Birth. – There shall be no cause of action or award of damages on behalf of any person based on a claim that, but for an action or omission of the defendant, a person once conceived would not or should not have been born. Nothing contained in this subsection shall be construed to provide a defense against any proceeding, charging a health care practitioner with intentional misrepresentation . . . , or any other act regulating the professional practices of health care practitioners.

(B) Wrongful Life. – There shall be no cause of action on behalf of any person based on a claim of that person, that, but for an action or omission of the defendant, the person would not have been conceived or once conceived, would or should have been aborted.

563 A.2d at 148. The court interpreted that statute as prohibiting the child's claim for wrongful life, but not the claim of the parents for their out-of-pocket expenses and pain and suffering. The court found that the provisions with regard to "wrongful birth" were ambiguous, and interpreted them as not posing a bar to the parents' wrongful conception claim arising out of the failed sterilization.

* *Page 40, add to footnote 2:*

The plaintiff child was born with profound defects and sought to recover on a claim of wrongful life against the defendants for their failure to inform the mother properly. Such information would have led her to terminate the pregnancy. The mother went to an osteopathic physician for obstetrical care. She contracted rubella during the first trimester. She claimed that the defendants failed to perform the appropriate laboratory tests which would have detected the measles, and further claimed that, upon learning of the risks to the fetus, she would have aborted the pregnancy. The Arizona Supreme Court discussed the various concepts of wrongful conception and wrongful birth claims in order to distinguish them from the wrongful life claim which was involved in this case. The wrongful life claim is one brought by the child against the physician or other health care provider responsible for the birth, in this case, of a profoundly impaired child. In Walker v. Mart, 164 Ariz. 37, 790 P.2d 735 (1990), the court held that the child had no viable wrongful life claim. The court found that, at least under these facts, the physician owed a duty to the mother and not to the child. Therefore, the parents had a wrongful birth claim, but the child had no tort claim against the physician. The court stated that the physician had the duty to inform the parents of the risk to the fetus and he could be held liable if the failure to detect the condition and to warn the mother was a breach of the standard of care.

In Keselman v. Kingsboro Medical Group, 156 A.D.2d 334, 548 N.Y.S.2d 287 (1989), the child was born with omphalecele, and died within a few hours after birth. The plaintiffs claimed that the genetic anomaly resulted in physical pain to the mother and child and emotional distress to the parents. The plaintiffs also claimed that, had they been advised that the child would have been genetically defective, they would have opted for other medical procedures. The court held that the plaintiffs failed to allege a viable cause of action for wrongful life. It found that the plaintiffs were not entitled to recover emotional distress damages because they sustained no independent physical harm. The fact that the mother had moderate bleeding subsequent to the birth was not a sufficient physical injury. The informed consent claims were rejected because they did not arise from a violation of the mother's physical integrity.

§ 3.2 Fetal Injuries

Page 40, add at the end of the section:

In *Singleton v. Ranz,* 534 So. 2d 847 (Fla. Dist. Ct. App. 1988), the plaintiffs brought a malpractice action following the stillbirth of their child. The appellate court reversed the lower court's grant of summary judgment for the defendant, holding that the mother had a valid cause of action for the negligent and/or intentional tortious injury to the fetus who at the time of the negligence qualified as living tissue within her body. The court also found that there was a question of material fact as to the existence of any medical negligence and a causal connection between any such acts and the stillbirth. The court recognized that the Florida Supreme Court has held that an unborn fetus is not a person for the purposes of a wrongful death action.

Elsewhere, in *Abdelaziz v. AMISUB of Florida, Inc. d/b/a Southeastern Medical Center,* 515 So. 2d 269 (Fla. Dist. Ct. App. 1987), the viable fetus was stillborn allegedly due to the negligence of the defendants. The mother was eight months pregnant and in labor. On the way to the hospital she was involved in a car accident. The plaintiffs contended that, due to the negligence of the defendants in their emergency room treatment, the viable fetus died. The trial court entered summary judgment for the defendant while awarding attorney's fees. The appellate court affirmed the summary judgment under the terms of the state wrongful death statute, but reversed the award of fees, as the plaintiffs were destitute. The court held that, under Fla. Stat. Ann. § 768.19 (West 1982), a fetus is not a person for wrongful death purposes. The court further rejected the allegation of negligent infliction of mental distress and an allegation of reckless conduct as failing to state claims cognizable under the statute.

The problem of the proper party plaintiff is often raised in the wrongful death scenario. *Giardina v. Bennett,* 111 N.J. 412, 545 A.2d 139 (1988), was a wrongful death action to recover for the stillbirth of a child. The trial court entered summary judgment for the defendant, which was affirmed by the appellate division. The supreme court affirmed, holding that the physician's negligence in causing the death of the fetus constituted a tort against the parents giving rise only to a standard malpractice claim. The unborn fetus was not a person within the scope of the wrongful death statute (N.J. Stat. Ann. § 2A:31-1 *et seq.* (West 1877)). The fact that some cases have held otherwise, and the legislature did not change the statute in response to those cases, does not constitute legislative approval of the those decisions.

In *Giardina,* the baby's due date was May 19. The mother had been regularly examined and was two weeks overdue at the time. On June 3, a nonstress test was performed which showed no problems. During the next nine days she had pain and contractions and was examined twice. The defendant allegedly refused to perform a cesarean. On June 12, the contractions were three minutes apart and the mother was told to go the hospital. At the hospital, the staff found no fetal heartbeat and the defendant determined that the fetus had died. A drug was administered to induce labor. The court extensively relied on *Berman v. Allen,* 80 N.J. 421, 404 A.2d 8 (1979), but the case was really one for deprivation of the right to terminate a pregnancy with a genetically defective child.

*

§ 3.3   Injuries at or after Birth

Page 41, add before last paragraph of section:

Wrongful death statutes may also affect the nature of the suit, the recoverable damages, and the parties plaintiff. In one such case, an infant died two days after birth. The plaintiff parents brought suit against the physician for wrongful death. The death was allegedly due to the negligence of the physician in the delivery of the child. There was also a claim for the mother's emotional distress. The trial court entered a summary judgment for the physician on the emotional distress claim, but the appellate court reversed. In *Ob-Gyn Associates v. Littleton,* 259 Ga. 663, 386 S.E.2d 146 (1989), the Georgia Supreme Court reversed the appellate decision. The supreme court determined that the mother and the child (even prior to its birth) are two separate persons. Therefore, the negligence directed toward the child did not constitute negligence toward the mother. Hence, the mother was not entitled to recover under the emotional distress claim when she suffered no physical injury. The court recognized the traditional rules applicable to claims for emotional distress. The court also noted that Georgia does not accept the *zone of danger rule,* which would permit recovery for witnessing physical injury to another, such as the infant. With respect to the wrongful death action, the court held that, under Ga. Code §§ 19-7-1, 51-4-1, 51-4-4, there could be a recovery without any deduction for the personal expenses which would have been incurred by the decedent. The wrongful death claim did not include recoveries for emotional distress suffered by the survivors.

In *Bulala v. Boyd,* 239 Va. 218, 389 S.E.2d 670 (1990), suit was brought against an obstetrician arising out of the failure to provide proper medical care during labor and the subsequent delivery. The mother went to the hospital and the nurse called the obstetrician at 4:00 a.m. to tell him of the mother's admission. The obstetrician told the nurse to monitor the plaintiff, and told the staff not to call him until labor reached the "crowning stage." The obstetrician was called again at 7:00 a.m. At 7:45, the staff determined that the fetal heart rate had dropped. Because there had been inadequate monitoring, the condition might have started an hour prior to discovery. The staff then called the obstetrician, who was still at home, and told him. The plaintiff was taken to the delivery room where she gave birth. The defendant arrived after the birth. The child was born with profound defects and lived for about three years. She died after the verdict was rendered in the case, but prior to the entry of judgment. The verdict provided $1.85 million to the child in compensatory damages and $1 million in punitive damages; to the mother, in the amount of $1.575 million in compensatory damages and $1 million in punitives; to the father, in the amount of $1.175 million in compensatory damages and $1.7 million for medical expenses until the child reached age 18. The defendant physician moved the court to reduce the verdicts to the $750,000 cap contained in Va. Code § 8.01-581.15.

The court held that the cap applied separately to the child's and mother's claims. The father's emotional distress claim and the claim for the parent's medical expenses were subject to the child's cap. The court held that the cap applied without regard to the number of legal theories sued upon; rather, the number of caps was determined by the number of patients. The mother was clearly a patient, and the court held that the child was a patient from the point of her birth. Where the caps were both reached by the awards of compensatory damages, there could be no punitive damage recovery. The court also held that the timing of the death of the child did not affect the awards and did not require the court to convert the action to one for wrongful death.

Page 41, add at the end of the section:

During the labor and birth process, the mother may also be injured. One plaintiff mother brought suit arising out of burns received in the course of an elective cesarean section. On the day after the procedure, a burn was discovered on the calf of the mother's right leg. The plaintiff claimed that the burn was caused during the procedure, and it was so severe that numerous skin grafts were required. The plaintiff was entitled to employ the doctrine of res ipsa loquitur in such a situation, and therefore expert testimony was not required. The court in *Dalley v. Utah Valley Regional Medical Center,* 791 P.2d 193 (Utah 1990), held that res ipsa loquitur was applicable and that the doctrine could be used to impose liability on multiple defendants. The plaintiff was not required to establish which defendant was negligent. While the patient was entitled to recover pain and suffering and other standard damages, she was not entitled to recover damages for emotional distress. Such a tort was not applicable under these facts, as emotional distress injuries are generally available only when the plaintiff witnesses the occurrence of the injury. In this case, she did not, because she was under anesthesia.

CHAPTER 4

STANDARD OF CARE

§ 4.1 Standard of Care in Malpractice Cases

Page 45, add before last paragraph of section:

Factual questions are also raised with regard to the standard of care and what actually transpired within the physician-patient relationship. *Baker v. Gordon,* 759 S.W.2d 87 (Mo. Ct. App. 1988), arose out of the alleged negligence of a physician in recommending an abortion. The trial court directed a verdict for the defendant, which was affirmed. Normally, a jury question is presented as to whether the physician actually recommended the abortion, if the accounts of the parties are contradictory. The plaintiff, however, failed to introduce expert testimony or to establish the standard of care required when the patient has an abnormal pap smear while pregnant. The cause of death of the fetus was not an element of such a claim based on the negligent recommendation of an abortion.

The defendant performed a colposcopy on the plaintiff, involving the cervix, but was unable to see lesions. The biopsies showed chronic cervicitis from endocervical scrapings and the canal showed slight dysplasia, which was later classified as mild to moderate. The plaintiff's pap smear showed no severe dysplasia. The plaintiff mother claimed that the defendant told her that an abortion was the best thing to treat her condition. The plaintiff testified that she would not have submitted to an abortion had not the physician recommended it.

A week after the physician received the pathology report, the abortion was performed. The plaintiff claimed that she sustained emotional problems which grew more serious after the birth of a child 14 months later. She claimed that such problems were due to the earlier abortion, but the plaintiff had never been treated by a psychologist or psychiatrist.

§ 4.2 The Measure of Duty – Generally

Page 46, add at the end of the section:

In *Scafidi v. Seiler,* 119 N.J. 93, 574 A.2d 398 (1990), the plaintiff parents brought a wrongful death action for the death of their infant child. They claimed that the defendant failed to treat the mother's early labor properly and arrest it. The child was born prematurely and this resulted in its death. At the time of the birth, the mother was in the seventh month of a difficult

17

pregnancy. On the day before the birth, the mother suffered severe bleeding and the physician prescribed bed rest. Later in the day, the mother spoke to an associate of the physician who prescribed vasodilian. She returned to the physician the next day and was hospitalized with a cervix that was dilated three centimeters. The physician began tocolytic therapy to arrest the labor but the plaintiff later gave birth to a child weighing two pounds, six ounces. The baby died of respiratory failure two days later. The claimed negligence on the part of the physician was the delay in starting tocolytic therapy and the prescription of the vasodilian, which did nothing to prevent the premature birth. The trial court entered judgment on the jury verdict for the defendant. The appellant court reversed and remanded. The Supreme Court of New Jersey modified and affirmed, holding that the trial court should have instructed the jury on the "increased risk" of injury caused by the alleged negligence of the defendant. Any damages which might be awarded should be measured by the loss of the chance for survival which was due to the negligence of the physician. The court also found that the jury should have been instructed that the physician was required to prove the extent to which the mother's preexisting condition of premature labor was responsible for the premature birth. This failure to so instruct was harmless because the court also failed to instruct the jury that the physician could not be held liable for damages caused by the mother's preexisting condition. Such an allocation of responsibility is consistent with the idea of the loss of a chance for the baby's survival, and presents the issue of whether the child would have died from the preexisting condition even if the physician had met the standard of care.

See also Bulger & Rostow, *Medical Professional Liability and the Delivery of Obstetrical Care,* 6 J. Contemp. Health L. & Pol'y 81 (Spring 1990); Gallup, *Can No-Fault Compensation of Impaired Infants Alleviate the Malpractice Crisis in Obstetrics?,* 14 J. Health Pol., Pol'y & L. 691 (Winter 1989); Freeman, *No-Fault Cerebral Palsy Insurance: An Alternative to the Obstetrical Malpractice Lottery,* 14 J. Health Pol., Pol'y & L. 707 (Winter 1989).

* ## § 4.4 – Standard of Care Related to Specialty

Page 49, add to footnote 11:

In many cases in which a patient goes to an HMO or to a clinic or practice group, the patient does not necessarily see the same physician on each visit to the clinic. In one such case, the plaintiff brought suit against the physicians arising out of injuries sustained in a debilitating stroke that occurred during a therapeutic abortion required by the administration of Depo-Testadiol. A defendant physician recommended the injection of the hormone after examining the plaintiff and hearing her problems. One month after the injection, the plaintiff went to the same obstetrics group and saw a second doctor, who determined that the plaintiff was pregnant and had conceived about the time of the injection. This, coupled with the fact that the plaintiff had contracted a mild case of chicken pox, posed a risk of birth defects to the unborn fetus. The physician advised the plaintiff to undergo a therapeutic abortion. A third physician performed the abortion and prescribed birth control pills. The last physician failed to notify the plaintiff that the laboratory analysis indicated that the abortion procedure had been unsuccessful. She was again referred to the second physician. By this time, she had visited the emergency room and was diagnosed as having a pelvic inflammation. The second physician performed a second abortion procedure on the plaintiff, and that evening she suffered a serious stroke that left her permanently impaired. The trial court entered judgment against the second physician, but granted judgment n.o.v. for the original physician who administered the hormone. The appellate court, in Coleman v. Atlanta Obstetrics & Gynecology Group, P.A., 194 Ga. App. 508, 390 S.E.2d 856 (1990), reversed in part and affirmed in part. The court held that the original physician could be held liable for any treatment by the other physicians which was foreseeable from the original negligent act of injecting the hormone without properly testing the plaintiff for pregnancy. The original physician was therefore liable for all resulting damages, including the unskillful performance of the first abortion and the second procedure that led to the stroke.

In another case, the plaintiffs sued the physician and the university hospital for negligence and the intentional infliction of emotional distress arising out of the defendants' failure to test the plaintiff parents for Tay-Sachs disease. The mother consulted with the defendants when she was 37 years old and pregnant with her second child. Due to the increased risk of Down's Syndrome, the plaintiff mother was referred for genetic counseling, during which a family history was taken. The plaintiff mother indicated that none of her family or her husband's family was Jewish. (There is an extremely low incidence of Tay-Sachs disease in non-Jews.) Therefore, the genetic counselor did not recommend genetic testing for that disease, although it was performed for other conditions. At the time of the initial counseling, the physician was aware of a greater risk for Tay-Sachs among a certain group of French Canadians. The child was subsequently born and, one year after birth, was diagnosed as suffering from Tay-Sachs. At that time, the plaintiffs learned that the plaintiff father's maternal grandfather's parents were French Canadian. The trial court granted the defendants' motion for summary judgment. The court, in Munro v. Regents of Univ. of Cal., 215 Cal. App. 3d 977, 263 Cal. Rptr. 879 (1989), affirmed the judgment. The court held that the plaintiffs failed to establish when genetic testing for Tay-Sachs is indicated. This must be done through the use of expert testimony, which requires an evaluation of the standard of care. The defendants presented sufficient evidence to show that the plaintiffs, as per the medical and family history given by the mother, did not meet any of the profiles which would indicate that such testing was appropriate. The court also held that there was no duty on the part of the defendants to inform the plaintiffs of the incidence of the disease in the general population and the nature and cost of the test, when administration of the test was not indicated on the information given.

Elsewhere, various pediatricians and attending physicians, as well as the hospital, were sued for the wrongful death of an infant child. In the trial court, the claims against all the defendants were either dismissed or a judgment entered in their favor pursuant to the jury verdict. The court of appeals, in Boyd v. Hicks, 774 S.W.2d 622 (Tenn. Ct. App. 1989), affirmed, centering its discussion on various jury instructions. Generally, although the court found that the language of the instructions was disfavored, it held that the instructions did not constitute reversible error. The challenged instructions involved the degree of proof, the trial court's definition of "probably true," and the fact that the jury could not presume negligence simply because a poor result was achieved. Another instruction stated that the failure of the physician to act in accord with the standard of practice constituted negligence. Such a statement was proper when the jury was also instructed that no liability could be imposed for a simple error in judgment. The court found that there was no reversible error in the trial court's four charges on the use of the physician's best judgment and the effect of errors in judgment. The degree of proof charge read as follows:

> Now, when I reach the end of that, I, of course, wonder, well, what does the jury think that means. And is there a better way to explain it? I'm not real sure. We deal in probabilities. And we say that to carry the burden of proof, the party having the burden must convince you that the claim is probably true. And there is always the question in the back of my mind, how probably true do you mean? And the only answer that I know of is, probably true enough that you are willing to accept it as being true as would a normal reasonable person. In other words, not that it's 51% true, but probably true enough that you can accept it as being true. Now if half of you believe that a point is true and half of you believe that it is not true, that is not an equipoise, or even balance, in the evidence. That's a hung jury. And you should debate further until you can reach a view that all of you can accept. It is when all of you find that a fact might be true, might even quite well be true, but on the other hand, it might just as well not be true, that's when you have an equipoise of evidence that would require your finding to be against the party having the burden of proving it.

774 S.W.2d at 625.

With regard to the issue of negligence being presumed from the occurrence of poor results, the court charged:

> One of the other rules I should not forget to reflect to you is you can't presume negligence merely from the happening of an unfortunate event. Bad things do happen even to good people. But the question is not whether a bad thing

happened, but whether it was caused by negligence or a failure, in this case, to live up to the standard of care upon which the particular physician should comply with.

774 S.W.2d at 626.

In Young v. Colligan, 560 So. 2d 843 (La. Ct. App. 1990), the plaintiff went to the defendant gynecologist with various symptoms. The physician performed an extensive examination and determined that she had a retroverted uterus. He recommended that she undergo an abdominal hysterectomy. While at the hospital prior to the procedure, the plaintiff informed the physician that it had been eight weeks since her last period. She had previously told the physician that her partner was sterile. When the defendant opened the plaintiff's abdomen, he discovered that she was pregnant and terminated the procedure. The plaintiff then terminated the pregnancy and had a hysterectomy performed by another physician. The plaintiff claimed that the physician was negligent in failing to perform a pregnancy test prior to scheduling the surgery. The medical review panel found that the physician breached the standard of care but that the plaintiff suffered no damage or injury. At trial, the jury answered "no" to the following interrogatory on the verdict form:

> Was Dr. John D. Colligan guilty of professional negligence which was a cause in fact of injuries to Ms. Connie Young, resulting from her being subject to elective surgery when she was pregnant?

560 So. 2d at 845. The appellate court affirmed the lower court judgment for the physician, holding that the verdict was supported by the evidence.

In another case, the plaintiffs sued the hospital for the death of their child two months after birth by cesarean section. They sued the physicians and the hospital. The trial court granted the defendants' motions for summary judgment. The appellate court reversed the summary judgment for the hospital. In Albain v. Flower Hosp., 50 Ohio St. 3d 251, 553 N.E.2d 1038 (1990), the Ohio Supreme Court reversed the appellate court's judgment. The plaintiff mother was visiting friends when she started bleeding, and was rushed to the hospital. Because her obstetrician did not have staff privileges at that particular hospital, he agreed to have the on-call obstetrician handle the situation. The mother was examined and the on-staff obstetrician was called. The on-staff physician was seeing patients in her office and gave care orders. She told the nurse that she would be at the hospital at 5:30. She went home and was called there and told that she had been expected. She arrived at the hospital at 8:00. She consulted with the plaintiff's obstetrician and transferred the plaintiff to another hospital which had a neonatologist. At 9:30, the plaintiff was examined by her regular obstetrician and the staff obstetrician, who determined that there was a possible abruptio placentae. The baby was delivered by cesarean section two hours later. The infant had suffered from neonatal asphyxia and died two months later. The court held that the hospital could not be held liable under the plaintiff's claims of negligence for the granting of staff privileges. The granting of staff privileges does not impart the necessary level of control over the physician so as to impose liability in respondeat superior. The court also rejected the claim that the hospital had a nondelegable duty to assure that physicians with staff privileges performed in a nonnegligent manner. The court found that hospitals only have a duty to assure that those with staff privileges are competent, and even a competent physician can be negligent in any given case. The hospital did not violate any duty owed to the plaintiff by failing constantly to supervise the actions of those physicians with staff privileges. The court further rejected an attempt to impose liability on theories of agency by estoppel or ostensible agency.

§ 4.5 – Standard of Care and the Locality Rule

Page 52, add at the end of the section:

Clearly, the developing trend is to find a broader, national standard of care with regard to treatment provided by specialists. In *Douzart v. Jones,* 528 So. 2d 602 (La. Ct. App. 1988), a child was injured at birth. The parents appealed from a judgment for the physician. The appellate court affirmed, holding that there was insufficient evidence to hold the defendant physician liable for failing to anticipate that there was a probability of shoulder dystocia which might have required the performance of a cesarean. Absent such evidence, the obstetrician could not be held liable for the child's mild Erb's palsy in his arm.

The court rejected the locality rule for establishing the standard of care for the obstetrician specialist and applied a national standard. The plaintiffs, however, failed to prove the essential elements of the case, and the defendant's actions were found to be a reasonable exercise of his professional judgment. The same mother's first child sustained shoulder dystocia, but the progress of the instant labor did not suggest the presence of the problem in this case. Shoulder dystocia occurs when one of the baby's shoulder is trapped behind the mother's pelvis during delivery, after exit of the infant's head. Such a situation often impairs the infant's breathing. In such a case, it is usually necessary to make a maximum incision on the back wall of the vagina to free the infant. The chances of recurring dystocia are extremely rare.

The court also found that the defendant's failure to use a fetal heart monitor was not a breach of the standard of care and, even if it were a breach, it did not have any causal connection to the injury in question.

§ 4.7 – Towards a "Universal" Standard of Care

Page 56, add before first full paragraph:

A universal standard of care most closely comports with the trend toward a national standard of care, which is and should always be used in evaluating the acts or omissions of specialist gynecologists and obstetricians. In *Bradford v. McGee*, 534 So. 2d 1076 (Ala. 1988), an infant allegedly contracted cerebral palsy due to the negligence of the defendant physician and hospital. The jury returned a verdict for the plaintiff in the amount of $950,000. The trial court denied the defendant's motion for j.n.o.v. and granted the motion for a new trial. The Alabama Supreme Court affirmed and remanded, pointing to possible prejudice from juror nonresponsiveness on voir dire with respect to material questions involving brain damage suffered by a relative in another personal injury case.

The applicable standard of care in such a case is established with regard to a national medical community. The plaintiff's expert testimony introduced some evidence that the physician breached the applicable standard of care by failing to conduct fetal testing at 42 weeks. The plaintiff failed to introduce sufficient evidence, however, that the delay in performing a cesarean section caused the cerebral palsy (CP).

The plaintiff presented evidence that the physician's breach of the standard of conduct potentially caused chronic hypoxia resulting in the CP, in relation to a further contention that the child was negligently allowed to remain in the womb for a dangerously protracted period of time. A plaintiff's evidence must have selective application to one theory of causation, proving it to a probability. In this case, the plaintiff introduced sufficient evidence that hypoxia can cause CP and that gestation periods greater that 42 weeks can deprive the fetus of essential oxygen. The case also contains extensive reporting of the expert examination.

§ 4.8 Standard of Care and the Need for Expert Testimony

Page 57, add to footnote 28:

In Montalbano v. North Shore Univ. Hosp., 154 A.D.2d 579, 546 N.Y.S.2d 408 (1989), the plaintiff parents sued the physician and hospital for malpractice arising out of the delivery of their child. The trial court's grant of summary judgment for the physician was reversed. The appellate court held that the physician's bare statements that he complied with the applicable standard of care, and that his actions were not the cause of the infant's injuries, were insufficient support for summary judgment in his favor. These statements were insufficient as a matter of law. The defendant physician also attempted to exculpate himself by claiming that he did not examine the child after the birth. This was also insufficient to support the summary judgment, particularly since the parents alleged that the failure to examine the infant constituted additional malpractice.

§ 4.9 Standard of Care Experts – The School of Practice

Page 59, add at the end of the section:

Even though, in prior sections, it has been stated that the trend is toward a national standard of care, such a standard is only applicable as respects practitioners of the same specialty. We have noted in this section of the main text that different standards may be applicable to different "schools of practice." It is also to be noted that there can be different schools of thought among obstetricians and gynecologists as to the preferred treatment of a particular condition. In such a situation, the physician is generally exonerated if he or she follows an accepted course of treatment, even if that course is accepted only by a respected minority of the profession.

For example, in *D'Angelis v. Zakuto,* 383 Pa. Super. 65, 556 A.2d 431 (1989), an infant died from undiagnosed pneumonia and the treating physician was sued. Judgment was entered for the defendant, but was reversed on appeal because the trial court improperly gave an instruction on the "two schools of thought" doctrine, which was reversible error.

There had been medical evidence for and against the physician's decision not to use x-ray testing on a child who had been febrile for several days, coughing up mucus, and had swollen glands and diarrhea. The instruction in question (556 A.2d at 433) provided:

> A physician may rightfully choose to practice his profession in accordance with a school of thought which differs in its concepts and procedures from another school of thought. Even though the school that he follows is a minority one, he will not be deemed to be negligent or practicing improperly so long as it is reputable and respected by reasonable medical experts.

§ 4.15 Standard of Care – Special Circumstances

Page 65, add at the end of the section:

The plaintiff went to the defendant physician complaining of urinary incontinence. The physician diagnosed the presence of a rectocele, a cystocele, stress incontinence, and a prolapsed uterus. He recommended repair of the conditions and a vaginal hysterectomy. The plaintiff consented to these procedures. During the procedure, the physician lacerated the plaintiff's bladder and stitched it up. He advised the patient of the laceration and its repair after the operation. The plaintiff returned to the hospital in four days in severe pain, and it was determined that the bladder, fallopian tube, and sigmoid colon were adhering; suture material was found at the adhesion. The trial court entered judgment for the defendant on the jury verdict. The court, in *Russell v. Kanaga,* 571 A.2d 724 (Del. 1990), held that there was no malpractice in the repair surgery, particularly where the plaintiff's experts gave the opinion that it was not malpractice to cause the adhesions and there was no evidence that the physician sutured the bladder to the colon during the repair of the laceration. The trial court refused to admit the medical malpractice review panel's written report. Such a ruling was harmless error when the report supported the defendant's position.

§ 4.16   – Obvious Acts of Negligence

Page 66, add after second paragraph:

Generally, counsel should not assume that the negligence is so obvious that expert testimony will not be required. The case of *Boyd v. Bulala,* 877 F.2d 1191 (4th Cir. 1989), applying Virginia law, was a claim for birth defects arising out of the failure to provide adequate medical care during labor and delivery. The trial court entered judgement for the plaintiff. The circuit court affirmed in part and reversed in part, holding that the statutory cap on recoverable damages in malpractice actions (Va. Code Ann. § 8.01-581.15 (1984)) was constitutional. A verdict was entered for the child in the amount of $1.85 million compensatory damages and $1 million punitive damages, for the mother in the amount of $1.575 million compensatory and $1 million punitive, and for the father in the amount of $1.175 million compensatory.

A jury question was presented as to the physician's liability for the negligence of nurses. There was evidence of the physician's control over the delivery room, and the nurses could have been found to have been agents of the physician. Therefore, this was another ground for the liability imposed on the physician.

Punitive damages were appropriate because they were supported by evidence of willful and wanton conduct, in that the physician diagnosed the plaintiff's condition over the telephone. The physician also failed to get the nurse's assessment of the stage of labor. The nurse was ordered not to call him until crowning occurred, which posed risks to the health of both the mother and child. There was expert testimony that this violated the applicable standard of care. The physician lowered his standard of care at night so that he could get his rest. Even in such a case, involving blatant disregard for the applicable standard of care, expert testimony was effectively used.

*

§ 4.17 – Res Ipsa Loquitur

Page 68, add to footnote 53:

During the labor and birth process, the mother may also be injured. One plaintiff mother brought suit arising out of burns received in the course of an elective cesarean section. On the day after the procedure, a burn was discovered on the calf of the plaintiff's right leg. The plaintiff claimed that the burn was caused during the procedure, and it was so severe that numerous skin grafts were required. The plaintiff was entitled to employ the doctrine of res ipsa loquitur in such a situation, and therefore expert testimony was not required. The court, in Dalley v. Utah Valley Regional Medical Center, 791 P.2d 193 (Utah 1990), held that res ipsa loquitur was applicable and that the doctrine could be used to impose liability on multiple defendants. The plaintiff was not required to establish which defendant was negligent. While the patient was entitled to recover pain and suffering and other standard damages, she was not entitled to recover damages for emotional distress. Such a tort theory was not applicable under these facts, because emotional distress injuries are generally available only when the plaintiff witnesses the occurrence of the injury. In this case, she did not; she was under anesthesia.

*

§ 4.18 Standard of Care of
Hospitals – Generally

Page 69, add to footnote 55:

The patient was terminally ill with cancer and was pregnant. At the time, she was over 26 weeks pregnant and the fetus was viable. The hospital sought a court order to permit it to perform a cesarean. The court ordered the cesarean and the patient's attempt to stay the order was denied. The cesarean was performed but the child died within two and one-half hours. The mother died two days later. The court in the case of *In re* A.C., 573 A.2d 1235 (D.C. 1990), vacated the prior judgment. The court held that, under the facts of the case, the decision of what action should have been taken was up to the patient, who was competent to give informed consent. The court decided these issues despite the fact that they were moot, since the court recognized that this problem would probably be faced in other cases. The court found that it was error for the trial court to order the procedure without obtaining the consent of the patient if she were competent or without proceeding via substituted judgment and the appointment of a guardian or similar procedure.

Elsewhere, a baby was born at an Indian Health Service hospital. The plaintiffs claimed that the baby was injured due to the failure of the hospital to treat the mother's hypertension and preeclampsia. It was alleged that these conditions resulted in oxygen deprivation to the fetus, thereby causing profound brain damage. The issue was raised as to the ability of the hospital to provide the mother and infant with proper care. The hospital was classified as a "level one" birth center; level one is the lowest level of care available and means that the hospital is equipped to handle only low-risk births. The protocols of the Indian Health Service require that, when it is determined that more intensive medical care is required, the patient should be taken to a hospital that can provide such care. This was the crux of the case. The court held that the plaintiff could recover only if she could establish that she had the warning signs of hypertension and preeclampsia and that the hospital failed to recognize these signs and act pursuant to its protocols. Additionally, it would be necessary to establish that the violation of the protocols was the cause of the child's brain damage. The court detailed the facts of the pregnancy and the treatment plus the lack of facilities at the Indian Health Service hospital in question. The court held that the hospital was negligent in failing properly to monitor and treat the mother, and that that negligence was the cause of the injuries sustained by the child. The plaintiffs were awarded $2.5 million for the cost of caring for the child, $760,000 for lost earning capacity, and $160,000 for medical expenses already incurred. The court further awarded the grandmother the sum of $525,000 for the loss of consortium with her grandchild. The mother, on the other hand, was not entitled to any such award, since she had effectively abandoned the child, leaving it with the grandmother. Anderson v. United States, 731 F. Supp. 391 (D.N.D. 1990).

In another case, the plaintiff parents alleged that their child was injured during birth. The child allegedly was in fetal distress prior to the delivery, and this resulted in oxygen deprivation and brain damage. The plaintiffs claimed that the defendants failed to conduct adequate fetal heart monitoring which could have prevented the injuries complained of. The court, in Gillis v. United States, 722 F. Supp. 713 (M.D. Fla. 1989), dismissed the case. The court recognized that the hospital had a duty to monitor the fetal heart rate. The mother had had an enema and was in the bathroom for a considerable period following her admission to the hospital. Upon admission, it was determined that the fetus was in stable condition. Subsequently, when the monitor was applied following the enema, the fetus was found to be experiencing late deceleration, and action was immediately taken. The question was presented as to whether the 50-minute delay in using the monitor after the initial examination constituted a breach of the duty of care. The court found that the standard of care required monitoring at least every 30 minutes. However, the bulk of the 50-minute period was taken up by the enema, during which time there could be no monitoring. The court found that there was no breach of duty; even if there was such a breach, it was not the cause of the oxygen deprivation which resulted in the injuries complained of.

In another case, the plaintiffs sued the family physician and the hospital's high-risk team for negligence in the care of their newborn, which resulted in severe neurological deficits. The defendants claimed that the deficits were due to a pre-birth brain malformation and accompanying birth defects. The birth was difficult, and shortly thereafter the child showed the characteristics of hypotonia and other symptoms of perinatal asphyxia. The child was born with club feet and dysmorphic physical features. The baby also suffered from hypoglycemia. The trial court entered judgment on the jury verdict (10-2) for the defendants. The court of appeals, in Richards v. Overlake Hosp. Medical Center, 59 Wash. App. 266, 796 P.2d 737 (1990), affirmed. The court held that the trial court committed harmless error in instructing the jury that the family physician was to be judged by the standard of a reasonably prudent family physician. The court properly rejected a plaintiffs' instruction seeking to base the standard of care on the expectations of society or of the patient. The court recognized that the jury found that the cause of the injuries was a prenatal event and not the care given after birth. An issue as to juror misconduct was also presented. One juror with a medical background reviewed the medical records which had been introduced into evidence, and came to the conclusion that the defects were due to the mother's contracting influenza 20 weeks into the pregnancy. This opinion was shared with other jurors. The court upheld the trial court's finding that this was not juror misconduct requiring a new trial.

The particular instructions given by the trial court were as follows:

> A physician who is a family practitioner has a duty to exercise the degree of skill, care and learning of a reasonably prudent family practitioner in the State of Washington acting in the same or similar circumstances at the time of the care or treatment in question. Failure to exercise such skill, care and learning is negligence.
>
> If a family practitioner holds himself out as qualified to provide pediatric care, or assumes the care or treatment of a condition which is ordinarily treated by a pediatrician, he has a duty to possess and exercise the degree of skill, care and learning of a reasonably prudent family practitioner in the State of Washington acting in the same or similar circumstances at the time of the care and treatment in question. Failure to exercise such skill, care and learning is negligence.
>
> The degree of care actually practiced by members of the medical profession is some evidence of what is reasonably prudent – it is not dispositive.
>
> The evidence must rise to the degree of proof that any injury plaintiffs claim occurred to Michelle Richards probably would not have occurred but for defendants' conduct, to establish a causal relationship.

796 P.2d at 740.

In Bulala v. Boyd, 239 Va. 218, 389 S.E.2d 670 (1990), suit was brought against an obstetrician arising out of the failure to provide proper medical care during labor and the subsequent delivery. The mother went to the hospital, and the nurse called the obstetrician at 4:00 a.m. to tell him of the mother's admission. The obstetrician told the nurse to monitor the plaintiff, and told the staff not to call him until labor reached the "crowning stage." The obstetrician was called again at 7:00. At 7:45, the staff determined that the fetal heart rate had dropped. Because there had been inadequate monitoring, the condition might have started an hour prior to discovery. The staff then called the obstetrician, who was still at home, and told him. The plaintiff was taken to the delivery room where she gave birth. The defendant arrived after the birth. The child was born with profound defects and lived for about three years. She died after the verdict was rendered in the case but prior to the entry of judgment. Substantial verdicts were returned by the jury. These verdicts were ultimately reduced on appeal through the application of the statutory cap on damages contained in Va. Code § 8.01-581.15.

§ 4.20 – Rules and Regulations

Page 73, add to footnote 71:

See also Bell v. Maricopa Medical Center, 157 Ariz. 192, 755 P.2d 1180 (Ct. App. 1988). This case involved the propriety of the court's refusal to give a jury instruction that if the jury found that the hospital broke its protocols, such a breach constituted negligence. The mother was having premature labor contractions while approximately 25 weeks pregnant. At the hospital she was given terbutaline to stop the contractions. The contractions stopped and she was released. She later experienced another bout of premature contractions and was treated with morphine sulfate. She was sent home, had strong contractions on the same day, and was again given terbutaline. The treating physician decided to deliver early, as there was a life-treatening infection in the amniotic sac. Excessive oxygen administered to the premature infant resulted in retrolental fibroplasia.

Such a course of treatment was contrary to established hospital protocols. In a malpractice case, the plaintiff must establish the standard of care, its breach, and causation, generally through expert testimony. The proffered instruction was an innocent statement of the law, as the jury could find that the violation of the protocol was evidence of negligence only after receiving proof that the protocol embodied the applicable standard with which the hospital should have compiled.

* *Page 73, add to footnote 73:*

The plaintiff adolescent sued a hospital which sent her to another hospital 200 miles away, while she was in labor, because she was indigent. The suit was brought pursuant to the Anti-Dumping Act, 42 U.S.C. § 1395dd. The plaintiff had been admitted, taken to a delivery room, and examined by a physician who was under contract with the hospital to provide obstetric care to indigent women. The physician, however, discharged the plaintiff, telling her to go to the distant hospital. That evening, the plaintiff obtained a temporary restraining order (TRO) against the hospital requiring them to admit the plaintiff. Four days later, after the issuance of the TRO, the plaintiff was admitted to the hospital, where the baby was delivered. The court, in Owens v. Nacogdoches County Hosp. Dist., 741 F. Supp. 1269 (E.D. Tex. 1990), held that the defendant hospital violated the Anti-Dumping Act and that the plaintiff had standing to obtain permanent injunctive relief. The court rejected the defendant hospital's claim that the transfer was required because the transferee had a neonatal unit which would be required.

In another case, the plaintiffs brought a wrongful death action for the death of their 16-week-old infant. The parents sued the physician who examined the infant in the emergency room. After that examination, the parents took the infant to another hospital, where the infant died. The plaintiffs also brought a claim under the Anti-Dumping Act (42 U.S.C. § 1395dd). The court, in Nichols v. Estabrook, 741 F. Supp. 325 (D.N.H. 1989), granted the defendant's motion to dismiss in part and for partial summary judgment. The court noted that the parents could not recover for their own emotional distress, under the terms of New Hampshire law. Further, there could be no recovery for the loss of the child's services and society. Under the wrongful death statute, the only recovery could be for pecuniary loss. Therefore, there could be no recovery for damages such as those for the loss of enjoyment of continued life. The court held that, under state law, no damages were recoverable for the death of the infant, and rejected claims for even nominal damages.

CHAPTER 5

PROXIMATE CAUSE IN MALPRACTICE

§ 5.1 The Need for an Expert Witness

* *Page 76, add to footnote 2:*

The plaintiff went to the defendant physician complaining of urinary incontinence. The physician diagnosed the presence of a rectocele, a cystocele, stress incontinence, and a prolapsed uterus. He recommended repair of the conditions and a vaginal hysterectomy, and the plaintiff consented to these procedures. During the procedure, the physician lacerated the plaintiff's bladder and stitched it up. He advised the patient of the laceration and its repair after the operation. The plaintiff returned to the hospital in four days in severe pain, and it was determined that the bladder, fallopian tube, and sigmoid colon were adhering; suture material was found at the adhesion. The trial court entered judgment for the defendant on the jury verdict. The court, in Russell v. Kanaga, 571 A.2d 724 (Del. 1990), held that there was no malpractice in the repair surgery, particularly where the plaintiff's experts gave the opinion that it was not malpractice to cause the adhesions and there was no evidence that the physician sutured the bladder to the colon during the repair of the laceration. The trial court refused to admit the medical malpractice review panel's written report. Such a ruling was harmless error when the report supported the defendant's position.

Elsewhere, the plaintiffs (child and parents) sued an obstetrician for injuries sustained by the child during delivery (brachial plexus palsy). The defendant physician's expert witness admitted that the injuries were caused by the defendant's acts during the delivery. The physician attempted to turn the baby's head to rotate the shoulders after discovering shoulder dystocia. The issue was whether the application of pressure to the head constituted a breach of the duty of care. The appellate court upheld the trial court's judgment for the physician on the jury verdict. The court found that the evidence supported the verdict. Dunne v. Somoano, 550 So. 2d 5 (Fla. Dist. Ct. App. 1989).

A plaintiff was allegedly injured during the course of an abortion. She sued the clinic. The trial court granted the clinic's summary judgment motion. This was affirmed on appeal by the court in Sorina v. Armstrong, 51 Ohio App. 3d 113, 554 N.E.2d 943 (1988). The court held that the patient's failure to follow the advice of the clinic, that she should go to her personal physician or to the clinic for a follow-up examination, was the cause of her injuries. The plaintiff's disregard for her own health was the cause of the injuries complained of. The defendant called the plaintiff several times to attempt to follow up, but the plaintiff never went for an examination. She cancelled an appointment and then stated that she was feeling better. Her failure to follow up resulted in complications remaining untreated, and ultimately a complete hysterectomy was required.

Page 77, add to footnote 7:

In Scafidi v. Seiler, 225 N.J. Super. 576, 543 A.2d 95 (App. Div. 1988), the plaintiffs claimed that the negligence of the defendant physician resulted in the premature birth and subsequent death of their baby. The complaint sought recovery of wrongful death damages for the injuries sustained during the life of the child. The jury found that the physician was negligent in treating the infant and mother, but that any such negligence was not the cause of the injuries and death. The appellate court reversed and remanded for a new trial, holding that a jury question was presented as to whether the risk of premature birth was increased by the defendant's negligence and whether this was a substantial factor in producing the death. The court recognized that, in such cases, the plaintiff has the burden of proving the standard of care, its breach, and causation. An increased risk of harm can satisfy the causation requirement. In *Scafidi*, mother was seven months pregnant when she visited the obstetrician because of heavy bleeding. The obstetrician told her to rest. The next day, the mother had cramping, but the obstetrician was unavailable. A covering physician prescribed medicine and told to keep her appointment with the obstetrician on the next day. The medicine, taken orally, is ineffective to arrest premature labor. The next day, the defendant obstetrician tried to arrest the labor, but used unacceptable therapy with the same drug. There was a deviation from the proper standard of care in not immediately hospitalizing the mother. The case was remanded for proof of damages.

In Blood v. Lea, 403 Mass. 430, 530 N.E.2d 344 (1988), the parents brought a malpractice action against the physician and hospital arising out of the care of the mother before, during, and after delivery. The medical review panel found that there was insufficient evidence to raise a question of liability. The trial court agreed and entered judgment against the plaintiff. The Supreme Judicial Court of Massachusetts vacated the judgment, finding that there was sufficient evidence to raise a question suitable for judicial resolution. The fact that the medical opinion obtained by the parents used the word "probably" did not mean that there would be insufficient proof of causation. The opinion letter was from an obstetrician-gynecologist and outlined the requirements of proper medical care for pregnancy-induced hypertension and intrauterine growth retardation. The expert stated that "delay in rescuing the fetus from its dangerous predicament probably contributed to the damage to this baby's brain." The plaintiff introduced this evidence in an offer of proof that included the physician's office records, a discharge summary, the labor and delivery summary, the labor progress sheet from the defendant hospital, and two opinion letters from physicians.

* *Page 77, add to footnote 8:*

Nickerson v. G.D. Searle & Co., 900 F.2d 412 (1st Cir. 1990) (applying Massachusetts law), was an IUD products liability claim. The plaintiff alleged that she was rendered infertile by use of an IUD. The appellate court affirmed the trial court judgment for the defendant IUD manufacturer. The court found that there was sufficient evidence to support a lower court finding that the cause of the infertility was a sexually transmitted disease. Although that portion of the decision is straightforward, the court held that the plaintiff was not entitled to a new trial on the basis of subsequently discovered evidence. The plaintiff later found a trial transcript from another case in which the manufacturer had disclosed the rate of infection attendant to the use of the IUD. No new trial was warranted, as such evidence is admissible only for impeachment purposes. The court also found that there was no error in failing to tell the jury that defense counsel had agreed that pelvic inflammatory disease was also a cause of infertility, despite the fact that such an admission was relevant to the sufficiency of the manufacturer's product warning.

In a Bendectin case, the plaintiff children, who were exposed to the drug in utero, sued the manufacturer of the drug on claims arising out of their birth defects (limb reductions). The court, in Daubert v. Merrell Dow Pharmaceuticals, Inc., 727 F. Supp. 570 (S.D. Cal. 1989), granted the manufacturer's motion for summary judgment. The court held that the plaintiffs failed to provide any evidence of a causal connection between the injuries suffered and use of the drug by their mothers. The plaintiffs had introduced expert testimony in support of their claims. The court rejected that testimony on the basis that the conclusions were based on in vitro, chemical, and animal studies. The court found that the testimony was insufficient, as experts in the field would have relied upon human epidemiological studies. The court also rejected the authority of an unpublished study which failed to conduct its own research but only reinterpreted prior studies. The court reviewed Federal Rule of Evidence 703 and found that the plaintiff's expert testimony failed to establish that the opinion was based on methodology usually relied upon by experts in the field. The court bolstered its decision by citing numerous other Bendectin cases which also held that there was a lack of sufficient scientific proof of causation. For a discussion of similar issues, *see* Cadarian v. Merrell Dow Pharmaceuticals, Inc., 745 F. Supp. 409 (E.D. Mich. 1989).

In another Bendectin case, a child was born with one finger missing on each hand. The court, in Wilson v. Merrell Dow Pharmaceuticals, Inc., 893 F.2d 1149 (10th Cir. 1990), applying Oklahoma law, affirmed the judgment on the jury verdict for the defendant drug company. The issue was whether the trial court should have given a missing-witness instruction where the manufacturer failed to call a geneticist to testify on causation. The appellate court held that the lower court properly exercised its discretion, as such testimony would have been cumulative. The trial court also properly permitted the use of sales charts which had graphs dealing with the frequency of birth defects in the general population as compared with sales of the drug, since this was a basis for the witness's expert opinion. Any defects in the charts were directed to the weight of such evidence and not its admissibility. The appellate court recognized the vast amount of scientific data which failed to establish a causal connection between the use of the drug and the occurrence of birth defects.

In Bernhardt v. Richardson-Merrell, Inc., 892 F.2d 440 (5th Cir. 1990) (applying Mississippi law), suit was brought for injuries sustained by a child as a result of in utero exposure to Bendectin taken by the mother during pregnancy. The child was born without fingers on one hand. In this case, the mother did not take the drug until the 54th or 55th day of her pregnancy. Medical evidence was introduced to the effect that fingers are found on the human fetus by the 44th day after conception. Therefore, fingers should have been present prior to the mother's use of the drug. Clearly, this destroyed the attempt to establish the required element of causation. The plaintiffs had submitted certified interrogatory answers, but these did not qualify as expert affidavits, which would have been required to counter the defendant's expert evidence. The answers to the interrogatories were, at best, only hearsay references to expert opinions. Such being the case, this court affirmed the trial court's grant of summary judgment for the defendant.

Elsewhere, the plaintiffs brought suit arising out of the death of a fetus in utero. The plaintiff mother was under the care of the defendants, and claimed that the defendant clinic failed promptly and properly to notify the obstetrician that fetal distress was occurring. The court granted the defendants' motion for summary judgment, holding that there was no evidence that any delay in alerting the physician to the loss of fetal heart tones was the cause of the fetus's death. There was evidence that the child was brain dead within a few minutes of the loss of heart tone, and substantially before a cesarean section could have been performed. Switzer v. Newton Health Care Corp., 734 F. Supp. 954 (D. Kan. 1990).

§ 5.2 Proximate Cause and Statistical Evidence

Page 79, add at the end of the section:

Clearly, birth defects can be due to natural occurrences, unrelated to the medical treatment. The probability of such a cause must be determined by expert testimony in order properly to assess fault arising out of the treatment. In *Willey v. Ketterer,* 869 F.2d 648 (1st Cir. 1989), applying New Hampshire law, suit was brought for damages suffered by a child born with cerebral palsy, claiming that the defendant hospital and obstetrician were negligent in delivery. The trial court entered judgment on the verdict for the defendant. The court of appeals reversed, ordering a new trial. The court held that the erroneous admission of evidence of febrile seizures suffered by the baby's sister and the uncle's Down's Syndrome constituted reversible error. Such evidence is not linked to cerebral palsy or used to show a genetic predisposition. Such a connection was promised by the defendant and the court admitted the evidence subject to the connection, which was never made.

The plaintiff moved to strike all references to the conditions at the close of all the evidence as it was obvious that no link had been established. The defendant agreed, but the evidence had already been heard by the jury. There had been extensive discovery, and the defendant should have known that no connection could be demonstrated.

    *   The plaintiffs sued a physician and a university hospital for negligence and the intentional infliction of emotional distress arising out of the defendants' failure to test the plaintiff parents for Tay-Sachs disease. The mother consulted with the defendants when she was 37 years old and pregnant with her second child. Because of the increased risk of Down's Syndrome, the plaintiff mother was referred for genetic counseling. A family history was taken, in which the plaintiff mother indicated that none of her family or her husband's family was Jewish. (There is an extremely low incidence of Tay-Sachs disease in non-Jews.) Therefore, the genetic counselor did not recommend genetic testing for that disease, although it was performed for other conditions. At the time of the initial counseling, the physician was aware of a greater risk for Tay-Sachs among a certain group of French Canadians. The child was subsequently born and, one year after birth, was diagnosed as suffering from Tay-Sachs. At that time, the plaintiffs learned that the plaintiff father's maternal grandfather's parents were French Canadian. The trial court granted the defendants' motion for summary judgment. The court, in *Munro v. Regents of University of California,* 215 Cal. App. 3d 977, 263 Cal. Rptr. 879 (1989), affirmed the judgment. The court held that the plaintiffs failed to establish when genetic testing for Tay-Sachs is indicated. This must be done through the use of expert testimony, which requires an evaluation of the standard of care. The defendants presented sufficient evidence to show that the plaintiffs, as per the medical and family history given by the mother, did not meet any of the profiles that would indicate that such testing was appropriate. The court also held that there was no duty on the part of the defendants to inform the plaintiffs of the incidence of the disease in the general population and the nature and cost of the test, when the administration of the test was not indicated by the information given.

When a plaintiff claims that injury arose from the ingestion of a drug or similar product, it is necessary to establish causation between the named defendant's product and the injury. This may require that the plaintiff establish the indentity of the product or otherwise invoke an available theory of alternative liability. *Smith v. Eli Lilly & Co.,* 173 Ill. App. 3d 1, 527 N.E.2d 333 (1988), was a diethylstilbestrol (DES) case; the trial court granted in part and denied in part the defendants' motions for summary judgment. On appeal, this court affirmed in part and reversed in part. The apellate court held that, even without a strict indentification of the manufacturer of the particular DES, the plaintiff could recover via a market-share liability theory. The manufacturers would then have the burden of exculpating themselves by proving that they did not distribute the drug in the area, that they did not manufacture the drug at the relevant times, or that they did not manufacture the drug in the particular form taken by the plaintiff's mother.

It should be noted that proof of the source or possible source of the drug is part of the required element of causation. The court held that a plaintiff may bring the claim against any manufacturer or marketer of DES in the form taken by the mother. Clearly, the plaintiff must also establish the exposure to the drug, that the drug caused the injuries complained of, and that the defendants breached duties owed to the plaintiff while she was still in utero.

Under a market-share liability theory, manufacturers are assessed their pro rata portion of the plaintiff's damages. Thus, if there are five manufacturers, each will be assessed one-fifth of the damages. The manufacturers may reduce their percentage liability by proof that they had a smaller share of the market. This may result in the plaintiff recovering less than 100 percent of the damages. Accurate market data on statewide or nationwide distribution of the drug may be used if there are no such figures for the particular locality.

In the decision, the court extensively discussed the history of DES, DES litigation, and the variety of legal theories. The court cited with approval *Martin v. Abbott Laboratories,* 102 Wash. 2d 581, 689 P.2d 268 (1984), which announced a modified market-share liability theory.

* The plaintiffs sued Eli Lilly & Co. for DES injuries. Two plaintiffs had cancer and another had a precancerous condition. They asserted enterprise liability, concerted action, market share, and alternative liability claims in addition to more traditional product liability theories. The court held that Florida law required dismissal of the claims where the plaintiffs were unable to identify the manufacturer of the actual drugs purchased and taken by their mothers. Another issue presented to the court was the application of the Florida statute of repose (Fla. Stat. Ann § 95.031). The statute provides a defense to product liability suits filed more than 12 years after the product was sold. By its terms, the statutory prohibition applies despite the date when the claim arose. The court, in *Wood v. Eli Lilly & Co.,* 723 F. Supp. 1456 (S.D. Fla. 1989), held that the statute violates Article I, § 21 of the

Florida Constitution, in that it eliminates access to the courts before the claim ever arises. It should be noted that the Florida legislature amended the statute of repose to render it inapplicable in product liability actions. However, that amendment was not retroactively applied to this claim.

* In *Winje v. Upjohn Co.*, 156 A.D.2d 987, 549 N.Y.S.2d 280 (1989), the plaintiff sued a physician who prescribed Delalutin to prevent premature labor. The plaintiffs conceded that the drug did not cause the infant's birth defects, but claimed that the defects were caused by the use of Provera or Premarin ingested by the mother. The medical records established that the physician did not prescribe either drug. The court held that this was sufficient evidence to entitle the defendant physician to the summary judgment which was denied by the trial court. Therefore, the appellate court reversed the trial court's denial of the motion.

*

§ 5.3 Proximate Cause – Loss of a Chance and Increased Risk

Page 83, add at the end of the section:

In *Scafidi v. Seiler*, 119 N.J. 93, 574 A.2d 398 (1990), the plaintiff parents brought a wrongful death action for the death of their infant child. They claimed that the defendant failed properly to treat the mother's early labor and arrest it. The child's premature birth resulted in its death. At the time of the birth, the mother was in the seventh month of a difficult pregnancy. On the day before the birth, the mother suffered severe bleeding, and the physician prescribed bed rest. Later in the day, she spoke to an associate of the physician who prescribed vasodilian. She returned to the physician the next day and was hospitalized with a cervix that was dilated three centimeters. The physician began tocolytic therapy to arrest the labor, but the plaintiff later gave birth to a child weighing two pounds, six ounces. The baby died of respiratory failure two days later. The claimed negligence on the part of the physician was the delay in starting tocolytic therapy and the prescription of the vasodilian, which did nothing to prevent the premature birth. The trial court entered judgment on the jury verdict for the defendant. The appellant court reversed and remanded. The Supreme Court of New Jersey modified and affirmed, holding that the trial court should have instructed the jury on the increased risk of injury caused by the alleged negligence of the defendant. Any damages which might be awarded should be measured by any loss of the chance for survival which was due to the negligence of the physician. The court also found that the jury should have been instructed that the physician was required to prove the extent to which the mother's preexisting condition of premature labor was responsible for the premature birth and the child's fatal condition. This failure to so instruct was harmless, though, because the court also failed to instruct the jury that the physician could not be held liable for damages caused by the mother's preexisting condition. Such an allocation of responsibility is consistent with the idea of the loss of a chance for the baby's survival, and presents the issue of whether the child would have died from the preexisting condition even if the physician's conduct had not been negligent.

With regard to the instructions, the plaintiffs requested the following charge:

> Once the plaintiffs in this case have produced evidence of a negligent act or failure to act which increased the risk that plaintiffs' child would be born prematurely and thereafter die of the complications of that premature birth, and that the premature birth and subsequent death of the child in fact occurred, you will then consider whether such increased risk was a substantial factor in that result. If you so find, you will proceed to a calculation of damages.

The court gave the following instruction instead:

> The plaintiff has the burden of proving that the injuries for which he seeks to be compensated were proximately caused by the accident in question.
>
> Now, I've used the term proximate cause. By proximate cause, we mean that the negligence of a particular party was a subsequent [sic] cause of the injury. That is, a cause which necessarily set the other causes in motion and was a substantial factor in bringing the injury complained of. It is a cause which naturally and probably led to, and might have been suspected to produce the injury complained of.

574 A.2d at 401.

In *Young v. Colligan*, 560 So. 2d 843 (La. Ct. App. 1990), the plaintiff went to the defendant gynecologist with various symptoms. The physician performed an extensive examination and determined that she had a retroverted uterus. He recommended that she undergo an abdominal hysterectomy. While at the hospital prior to the procedure, the plaintiff informed the physician that it had been eight weeks since her last period. She had previously told the physician that her partner was sterile. When the defendant opened the plaintiff's abdomen, he discovered that she was pregnant. The plaintiff then terminated the pregnancy and had a hysterectomy performed by another physician. The plaintiff claimed that the first physician was negligent in failing to perform a pregnancy test prior to scheduling the surgery. The medical review panel found that the physician breached the standard of care but that the plaintiff suffered no damage or injury. At trial, the jury answered "no" to the following interrogatory on the verdict form:

> Was Dr. John D. Colligan guilty of professional negligence which was a cause in fact of injuries to Ms. Connie Young, resulting from her being subject to elective surgery when she was pregnant?

560 So. 2d at 845. The appellate court affirmed the lower court judgment for the physician, holding that the verdict was supported by the evidence.

In another case, the plaintiffs sued the family physician and a hospital's high-risk team for negligence in the care of their newborn, which resulted in severe neurological deficits. The defendants claimed that the deficits were due to a pre-birth brain malformation and accompanying birth defects. The birth was difficult, and shortly thereafter the child showed the characteristics of hypotonia and other symptoms of perinatal asphyxia. The child was born with club feet and dysmorphic physical features. The baby also suffered from hypoglycemia. The trial court entered judgment on the jury verdict (10-2) for the defendants. The court of appeals, in *Richards v. Overlake Hospital Medical Center,* 59 Wash. App. 266, 796 P.2d 737 (1990), affirmed. The court held that the trial court committed harmless error in instructing the jury that the family physician was to be judged by the standard of a reasonably prudent family physician. The court properly rejected a plaintiffs' instruction seeking to base the standard of care on the expectations of society or of the patient. The court recognized that the jury found that the cause of the injuries was a prenatal event rather than the care given after birth. An issue was also presented as to juror misconduct. One juror with a medical background reviewed the medical records which had been introduced into evidence and came to the conclusion that the defects were due to the mother's contracting influenza 20 weeks into the pregnancy. This opinion was shared with other jurors. The court upheld the trial court's finding that this was not juror misconduct requiring a new trial.

In *Banks v. Hospital Corp.,* 566 So. 2d 544 (Fla. Dist. Ct. App. 1990), a premature infant required the insertion of an umbilical artery catheter in her aorta. Part of the catheter was left in the infant and a surgical procedure had to be performed to remove it. The defendants admitted that they were negligent in leaving the portion of the catheter in the child. They alleged, however, that their negligence was not the cause of the child's learning disabilities and other medical problems. The court found that the evidence supported the giving of a jury instruction on concurrent causes. The failure to give the instruction constituted reversible error. The standard jury instruction on the subject provides:

> In order to be regarded as a legal cause of [loss] [injury] [or] [damage], negligence need not be the only cause. Negligence may be a legal cause of [loss] [injury] [or] [damage] even though it operated in combination with [the act of another] [some natural cause] [or] some other cause if such other cause occurs at the same time as the negligence and if the negligence contributes substantially to producing such [loss] [injury] [or] [damage].

CHAPTER 6

DAMAGES RECOVERABLE IN BIRTH TRAUMA CASES

§ 6.2 Damages Recoverable by Parents of an Injured Child

Page 87, add at the end of the section:

Clearly, the amount of the recovery depends on the legal theory or statutory authority sought to support the imposition of liability. *Reilly v. United States,* 665 F. Supp. 976 (D.R.I. 1987), was a Federal Tort Claims Act (FTCA) suit arising out of the negligence of the defendant naval obstetrician in the delivery of the child. The court held that liability could be imposed on the government for the failure of the obstetrician to meet the requisite standard of care, which breach resulted in the injuries sustained. Rhode Island law was applied to determine the standard of care. The court ordered that amounts recovered for the child's lost earnings ($1.1 million) and for future medical and other care ($8.93 million) be placed in a reversionary trust. The court, however, refused to award noneconomic damages in addition to the child's pain and suffering ($1 million) without an answer from the Rhode Island Supreme Court on what noneconomic damages were available; that is, whether the parents could recover for their emotional distress, loss of consortium, and loss of the child's society.

The evidence established that the defendant was negligent in the failure to perform a cesarean section even though the baby was clearly asphyxiated. There was negligence in failing to take measures to terminate the labor and in failing to use a heart monitor to track the progress of the fetus. The defendant was further negligent in using a vacuum suction technique on the baby's head while the baby was in such distress. At 3:35, the mother was admitted to the hospital. At 9:00, there was a deceleration of the fetal heart rate. The mother was not responsive to therapy, and labor was going on for an extended period. The baby was large and in the occiput position, all of which pointed to asphyxia. The defendant called for an operating room to perform a cesarean section, but then abandoned the idea. The defendant tried to have the mother push before the cervix was fully dilated. At 10:15, the defendant removed the fetal monitor, an absolute breach of the standard of care. Shortly thereafter, there was further dramatic deceleration. This case also contains an extensive discussion of various damage elements.

In *C.S. v. Nielson,* 767 P.2d 504 (Utah 1988), a normal, healthy baby was born after the defendant performed a tubal ligation that failed. The mother claimed that the defendant failed to tell her that the prior sterilization procedure was not absolute and that there were alternative procedures with varying success rates. The district court certified, to the Utah Supreme Court, the question of whether there is a viable claim for wrongful pregnancy and what would be the applicable measure of damages for such a tort. The parents sought monetary and emotional damages for the birth of a healthy but unwanted child arising out of the negligent sterilization.

A wrongful birth claim exists where there is a risk of an impaired child who if the risk were disclosed, would have been aborted. A wrongful life claim is generally brought by an impaired child for his or her injuries or impairments. The claim in *C.S.* was of the wrongful pregnancy variety. Wrongful pregnancy damages include medical expenses, the cost of another sterilization procedure, prenatal care, childbirth and postnatal care, physical and mental pain during pregnancy, lost income, and punitives, if applicable. It is not necessary to attempt to mitigate damages through submitting to an abortion or an adoption. Such a claim does not violate Utah Code Ann. §§ 78-11-23 to 78-11-25 (1986), which are decidedly in favor of a right to life and state that an act or omission preventing abortion is not actionable. The court noted that the benefits of having a child greatly outweigh the expenses of child rearing.

The following statutes were relied upon by the court in evaluating the available tort claims:

78-11-23. Right to life – State policy.

The Legislature finds and declares that it is the public policy of this state to encourage all persons to respect the right to life of all persons, regardless of age, development, condition or dependency, including all handicapped persons and all unborn persons.

78-11-24. Act or omissions preventing abortion not actionable.

A cause of action shall not arise, and damages shall not be awarded, on behalf of any person, based on the claim that but for the act or omission of another, a person would not have been permitted to have been born alive but would have been aborted.

78-11-25. Failure or refusal to prevent birth not a defense.

The failure or refusal of any person to prevent the live birth of a person shall not be a defense in any action, and shall not be considered in awarding damages or child support, or in imposing a penalty, in any action.

The court also reviewed the informed consent statute, Utah Code Ann. § 78-14-5(1) (1987), with regard to disclosing the nature and potential for failure of the procedure to the plaintiff.

* *Burke v. Rivo,* 406 Mass. 764, 551 N.E.2d 1 (1990), was a case brought for the birth of a healthy child following a failed sterilization operation. The

defendant physician recommended a bipolar cauterization after the plaintiff expressed her desire not to have any more children. The procedure was performed. Sixteen months later, a pregnancy test confirmed that she was pregnant, and she later gave birth to her fourth child. The day after the birth, she underwent a bilateral salpingectomy sterilization procedure. The plaintiffs alleged that, had they been told of the risk of canalization from the bipolar cauterization, they would have chosen another form of sterilization procedure. The trial court reported questions to the appellate court, which transferred the case to the Massachusetts Supreme Court. The court held that the parents could recover the cost of raising the child to adulthood. The court reasoned that this was proper where the parents sought the sterilization to avoid additional children for economic reasons. The court held that this was the proper measure of damages in a case wherein a sterilization is negligently performed or in which the physician fails to disclose the chance of failure of a procedure so that another procedure might have been selected. In addition to the costs associated with raising the child, the plaintiffs could recover the loss of the wife's earning capacity, medical expenses for the delivery, the cost of another sterilization procedure, and other consequential expenses. The husband could recover for the loss of consortium. The wife could recover for the pain and suffering which is attendant to being pregnant and giving birth. There were also valid claims for emotional distress arising from the fact of the unwanted pregnancy.

* It should be noted that this case runs counter to most decisions in other states. Most courts would allow the recovery of damages for these elements with the exception of the cost of raising the healthy child. It is generally held that, as a matter of public policy, the benefits of having such a child greatly outweigh the attendant costs.

* On the same day that it decided the *Burke* case, the Massachusetts Supreme Court decided *Viccaro v. Milunsky,* 406 Mass. 777, 551 N.E.2d 8 (1990). In that case, the child was born with anhidrotic ectodermal dysplasia. The child brought a wrongful life claim against the physician for negligence in the genetic counseling of the parents. The parents also brought a claim for wrongful birth. The parents had consulted with the defendant genetics specialist to determine the possibility that the wife was a carrier of the genetic disorder ectodermal dysplasia. The defendant determined that she was not a carrier and had no risk of giving birth to children afflicted with the disease. The parents had one child who was healthy. This case arose from the birth of their second child, who was severely afflicted. This decision was the result of a question certified to the court from the United States district court. The court held that Massachusetts recognizes the tort of wrongful birth arising under the facts of this case. The damages in such a case were the extraordinary expenses attendant to raising a child suffering from such a condition. The parents could recover such costs beyond the time the child

reached the age of majority upon a showing that the child would still be dependent on them and they would still be liable for his support. The court held that the parents were entitled to recover for their emotional distress, but that any such amounts could be subject to an offset for the emotional benefits attributable to the first child and any emotional benefits attributable to the affected child. The court rejected the claim for wrongful life, however. This case follows the decision in the *Burke* case, and is also consistent with decisions in many other jurisdictions which allow the recovery of extraordinary costs associated with raising a child with genetic defects.

    *   In *Atlanta Obstetrics & Gynecology Group, P.A. v. Abelson,* 195 Ga. App. 274, 392 S.E.2d 916 (1990), the parents sued the physicians for wrongful birth arising out of the birth of a child afflicted with Down's Syndrome. The plaintiffs claimed that the physicians were negligent in failing to advise them of the increased risk of genetic defects associated with bearing children at age 36. They also claimed that the defendants should have performed amniocentesis which would have detected the genetic defect. The plaintiffs alleged that, had there been amniocentesis, it would have detected the defect, and they would have aborted the pregnancy. The trial court denied the defendants' motion to dismiss. The appellate court affirmed in part and reversed in part. The court held that the plaintiffs had a valid wrongful birth claim pursuant to Ga. Code § 51-1-27 because they could demonstrate that they would have had a legal abortion upon learning the results of amniocentesis. The damages available for such a claim are the extraordinary costs of raising a defective child. The plaintiffs could only recover the additional costs attributable to the defect for the period of the child's life expectancy, which corresponded to the remaining life expectancy of the parents. The court further held that any emotional benefits derived from the child were not to be offset against the other recoverable damages. However, the parents' emotional distress arising from the pregnancy and birth was not compensable.

    *   In another case, a baby was born at an Indian Health Service hospital. The plaintiffs claimed that the baby was injured by the failure of the hospital to treat the mother's hypertension and preeclampsia. It was alleged that these conditions resulted in oxygen deprivation to the fetus, thereby causing profound brain damage. The issue was raised as to the ability of the hospital to provide the mother and infant with proper care. The hospital was classified as a "level one" birth center; level one is the lowest level of care available, and means that the hospital is equipped to handle only low-risk births. The protocols of the Indian Health Service require that when it is determined that more intensive medical care is required, the patient should be taken to a hospital that can provide such care. This was the crux of the case. The court held that the plaintiff could recover only if she could establish that she had the warning signs of hypertension and preeclampsia and that the hospital failed to recognize these signs and act pursuant to its

protocols. Additionally, it would be necessary to establish that the violation of the protocols was the cause of the child's brain damage. The court detailed the facts of the pregnancy and the treatment plus the lack of facilities at the Indian Health Service hospital in question. The court held that the hospital was negligent in failing properly to monitor and treat the mother, and that that negligence was the cause of the injuries sustained by the child. The plaintiffs were awarded $2.5 million for the cost of caring for the child, $760,000 for lost earning capacity, and $160,000 for medical expenses already incurred. The court further awarded the grandmother the sum of $525,000 for the loss of consortium with her grandchild. The mother, on the other hand, was not entitled to any such award, since she had effectively abandoned the child, leaving it with the grandmother. *Anderson v. United States,* 731 F. Supp. 391 (D.N.D. 1990).

§ 6.5 – Medical Expenses: Parental Care

Page 91, add after carryover paragraph:

Many cases arise out of the failure of sterilization procedures. In such cases, the measure of damages should be determined by the health of the child and the reasons behind the plaintiffs' desire for the procedure which was unsuccessful. In *Owens v. Foote,* 773 S.W.2d 911 (Tenn. 1989), the baby was born with Down's Syndrome. The parents sued the surgeon who had previously performed a vasectomy on the husband. They sought to recover the costs attendant to the pregnancy, the delivery, and accompanying medical expenses, as well as, the cost of another vasectomy. The plaintiffs also sought to recover the additional expenses of raising such a child and for their emotional distress attendant to the birth of the Down's Syndrome child. The Tennessee Supreme Court held that damages could be recovered for emotional distress, despite the lower court holding that the emotional distress and cost of child rearing were not compensable. The supreme court recognized that the plaintiffs were required to prove causation between any act or omission on the part of the defendant and the damages sustained. The instant complaint, however, failed to state such elements of proximate causation, but such a lack could be remedied by a proper amendment to the complaint. The claim was essentially one for wrongful pregnancy, which is recognized in most jurisdictions.

The normal type of case, however, involves the failure of a tubal ligation or similar procedure performed on the mother. In *Goforth v. Porter Medical Associates,* 755 P.2d 678 (Okla. 1988), the plaintiffs brought suit arising out of a failed sterilization procedure. The plaintiff was sterilized in August 1980 and was assured that she was sterile. She delivered the child in October 1981. They sought the recovery of their medical expenses and the expenses of raising the child incurred because of the defendants' negligence in performing the procedure. The Oklahoma Supreme Court held that the plaintiffs could recover the medical costs associated with the pregnancy, lost wages, and similar damages. They were not entitled to recover for the cost of raising the healthy, normal, but unwanted child who was born. The Oklahoma court followed its prior decision in *Morris v. Sanchez*, 746 P.2d 184 (Okla. 1987), which adopted the reasoning of *Byrd v. Wesley Medical Center*, 237 Kan. 215, 699 P.2d 459 (1985).

In *Marciniak v. Lundborg*, 147 Wis. 2d 556, 433 N.W.2d 617 (Ct. App. 1988), the plaintiff parents sued the defendant clinic over a failed sterilization procedure. On such a claim, the court of appeals reversed the lower court holding in favor of the plaintiffs. The appellate court, consistent with other jurisdictions, held that, in such a situation, the plaintiffs could not recover the cost of raising a healthy child. This is consistent with a majority view of public policy and a recognition of the wide-ranging benefits attendant to raising a child. The court recognized that it would not be proper to "exonerate a physician who negligently diagnoses pregnancy thus preventing an abortion, while holding another physician liable for failing to prevent a pregnancy through sterilization." 433 N.W.2d at 618. The plaintiffs should, however, be entitled to recover the medical and similar expenses incurred related to the pregnancy and delivery.

In *Wofford v. Davis*, 764 P.2d 161 (Okla. 1988), the plaintiff parents sought to sue the physician for negligence in the performance of a sterilization followed by the birth of a healthy but unwanted child. The trial court dismissed the claim for the cost of raising the child, and that holding was affirmed by the Oklahoma Supreme Court. The court found that such claims for the cost of raising a healthy child would be contrary to public policy. Citing *Morris v. Sanchez*, 746 P.2d 184 (Okla. 1987), the *Wofford* court stated (764 P.2d at 162):

> As a matter of public policy, the birth of a normal and healthy child does not constitute a legal harm for which damages are recoverable. We recognize wrongful death actions because of the great value we place on human life. Conversely, we cannot recognize actions for wrongful birth or wrongful conception of a normal, healthy child. The birth of a normal, healthy child may be one of the consequences of a negligently performed sterilization, but we hold that it is not a legal wrong for which damages should be or may be awarded.

The court further held that the three-year statute of limitations in the medical malpractice statute was unconstitutional, based on the fact that the special statute of limitations for malpractice was an impermissible special law in contravention of Okla. Const. art. 5, §§ 46, 59.

Elsewhere, in the case of *Pitre v. Opelousas General Hospital*, 530 So. 2d 1151 (La. 1988), the daughter was born with albinism, and suit was brought against the physician for failing to prevent conception. The trial court denied the defendant's motion to dismiss. The appellate court dismissed the child's wrongful life claim and the plaintiff parents' individual claims, except for expenses associated with the pregnancy and delivery. The Supreme Court of Louisiana reversed in part and affirmed in part, holding that the physician had a duty to warn of the potential failure of the tubal ligation. The physician, however, had no duty to protect the child from the risk of albinism; thus, the plaintiff parents could not recover the costs associated with the albinism. The amount of the recovery was the same as in cases in which the child was born normal. The court defined the terms *wrongful birth* (risk of birth defects), *wrongful life* (the child's claim), and *wrongful pregnancy* (child born healthy but unwanted).

The standard of care for the performance of the tubal ligation was determined by the physician's specialty. The defendant owed the duty to inform the plaintiffs if the object of the sterilization was not achieved if the physician was so aware. The defendant was found not to have violated any duty in performing the ligation, but his failure to warn could constitute negligence. The ligation was performed on April 25, 1984. On April 30, 1984, the pathology report showed the defendant had severed fibro-muscular-vascular tissue and not the tubes, but the defendant never told this to the plaintiff. The defendant also owes a duty to the child if the defendant is aware of an unreasonable risk to the child. However, albinism cannot be easily predicted or foreseen; therefore, no obligation was owed to the child. The court reviewed other decisions from a variety of jurisdictions and stated that it might impose a duty on the physician for the protection of the child in certain situations.

§ 6.6 – Loss of Society and Companionship

Page 92, add at the end of the section:

Questions often arise as to the effect of the death of the fetus as related to the damages recoverable by the surviving parents. The parents sought to recover for the loss of society of the unborn child in *Denham v. Burlington Northern Railroad,* 699 F. Supp. 1253 (N.D. Ill. 1988). This was a wrongful death case arising from the collision of a railroad engine with a car carrying the pregnant motorist. The defendant moved for summary judgment. The court held that the father could recover for the death of the unborn baby, but could not recover for the loss of the baby's society because the fetus was not born at the time of the accident. The court quoted from *Hunt v. Chettri,* 158 Ill. App. 3d 76, 110 Ill. Dec. 293, 295, 510 N.E.2d 1324, 1326 (1987):

> The court's rationale for recognizing loss-of-society damages in the above cases is dependent upon the relationship of parent and child. In the death of an unborn fetus, no guidance, love, affection or security have been exchanged. While parents may love and have affection for an unborn child, the child cannot be said

to have returned such affection. To allow damages for the loss of society of a stillborn fetus confuses loss of society with recovery for the parents' grief over their unborn child's death. The [Illinois] supreme court has rejected recovery for mental anguish or bereavement as an element of loss of society. Undoubtedly, it could be claimed that there is virtually no difference between the loss suffered by a parent where a child is born but remains alive only momentarily and where the child is stillborn. However, the initial bonding which takes place cannot be dismissed so easily. The length, intensity and quality of the parent-child relationship are determinative of the loss experienced by the parent. Certainly, birth is a proper point at which to begin to measure the loss of a child's society.

* The plaintiffs brought a wrongful death action for the death of their 16-week-old infant. The parents sued a physician who examined the infant in an emergency room. The parents later took the infant to another hospital where the infant died. The plaintiffs also brought a claim under the Anti-Dumping Act (42 U.S.C. § 1395dd). The court, in *Nichols v. Estabrook*, 741 F. Supp. 325 (D.N.H. 1989), granted the defendant's motion to dismiss in part and for partial summary judgment. The court noted that the parents could not recover for their own emotional distress under the terms of New Hampshire law. Further, there could be no recovery for the loss of the child's services and society. Under the wrongful death statute, the only recovery could be for pecuniary loss. Therefore, there could be no recovery for damages such as those for the loss of enjoyment of continued life. The court held that, under state law, no damages were recoverable for the death of the infant, and it rejected claims for even nominal damages.

§ 6.7 – Mental Anguish

Page 93, add after first paragraph:

Such a situation arose in the case of *Sceusa v. Master,* 135 A.D.2d 117, 525 N.Y.S.2d 102 (1988). The plaintiff mother brought suit for mental distress arising from the birth of twins, one of whom was stillborn and the other died shortly after birth. The appellate court affirmed the lower court's dismissal of the action. There could be no recovery for the plaintiff's emotional distress when she did not personally sustain a separate physical injury. The court rejected the argument that by virtue of the performance of a cesarean section, the plaintiff sustained such a physical injury necessary to support a recovery for emotional distress. The court further rejected the argument that the plaintiff could recover such emotional injury damages under the zone-of-danger theory, as such a theory was not intended to apply to this type of fact pattern. The court recognized that there is prior authority holding that "a mother may not recover for the psychic injury caused by the negligence of a doctor resulting in the death or injury to a child either in utero or post partum where the mother sustains no physical injury." 525 N.Y.S.2d at 102.

Page 94, add before second full paragraph:

Clearly, there must be some unusual event or other evidence supportive of a finding that the plaintiff actually sustained emotional distress of a nature that would be compensable. In *Bubendey v. Winthrop University Hospital,* 151 A.D.2d 713, 543 N.Y.S.2d 146 (1989), the plaintiff mother sued the hospital arising out of her treatment during childbirth, seeking recovery for emotional distress. The appellate court affirmed dismissal of the suit, because the plaintiff failed to allege that she sustained any independent physical injury attendant to the hospital's conduct relating to the birth. The only alleged injury was that she suffered extensively through the labor, which continued for many hours. She also claimed that the failure to admit her to the hospital resulted in alleged brain damage to the child, who died four months later, and she claimed to have sustained "severe psychological trauma" as a result of the harm inflicted on her child. However, the court found that she could not recover for any distress normally attendant to birthing and extended labor in such a situation.

Emotional distress damages were claimed with regard to the effects of ingestion of diethylstilbestrol (DES) during pregnancy. In the unusual three-generation case of *Enright v. Eli Lilly & Co.,* 141 Misc. 2d 194, 533 N.Y.S.2d 224 (Sup. Ct. 1988), the plaintiff child sustained birth defects allegedly due to the grandmother's ingestion of DES while pregnant with the child's mother. The trial court held that such a child could not maintain a claim against the manufacturer. The manufacturer, however, was not entitled to summary judgment on the mother's claims for injuries caused by her direct exposure to the drug in utero. The revival portion of the statute of limitations dealing with DES cases permitted the filing of the mother's claim, but there was no viable claim for her emotional distress arising out of the birth of her handicapped child. There is no cause of action for injuries to a child conceived after the original tort injury to the parent. In order for the mother to recover on her own claim, she must introduce evidence of the identity of the pharmacy, prescription, or some similar proof of the drug actually ingested, that is, the particular substance and the manufacturer. Without identifying the substance, there can be no recovery, even under a market-share theory.

The grandmother took DES from 1959-1960. The mother was born in January, 1960. The grandchild was born premature, with cerebral palsy and with grand mal seizures, among other defects. Such a third-generation claim is not available, under the authority of *Albala v. City of New York,* 54 N.Y.2d 269, 429 N.E.2d 786, 445 N.Y.S.2d 108 (1981). The court also looked to "commonly known categories of victims" of exposure to the drug.

The plaintiffs sued six major manufacturers, but not all manufacturers, or even the twelve manufacturers who comprised a committee to the FDA were made defendants; therefore, there could be no alternative liability or market-share liability.

* Wrongful death statutes may also affect the nature of the suit and the recoverable damages. In one such case, an infant died two days after birth. The plaintiff parents brought suit against the physician for wrongful death. The death was allegedly due to the negligence of the physician in the delivery of the child. There was also a claim for the mother's emotional distress. The trial court entered summary judgment for the physician on the emotional distress claim. The appellate court reversed. In *Ob-Gyn Associates v. Littleton,* 259 Ga. 663, 386 S.E.2d 146 (1989), the Georgia Supreme Court reversed the appellate decision. The supreme court determined that the mother and the child (even prior to its birth) are two separate persons. Therefore, the negligence directed toward the child did not constitute negligence toward the mother. Hence, the mother was not entitled to recover under the emotional distress claim, because she suffered no physical injury. The court recognized the traditional rules applicable to claims for emotional distress. The court also noted that Georgia does not accept the *zone of danger rule,* which would permit recovery for witnessing physical injury to another, such as the infant. With respect to the wrongful death action, the court held that, under Ga. Code §§ 19-7-1, 51-4-1, and 51-4-4, there could be recovery without any deduction for the personal expenses which would have been incurred by the decedent. The wrongful death claim did not include recoveries for emotional distress suffered by the survivors.

* The wife was allegedly injured during the course of the defendants' performance of an amniocentesis procedure. She contracted a staphyloccus infection, which resulted in a spontaneous abortion. The trial court granted the defendants' motion for summary judgment dismissing the claims seeking recovery for emotional distress damages. The court, in *Buzniak v. County of Westchester,* 156 A.D.2d 631, 549 N.Y.S.2d 130 (1989), affirmed in part and reversed in part. The court held that the wife could recover for her emotional distress, as such was supported by the requisite personal injury, namely, the infection.

* In *Keselman v. Kingsboro Medical Group,* 156 A.D.2d 334, 548 N.Y.S.2d 287 (1989), a child was born with omphalecele. The child died within a few hours after birth. The plaintiffs claimed that the genetic anomaly resulted in physical pain to both the mother and child and emotional distress to the parents. The plaintiffs also claimed that, had they been advised that the child was genetically defective, they would have opted for other medical procedures. The court held that the plaintiffs failed to allege a viable cause of action for wrongful life. The court also held that the plaintiffs were not entitled to recover emotional distress damages, because they sustained no independent physical harm. The fact that the mother had moderate bleeding subsequent to the birth did not constitute a sufficient physical injury. The informed consent claims were rejected, as they did not arise from a violation of the mother's physical integrity.

§ 6.8 Damages Recoverable by the Injured Child

Page 95, add at the end of the section:

The nature of the damages awarded to the plaintiff child can vary according to the nature of the claim, as in the difference between wrongful life and wrongful birth claims. But the major determinant in most cases, however, will be the nature and extent of the injuries sustained by the child. *McCarthy v. United States,* 870 F.2d 1499 (9th Cir. 1989), applying Washington law, involved negligent treatment during a birth which resulted in injury to the baby. The trial court entered judgment for the plaintiff, which the circuit court affirmed in part while reversing in part. The trial court verdict awarded $2.2 million for past and future pain and suffering; the circuit court found this excessive and reduced it to $1.1 million.

There was sufficient medical expert testimony to support the determination of future medical expenses. The real interest rate should have been used to establish the present value of lost income, and historical growth rates could have been used to calculate the present value of medical services discounted by the market rate of interest. The substandard treatment resulted in severe mixed spastic athetoid quadriparesis, microcephaly, severe developmental delays, and seizure disorders. The plaintiff's condition was stable but consisted of significantly diminished capacity. The mother was awarded $150,000 for loss of love; $4.28 million was awarded for economic losses.

* In *Sastoque v. Maimonides Medical Center,* _____ A.D.2d _____, 556 N.Y.S.2d 108 (1990), an infant sustained brain damage due to oxygen deprivation which occurred during and immediately after birth. The jury returned a verdict for the plaintiff in the amount of $300,000 for lost earning capacity; $250,000 for future medical therapy; $75,000 for custodial care at home until age 21; $900,000 for residential care for the remainder of the child's life; $675,000 for past pain, suffering, and loss of the enjoyment of life; and $2 million for future pain, suffering, and loss of the enjoyment of life. The defendants appealed the amounts for pain, suffering, and loss of enjoyment of life as excessive. The court held that those amounts were excessive, affirmed the judgment as modified, and alternatively ordered a new trial if the plaintiff refused to accept the reduction. The court reduced the claim for past pain, suffering, and loss of enjoyment to $375,000 and for future pain, suffering, and loss of enjoyment of life to $1,375,000. The court cited

Kavanaugh v. Nussbaum, 129 A.D.2d 559, 514 N.Y.S.2d 55 (1987), in which it also reduced pain and suffering damages from $2.5 million to $1.5 million.

* In *Bulala v. Boyd*, 239 Va. 218, 389 S.E.2d 670 (1990), suit was brought against an obstetrician arising out of a failure to provide proper medical care during labor and the subsequent delivery. The mother went to the hospital, and the nurse called the obstetrician at 4:00 a.m. to tell him of the mother's admission. The obstetrician told the nurse to monitor the plaintiff, and told the staff not to call him until labor reached the "crowning stage." The obstetrician was called again at 7:00. At 7:45, the staff determined that the fetal heart rate had dropped. Because there had been inadequate monitoring, the condition might have started an hour prior to discovery. The staff then called the obstetrician, who was still at home, and told him. The plaintiff was taken to the delivery room, where she gave birth. The defendant arrived after the birth. The child was born with profound defects and lived for about three years. She died after the verdict was rendered in the case but prior to the entry of judgment. The verdict provided $1.85 million to the child in compensatory damages and $1 million in punitive damages; to the mother, in the amount of $1.575 million in compensatory damages and $1 million in punitives; to the father, in the amount of $1.175 million in compensatory damages and $1.7 million for medical expenses until the child reached age 18. The defendant physician moved the court to reduce the verdicts to the $750,000 cap contained in Va. Code § 8.01-581.15.

* The Virginia Supreme Court was required to determine whether the cap was to be applied to the individual recoveries of each plaintiff, or to the case as a whole. It was also necessary to determine whether the cap applied to claims of emotional distress and whether it applied to the punitive damage award. The court was also faced with the problem of determining the effect of the death of the child on the damage cap. The court held that the cap applied separately to the child's and mother's claims. The father's emotional distress claim and the claim for the parents' medical expenses were subject to the child's cap. The court held that the cap applied without regard to the number of legal theories sued upon; the number of caps was determined by the number of patients. The mother was clearly a patient, and the court held that the child was also a patient from the point of its birth. Where the caps were both reached by the awards of compensatory damages, there could be no punitive damage recovery. The court also held that the timing of the death of the child did not affect the awards and did not require the court to convert the action to one for wrongful death.

§ 6.11 – Intangible Damages

Page 98, add after first full paragraph:

Pain and suffering and attendant emotional distress constitute the vast majority of the recoverable intangible damages in most cases. In *Scott v. United States*, 884 F.2d 1280 (9th Cir. 1989), applying Alaska law, the child was injured prior to and during his birth at a military hospital. The district court entered judgment for the plaintiffs. The circuit court affirmed in part and reversed in part, holding that the trial court properly permitted the recovery of damages arising from the effect of the child's spastic quadriplegia (cerebral palsy) on the parent-child relationship. The appellate court upheld that award of separate amounts for the child's past and future pain and suffering, as distinguished from an award of his past and future impairment. The trial court was required, however, to recalculate the discount rate for the economic losses comprising lost income and medical expense. Alaska law applied to determine the discount rate in this Federal Tort Claims Act case. The child was properly awarded $2 million for the injuries which rendered him incapable of any form of an independent life and required around-the-clock professional care. The trial jury awarded the child $8.75 million for future economic losses reduced to present value. The parents were awarded $350,000 for loss of the parent-child relationship. This case extensively discusses the damage perspective, but has no discussion of the underlying negligence on the part of the defendant which resulted in the injuries.

* An infant sued a hospital seeking damages arising from the severe burns sustained 11 days after the infant's premature birth. The burns caused serious and permanent damage to the child's feet. The trial court denied the defendant hospital's motion to set aside the verdict of $650,000 as excessive. The appellate court, in *Rivera v. City of New York*, _____ A.D.2d _____, 554 N.Y.S.2d 706 (1990), affirmed the amount of the verdict, holding that it was not shockingly excessive.

§ 6.14 Structured Settlements

Page 102, add at the end of the section:

Practice Note. The following is a sample structured settlement for a 6-year-old child with athetoid cerebral palsy proximately caused by hypoxia during labor. The structure has a present value of $4.1 million, with an up-front cash payment of $1,150,000. Attorney's fees are also structured on the 50 percent contingency contract.

JESSICA L

D.O.B.	10-1-1980	Proposal Date	12-10-86
Age	6.2 Years	Funding Date	1-1-87
Life Exp.	73.2 Years	Rates Expire	1-1-87

Benefits	Present Value	Guaranteed Yield	Lifetime Yield
Immediate Payment:			
$1,150,000	$1,150,000	$1,150,000	$1,150,000
Lifetime Monthly Income:			
$3,500 per month ($42,000/yr), increasing 3% per annum, for Life, guaranteed 30 years, commencing 3-1-87			
	$1,213,313	$1,998,167	$7,247,709
Future Certain Payments:			
$25,000 on 1-1-1990	$20,990	$25,000	$25,000
$50,000 on 1-1-93	$35,248	$50,000	$50,000
$75,000 on 1-1-96	$44,392	$75,000	$75,000
$100,000 on 1-1-99	$49,697	$100,000	$100,000
$150,000 on 1-1-02	$62,590	$150,000	$150,000
$20,000 on 9-1-00	$8,976	$20,000	$20,000
$20,000 on 9-1-01	$8,468	$20,000	$20,000
$20,000 on 9-1-02	$7,988	$20,000	$20,000
$20,000 on 9-1-03	$7,536	$20,000	$20,000
$40,000 on 9-1-04	$14,220	$40,000	$40,000
$20,000 on 9-1-05	$6,707	$20,000	$20,000
$20,000 on 9-1-06	$6,328	$20,000	$20,000
$20,000 on 9-1-07	$5,969	$20,000	$20,000
$20,000 on 9-1-08	$5,632	$20,000	$20,000

JESSICA L (*Continued*)

D.O.B.	10-1-1980	Proposal Date	12-10-86
Age	6.2 Years	Funding Date	1-1-87
Life Exp.	73.2 Years	Rates Expire	1-1-87

Benefits	Present Value	Guaranteed Yield	Lifetime Yield
Deferred Attorney's Fees:			
$10,000 per month for 36 months, commencing 2-1-87	$330,244	$360,000	$360,000
$500,000 on 1-2-88	$471,698	$500,000	$500,000
$250,000 on 7-1-88	$229,210	$250,000	$250,000
$250,000 on 7-1-89	$216,236	$250,000	$250,000
$250,000 on 7-1-90	$203,996	$250,000	$250,000
	$1,451,384	$1,610,000	$1,610,000
TOTAL:	**$4,099,439**	**$5,358,167**	**$10,607,709**

The legislatures of the following states have adopted statutes providing for periodic payments of damages in medical malpractice cases:

Alabama: 5 Ala. Code §§ 6-5-486 (1975); 6-11-3 *et seq.* (Supp. 1987)

Alaska: Alaska Stat. §§ 09.55.548 (1976); 09.17.040 (1986)

Arkansas: Ark. Stat. Ann. §§ 34-2619 (1979); 16-114-208 (1979)

California: Cal. Civ. Proc. Code § 667.7 (West 1975)

Delaware: 18 Del. Code Ann. § 6864 (1986 Supp.)

Forida: Fla. Stat. Ann. § 768.51 (West 1985)

Illinois: Ill. Stat. ch. 110, para. 2-1705 *et seq.* (Smith-Hurd 1987 Supp.)

Indiana: Ind. Code §§ 16-9.5-2-2.2 through 16-9.5-2-2-4 (Burns 1987 Supp.)

Kansas: Kan. Stat. Ann. § 60-3407 (1987 Supp.)

Louisiana: La. Rev. Stat. Ann. § 13:S114 (West Supp. 1988)

Maryland: Md. Ann. Code § 3-2A-08 (1976)

Michigan: Mich. Comp. Laws § 600-6309 (West 1986)

Montana: Mont. Code Ann. § 25-9-403 (1987)

New Hampshire: N.H. Rev. Stat. Ann. § 507-C.7 (1976) (held unconstitutional)

New Mexico: N.M. Stat. Ann. §§ 41-5-7 through 41-5-9 (1976)

North Dakota: N.D. Cent. Code § 26-40.1-16 (repealed), §§ 26-40.1-17, 26-40.1-18 (1977)

New York:	N.Y. Civ. Prac. L.&R. § 5041 (McKinney 1989)
Oregon:	Or. Rev. Stat. §§ 752.070, 752.090, 752.100 (1976)
Rhode Island:	R.I. Gen. Laws § 9-21-13 (Supp. 1987)
South Carolina:	S.C. Code Ann. § 38-59-188 (1976)
South Dakota:	S.D. Codified Laws § 21-3A-6 *et seq.* (1987)
Utah:	Utah Code Ann. § 78-14-9.5 (1986)
Washington:	Wash. Rev. Code § 4.56.240 (Supp. 1987)
Wisconsin:	Wis. Stat. Ann. §§ 655.015, 655.27 (West Supp. 1987)

Periodic payment statutes have fallen to constitutional attack in Florida, *Florida Medical Center v. Von Stetina,* 436 So. 2d 1022 (Fla. Dist. Ct. App. 1983); New Hampshire, *Carson v. Muru,* 424 F.2d 825 (N.H. 1980); and North Dakota, *Arneson v. Carlson,* 270 N.W.2d 125 (N.D. 1978), on the grounds that these statutes, by singling out medical malpractice victims and treating them differently from other tort victims, violate equal protection and deny substantive due process. The statutes have survived constitutional attack, however, in California, *Americas Bank & Trust Co. v. Community Hospital of Los Gatos-Saratoga, Inc.,* 36 Cal. 3d 359, 683 P.2d 670, 204 Cal. Rptr. 671 (1984); and Wisconsin, *State ex rel. Strykowsky v. Wilkie,* 81 Wis. 2d 491, 261 N.W.2d 434 (1978).

Practice Note. *See* D. Hindent, J. Dehner, & P. Hindent, *Structured Settlement and Periodic Payment Judgments* (1986) for the most thorough, comprehensive, and readable analysis available in this complicated field.

CHAPTER 7

STATUTORY HURDLES

§ 7.1 Special Problems of Malpractice Litigation

Page 106, add before first full paragraph:

Among these hurdles to be overcome is proof of the element of causation. By statute, it may be necessary to obtain an expert's affidavit to the effect that there is a viable malpractice claim. Such an affidavit may be required to be filed contemporaneously with or shortly after filing of the complaint. In the case of *Blood v. Lea*, 403 Mass. 430, 530 N.E.2d 344 (1988), the parents brought a malpractice action against the physician and hospital arising out of the care of the mother before, during, and after delivery. The medical review panel found that there was insufficient evidence to raise a question of liability. The trial court agreed and entered judgment against the plaintiff. The Supreme Judicial Court of Massachusetts vacated the judgment, finding that there was sufficient evidence to raise a question suitable for judicial resolution. The fact that the medical opinion obtained by the parents used the word "probably" did not mean that there would be insufficient proof of causation. The opinion letter was from an obstetrician-gynecologist, and outlined the requirements of proper medical care for pregnancy-induced hypertension and intrauterine growth retardation. The expert stated that "delay in rescuing the fetus from its dangerous predicament probably contributed to the damage to this baby's brain." The plaintiff introduced this evidence in an offer of proof that included the physician's office records, a discharge summary, the labor and delivery summary, the labor progress sheet from the defendant hospital, and two opinion letters from physicians.

*   In *Premo v. Falcone*, 197 Ill. App. 3d 625, 554 N.E.2d 1071 (1990), the plaintiff brought suit against a physician, a gynecological service, and a hospital. The plaintiff mother was admitted to the hospital where she gave birth. The child was then transferred to another hospital, where she died four days later. The trial court dismissed the case with prejudice for the failure of the plaintiffs to file a certificate of merit as required by Ill. Rev. Stat. ch. 110, para. 2-622. The appellate court affirmed the trial court's dismissal. The statute provides that defendants are not required to answer a complaint or otherwise plead until 30 days after being served with an affidavit of consultation. In this case, the plaintiffs failed to file a certificate of merit under the statute. This failure allowed the judge the discretion as to whether to dismiss the claim. The court found that the original report

prepared by the physician who reviewed the claim was insufficient to satisfy the statutory requirements, because it failed to discuss the actions which allegedly constituted negligence and only gave a bare conclusion of negligence. This defect was fatal to the attempt. The court also found that an amended report dealing with errors in medications was insufficient because it failed to identify persons responsible for the errors. Such an identification would be required in order to hold the hospital liable.

§ 7.2 Statutes of Limitations

Page 108, add to footnote 3:

Wilsman v. Sloniewicz, 172 Ill. App. 3d 492, 526 N.E.2d 645 (1988), arose out of a failed tubal ligation. Suit was filed in March 1983. The negligent tubal ligation resulted in severe abdominal pain for four years. The defendant allegedly deviated from the standard of care by using clamps, resulting in severe scar tissue which caused the stomach pain. However, the scars could have been caused by previous surgery. The trial court entered a directed verdict for the defendant physician, which judgment was reversed on appeal. The appellate court held that there were sufficient factual questions for jury determination created by the plaintiff's expert testimony of community medical standards. There were similar factual questions for the jury to determine whether the suit was barred by the statute of limitations.

An expert must testify as to the appropriate standard of care, its breach, and causation; it is not sufficient to state that the expert would have done things differently. Generally, this presents jury questions when an expert establishes that the procedure was not used by other skilled physicians.

Similarly, in *Wilsman* there was a fact question as to whether there was a continuous course of treatment extending from 1977 to 1981, during which period the defendant claimed he provided no services. The defendant had said that he would see patients who had not paid their bills only on an emergency basis, unless arrangements for payment were made, but the plaintiff made no such arrangement. The plaintiff claimed that she saw the defendant during the period and that he concealed relevant facts.

In Spruill v. Barnes Hosp., 750 S.W.2d 732 (Mo. Ct. App. 1988), the plaintiff brought suit arising out of a failed sterilization. The trial court dismissed the complaint as barred by the statute of limitations. The appellate court dismissed the appeal, holding that the characterization of the claim as one in contract was specious and that the malpractice limitation period under Mo. Stat. Ann. § 516.105 (Vernon 1978) applied. The plaintiffs claimed that they contracted for a tubal ligation but the defendant physician instead performed a laparoscopic fulgration. The court quoted from Barnhoff v. Aldridge, 327 Mo. 767, 38 S.W.2d 1029, 1030 (1931):

The improper performance by a physician or surgeon of the duties devolved and incumbent upon him and the services undertaken by him, whether same be said to be under a contractual relationship with the patient arising out of either an express or implied contract or the obligation imposed by law under a consensual relationship, whereby the patient is injured in body and health is malpractice, and any action for damages, regardless of the form thereof, based upon such improper act, comes within the inhibition of the two-year statute of limitation.

750 S.W.2d at 733.

Page 108, add at the end of the section:

Clearly, numerous wrinkles must be considered when applying statues. In *Jones v. Salem Hospital,* 93 Or. App. 252, 762 P.2d 303 (1988), the trial court granted summary judgment for the defendant on the statute of repose. The appellate court affirmed in part and reversed in part. The statute of repose (Or. Rev. Stat. § 12.110(4) (1987)) was found not to violate the equal protection clause, despite the fact that it provides a shorter limitations period for minor victims of medical malpractice than for those suffering from other torts. The court found that one physician's misrepresentation does not toll the statute with regard to claims against other defendants. Similarly, unintended misrepresentations do not toll the statute, nor does one physician's misrepresentations with regard to the negligence of other physicians. Nondisclosure does not toll the statute, nor does the failure to disclose the results of diagnostic tests. Any nondisclosure on tangential issues is irrelevant. However, misrepresentations made two years after the birth does toll the running of the statute. The child was the victim of fetal stress after amniocentesis punctured the umbilical cord and caused heavy bleeding. The diagnostic tests performed after birth demonstrated that the newborn experienced respiratory acidosis, but such did not go to the gravamen of the complaint, which involved negligence in the administration of oxygen and the failure to take blood samples for the assessment of blood gases. There were misrepresentations of good care during the pregnancy, delivery, and neonatal care. The child's disabilities were caused by negligence and not by the child's prematurity.

* *Cosgrove v. Merrell Dow Pharmaceuticals, Inc.,* 117 Idaho 470, 788 P.2d 1293 (1989), is yet another Bendectin suit. In this case, strict liability and negligence claims were brought by the plaintiffs. The trial court entered judgment on the jury verdict, which was affirmed on appeal. The mother brought a claim against the manufacturer, but the manufacturer was properly granted summary judgment on that claim, as the suit was filed after the two-year statute of limitations (Idaho Code § 5-219) had run. The child was born without a portion of one arm and hand. The trial court gave the jury a list of special verdict questions. The first question on the list related to causation. The order of questions was not error even though most such lists start with issues of strict liability or negligence.

* In another case, the plaintiffs sued Eli Lilly & Co. for DES injuries. Two plaintiffs had cancer and another had a precancerous condition. They asserted enterprise liability, concerted action, market share, and alternative liability claims, in addition to more traditional product liability theories. The court held that Florida law required dismissal of the claims because the plaintiffs were unable to identify the manufacturers of the actual drugs purchased and taken by their mothers. Another issue presented to the court was the application of the Florida statute of repose (Fla. Stat. Ann. § 95.031). The statute provides a defense to product liability suits filed more than 12 years after the product was sold. By its terms, the statutory prohibition applies despite the date the claim arises. The court, in *Wood v. Eli Lilly & Co.*, 723 F. Supp. 1456 (S.D. Fla. 1989), held that the statute violates Article I, § 21 of the Florida Constitution, in that it eliminates access to the courts before the claim ever arises. It should be noted that the Florida legislature amended the statute of repose to render it inapplicable in product liability actions. However, that amendment was not retroactively applied to this claim.

* In *Menendez v. Public Health Trust*, 566 So. 2d 279 (Fla. Dist. Ct. App. 1990), a child sustained profound nerve and brain damage, allegedly because of the defendants' negligent obstetrical care. The application of the statute of limitations and the statute of repose raised issues of material fact precluding a grant of summary judgment. The mother was first admitted to the hospital on June 8, 1981. On July 14, she was again admitted for hemorrhaging. She was also suffering from gestation diabetes. A cesarean was performed on July 18. The baby was 10 weeks premature. The infant was ventilated and had low Apgar scores. In April 1982, the child was diagnosed as having congenital brain damage and cerebral palsy, with other complications. In January 1984, a therapist working with the child offered the opinion to the mother that the problems could have been caused by the mother's hemorrhaging during pregnancy. In July 1985, the plaintiffs consulted a lawyer, and suit was filed in September 1985. The limitation period applicable to claims against public hospitals was four years (Fla. Stat. Ann. § 95.11(4)). The court found that factual issues arose as to when the plaintiffs knew or should have known of the injury and negligence. Such a determination would be essential to a determination of when the cause of action accrued and when the limitations period commenced. The parents also claimed that there was concealment of negligence; however, the court found that, even had there been concealment, the parents still should have discovered the alleged negligence within the four-year statute of repose.

§ 7.3 – The Discovery Rule

Page 109, add to footnote 6:

Holder v. Eli Lilly & Co., 708 F. Supp. 672 (E.D. Pa. 1989), involved in utero exposure to diethylstilbestrol (DES). The suit was filed against various manufacturers. Summary judgment was granted for the manufacturers on the basis of the statute of limitations. In granting the motion, the court held that the cause of action accrued when the plaintiff learned that she had been exposed to DES and that it had injured her (creating cervical abnormalities), not at the time she learned of the specific risk of a deformed uterus. The deformed uterus allegedly placed the plaintiff at risk during her own pregnancy and created a risk of premature delivery. In 1982, a gynecologist determined that the plaintiff had an enlarged cervical hood, and a pap smear showed abnormal cells with an increased risk of cancer. The gynecologist told the plaintiff that this was due to exposure to DES, after reviewing the mother's medical records. Suit was not filed, however, until 1982. The limitations period was two years under 42 Pa. Cons. Stat. Ann. § 5524(2) (Supp. 1989), and therefore the suit was untimely.

In Kohnke v. St. Paul Fire & Marine Ins. Co., 144 Wis. 2d 352, 424 N.W.2d 191 (1988), the trial court granted summary judgment for the defendant physician, which judgment was reversed by the appellate court. The reversal was affirmed by the Wisconsin Supreme Court. This was a claim for injuries sustained when the plaintiff infant was five months old. The claim, for statute of limitations purposes, accrued at discovery 22 years later. The injury was the sterility of the plaintiff arising from the prior malpractice when the defendant allegedly negligently performed a bilateral hydrocele repair. The plaintiff only discovered the sterility when he was trying to have a child with his wife and thought that there was a potential fertility problem. The suit was timely filed when it was brought within five years of the plaintiff's reaching the age of majority and within one year of the date of discovery. Normally, without the tolling provisions, the statute of limitation was three years for such a claim.

§ 7.4 – Tolling Provisions

Page 111, add to footnote 8:

In Myer v. Dyer, 542 A.2d 802 (Del. Super. Ct. 1987), the plaintiff alleged negligence in the delivery of a child. The court, in response to the defendant physician's motion to dismiss the complaint, held that while the allegations of the complaint were made with the necessary degree of specificity, the parents' claims were time barred, whereas the child's claim was viable due to the tolling provisions of the statute. In pleading, it is not necessary to allege the appropriate standard of care with specificity; that need only be established at trial through the use of expert testimony. In this case, suit was filed in May 1986, arising out of the treatment of the child from birth in June 1982 through September 1982. The complaint contained specific allegations of oxygen deprivation, failure to monitor, improper termination of CPAP, and other specific acts which allegedly resulted in the child's brain damage and cerebral palsy. For the child's claim, the statute of limitations was tolled.

Page 111, add at the end of the section:

The period for bringing suit may be tolled by a special statute applicable to certain types of claims. Typical of such a situation is *Sandberg v. White Laboratories,* 871 F.2d 5 (2d Cir. 1989), applying New York law. The mother had been injected with diethylstilbestrol (DES) while she was pregnant during 1951-1952. Years later she became sterile from a damaged cervix uteri. New York Civ. Prac. L.&R. § 214 (1986), which extends the limitations period for claims such as those involving the taking of DES, was held inapplicable to the instant claim. The court chose to construe the term of the statute narrowly, and dismissed the action.

§ 7.8 Limitations on Damages

Page 116, add at the end of the section:

Wrongful death statutes may also affect the nature of the suit and the recoverable damages. In one such case, an infant died two days after birth. The plaintiff parents brought suit against the physician for wrongful death. The death was allegedly due to the negligence of the physician in the delivery of the child. There was also a claim for the mother's emotional distress. The trial court entered summary judgment for the physician on the emotional distress claim. The appellate court reversed. In *Ob-Gyn Associates v. Littleton,* 259 Ga. 663, 386 S.E.2d 146 (1989), the Georgia Supreme Court reversed the appellate decision. The supreme court determined that the mother and the child (even prior to its birth) are two separate persons. Therefore, the negligence directed toward the child did not constitute negligence toward the mother. Hence, the mother was not entitled to recover under the emotional distress claim, because she suffered no physical injury. The court recognized the traditional rules applicable to claims for emotional distress. The court noted that Georgia does not accept the *zone of danger rule,* which permits recovery for witnessing physical injury to another, such as the infant. With respect to the wrongful death action, the court held that, under Ga. Code §§ 19-7-1, 51-4-1, and 51-4-4, there could be recovery without any deduction for the personal expenses which would have been incurred by the decedent. The wrongful death claim did not include recovery for emotional distress suffered by the survivors.

§ 7.11 – Statutes Fixing a Ceiling on Damages

Page 118, add to footnote 33:

Boyd v. Bulala, 877 F.2d 1191 (4th Cir. 1989), applying Virginia law, was a claim for birth defects arising out of the failure to provide adequate medical care during labor and delivery. The trial court entered judgment for the plaintiff. The circuit court affirmed in part and reversed in part, holding that the statutory cap on recoverable damages in malpractice actions (Va. Code Ann. § 8.01-581.15 (1984)) was constitutional. A verdict was entered for the child in the amount of $1.85 million in compensatory damages and $1 million punitive damages, for the mother in the amount of $1.575 million compensatory and $1 million punitive, and for the father in the amount of $1.175 million in compensatories. The Virginia statutory cap of $750,000 applied per claim exclusive of any punitive damage award. In support of its decision, the court cited Etheridge v. Medical Center Hosp., 237 Va. 87, 376 S.E.2d 525 (1989).

In *Boyd*, a jury question was presented as to the physician's liability for the negligence of nurses. There was evidence of the physician's control over the delivery room, and the nurses could have been found to have been agents of the physician. Therefore, this was another ground for liability imposed on the physician. Punitive damages were appropriate because supported by evidence of willful and wanton conduct, in that the physician diagnosed the plaintiff's condition over the telephone. The physician also failed to get the nurse's assessment of the stage of labor. The nurse was ordered not to call him until crowning occurred, which posed risks to the health of the mother and child. There was expert testimony that this violated the applicable standard of care. The physician lowered his standard of care at night so that he could get his rest.

* In Bulala v. Boyd, 239 Va. 218, 389 S.E.2d 670 (1990), the defendant physician moved the court to reduce the verdicts to the $750,000 cap contained in Va. Code § 8.01-581.15. The Virginia Supreme Court was required to determine whether the cap was to be applied to the individual recoveries of each plaintiff, or to the case as a whole. It was also necessary to determine whether the cap applied to claims of emotional distress and whether it applied to the punitive damage award. The court was also faced with the problem of determining the effect of the death of the child on the damage cap. The child died after the verdict was rendered in the case but prior to the entry of judgment. The court held that the cap applied separately to the child's and mother's claims. The father's emotional distress claim and the claim for the parents' medical expenses were subject to the child's cap. The court held that the cap applied without regard to the number of legal theories sued upon; the number of caps was determined by the number of patients. The mother was clearly a patient, and the court held that the child was also a patient from the point of its birth. Where the caps were both reached by the awards of compensatory damages, there could be no punitive damage recovery. The court also held that the timing of the death of the child did not affect the awards and did not require the court to convert the action to one for wrongful death, which might otherwise change the measure of damages. However, even in such a situation, the statutory cap would be applied.

* In Surratt v. Prince George's County, 320 Md. 439, 578 A.2d 745 (1990), the parents brought wrongful death and survival actions arising out of the death of their child 14 days after his birth. The parents claimed that the child died due to negligent prenatal treatment provided at the county hospital where the child was ultimately born. A health claims arbitration panel rejected the parents' claim. In determining the extent of governmental immunity, the court was required to look to the county's actions. The courts effectively limited the county's liability to $250,000 for each individual per occurrence, but greater recovery could be had to the limit of insurance coverage if in excess of $250,000. The court held that this effectively limited the county's liability to $250,000 or the limit of liability insurance for this claim.

In 1988, Florida enacted the Florida Birth Related Neurological Injury Compensation Plan, Fla. Stat. Ann. § 766.301 *et seq.* (West Supp. 1989). This statutory scheme provides special treatment for certain obstetrical injuries, in recognition of the tremendous increases in medical malpractice insurance of such practitioners vis-à-vis other physicians. The legislature also recognized that the costs of birth-related neurological injuries are great. The statutory plan is the exclusive remedy for the child, parents, and other plaintiffs, and applies except where there is willful or wanton conduct. The statute of limitation is tolled by filing a claim with the compensation plan, but such must be filed within seven years of the birth. The claim is heard by a medical advisory panel. Upon finding that a neurological birth injury has occurred, the board shall make an award for medical and hospital expenses, including custodial care, but there can be no recovery for the benefits receivable for the government and certain insurance benefits. Additionally, there can be a periodic payment recovery to the parent which shall not exceed $100,000. Past expenses are to be paid immediately, and future expenses will be paid as they accrue. The plan is applicable to the patients of hospitals and participating physicians, who must notify their patients of their participation in the plan. The physicians participate in the plan through the payment of assessments.

Page 119, add at the end of the section:

The following is a table of statutory authority regarding damages:

Alabama Code § 6-5-544 (1988 Supp.) (noneconomic); § 6-5-547 (general limit); § 6-11-21 (punitives)

STATUTORY HURDLES

Alaska Stats. § 09.17.010 (1986) (noneconomic); § 09.17.020 (punitives)

California Civ. Code § 333.2 (West 1988) (noneconomic)

Colorado Rev Stat. § 13-21-102 (1988 Supp.) (punitives); § 13-21-102.5 (noneconomic)

Florida Stat. Ann. § 768.73 (1988 Supp.) (punitives); § 768.80 (noneconomic)

Georgia Code Ann. § 105-2002.1 (Harrison Supp. 1988) (punitives)

Idaho Code § 6-1603 (1988 Supp.) (noneconomic); § 6-1604 (punitives)

Illinois Rev. Stat. ch. 110, para. 2-1115 (Smith-Hurd 1987) (punitives)

Indiana Code Ann. § 16-9.5-2.2 (Burns Supp. 1988)

Kansas Stat. Ann. § 30-3402 (1985) (punitives); § 60-3407 (compensatory)

Louisiana Rev. Stat. Ann. § 1299.39 (West Supp. 1989) (liability of state); § 1299.42 (general)

Maryland Cts. & Jud. Proc. Code § 11-108 (1986) (noneconomic)

Massachusetts Gen. Laws Ann. ch. 231, § 60H (West 1986) (noneconomic)

Michigan Comp. Laws § 1483 (1986) (noneconomic)

Minnesota Stat. Ann. § 599.23 (West 1986) (noneconomic)

Missouri Ann. Stat. § 538.210 (Vernon 1986) (noneconomic and punitive)

Montana Code Ann. § 2-9-108 (1987) (government liability)

Nebraska Rev. Stat. § 44-2825 (Supp. 1988) (all damages)

New Hampshire Rev. Stat. Ann. § 508:4d (1986) (noneconomic)

New Jersey Stat. Ann. § 2A:53A-7 (West 1987) (charitable health-care providers)

New Mexico Stat Ann. § 41-5-6 (1987) (noneconomic)

North Dakota Cent. Code § 26.1-14-11 (Supp. 1988) (limit for insured providers)

Ohio Rev. Code Ann. § 2307.43 (Page 1981) (general damages); § 2307.80 (Page 1988) (punitive)

Oklahoma Stat. Ann. tit. 23, § 9 (1987) (punitive)

Oregon Rev. Stat. § 752.040 (1985) (insured health-care providers); § 30.927 (1988) (punitives)

Pennsylvania Stat. Ann. § 8528 (Purdon 1985) (total damages)

South Dakota Codified Laws Ann. § 21-3-11 (1986) (general damages)

Texas Civ. Prac. & Rem. Code Ann. § 41.007 (Vernon Supp. 1989); Texas Rev. Civ. Stat. Ann. § 81.003 (1987) (punitives)

Utah Code Ann. § 78-14-7.1 (Supp. 1988) (noneconomic)

Virginia Code Ann. § 8.01-581.15 (1984) (total limit)

Washington Rev. Code Ann. § 4.22.301 (1986) (noneconomic)

West Virginia Code § 55-7B-8 (1986) (noneconomic)

Wisconsin Stat. Ann. § 893.55 (West Supp. 1988)

CHAPTER 8

OTHER ACTIONS

§ 8.1 Breach of Contract

Page 122, add to footnote 2:

In Spruill v. Barnes Hosp., 750 S.W.2d 732 (Mo. Ct. App. 1988), the plaintiff brought suit arising out of a failed sterilization. The trial court dismissed the complaint as barred by the statute of limitations. The appellate court dismissed the appeal, holding that the characterization of the claim as one in contract was specious and that the malpractice limitation period under Mo. Stat. Ann. § 516.105 (Vernon 1978) applied. The plaintiffs claimed that they contracted for a tubal ligation but the defendant physician instead performed a laparoscopic fulgration. The court quoted from Barnhoff v. Aldridge, 327 Mo. 767, 38 S.W.2d 1029, 1030 (1931):

> The improper performance by a physician or surgeon of the duties devolved and incumbent upon him and the services undertaken by him, whether same be said to be under a contractual relationship with the patient arising out of either an express or implied contract or the obligation imposed by law under a consensual relationship, whereby the patient is injured in body and health is malpractice, and any action for damages, regardless of the form thereof, based upon such improper act, comes within the inhibition of the two-year statute of limitation.

750 S.W.2d at 733.

*   A plaintiff mother was injured in the course of delivery and sued a hospital and private diagnostic clinic for damages. Two months prior to delivery, she consulted with her physician at the clinic, and received assurances that, if in the course of the delivery she required epidural anesthesia, it would be administered by that particular physician or by an anesthesiologist who would insert the catheter. She was admitted to the hospital as a private patient of the clinic and its physicians. She was given an epidural anesthetic block to the epidural space of the spinal cord. The anesthesia was administered by a resident of the hospital. The first attempt to insert the catheter failed and punctured the layers covering the spinal cord, releasing spinal fluid. The second attempt struck a blood vessel. The third attempt was successful. Following the delivery, the plaintiff suffered various problems attributable to the puncture of the spinal cord covering and the loss of fluid. The trial court entered summary judgment for the defendants. That judgment was affirmed by the court in Labarre v. Duke Univ., 99 N.C. App. 563, 393 S.E.2d 321 (1990). The plaintiff's breach of contract claim also failed, because there was no consideration supporting the promise that the physician or an anesthesiologist would administer the anesthetic. The tort claim of the plaintiff was rejected because she failed to allege that the resident who administered the anesthetic was negligent. Therefore, liability for those acts could not be imputed to the hospital.

§ 8.2 Informed Consent

Page 124, add to footnote 5:

In Madsen v. Park Nicollet Medical Center, 431 N.W.2d 855 (Minn. 1988), the plaintiff father sued the medical center and the physician for injuries sustained by the plaintiff's premature son. The judgment was entered for the defendants, but on appeal was reversed and remanded. The court held that informed consent does not require that the attending physician disclose the availability of similar treatment or all of the potential risks of injury arising out of the rejection of supplemental treatments. The defendant physician decided to manage the pregnancy in the home setting as opposed to a hospital setting, and did not insist that the mother undergo hospitalization three days before the premature birth. The court found that this was not a choice between alternative treatments, and therefore there was no duty to disclose the risk of additional or alternative treatments. There was also a claim that the defendant failed to disclose the risk of a premature birth, which disclosure would have affected the mother's decisions.

The child was born with severe and permanent disabilities. It had been detected that the mother was leaking amniotic fluid and an ultrasound had been taken. The mother started bleeding and was sent to a hospital which had no neonatal unit (no hospitals with the necessary neonatal units existed in the area). She was then taken by air ambulance to a hospital with appropriate facilities. The child was born blind in one eye and had spastic quadriplegia, cerebral palsy, and neurological disorders. The court separated the informed consent issue from the claims of negligence in treatment or failure to diagnose, while remanding on the former issue.

In Grasser v. Kitzis, 230 N.J. Super. 216, 553 A.2d 346 (App. Div. 1988), the plaintiff was injured when the physician performed a dilation and evacuation (D&E) procedure for the removal of dead fetal tissue from her uterus. The court reversed the judgment of the trial court in favor of the physician. While the court found that there was sufficient evidence to support the jury verdict that the defendant was not negligent in performing the procedure, the physician could be held liable for failing properly to inform the plaintiff patient of the nature and extent of the procedure, in violation of her right to informed consent.

During the procedure, the plaintiff's uterus and small bowel were seriously injured. These injuries required surgical repair, which was performed by extending the procedure of the D&E under general anesthetic. There were other alternative treatments which were never discussed with the patient. The evidence supported the finding of a lack of informed consent, despite the fact that the defendant claimed he disclosed the alternatives to the D&E procedure, which carries an inherent risk of uterine perforation. The plaintiff signed a consent form without reading it and without being given an explanation. She had been given a sedative prior to presentation of the form. The court entered judgment on liability for the plaintiff and remanded for a determination of damages.

* In Atlanta Obstetrics & Gynecology Group, P.A. v. Abelson, 195 Ga. App. 274, 392 S.E.2d 916 (1990), the parents sued the physicians for wrongful birth arising out of the birth of a child afflicted with Down's Syndrome. The plaintiffs claimed that the physicians were negligent in failing to advise them of the increased risk of genetic defects associated with bearing children at age 36. They also claimed that the defendants should have performed amniocentesis, which would have detected the genetic defect. The plaintiffs alleged that, had there been an amniocentesis, it would have detected the defect and they would have aborted the pregnancy. The trial court denied the defendants' motion to dismiss. The appellate court affirmed in part and reversed in part. The court held that the plaintiffs had a valid wrongful birth claim pursuant to Ga. Code § 51-1-27, because they could demonstrate that they would have had a legal abortion upon learning the results of amniocentesis. The damages available for such a claim are the extraordinary costs of raising a defective child. The plaintiffs could only recover the additional costs attributable to the defect for the period of the child's life expectancy, which corresponded to the remaining life expectancy of the parents. The court further held that any emotional benefits derived from the child were not to be offset against the other recoverable damages. However, the parents' emotional distress arising from the pregnancy and birth was not compensable.

* In another case, the pregnant patient was terminally ill with cancer. At the time, she was over 26 weeks pregnant, and the fetus was viable. The hospital sought a court order to permit it to perform a cesarean. The court ordered the cesarean and the patient's attempt to stay the order was denied. The cesarean was performed, but the child died within two and one-half hours. The mother died two days later. The court, in the case of In re A.C., 573 A.2d 1235 (D.C. 1990), vacated the prior judgment. The court held that, under the facts of the case, the decision of what action should have been taken was up to the patient, who was competent to give informed consent. The court made this decision despite the fact that the issue was moot, since it recognized that this problem would likely be faced in other cases. The court found that it was error for the trial court to order the procedure without obtaining the consent of the patient if she was competent, or without proceeding via substituted judgment and the appointment of a guardian or similar procedure.

*   In Azarbal v. Medical Center, 724 F. Supp. 279 (D. Del. 1989), the plaintiff parents sued the medical center and physicians under claims of a lack of informed consent. The physician performed amniocentesis on the plaintiff wife. It was alleged that, during the procedure, the needle penetrated the skull of the fetus and damaged the baby's brain. Immediately following the birth by cesarean section, the physician performed a tubal ligation. The baby died less than eight months after birth due to the brain damage. Suit was filed exactly two years after the date of amniocentesis. The complaint sounded in negligence in the performance of the amniocentesis procedure. The plaintiffs later attempted to amend the complaint to include claims for lack of informed consent relating to the amniocentesis and to the sterilization procedure. They also sought to add counts against the hospital for post-birth negligence in failing to detect and treat the baby's condition. The court granted the motion to amend the complaint. The issue presented was whether the statute of limitations had run on the informed consent claims so as to defeat the attempt to amend the complaint to allege the new causes of action. The court held that the two-year limitations period (Del. Code Ann. tit. 18, § 6856) was applicable to the informed consent claim and that the period began to run on the date of the amniocentesis. The court found that the informed consent claims related back to the date of the filing of the complaint and therefore were not time barred. The court held that the original complaint gave sufficient notice to the defendant that the claims arose from the amniocentesis. The court further found that the claim for punitive damages arising from the defendant's actual or constructive knowledge of the fetal injury prior to performance of the tubal ligation was sufficient, if proved, to support the imposition of punitive damages.

*   *Page 124, add to footnote 6:*

Burke v. Rivo, 406 Mass. 764, 551 N.E.2d 1 (1990), was a case brought for the birth of a healthy child following a failed sterilization operation. The defendant physician recommended a bipolar cauterization after the plaintiff expressed her desire not to have any more children. The procedure was performed. Sixteen months later, a pregnancy test confirmed that the plaintiff was pregnant, and she later gave birth to her fourth child. The day after the birth, she underwent a bilateral salpingectomy sterilization procedure. The plaintiffs alleged that, had they been told of the risk of canalization from the bipolar cauterization, they would have chosen another sterilization procedure. The trial court reported questions to the appellate court, which transferred the case to the Massachusetts Supreme Court. The court held that the parents could recover the cost of raising the child to adulthood. The court reasoned that this was proper because the parents had sought the sterilization to avoid additional children for economic reasons.

The court held that this was the proper measure of damages in a case in which a sterilization is negligently performed, or in which a physician fails to disclose the chance of failure of the procedure so that another procedure might be selected. In addition to the costs associated with raising the child, the plaintiffs could recover the loss of the wife's earning capacity, medical expenses for the delivery, the cost of another sterilization procedure, and other consequential expenses. The husband could recover for the loss of consortium. The wife could recover for pain and suffering attendant to being pregnant and giving birth. There were also valid claims for emotional distress arising from the fact of the unwanted pregnancy.

In Moore v. Raeuchele, 386 Pa. Super. 438, 563 A.2d 1217 (1989), the plaintiff patient brought suit claiming a lack of informed consent. The plaintiff was unmarried, but she and her boyfriend intended to marry and have children. The plaintiff sought to have the defendant determine whether she was fertile. After a pelvic examination, the physician recommended testing to determine whether her tubes were open. The physician informed her of the nature of the laparoscopy test and the plaintiff gave her consent, although she insisted that the procedure be only explorative and did not consent to any corrective surgery. During the procedure, the physician discovered that the plaintiff's tubes were closed. The plaintiff's condition was not life-threatening, but the physician proceeded to perform reconstructive surgery on the tubes, removing part of the tube which he thought was diseased. The trial court entered judgment for the defendant. On appeal, that judgment was reversed. The court held that the performance of the reconstructive surgery without any warning as to the risks and effects on fertility was a violation of informed consent, and supported a claim for the plaintiff. The court held that the plaintiff's motion for judgment n.o.v. should have been granted.

Gunn v. Sison, 552 So. 2d 60 (La. Ct. App. 1989), is another informed consent case. The postmenopausal plaintiff sued the physician over exploratory abdominal surgery during which the defendant removed her left tube and ovary. The jury found that there was no malpractice and found that the plaintiff consented to the surgery. The appellate court reversed. Upon examining the plaintiff, it was determined that she had indications of possible colon cancer. She authorized the performance of an abdominal exploration with a possible colonoscopy and possible colectomy. The exploratory revealed no colon cancer, but found a diaphragmatic hernia, an inflammation of the diverticulum, and adhesions on the tube and ovary. During the exploratory surgery, the defendant removed the inflamed diverticulum and removed the tube and ovary after he determined that these contributed to the plaintiff's pain. The physician stated that he did this knowing that the tube and ovary were nonfunctional. The court held that because the patient's life was not threatened and she had not given her permission for such a procedure, the actions of the physician constituted a medical battery for which recovery could be had. The court held that an award of $1,000 was adequate under the circumstances.

Page 124, add to footnote 7:

Dohn v. Lovell, 187 Ga. App. 523, 370 S.E.2d 789 (1988), arose from the performance of an unsuccessful voluntary postpartum sterilization. On the physician's motion for summary judgment, the trial court denied the motion. The appellate court affirmed in part and reversed in part, and reviewed the terms of the Georgia Voluntary Sterilization Act (Ga. Code Ann. § 31-20-2 (Michie 1988)). Under the terms of the statute, as applied to this situation, the physician could be held liable for informing the patient only that the result of the procedure would be to render her unable to have children. The Act requires that the patient be given "a full and reasonable medical explanation . . . by such physician . . . as to the meaning and consequence of such operation." It should be necessary to explain the method of the sterilization, and not just the intended result. The plaintiff stated that she wanted her tubes "cut, tied and burnt." The physician represented that the Blier clip was 99.9% effective, but there was actually a 10% failure rate not known to the physician. The defendant, however, did not have the duty to disclose the risk and complications of the procedure. There was insufficient evidence to support the imposition of liability on other claims for the physician's lack of knowledge of the high failure rate of Blier clips at the time of the procedure.

In Pitre v. Opelousas General Hosp., 530 So. 2d 1151 (La. 1988), the plaintiffs' daughter was born with albinism, and suit was brought against the physician for failing to prevent conception. The trial court denied the defendant's motion to dismiss. The appellate court dismissed the child's wrongful life claim and the plaintiff parents' individual claims, except for expenses associated with pregnancy and delivery. The Supreme Court of Louisiana reversed in part and affirmed in part, holding that the physician had a duty to warn of the potential failure of the tubal ligation. The physician, however, had no duty to protect the child from the risk of albinism. The plaintiff parents could not recover the costs associated with albinism; the amount of the recovery was the same as in a case in which the child was born normal.

The defendant owed the duty to inform the plaintiffs if the object of the sterilization was not achieved, provided that the physician was so aware. The defendant was found not to have violated the duty in performing the ligation, but his failure to warn could constitute negligence. The ligation was performed on April 25, 1984. On April 30, 1984, the pathology report showed that the defendant had severed fibro-muscular-vascular tissue and not the tubes, but he never told this to the plaintiff. The defendant owes a duty to the child if the defendant is aware of an unreasonable risk to the child. Albinism cannot be easily predicted or foreseen; therefore, no obligation was owed to the child.

In Laubach v. Franklin Square Hosp., 79 Md. App. 203, 556 A.2d 682 (1989), a husband and wife sued a hospital for fraud and a violation of statute. The trial court entered summary judgment for all defendants except the hospital, granted summary judgment for the hospital on the fraud and civil conspiracy claims, and awarded $1 million compensatory and punitive damages on the remaining claims. The appellate court affirmed the compensation for emotion distress. There was evidence that the hospital violated the disclosure statute, Md. Health-Gen. Code Ann. § 4-302(d)(2) (1982), which provides:

> If a facility refuses to disclose a medical record within a reasonable time after a person in interest requests the disclosure, the facility is, in addition to any liability for actual damages, liable for punitive damages.

The hospital in *Laubach* refused to disclose fetal monitoring tracings as required by the statute. The tracings qualified as medical records for the statutory purpose, where the tracings showed the administration of pitocin and therefore were a record of medical care. The child died shortly after birth. For the violation of statute, the plaintiff was also entitled to recover litigation costs.

Wilson v. Kuenzi, 751 S.W.2d 741 (Mo. 1988), was a wrongful life and wrongful birth suit arising from the defendant's failure to inform the parents of the possible use of amniocentesis to determine the presence of Down's Syndrome in their unborn child. The trial court dismissed the claim and was affirmed on appeal. The Missouri Supreme Court again affirmed, holding that, even though the statute (Mo. Ann. Stat. § 188.130(1) (Vernon 1986)) precluding claims for wrongful life and wrongful birth did not apply retroactively, the causes of action were not recognized in the state prior to the statute.

The mother was age 36 at conception, and there is a 1 in 300 risk of a Down's Syndrome child for women that age. The plaintiff claimed that if she had been told of the test and if the test had been performed, she would have had the opportunity to abort the fetus, which she would have done. The court assumed that it would be proper practice to advise of the test, but still found no enforceable cause of action. The relevant statute provides:

> 1. No person shall maintain a cause of action or receive an award of damages on behalf of himself or herself based on the claim that but for the negligent conduct of another, he or she would have been aborted.
>
> 2. No person shall maintain a cause of action or receive an award of damages based on the claim that but for the negligent conduct of another, a child would have been aborted.

The court discussed the difference between the wrongful life and wrongful birth causes of actions, and recognized the multiplicity of authority for such claims, but chose to disregard such authority. The court cited Note, *Wrongful Birth Actions: The Case Against Legislative Curtailment,* 100 Harv. L. Rev. 2017 (1987), which lists authority in the following jurisdictions as recognizing a cause of action for wrongful birth: Alabama, California, Florida, Illinois, Maine, Michigan, New Hampshire, New Jersey, New York, North Carolina, Pennsylvania, South Carolina, Texas, Virginia, Washington, West Virginia, and Wisconsin.

In Spencer v. Seikel, 742 P.2d 1127 (Okla. 1987), a child was born suffering from hydrocephalus. Suit was brought on a theory that the defendants were negligent in failing to disclose the possibility of an abortion when the fetus was 23 weeks old and it was determined that the hydrocephalus was present. The trial court entered judgment for the defendant and the intermediate appellate court affirmed. The Oklahoma Supreme Court affirmed the trial court judgment for the defendant, holding that the defendant had no duty to disclose the possibility of an abortion when the life or health of the mother were not in danger. At the time of discovery of the condition, the child was viable and thus state statutes prohibited the performance of an abortion (Okla. Stat. tit. 63, § 1-732(A) (1981)). The physician was also found not to have had a duty to inform the mother that other states would permit an abortion at that stage. The record established that the mother in fact knew that abortion was a possible alternative course of treatment. The court looked to the nature of the informed consent doctrine and found that the patient's subjective feelings were determinative of the issue of materiality of the nondisclosure. The court held that since the patient had previously consulted with the defendant about aborting another pregnancy, even though she decided not to have the abortion, she was aware of her alternatives.

In Begin v. Richmond, 150 Vt. 517, 555 A.2d 363 (1988), the plaintiff underwent a vasectomy and was not informed of the risk of failure through recanalization. The plaintiff was told that there was no risk of failure of the vasectomy if the eight-month specimen showed no live sperm. The tests at eight weeks and eight months showed no live sperm, but two and one-half years later, his wife became pregnant. The trial court denied motions for a directed verdict. The supreme court held that there was a jury question as to the negligence of the urologist, but that the patient's claim was not governed by the informed consent statute (Vt. Stat. Ann. tit. 12, §§ 1908, 1909). The trial court determination of the cost of raising the resultant child was not a final judgment which could be reversed on appeal. The court discussed authority from other wrongful conception cases and cited Jackson v. Bumgarden, 318 N.C. 172, 347 S.E.2d 743 (1986).

§ 8.5 – Medicines and Medical Equipment

Page 129, add to footnote 19:

In Lynch v. Bay Ridge Obstetrical & Gynecological Assocs., 72 N.Y.2d 632, 532 N.E.2d 1239, 536 N.Y.S.2d 11 (1989), the claim sounded in the negligence of the defendant gynecologist for failing to diagnose the defendant's pregnancy. He prescribed a drug for her without warning of risks to the baby if she were pregnant when the drug was taken. The drug resulted in a congenitally defective child. The failure to warn of the risks deprived the plaintiff of the choice of whether to continue or terminate the pregnancy. The trial court and intermediate appellate court dismissed the complaint. The New York Court of Appeals held that there was a viable claim other than that stated for injuries inflicted on a fetus, which would normally not be recoverable. The plaintiff's choice to have an abortion was not a superseding cause. The hormonal drugs forced the plaintiff to risk a congenitally defective child or submit to an abortion in violation of her personal, moral, and religious convictions. This left her with a cause of action for physical and emotional injuries.

In Brecher v. Cutler, _____ Pa. Super. _____, 578 A.2d 481 (1990), the plaintiff sued the manufacturer of a Copper-seven (Cu-7) IUD, which allegedly rendered her sterile from pelvic infections and adhesions caused by use of the IUD. The trial court granted summary judgment to the manufacturer. That judgment was affirmed on appeal. The court held that the manufacturer's package insert was sufficient to warn of the potential risks of using the IUD. The manufacturer could therefore use the learned intermediary rule to defeat claims based on an alleged failure to warn, since the prescribing physicians were given sufficient warnings. The physician in question testified that he had read the insert and was aware of the contents of the warning and the potential side effects of using the IUD. The following warning was given by the manufacturer (578 A.2d at 484):

WARNINGS

Pelvic Infection: An increased risk of pelvic inflammatory disease associated with use of IUDs has been reported. While unconfirmed, this risk appears to be greatest for young women who are nulliparous and/or who have a multiplicity of sexual partners. Salpingitis can result in tubal damage and occlusion thereby threatening future fertility. Therefore it is recommended that patients be taught to look for symptoms of pelvic inflammatory disease. The decision to use an IUD in a particular case must be made by the physician and the patient with the consideration of a possible deleterious effect on future fertility. Pelvic infection may occur with a Cu-7 in situ and at times result in the development of tubo-ovarian abscesses or general peritonitis. The symptoms of pelvic infection include: new development of menstrual disorders (prolonged or heavy bleeding), abnormal vaginal discharge, abdominal or pelvic pain, dyspareunia, fever. The symptoms are especially significant if they occur following the first two or three cycles after insertion. Appropriate aerobic and anaerobic bacteriologic studies should be done and antibiotic therapy initiated promptly. If the infection does not show marked clinical improvement within 24 to 48 hours, the Cu-7 should be removed and the continuing treatment reassessed on the basis of the results of culture and sensitivity tests.

ADVERSE REACTIONS

Pelvic infection including salpingitis with tubal damage or occlusion has been reported. This may result in future infertility.

*   In another case, the issue of the application of strict liability with respect to unavoidably unsafe products was presented, again involving the use of an IUD. The plaintiff used the Cu-7 device manufactured by Searle. Three years after the IUD was implanted, the plaintiff gave birth. The day after the birth, she had a tubal ligation. In the course of the procedure, it was determined that the IUD had perforated her uterus and was embedded in her small bowel. The trial court granted summary judgment for the manufacturer, holding that the IUD was an unavoidably unsafe product under the terms of comment k of Restatement (Second) of Torts § 402A. The court, in Hill v. Searle Laboratories, 884 F.2d 1064 (8th Cir. 1989), applying Arkansas law, reversed the summary judgment. The court held that the plaintiff was entitled to a warning of the dangers of using the Cu-7, and that a factual question had been presented as to whether she was given such a warning. The court stated that the learned intermediary rule was inapplicable where the physician was not a party intervening between the relationship of manufacturer and user. The court also noted that a warning in the form of package inserts was required by the FDA. The plaintiff's physician was aware of the risk of perforation, but there was a question as to whether any warning had been given to the plaintiff, who stated that she never received the patient brochure.

*   Nickerson v. G.D. Searle & Co., 900 F.2d 412 (1st Cir. 1990) (applying Massachusetts law), was an IUD products liability claim. The plaintiff alleged that she was rendered infertile by use of an IUD. The appellate court affirmed the trial court judgment for the defendant IUD manufacturer. The court found that there was sufficient evidence to support a lower court finding that the cause of the infertility was a sexually transmitted disease. While that portion of the decision is straightforward, the court held that the plaintiff was not entitled to a new trial on the basis of subsequently discovered evidence. The plaintiff later found a trial transcript from another case in which the manufacturer had disclosed the rate of infection attendant to use of the IUD. No new trial was warranted, as such evidence was admissible only for impeachment purposes. The court also found that there was no error in failing to tell the jury that defense counsel had agreed that pelvic inflammatory disease was also a cause of infertility, despite the fact that such an admission was relevant to the sufficiency of the manufacturer's product warning.

*   Lacy v. G.D. Searle & Co., 567 A.2d 398 (Del. 1989), was another IUD case. The device was implanted in the plaintiff too soon following her delivery of a child. The manufacturer's warnings to physicians disclosed a heightened risk of uterine perforation if the Cu-7 were implanted sooner than two months after the patient had been pregnant. This is because, at such time, the uterus would not have had an opportunity to return to its normal size. Nevertheless, the plaintiff's physician installed her IUD six weeks after the plaintiff's delivery. The IUD perforated the uterus and became embedded. To correct the problems, the plaintiff's tubes were tied and her ovaries were removed. The plaintiff recovered damages from the physician and the medical center. This case also involved the liability of the manufacturer of the IUD. The court affirmed summary judgment for the manufacturer, holding that the manufacturer had properly warned physicians of this risk of injury and satisfied its obligations under the learned intermediary rule. The fact that the physician never conveyed the warnings to the plaintiff did not affect the manufacturer's satisfaction of its duties.

Page 129, add at the end of the section:

DES Cases

Enright v. Eli Lilly & Co., 141 Misc. 2d 194, 533 N.Y.S.2d 224 (Sup. Ct. 1988). The plaintiff child sustained birth defects allegedly due to the grandmother's ingestion of diethylstilbestrol (DES) while pregnant with the child's mother. The trial court held that such a child could not maintain a claim against the manufacturer. There is no cause of action for injuries to a child conceived after the original tort injury to the parent.

The grandmother took DES from 1959-1960 before the mother's birth in January 1960. The grandchild was born premature, with cerebral palsy and grand mal seizures, among other defects. Such a third-generation claim is not available under the authority of *Albala v. City of New York,* 54 N.Y.2d 269, 429 N.E.2d 786, 445 N.Y.S.2d 108 (1981). The court also looked to "commonly known categories of victims" of the exposure to the drug.

The manufacturer, however, was not entitled to summary judgment on the mother's claims for injuries caused by her direct exposure to the drug in utero. The revival portion of the statute of limitations dealing with DES cases permitted the filing of the mother's claim, but there was no viable claim for her emotional distress arising out of the birth of her handicapped child. In order for the mother to recover on her own claim, she must establish the pharmacy that supplied the drug, the prescription, or some similar proof of the drug taken, that is, the particular substance and the manufacturer. Without identifying the substance, there can be no recovery, even under a market-share theory. The plaintiffs sued six major manufacturers, but not all manufacturers, or even the twelve manufacturers who formed a committee to the FDA, were made defendants; therefore, there could be no alternative liability or market-share liability.

Holder v. Eli Lilly & Co., 708 F. Supp. 672 (E.D. Pa. 1989). This case involved in utero exposure to DES. The suit was filed against various manufacturers. Summary judgment was granted for the manufacturers on the basis of the statute of limitations. In granting the motion, the court held that the cause of action accrued when the plaintiff learned that she had been exposed to DES and that it had injured her (creating cervical abnormalities), and not when she learned of the specific risk of the deformed uterus. The deformed uterus allegedly placed the plaintiff at risk during her own pregnancy and created a risk of premature delivery.

In 1982, a gynecologist determined that the plaintiff had an enlarged cervical hood, and a pap smear showed abnormal cells with an increased risk of cancer. The gynecologist told the plaintiff that this was due to exposure to DES, after reviewing the mother's medical records. Suit was not filed, however, until 1982. The limitations period was two years under 42 Pa. Cons. Stat. Ann. § 5524(2), and therefore the suit was untimely.

Smith v. Eli Lilly & Co., 173 Ill. App. 3d 1, 527 N.E.2d 333 (1988). In this DES case, the trial court granted in part and denied in part the defendants' motions for summary judgment. On appeal, the appellate court affirmed in part and reversed in part, holding that even without a strict identification of the manufacturer of the particular DES, the plaintiff could recover via a market-share liability theory. The manufacturers would then have the burden of exculpating themselves by proving that they did not distribute the drug in the area, that they did not manufacture the drug at the relevant times, or that they did not manufacture the drug in the particular form taken by the plaintiff's mother.

It should be noted that proof of the source or possible source of the drug is part of the required element of causation. The court held that the plaintiff could bring a claim against any manufacturer or marketer of DES in the form taken by the mother. Clearly, the plaintiff must also establish the exposure to the drug, that the drug caused the injuries complained of, and that the defendants breached duties owed to the plaintiff while she was still in utero.

Under the market-share theory, manufacturers are assessed their pro rata portion of the plaintiff's damages; if there are five manufacturers, each will be assessed one-fifth of the damages. The manufacturers may reduce their percentage liability by proof that they had a smaller share of the market, even though the plaintiff may thus recover less than 100 percent of the damages. Accurate market data on statewide or nationwide distribution of the drug may be used if there are no such figures for the particular locality. In the decision, the court extensively discussed the history of DES, DES litigation, and the variety of legal theories. The court cited with approval *Martin v. Abbott Laboratories,* 102 Wash. 2d 581, 689 P.2d 268 (1984), which announced a modified market-share liability theory.

Castrigano v. E.R. Squibb & Sons, 546 A.2d 775 (R.I. 1988). This was another DES case, in which the district court held the manufacturer strictly liable and liable for a breach of the warranty of merchantability. After the verdict, however, it certified the question to the Rhode Island Supreme Court. The Supreme Court held that Rhode Island law recognizes the viability of claims arising while the plaintiff is in utero as a result of DES ingested by the mother. The exemption from strict liability is available for unavoidably unsafe drugs, which is a defense to a claim based on a design defect but which is not a defense to a claim for failure to warn. Similarly, there is an exemption for unavoidably unsafe drugs under contract theories. The court recognized that the public policy interest in developing drugs that are safe is served by a case-by-case analysis to determine the defective design claim. For a drug to be exempt from a no-fault strict liability claim, the benefits of the drug must exceed the risks, as known at the time the drug was marketed. The court extensively reviewed the nature of strict liability per § 402A of the *Restatement (Second) of the Law of Torts* (1969), stating (546 A.2d at 778):

1. Based on the facts of this case Rhode Island law recognized actions for damages for personal injury based on theories of strict liability in tort and breach of implied warranty of merchantability.
2. In a tort action comment k is a defense to an allegation of design defect. Comment k, however, is not a defense to an allegation of failure to warn. Comment k also is a defense for liability under contract theory of breach of implied warranty of merchantability.
3. The application of comment k is a mixed question of law and fact. The defendant who uses comment k as a defense bears the burden of proving that the comment applies. If reasonable minds could only reach one conclusion, the judge may rule on comment k's application. Otherwise, the question should be submitted to the jury.

The court set out the text of comment k to *Restatement* § 402A (546 A.2d at 779):

Unavoidably unsafe products. There are some products which, in the present state of human knowledge, are quite incapable of being made safe for their intended and ordinary use. These are especially common in the field of drugs. An outstanding example is the vaccine for the Pasteur treatment of rabies, which not uncommonly leads to very serious and damaging consequences when it is injected. Since the disease itself invariably leads to a dreadful death, both the marketing and the use of the vaccine are fully justified, notwithstanding the unavoidable high degree of risk which they involve. Such a product, properly prepared, and accompanied by proper directions and warning, is not defective, nor is it *unreasonably* dangerous. . . . It is also true in particular of many new or experimental drugs as to which, because of lack of time and opportunity for sufficient medical experience, there can be no assurance of safety, or perhaps even of purity of ingredients, but such experience as there is justifies the marketing and use of the drug notwithstanding a medically recognizable risk. The seller of such products, again with the qualification that they are properly prepared and marketed, and proper warning is given, where the situation calls for it, is not to be held to strict liability for unfortunate consequences attending their use, merely because he has undertaken to supply the public with an apparently useful and desirable product, attended with a known but apparently reasonable risk.

Hymowitz v. Eli Lilly & Co., 73 N.Y.2d 487, 539 N.E.2d 1069, 541 N.Y.S.2d 941 (1989). Multiple actions raised certified questions to the court of appeals. The court held that the market-share theory is appropriate for determining liability and apportioning damages where identification of the particular manufacturer of the drug actually ingested is impossible. The court held that alternative liability theory is not available where there is a chance of identifying the manufacturer. The court rejected the concerted action doctrine where there was no parallel activity, identification was unlikely, and there was no agreed-upon conduct among the manufacturers. The court held that, under the market-share theory, it is proper to use a nationwide market standard where identification of the particular manufacturer is impossible. The court recognized that the liability of the producers of DES was several but could not be imposed where all manufacturers were not before the court. Such a nationwide market would be applied for practical reasons. The court stated (539 N.E.2d at 1075):

> Indeed, it would be inconsistent with the reasonable expectations of a modern society to say to these plaintiffs that because of the insidious nature of an injury that long remains dormant, and because so many manufacturers, each behind a curtain, contributed to the devastation, the cost of injury should be borne by the innocent and not the wrongdoers. This is particularly so where the Legislature consciously created these expectations by reviving hundreds of DES cases. Consequently, the ever-evolving dictates of justice and fairness, which are the heart of our common-law system, require formulation of a remedy for injuries caused by DES.

The court looked extensively to the case of *Bichler v. Eli Lilly & Co.,* 55 N.Y.2d 571, 436 N.E.2d 182, 450 N.Y.S.2d 776 (1982), while rejecting in part the reasoning of the landmark case of *Sindell v. Abbott Laboratories,* 26 Cal. 3d 588, 607 P.2d 924, 163 Cal. Rptr. 132 (1980).

Shields v. Eli Lilly & Co., 697 F. Supp. 12 (D.D.C. 1988). The defendant drug manufacturer moved for summary judgment, which was granted because the court found insufficient evidence to establish a causal connection between the plaintiff's injuries and the mother's ingestion of DES while pregnant with the plaintiff. The plaintiff's pathologist-expert could only state that it was likely that the use of DES or its congeners was a cause of the injury. There was insufficient proof of causation where the plaintiff's mother could only testify that she ingested a small red pill, prescribed because she was straining early in her pregnancy and her obstetrician hoped that the drug would prevent miscarriage. She took the drug twice daily for one month. She had a problem recalling the description of the drug and only did so after a 25-pill line-up. There was no evidence that her particular obstetrician prescribed DES for her bleeding. The plaintiff's vaginal tract was deformed and abnormal, but there could be no recovery where there was no evidence that DES or any similar drug in the 1950s came in small red pills such as those taken by the mother.

*   The plaintiffs sued Eli Lilly & Co. for DES injuries. Two plaintiffs had cancer and another had a precancerous condition. They asserted enterprise liability, concerted action, market share, and alternative liability claims, in addition to more traditional product liability theories. The court held that Florida law required dismissal of the claims, because the plaintiffs were unable to identify the manufacturers of the actual drugs purchased and taken by their mothers. Another issue presented to the court was the application of the Florida statute of repose (Fla. Stat. Ann § 95.031). The statute provides a defense to product liability suits filed more than 12 years after the product was sold. By its terms, the statutory prohibition applies despite the date when the claim arises. The court, in *Wood v. Eli Lilly & Co.,* 723 F. Supp. 1456 (S.D. Fla. 1989), held that the statute violates Article I, § 21 of the Florida Constitution, in that it eliminates access to the courts before the claim can ever arise. It should be noted that the Florida legislature amended the statute of repose to render it inapplicable in product liability actions. However, that amendment was not retroactively applied to this claim.

*   *Krist v. Eli Lilly & Co.,* 897 F.2d 293 (7th Cir. 1990), applying Wisconsin law, was also a DES case. Product liability cases of this nature generally require that the plaintiff establish that her mother took DES when pregnant with the plaintiff; that the injuries complained of were caused by the DES; and that, at the time in question, the manufacturer produced the type of DES taken by the mother. At trial, the mother repeatedly testified that she took little red pills. At the time in question, manufacturer Lilly did not produce or market any red pills. The mother further testified that the pills were coated, and Lilly produced no coated pills during the relevant period. The plaintiff failed to sue other manufacturers and, even though Lilly impleaded other manufacturers, the statute of limitations had run, thereby barring any attempt on the part of the plaintiff to sue those manufacturers. Summary judgment in favor of Lilly was affirmed on appeal. The court noted that the plaintiff's attorney never sought to impeach the mother's testimony or otherwise question the reliability of her recollection. This tactical decision, made by the plaintiff, virtually required the judgment for Lilly.

Depo-Provera

Upjohn Co. v. MacMurdo, 536 So. 2d 337 (Fla. Dist. Ct. App. 1988). The trial court granted summary judgment for the manufacturer in this products liability suit. The appellate court reversed on the issue of failure to warn of the risks inherent in the use of the drug. On remand, the manufacturer was found liable, but the plaintiff was also assessed 49 percent comparative fault. The appellate court, in this opinion, found that there was a jury question as to the manufacturer's failure to warn, and that the plaintiff could not be assessed a percentage of comparative fault for requesting a hysterectomy to control bleeding (caused by the injection of the drug) without exploring alternative treatments. The treatment was initiated due to excessive bleeding during menstruation, caused by Depo-Provera that was being used as a contraceptive. As opposed to a total hysterectomy, a tubal ligation would have been a reasonable alternative, but the plaintiff was not required to determine whether the hysterectomy was a proper treatment. Even if she did request the hysterectomy which was a contributory cause of the injury, the court found that such was not a legal cause of the injury. The court stated (536 So. 2d at 340):

> Public policy dictates, and other jurisdictions have held, that a patient does not have an obligation or duty to determine whether an injury is being properly treated by a physician. Any other rule would offend common sense by requiring the patient to be the judge of a physician's professional competence.

Anesthetic

Ramon v. Farr, 770 P.2d 131 (Utah 1989). The defendant physician injected the mother's cervix with an anesthetic one hour before birth. The child sustained serious physical and mental defects. The trial court entered judgment for the defendant. The appellate court held that a manufacturer's package insert does not per se establish the standard of care for physicians.

The question was presented as to whether the physician directly injected the child with the Marcaine. The plaintiffs did not introduce sufficient evidence to support the claim that an injection to the mother without injecting the child would have not affected the child. Such a use of the anesthetic was not recommended by the manufacturer, and the court held that such could be prima facie evidence of negligence. The package insert was evidence that should be considered by the jury.

An issue was also raised as to the refusal of the court to give an offered instruction. It was harmless error to refuse to give the instruction that the parents were entitled to recovery if the physician failed to give information on a paracervical block procedure. The refused instruction read as follows:

> You are instructed that the manufacturers of Marcaine included a package insert which stated that "Until further clinical experience is gained, paracervical block with Marcaine is not recommended. Fetal bradycardia frequently follows paracervical block with some amide-type local anesthetics and may be associated with fetal acidosis," and that the *Physician's Desk Reference* contained an identical warning. The Defendants either knew or should have known of such

warning. If you find that the Defendants nevertheless proceeded to use Marcaine as a paracervical block and that such use was a proximate cause of Plaintiffs' injuries, then, the fact that Defendants used Marcaine for a paracervical block contrary to written warning would be prima facie evidence of negligence by the Defendants. Prima facie means that such action by Defendants would not be conclusive, but that in the absence of other evidence which is convincing in repudiating the assumption, that such actions were reasonable and prudent, you should find in favor of the Plaintiffs and against one or both of the Defendants.

Other rejected instructions provided:

In connection with the use of the drug Marcaine by the Defendants and your determination as to whether or not the Defendants were negligent by its use and/or whether or not the Defendant had a duty to inform Plaintiff . . . of its use, you may take into consideration the fact that the manufacturer of Marcaine inserted a package insert with the drug . . . warning that "Until further clinical experience is gained, paracervical block with Marcaine is not recommended. Fetal bradycardia frequently follows paracervical block with some amide-type local anesthetics and may be associated with fetal acidosis," and that the *Physician's Desk Reference* for 1980 contained exactly the same warning and that both Defendants were aware of such warning at the time Marcaine was used upon [the plaintiff], but that neither Defendant informed [the plaintiff] of such warning or told her that Marcaine would be used for a paracervical block.

It is the settled general rule that in the absence of an emergency or unanticipated condition, a physician must first obtain the consent of the patient before treating or operating upon him or her.

The relationship between a physician and his patient creates a duty in the physician to disclose to his patient any material information concerning the patient's physical condition and treatment. This duty to inform stems from the fiduciary nature of the relationship and the patient's right to determine what shall or shall not be done with his or her body. The scope of the duty is defined by the materiality of the information in the decisional process of an ordinary individual. If a reasonable person in the position of the patient would consider the information important in choosing a course of treatment, then the information is material and disclosure is required. Once the duty to disclose certain information is established, then the physician's total breach of that duty presents to the jury the question of what damages were proximately caused by the breach of the duty.

Under Utah law, it shall be presumed that what the physician did to or for a patient was either expressly or impliedly authorized to be done. However, this is a rebuttable presumption and a patient may recover damages from a physician based upon the physician's failure to obtain the informed consent of the patient, upon showing [the elements of Utah Code Ann. § 78-14-5(1)].

Bendectin

Hagen v. Richardson-Merrell, Inc. 697 F. Supp. 334 (N.D. Ill. 1988). This suit resulted from a birth defect to the child's hand allegedly caused by exposure of Bendectin while in utero. The defendant moved for summary judgment. The court held that there were material issues of fact as to the cause of the child's ectrodactyly and therefore denied the motion.

The Bendectin was prescribed in June 1976 and was taken by the mother through the fourth month of the pregnancy. The defendant contended that the defect was genetic in nature and that it could not be held liable, as the drug is not a mutagen. The plaintiff contended that the drug was a teratogen which affected limb development.

The court recognized that the plaintiff failed to establish fraud regarding the manufacturer's labeling the drug as safe and destroying fetal specimens, and held that punitive damages were not recoverable. The court determined that the failure of the manufacturer to use premarketing testing was not relevant to such a fraud claim. Falsifying test results was similarly irrelevant when the FDA investigated and concluded that variances in testing were justifiable and further testing was conducted. The court further held that the claim for breach of warranty was time barred. The plaintiff had waited five years after the eight-year statute of repose was adopted before filing the strict liability claims. The eight-year statute was effective to bar such claims.

Hull v. Merrell Dow Pharmaceuticals, 700 F. Supp. 28 (S.D. Fla. 1988). This case involved a defect allegedly caused by the mother's use of Bendectin during pregnancy. The case was removed from state to federal court. The defendant manufacturer then moved for summary judgment, which was granted. The court noted 30 human epidemiological studies finding that Bendectin is not teratogenic, and held that, even if the drug could cause birth defects, its use seven weeks into the pregnancy did not cause the child's extensive leg and foot deformities. The manufacturer claimed that such ingestion was too late in the plaintiff's pregnancy to cause the deformity complained of. The court cited the case of *Lynch v. Merrill-National Laboratories,* 646 F. Supp. 856 (D. Mass. 1986), *aff'd,* 830 F.2d 1190 (1st Cir. 1987), which similarly granted summary judgment for the manufacturer in a case involving a similar limb defect.

Brock v. Merrell Dow Pharmaceuticals, 874 F.2d 307 (5th Cir. 1989), applying Texas law. The child was born with Poland's Syndrome (an absence of fingers or their shortening with a corresponding decrease of the pectoralis muscle) following in utero exposure to Bendectin. The trial court entered judgment for the plaintiff. The appellate court reversed for lack of sufficient epidemiological proof which would establish the essential element of causation, and held that the defendant was entitled to j.n.o.v.

In late July, the mother ingested the drug; the birth occurred in late March. The court found that there is no medical consensus that Bendectin is teratogenic, and also found that the plaintiff failed to trace the etiology of the birth defect to the drug. The court looked to the manner in which causation was established in Agent Orange litigation and also to similar Bendectin cases such as *Richardson v. Richardson-Merrell, Inc.,* 857 F.2d 823

(D.C. Cir. 1988), which affirmed a j.n.o.v. granted for the defendant. The court did recognize, however, that while the lack of epidemiological proof was fatal to this case, that does not mean that such a lack would be fatal to all toxic tort cases.

St. Amand v. Merrell Dow Pharmaceuticals, 140 Misc. 2d 278, 530 N.Y.S.2d 428 (1988). The plaintiff child was born with Pierre-Robin Syndrome, allegedly due to in utero exposure to the defendant's drugs. The mother also claimed that the obstetrician's management of the labor and delivery, coupled with the mother's taking of Bendectin, was the cause of the child's injuries. The manufacturer sought discovery of the mother's medical and employment records in order to discover other potential causes of the condition. The manufacturer was entitled to obtain the medical history of the mother, family history, and genetic factors to determine the etiology of the child's condition and whether such factors caused the syndrome, as opposed to exposure to its drug.

* In a Bendectin case, the plaintiff children, who were exposed to the drug in utero, sued the manufacturer of the drug on claims arising out of their birth defects (limb reductions). The court, in *Daubert v. Merrell Dow Pharmaceuticals, Inc.,* 727 F. Supp. 570 (S.D. Cal. 1989), granted the manufacturer's motion for summary judgment. The court held that the plaintiffs failed to provide any evidence of a causal connection between the injuries suffered and use of the drug by their mothers. The plaintiffs had introduced expert testimony in support of their claims. The court rejected that testimony because the conclusions were based on in vitro, chemical, and animal studies. The court found that the testimony was insufficient, as experts in the field would have relied upon human epidemiological studies. The court also rejected the authority of an unpublished study which failed to conduct its own research but only reinterpreted prior studies. The court reviewed Federal Rule of Evidence 703 and found that the plaintiff's expert testimony failed to establish that the opinion was based on methodology usually relied upon by experts in the field. The court bolstered its decision by citing numerous other Bendectin cases which had also held that there was a lack of sufficient scientific proof of causation. To the same effect, and discussing the same issues, *see Cadarian v. Merrell Dow Pharmaceuticals, Inc.,* 745 F. Supp. 409 (E.D. Mich. 1989).

* In another Bendectin case, a child was born with one finger missing on each hand. The court, in *Wilson v. Merrell Dow Pharmaceuticals, Inc.,* 893 F.2d 1149 (10th Cir. 1990), applying Oklahoma law, affirmed the judgment on the jury verdict for the defendant drug company. The issue presented was whether the trial court should have given a missing-witness instruction, where the manufacturer failed to call a geneticist to testify on causation. The appellate court held that the lower court properly exercised its discretion, as such testimony would have been cumulative. The trial court also properly permitted the use of sales charts which had graphs dealing with the frequency of birth defects in the general population as compared with sales of the drug, since this was a basis for the witness's expert opinion. Any defects in the charts were directed to the weight of such evidence and not its admissibility. The appellate court recognized the vast amount of scientific data which failed to establish a causal connection between the use of the drug and the occurrence of birth defects.

* In *Bernhardt v. Richardson-Merrell, Inc.*, 892 F.2d 440 (5th Cir. 1990), applying Mississippi law, suit was brought for injuries sustained by a child as a result of in utero exposure to Bendectin taken by the mother during pregnancy. The child was born without fingers on one hand. In this case, the mother did not take the drug until the 54th or 55th day of her pregnancy. Medical evidence was introduced to the effect that fingers are found on the human fetus by the 44th day after conception. Therefore, fingers should have been present prior to the mother's use of the drug. Clearly, this destroyed the plaintiff's attempt to establish the required element of causation. The plaintiffs had submitted certified interrogatory answers, but these did not qualify as expert affidavits, which would have been required to counter the defendant's expert evidence. The answers to the interrogatories were, at best, only hearsay references to expert opinions. Thus, this court affirmed the trial court's grant of summary judgment for the defendant.

* *Cosgrove v. Merrell Dow Pharmaceuticals, Inc.*, 117 Idaho 470, 788 P.2d 1293 (1989), is yet another Bendectin suit. In this case, strict liability and negligence claims were brought by the plaintiffs. The trial court entered judgment on the jury verdict, which was affirmed on appeal. The mother brought a claim against the manufacturer, but the manufacturer was properly granted summary judgment on that claim because the suit was filed after the two-year statute of limitations (Idaho Code § 5-219) had run. The child was born without a portion of one arm and hand. The trial court gave the jury a list of special verdict questions. The first question on the list related to causation. The order of questions was not error even though most such lists start with issues of strict liability or negligence.

Accutane

Felix v. Hoffman-La Roche, Inc., 540 So. 2d 102 (Fla. 1989). The plaintiff mother ingested Accutane while pregnant. She sued the manufacturer, claiming that the fetus in utero was killed by her use of the drug. The trial court entered summary judgment for the manufacturer, which was affirmed on appeal (513 So. 2d 1319 (Fla. Dist. Ct. App. 1987)). On appeal to the Florida Supreme Court, the judgment was affirmed, the court holding that a question of law was presented as to the adequacy of the manufacturer's warning, since the warning was unambiguous. The court found that the warning given by the manufacturer to physicians, under the learned intermediary rule, of the dangers to the fetus posed by the use of the drug was sufficient. Even if the warning was inadequate, the use of the drug was not the cause of the defects and the subsequent death of the infant shortly after birth. The warning of the teratogenicity was clear to the physicians who would prescribe the drug, and the plaintiff's physician stated that he understood the nature of the warning. The labeling on the package insert stated that Accutane was for the treatment of cystic acne, and warned as follows:

CONTRAINDICATIONS: Teratogenicity was observed in rats at a dose of isotretinoin of 150 mg/kg/day. In rabbits a dose of 10 mg/kg/day was teratogenic and embryotoxic, and induced abortion. There are not adequate and well-controlled studies in pregnant women. Because teratogenicity has been observed in animals given isotretinoin, patients who are pregnant or intend to become pregnant while undergoing treatment should not receive Accutane. Women of childbearing potential should not be given Accutane unless an effective form of contraception is used, and they should be fully counseled on the potential risks to the fetus should they become pregnant while undergoing treatment. Should pregnancy occur during treatment, the physician and patient should discuss the desirability of continuing the pregnancy.

*   *   *

WARNINGS: Although no abnormalities of human fetus have been reported thus far, animal studies with retinoids suggest that teratogenic effects may occur. It is recommended that contraception be continued for one month or until a normal menstrual period has occurred following discontinuation of Accutane therapy.

*   *   *

PRECAUTIONS: INFORMATION FOR PATIENTS:

*   *   *

Women of childbearing potential should be instructed to use an effective form of contraception when Accutane therapy is required (See CONTRAINDICATIONS AND WARNINGS.)

*   *   *

PREGNANCY: Category X. See "CONTRAINDICATIONS" section.

*   In *Bealer v. Hoffman-La Roche, Inc.*, 729 F. Supp. 43 (E.D. La. 1990), the court granted the manufacturer's motion for summary judgment. The plaintiff had a therapeutic abortion after she learned she was pregnant, because she was taking the drug Accutane, which is associated with a high risk of birth defects. She sued the manufacturer on a claim that the drug was unreasonably unsafe. The court found that the warning was adequate, as a matter of law, where the manufacturer properly gave warnings and information to prescribing physicians. This court also cited other decisions upholding the sufficiency of thy warning. The warning provided (729 F. Supp. at 45):

WARNING TO FEMALE PATIENTS

YOU MUST NOT TAKE ACCUTANE IF YOU ARE OR MAY BECOME PREGNANT DURING TREATMENT

Severe birth defects are known to occur in infants of women taking Accutane during pregnancy. The possibility that you may become pregnant must be ruled out by you and your doctor before you start Accutane therapy. Wait until the second or third day of your next normal menstrual period before beginning Accutane therapy.

An effective form of contraception (birth control) should be discussed with your doctor. Contraception must be used for at least one month before beginning therapy and during therapy, and it must be continued for one month after Accutane treatment has stopped. Immediately stop taking Accutane if you become pregnant while you are taking the drug, and immediately contact your physician to discuss the desirability of continuing the pregnancy.

§ 8.7 – Wrongful Birth Causes of Action

Page 131, add after carryover paragraph:

In *C.S. v. Nielson*, 767 P.2d 504 (Utah 1988), a normal, healthy baby was born. The wife claimed that the defendant failed to tell her that a prior sterilization procedure (a tubal ligation that failed) was not absolute and that there were alternative procedures with varying success rates. The parents sought monetary and emotional damages for the birth of a healthy but unwanted child arising out of the negligent sterilization. The district court certified to the Utah Supreme Court the question of whether there is a viable claim for wrongful pregnancy and what would be the applicable measure of damages for such a tort.

A wrongful birth claim exists when there is a risk of an impaired child who, if the risk had been disclosed, would have been aborted. A wrongful life claim is generally brought by an impaired child for his or her injuries or impairments. This claim, however, was of the wrongful pregnancy variety. Such a claim does not violate Utah Code Ann. §§ 78-11-23 to 78-11-25 (1983), which are decidedly in favor of the right to life, and state that an act or omission preventing abortion is not actionable. Wrongful pregnancy damages include medical expenses, the cost of another sterilization procedure, prenatal care, childbirth and postnatal care, physical and mental pain during pregnancy, lost income, and punitives, if applicable. It is not necessary to attempt to mitigate damages through submitting to an abortion or an adoption. The court did note, though, that the benefits of having a child greatly outweigh the expenses of child bearing.

The following statutes were relied upon by the court in evaluating the available tort claims:

78-11-23. Right to life – State policy.

The Legislature finds and declares that it is the public policy of this state to encourage all persons to respect the right to life of all persons, regardless of age, development, condition or dependency, including all handicapped persons and all unborn persons.

78-11-24. Act or omissions preventing abortion not actionable.

A cause of action shall not arise, and damages shall not be awarded, on behalf of any person, based on the claim that but for the act or omission of another, a person would not have been permitted to have been born alive but would have been aborted.

78-11-25. Failure or refusal to prevent birth not a defense.

The failure or refusal of any person to prevent the live birth of a person shall not be a defense in any action, and shall not be considered in awarding damages or child support, or in imposing a penalty, in any action.

The court also reviewed the informed consent statute, Utah Code Ann. § 78-14-5(1) (1987), with regard to disclosing the nature and potential for failure of the procedure to the plaintiff.

Lininger v. Eisenbaum, 764 P.2d 1202 (Colo. 1988), involved claims for both wrongful birth and wrongful life. The child was born blind. The trial court dismissed the suit and the appellate court affirmed. The Supreme Court of Colorado affirmed in part and reversed in part, holding that the wrongful birth claim was viable whereas the wrongful life claim was properly dismissed. The plaintiff parents claimed that if the defendant physicians had not been negligent in failing to determine that the first child's blindness was hereditary, the parents would not have had this second child. This stated a claim for the recovery of extraordinary medical and educational expenses. The *Lininger* court overruled the decision in *Continental Casualty Co. v. Empire Casualty Co.,* 713 P.2d 384 (Colo. 1986), on the wrongful life claim.

In October 1981, the first child was born, and in March 1982 his vision problems were detected. A pediatric ophthalmologist, neuro-ophthalmologist, and another ophthalmologist each stated that the first child had congenital optic nerve hypoplasia. Therefore, the plaintiffs thought that the blindness might be genetic, but was assured by the defendants that it was not. The plaintiffs thought that another child could help the first child and sought further advice on the possibility that the second child would be born blind. The defendants again stated that the condition was not hereditary. In August 1983, the second child was born and, several months later, was diagnosed as being blind. It was then discovered that the blindness was due to Leber's congenital amaurosis, which is hereditary. The risk of the condition arising in the second child was one in four. The court looked at the blindness as the same type of monetary burden as would occur in any personal injury. There was an extensive review of these torts in other jurisdictions, but the court rejected the wrongful life claim, holding that the defendant's physicians did not owe a duty to the child.

Rinaud v. Biczak, 177 Mich. App. 287, 441 N.W.2d 441 (1989), arose out of the defendant's failure to diagnose the pregnancy of the plaintiff's daughter. The trial court entered judgment for the plaintiff. The court of appeals held that the cost of rearing a healthy, normal child was not recoverable. The plaintiffs were the grandparents and the child's adoptive parents; as such, they could not maintain any cause of action arising out of the alleged negligence. The court, however, recognized the right of appropriate parties to bring the cause of action. The term *wrongful birth* defines the nature of the claim sounding in the lack of diagnosis, the negligent failure to inform of the risk of birth, and the failure which precluded an informed decision on the continuation or termination of the pregnancy. Recovery on such a claim is limited to costs associated with the pregnancy and birth, pain and suffering, and lost wages.

Johnson v. University Hospital, 44 Ohio St. 3d 49, 540 N.E.2d 1370 (1989), was a wrongful pregnancy case arising out of a failed tubal ligation. The trial court granted the defendant's motion to dismiss. The appellate court held that the plaintiff's recovery was limited to the costs associated with the pregnancy. The supreme court affirmed, holding that parents need not take unreasonable steps to mitigate damages – that is, abortion or adoption – in order to retain the right to recover. However, there could be no recovery for the cost of rearing the unwanted but healthy child. The instant claim was different from a wrongful birth claim, which involves the birth of an impaired child, or a wrongful life action, which is brought by the child.

The plaintiff was allowed recovery for medical and hospital costs for prenatal and delivery care and the immediate care of the newborn. The plaintiff could also recover for pain and suffering and the cost of a subsequent sterilization. The arbitration panel recommended a finding for the plaintiff without the recovery for the cost of raising the child, as it is generally held that the cost of raising a child is outweighed by the value of the child's society, love, and so forth. The court cited a variety of cases, including *C.S. v. Nielson,* 767 P.2d 504 (Utah 1988).

Butler v. Rolling Hill Hospital, 382 Pa. Super. 317, 555 A.2d 205 (1989), arose out of the birth of an unwanted child. The plaintiff claimed that the defendant was negligent in failing to make a timely diagnosis that she was pregnant. The trial court granted summary judgment for the defendants, which decision was affirmed on appeal. The appellate court held that 42 Pa. Cons. Stat. Ann. § 8305 (1988) effectively precludes such a wrongful birth case sounding in the failure to detect a pregnancy which thereby destroys the mother's ability to have an abortion. The plaintiff's attempt to challenge the constitutionality of retroactive application of the statute was defeated by the failure to properly notify the attorney general of the constitutionality challenge.

The plaintiff, who had undergone a tubal ligation two years prior to the pregnancy, went to the family physician about a swelling in her breasts, an empty feeling, and weight gain. The physician did not order a pregnancy test either then or when she requested one two months later. The child was born healthy. The suit sought all the damages attendant to the pregnancy and delivery as well as child-rearing expenses.

The applicable statute provides:

> (a) *Wrongful birth.* – There shall be no cause of action or award of damages on behalf of any person based on a claim that, but for an act or omission of the defendant, a person once conceived would not or should not have been born. Nothing contained in this subsection shall be construed to prohibit any cause of action or award of damages for the wrongful death of a woman, or on account of physical injury suffered by a woman or child, as a result of an attempted abortion. Nothing contained in this subsection shall be construed to provide a defense against any proceeding charging a health care practitioner with intentional misrepresentations under [citations omitted], or any other act regulating the professional practices of health care practitioners.
>
> (b) *Wrongful life.* – There shall be no cause of action on behalf of any person based on a claim of that person, that, but for an act or omission of the defendant, the person would not have been conceived or, once conceived, would or should have been aborted.
>
> (c) *Conception.* – A person shall be deemed to be conceived at the moment of fertilization.

*   *Hatter v. Landsberg*, 259 Pa. Super. 438, 563 A.2d 146 (1989), was a wrongful conception case. The plaintiffs brought suit arising out of a failed tubal ligation procedure. The trial court granted summary judgment for the physician. On appeal, the court affirmed in part and reversed in part. The court was required to consider 42 Pa. Cons. Stat. § 8305. The court interpreted that statute as prohibiting the child's claim for wrongful life, but not the claim of the parents for their out-of-pocket expenses and pain and suffering. The court found that the statutory provisions with regard to wrongful birth were ambiguous, and interpreted them as not posing a bar to the parents' wrongful conception claim arising out of the failed sterilization.

In *Wofford v. Davis*, 764 P.2d 161 (Okla. 1988), the plaintiff parents sought to sue the physician for negligence in the performance of a sterilization followed by the birth of a healthy but unwanted child. The trial court dismissed the claim for the cost of raising the child. That holding was affirmed by the Oklahoma Supreme Court. The court further held that the three-year statute of limitations in the medical malpractice statute was unconstitutional, because the special statute of limitations for malpractice was an impermissible special law in contravention of Okla. Const. art. 5, §§ 46, 59. The court found that such claims for the cost of raising a healthy child would be contrary to public policy. Citing *Morris v. Sanchez*, 746 P.2d 184 (Okla. 1987), the court stated (764 P.2d at 162):

> As a matter of public policy, the birth of a normal and healthy child does not constitute a legal harm for which damages are recoverable. We recognize

89

wrongful death actions because of the great value we place on human life. Conversely, we cannot recognize actions for wrongful birth or wrongful conception of a normal, healthy child. The birth of a normal, healthy child may be one of the consequences of a negligently performed sterilization, but we hold that it is not a legal wrong for which damages should or may be awarded.

In *Goforth v. Porter Medical Associates,* 755 P.2d 678 (Okla. 1988), the plaintiffs brought suit arising out of a failed sterilization procedure. The plaintiff was sterilized in August 1980 and was assured that she was sterile. She delivered the child in October 1981. They sought recovery of their medical expenses and the expenses of raising the child due to the defendants' negligence in performing the procedure. The Oklahoma Supreme Court held that they could recover medical costs associated with the pregnancy, lost wages, and similar damages, but were not entitled to recover under the claim for the cost of raising the healthy, normal, but unwanted child who was born. The Oklahoma court followed its prior decision in *Morris v. Sanchez,* 746 P.2d 184 (Okla. 1987), which adopted the reasoning in *Byrd v. Wesley Medical Center,* 237 Kan. 215, 699 P.2d 459 (1985).

In *Owens v. Foote,* 773 S.W.2d 911 (Tenn. 1989), a baby was born with Down's Syndrome. The parents sued the surgeon who had previously performed a vasectomy on the husband. They sought to recover the costs attendant to the pregnancy and delivery, accompanying medical expenses, and the cost of another vasectomy. The plaintiffs also sought to recover the additional expenses of raising such a child and for their emotional distress attendant to the birth of the Down's Syndrome child. The Tennessee Supreme Court held that damages could be recovered for emotional distress, despite the lower court holding that the emotional distress and cost of child rearing were not compensable. The supreme court recognized that the plaintiffs were required to prove causation between any act or omission on the part of the defendant and the damages sustained. The instant complaint, though it failed to state such elements of proximate causation, could be remedied by a proper amendment. The claim was essentially one for wrongful pregnancy, which is recognized in most jurisdictions.

In *Marciniak v. Lundborg,* 147 Wis. 2d 556, 433 N.W.2d 617 (Ct. App. 1988), the plaintiff parents sued the defendant clinic over a failed sterilization procedure. The court of appeals reversed the lower court holding in favor of the plaintiffs. The appellate court, consistent with other jurisdictions, held that, in such a situation, the plaintiffs could not recover the cost of raising a healthy child. This is also consistent with a majority view of public policy and a recognition of the wide-ranging benefits attendant to raising a child. The court recognized that it would not be proper to "exonerate a physician who negligently diagnoses pregnancy thus preventing an abortion, while holding another physician liable for failing to prevent a pregnancy through sterilization." 433 N.W.2d at 618. The plaintiffs should be entitled, however, to recover the medical and similar expenses incurred related to the pregnancy and delivery.

* *Burke v. Rivo,* 406 Mass. 764, 551 N.E.2d 1 (1990), was a case brought for the birth of a healthy child following a failed sterilization operation. The defendant physician recommended a bipolar cauterization after the plaintiff expressed her desire not to have any more children. The procedure was performed. Sixteen months later, a pregnancy test confirmed that she was pregnant, and she later gave birth to her fourth child. The day after the birth, she underwent a bilateral salpingectomy sterilization procedure. The plaintiffs alleged that, had they been told of the risk of canalization from the bipolar cauterization, they would have chosen another sterilization procedure. The trial court reported questions to the appellate court, which transferred the case to the Massachusetts Supreme Court. The court held that the parents could recover the cost of raising the child to adulthood, reasoning that this was proper where the parents had sought the sterilization in order to avoid having additional children for economic reasons. The court held that this was the proper measure of damages in a case in which a sterilization is negligently performed, or in which a physician fails to disclose the chance of failure of the procedure so that another procedure might be selected. In addition to the costs associated with raising the child, the plaintiffs could recover the loss of the wife's earning capacity, medical expenses for the delivery, the cost of another sterilization procedure, and other consequential expenses. The husband could recover for the loss of consortium. The wife could recover for the pain and suffering attendant to being pregnant and giving birth. There also were valid claims for emotional distress arising from the fact of the unwanted pregnancy.

* It should be noted that this case runs counter to most decisions in other states. Most courts would allow the recovery of damages for these elements with the exception of the cost of raising the healthy child. It is generally held that, as a matter of public policy, the benefits of having such a child greatly outweigh the attendant costs.

* On the same day that it decided the *Burke* case, the Massachusetts Supreme Court decided *Viccaro v. Milunsky,* 406 Mass. 777, 551 N.E.2d 8 (1990). In that case, a child was born with anhidrotic ectodermal dysplasia. The child brought a wrongful life claim against the physician for negligence in genetic counseling of the parents. The parents also brought a claim for wrongful birth. The parents had consulted with the defendant genetics specialist to determine the possibility that the wife was a carrier of the genetic disorder ectodermal dysplasia. The defendant determined that she was not a carrier and had no risk of giving birth to children afflicted with the disease. The parents had one child who was healthy. This case arose from the birth of their second child, who was severely afflicted. The court held that Massachusetts recognizes the tort of wrongful birth arising under the

facts of this case. The damages in such a case were the extraordinary expenses attendant to raising a child with such a condition. The parents could recover such costs beyond the time the child would reach the age of majority, upon a showing that the child would still be dependent on them and they would still be liable for his support. The court held that the parents were entitled to recover for their emotional distress, but that any such amounts could be subject to an offset for the emotional benefits attributable to the first child and any emotional benefits which might be attributable to the affected child. The court rejected the claim for wrongful life, however. This case follows the decision in the *Burke* case and is consistent with decisions in many other jurisdictions, which allow the recovery of extraordinary costs associated with raising a child with genetic defects.

* In *Atlanta Obstetrics & Gynecology Group, P.A. v. Abelson,* 195 Ga. App. 274, 392 S.E.2d 916 (1990), the parents sued the physicians for wrongful birth arising out of the birth of a child afflicted with Down's Syndrome. The plaintiffs claimed that the physicians were negligent in failing to advise them of the increased risk of genetic defects associated with bearing children at age 36. They also claimed that the defendants should have performed an amniocentesis, which would have detected the genetic defect. The plaintiffs alleged that, had there been an amniocentesis, it would have detected the defect and they would have aborted the pregnancy. The trial court denied the defendants' motion to dismiss. The appellate court affirmed in part and reversed in part. The court held that the plaintiffs had a valid wrongful birth claim pursuant to Ga. Code § 51-1-27, because they could demonstrate that they would have had a legal abortion upon learning the results of the amniocentesis. The damages available for such a claim are the extraordinary costs of raising a defective child. The plaintiffs could only recover the additional costs attributable to the defect for the period of the child's life expectancy, which corresponded to the remaining life expectancy of the parents. The court further held that any emotional benefits derived from the child were not to be offset against the other recoverable damages. However, the parents' emotional distress arising from the pregnancy and birth were not compensable.

* In *Shelton v. St. Anthony's Medical Center,* 781 S.W.2d 48 (Mo. 1989), the plaintiff went to the defendants for ultrasound tests on her developing child. The plaintiff sued the defendants for their failure to properly read and interpret the ultrasound pictures. They failed to determine that the child was developing without arms and with other severe defects. The trial court dismissed the complaint, and that dismissal was affirmed on appeal. The Missouri Supreme Court reversed and remanded the case. The court held that Mo. Ann. Stat. §§ 188.130.2 and 516.105 applied to the case. The statute bars claims based on allegations that "but for the negligence of the defendant the child would not have been born." That statute was applicable where the child was conceived prior to the effective date of the statute but was born after the effective date. Section 188.130.2 provides: "No person shall maintain a cause of action or receive an award of damages based on the claim that but for the negligent conduct of another, a child would have been aborted." However, the mother, who could not bring a wrongful birth claim, could still pursue a claim for emotional distress arising out of the failure to inform. Such an emotional distress claim was not precluded by the statute.

§ 8.9   –Wrongful Life: Damages and Claimants

Page 134, add to footnote 30:

In Cowe v. Forum Group, 541 N.E.2d 962 (Ind. Ct. App. 1989), the plaintiff child brought a wrongful life suit alleging negligence and other prenatal torts against the nursing home responsible for the care of his mother. The trial court granted summary judgment for the defendant. The appellate court reversed, finding that there were genuine issues of material fact which required jury determination.

The child sought to recover cost of his support. The court found that such might be reasonable in a wrongful life suit, but only for the period from the date of birth until the date of the child's adoption. Once adopted, the adoptive parents were responsible for the child's support. The wrongful life claim alleged that, but for the negligence in a procedure other than an abortion, which was intended to prevent the birth of a defective child, the child would not have been born to experience pain and suffering arising out of his deformity. The court stated that there could be no wrongful life recovery for the negligent performance of an abortion. However, the wrongful life claim existed where the mother, who allegedly was raped by another patient, was so severely mentally and physically impaired that she could not affirmatively decide to have or care for the child. The private nursing home had the duty to provide reasonable care for the woman and prevent her rape and subsequent pregnancy. This, however, raised questions of fact as to the existence and breach of such a duty and the existence of a causal connection to the child plaintiff.

The child, who was suffering from fetal hydantoin syndrome, could potentially have recovered the cost of his support had he not been adopted less than one year after his birth. There was also a question of fact as to whether the child was physically injured due to the negligence of the defendant, arising out of the administration of the drug Dilantin to the mother while the child was in utero. The claim also sounded in the failure of the defendant to provide prenatal care in the first five months of fetal life. The court recognized that although the tort of wrongful life has not yet been recognized in Indiana, courts previously had only reviewed such claims in the context of ineffective abortions. The court cited with approval the cases

of Harbeson v. Parke-Davis, 98 Wash. 2d 460, 656 P.2d 483 (1982) and
Procanik v. Cillo, 97 N.J. 339, 478 A.2d 755 (1984).

* The plaintiff child was born with profound defects, and sought to recover
on a claim of wrongful life against the defendants for their failure to inform
the mother properly. Such information would have led her to terminate the
pregnancy. The mother went to an osteopathic physician for obstetrical care.
She contracted rubella during the first trimester. She claimed that the
defendants failed to perform the appropriate laboratory tests which would
have detected the measles; upon learning that she had rubella, she would
have been informed of the risks to the fetus and would have aborted the
pregnancy. The Arizona Supreme Court discussed the various concepts of
wrongful conception and wrongful birth claims in order to distinguish them
from the wrongful life claim involved in this case. The wrongful life claim is
one brought by the child against the physician or other health care provider
responsible for the birth, in this case, of a profoundly impaired child. In
Walker v. Mart, 164 Ariz. 37, 790 P.2d 735 (1990), the court held that the
child had no viable wrongful life claim. The court found that, at least under
these facts, the physician owed a duty to the mother and not to the child.
Therefore, the parents had a wrongful birth claim, but the child had no tort
claim against the physician. The court recognized that the physician had the
duty to inform the parents of the risk to the fetus, and that he could be held
liable if the failure to detect the condition and so warn the mother was a
breach of the standard of care.

* In Keselman v. Kingsboro Medical Group, 156 A.D.2d 334, 548 N.Y.S.2d
287 (1989), a child was born with omphalecele, and died within a few hours
after birth. The plaintiffs claimed that the genetic anomaly resulted in
physical pain to both mother and child and emotional distress to the parents.
The plaintiffs also claimed that, had they been advised that the child was
genetically defective, they would have opted for other medical procedures.
The court held that the plaintiffs failed to allege a viable cause of action for
wrongful life. The court held that the plaintiffs were not entitled to recover
emotional distress damages, because they sustained no independent physical
harm. The fact that the mother had moderate bleeding subsequent to the
birth did not constitute a sufficient physical injury. The informed consent
claims were rejected because they did not arise from a violation of the
mother's physical integrity.

CHAPTER 9

PRENATAL CARE

§ 9.1 Introduction

Page 139, add after first paragraph:

Care must be taken in such examinations, as the health of both mother and child is at stake. In *Henderson v. North,* 545 So. 2d 486 (Fla. Dist. Ct. App. 1989), the plaintiffs brought a malpractice action against the physician and hospital for negligence in the diagnosis of the wife's condition, which resulted in the performance of allegedly unnecessary surgery that caused the termination of her pregnancy. The trial court granted the defendants' motion for summary judgment. The appellate court affirmed in part and reversed in part, holding that the allegations of negligence resulting in the termination of the pregnancy were essentially a claim for the wrongful death of a fetus, which is not recognized by Florida law. The erroneous diagnosis involved discovery of a tumor in the womb, and the pregnancy was terminated due to the performance of a biopsy. The plaintiff parents had no viable claim for their pain and suffering associated with the termination of the pregnancy, but could properly pursue a traditional malpractice claim for the pain suffered by the patient and the associated mental suffering, coupled with medical expenses and amounts for loss of consortium on the part of the husband.

§ 9.6 Subsequent Prenatal Examinations

Page 146, add at the end of the section:

In *Madsen v. Park Nicollet Medical Center,* 431 N.W.2d 855 (Minn. 1988), the plaintiff father sued the medical center and the physician for injuries sustained by his premature son. Judgment was entered for the defendants, but on appeal was reversed and remanded. The court held that informed consent does not require the attending physician to disclose the availability of similar treatment or all of the potential risks of injury arising out of the rejection of supplemental treatments. The defendant physician decided to manage the pregnancy in the home setting as opposed to a hospital setting, and did not insist that the mother undergo hospitalization three days before the premature birth. The court found that this was not a choice between alternative treatments, and therefore there was no duty to disclose the risk of additional or alternative treatments.

There was also a claim that the defendant failed to disclose the risk of a premature birth which would have affected the mother's decisions. It had been detected that the mother was leaking amniotic fluid, and an ultrasound had been taken. The mother started bleeding and was sent to a hospital which had no neonatal unit (no hospitals with the necessary neonatal units existed in the area). She was then taken by air ambulance to a hospital with appropriate facilities. The child was born with severe and permanent disabilities: blindness in one eye, spastic quadriplegia, cerebral palsy, and neurological disorders. The court separated the informed consent issue from the claims of negligence in treatment or the failure to diagnose, while remanding on the former issue.

Often serious conditions can be prevented, or their effect mitigated, with proper prenatal examinations and treatment. *Footit v. Monsees,* 26 Mass. App. Ct. 173, 525 N.E.2d 423 (1988), was a wrongful death action for the death of the mother and the unborn child. The trial court entered judgment on the verdict for the defendant, which judgment was affirmed on appeal. The jury answers (that neither physician was negligent in the treatment of the mother or unborn child) were dispositive as to the physicians' liability and rendered immaterial confusing answers to other special questions. The defendants were two board-certified obstetrician-gynecologists who practiced as a professional corporation. The suit claimed that they failed to diagnose the mother's medical condition properly and failed to perform appropriate tests or refer the patient to an internist or cardiologist for treatment.

The mother, who suffered from coronary artery disease, had regular prenatal examinations. The child was due in April 1983. In late December 1982, she had severe nausea and vomiting, but otherwise the pregnancy was normal. In early April, she had difficulty breathing and severe nausea and diarrhea. Three days later, she had further difficulty breathing, and was examined by the defendant who listened to the baby's heart and the mother's lungs and performed a pelvic exam, but never listened to the mother's heart. The defendant said that she had flu-like symptoms. Four days later, an exam showed that labor was imminent, but the defendant did not consider performing a cesarean, as the pelvic exam showed favorable for a vaginal delivery. Two days later, the mother was taken to the hospital with severe breathing problems. The fetus died and was removed by cesarean section. The wife encountered severe heart problems and died.

Such facts presented issues for the jury to consider with regard to liability. The jury questions were straightforward and dealt with the liability of each physician. With respect to each physician, the questions were:

Was the defendant Dr. _____, negligent with respect to his duty to . . . [Mrs. Footit]?
Was the negligence, if any, of Dr. _____ the proximate cause of the illness and death of . . . [Mrs. Footit]?

> Was the defendant Dr. _____, negligent with respect to the unborn child of . . . [Mrs. Footit]?
>
> Was the negligence, if any, of Dr. _____ the proximate cause of the death of the unborn child of . . . [Mrs. Footit]?

The jury answered "no" to all questions, and judgment was entered on the verdict for the defendants. The court ignored the answers to allegedly confusing special questions.

In *Scafidi v. Seiler*, 225 N.J. Super. 576, 543 A.2d 95 (App. Div. 1988), the plaintiffs claimed that the negligence of the defendant physician resulted in the premature birth and subsequent death of the baby. The complaint sought recovery of wrongful death damages for the injuries sustained during the life of the child. The jury found that the physician was negligent in treating the infant and mother but that any such negligence was not the cause of the injuries and death. The appellate court reversed and remanded for a new trial, while holding that a jury question was presented as to whether the risk of premature birth was increased by the defendant's negligence and whether this was a substantial factor in producing the death. The court recognized that, in such cases, the plaintiff has the burden of proving the standard of care, its breach, and causation. The increased risk of harm can satisfy the causation requirement.

In this case, the mother was seven months pregnant. She visited the obstetrician because of heavy bleeding. The obstetrician told her to rest. The next day, the mother had cramping but the obstetrician was unavailable. A covering physician prescribed medicine and told her to keep her appointment with the obstetrician on the next day. The medicine, taken orally, is ineffective to arrest premature labor. The next day, the defendant obstetrician tried to arrest the labor but used unacceptable therapy with the same drug. There was a deviation from the proper standard of care in not immediately hospitalizing the mother. The case was remanded for proof of damages.

In *Shelton v. St. Anthony's Medical Center*, 781 S.W.2d 48 (Mo. 1989), the plaintiff went to the defendants for ultrasound tests on her developing child. The plaintiff sued the defendants for their failure to properly read and interpret the ultrasound pictures. They failed to determine that the child was developing without arms and with other severe defects. The trial court dismissed the complaint, and that dismissal was affirmed on appeal. The Missouri Supreme Court reversed and remanded the case. The court held that Mo. Ann. Stat. §§ 188.130.2 and 516.105 applied to the case. One statute bars claims based on allegations that "but for the negligence of the defendant the child would not have been born." That statute was applicable when the child was conceived prior to the effective date of the statute but born after the effective date. However, the mother, who could not bring a wrongful birth claim, could still pursue a claim for emotional distress arising out of the failure to inform. Such an emotional distress claim was not precluded by the statute, § 188.130.2, which provides: "No person shall maintain a cause of action or receive an award of damages based on the claim that but for the negligent conduct of another, a child would have been aborted."

* Elsewhere, a plaintiff sued a hospital and physicians arising out of alleged negligent management of the plaintiff's pregnancy which resulted in a miscarriage. The plaintiff suffered from hypertension, which condition required special treatment and attention. The trial court dismissed the complaint as failing to state a claim. The appellate court, in *Coughling v. George Washington University Health Plan, Inc.*, 565 A.2d 67 (D.C. 1989), reversed. The court held that the plaintiff was entitled to be treated in a nonnegligent manner. The failure of the defendants to exercise the appropriate standard of care could support recovery without regard to whether there was a cause of action for the negligence that resulted in the injury to a viable fetus. The plaintiff's complaint alleged injuries that she actually sustained and not a wrongful death claim for loss of the fetus. The court further held that the plaintiff properly alleged a physical impact so as to support a claim for negligent infliction of emotional distress. The negligent treatment resulted in preeclampsia, which increased the plaintiff's risk of injury and destroyed her placenta. As a result of the negligence, she was required to submit to two painful procedures to remove the dead fetus from her uterus. Such allegations were sufficient to state a claim.

§ 9.8 Genetic Counseling

Page 152, add after third full paragraph:

Similarly, the presence of a genetic defect in a first child must be considered by the physician and disclosed to the parents who are concerned about the possibility of recurrence of the defect in a subsequently conceived child. In *Pratt v. University of Minnesota Affiliated Hospitals*, 414 N.W.2d 399 (Minn. 1987), the genetically defective child sued the hospitals for negligent nondisclosure occurring in the course of genetic counseling given to the parents. The trial court granted summary judgment for the defendant. The appellate court reversed at 403 N.W.2d 865 (Minn. Ct. App. 1987). The Minnesota Supreme Court reversed the appellate court, holding that the diagnosis of a genetic condition following the performance of tests does not trigger a duty to disclose the risks attendant to other conditions which were not diagnosed. The defendants could not be held liable where they had properly employed all available tests, exercised the requisite standard of care in making their diagnosis, and then fully disclosed their findings to the parents. There was no expert testimony as to whether the defendants violated the standard of care or as to whether the failure to disclose the undiagnosed condition was a breach of the standard of care.

The plaintiff parents sought genetic counseling to see if the birth defects of their third child were genetic. Their other children were normal. The plaintiffs wanted to find out if there was a risk of conceiving other genetically defective children. Two physicians examined the child and determined that the third child did not fit into a defined syndrome. The chromosome study was normal. The defendants concluded that the birth defects were of unknown origin and were unlikely to recur. The plaintiffs were told that their chance of conceiving another defective child was the same as that of other parents in the general public. The defendants failed to diagnose the child's autosomal recessive condition which had a 25 percent chance of recurrence. The subsequent child was also genetically defective. The court looked to the case of *Karlson v. Guerinat*, 57 A.D.2d 73, 394 N.Y.S.2d 933 (1977), which addressed the same issue. This court applied the general rule enunciated in that case.

Page 154, add after carryover paragraph:

In *Corley v. Commonwealth Edison Co.*, 703 F. Supp. 748 (N.D. Ill. 1989), the plaintiffs sued their employer for severe birth defects suffered by the plaintiffs' children. The defendant employer moved for summary judgment, claiming that the essence of the claim was one not recognized by Illinois law. The tort of wrongful birth is only available when the negligence results in depriving the parents of a meaningful, informed decision between abortion or birth of a genetically defective baby. The birth defects in question were allegedly caused by the employee's exposure to chemical and radiation leaks. The claim was not viable where the employer did not provide genetic testing or counseling. However, the court recognized the viability of such a claim upon proper circumstances, which were absent in this case.

CHAPTER 10

TECHNIQUES TO EVALUATE FETAL HEALTH

§ 10.2 Antepartum Assessment of Fetal Well-Being

Page 159, add after the third full paragraph:

Many obstetricians prefer nipple stimulation to oxytocin as a means of stimulating the uterus to contract for purposes of evaluation of the fetal status. Nipple stimulation avoids the potentially stressful effects of oxytocin, which is especially important if the body is already in a sick uterine environment (a condition of borderline fetal oxygenation). The contraction stress test (nipple or oxytocin stimulation) is considered to be positive if persistent late deceleration occurs; late decelerations indicate fetal distress and mandate as expeditious a delivery of the fetus as is medically permissible. A negative CST is reassuring, but the reassurance is only temporary in a high risk pregnancy–that is, the test should be repeated weekly.

§ 10.4 – Amniocentesis: Uses

Page 165, add at the end of "Genetic Aberrations" subsection:

The importance of amniocentesis was discussed in *Wilson v. Kuenzi*, 751 S.W.2d 741 (Mo. 1988), a wrongful life and wrongful birth suit arising from the defendant's failure to inform the parents of the possible use of amniocentesis to determine the presence of Down's Syndrome in their unborn child. The trial court dismissed the claim and was affirmed on appeal. The Missouri Supreme Court also affirmed, holding that the statute (Mo. Ann. Stat. § 188.130(1) (Vernon 1986)), precluding claims for wrongful life and wrongful birth, did not apply retroactively and that the causes of action asserted were not recognized in the state prior to the statute.

The mother was age 36 at conception; there is a 1 in 300 risk of a Down's Syndrome child for women that age. The plaintiffs claimed that if she had been told of the test or if the test had been performed, she would have had the opportunity to abort the fetus, which she would have done. The court assumed that it would be proper practice to advise of the test, but still found that no enforceable cause of action. The relevant statute provides:

1. No person shall maintain a cause of action or receive an award of damages on behalf of himself or herself based on the claim that but for the negligent conduct of another, he or she would have been aborted.

2. No person shall maintain a cause of action or receive an award of damages based on the claim that but for the negligent conduct of another, a child would have been aborted.

The court discussed the difference between the wrongful life and wrongful birth causes of actions, and recognized the multiplicity of authority for such claims, but chose to disregard such authority. It cited Note, *Wrongful Birth Actions: The Case Against Legislative Curtailment,* 100 Harv. L. Rev. 2017 (1987), which lists authority in the following jurisdictions as recognizing a cause of action for wrongful birth: Alabama, California, Florida, Illinois, Maine, Michigan, New Hampshire, New Jersey, New York, North Carolina, Pennsylvania, South Carolina, Texas, Virginia, Washington, West Virginia, and Wisconsin.

*

§ 10.5 – Amniocentesis: Safety

Page 168, add after carryover paragraph:

In *Azarbal v. Medical Center,* 724 F. Supp. 279 (D. Del. 1989), the plaintiff parents sued the medical center and physicians under claims of a lack of informed consent. The physician performed amniocentesis on the plaintiff wife. It was alleged that, during the procedure, the needle penetrated the skull of the fetus and damaged the baby's brain. Immediately following the birth by cesarean section, the physician performed a tubal ligation. The baby died less than eight months after the birth, because of the brain damage. Suit was filed exactly two years after the date of amniocentesis. The complaint sounded in negligence in the performance of the amniocentesis procedure. The plaintiffs later attempted to amend the complaint to include claims for a lack of informed consent relating to the amniocentesis and to the sterilization procedure. They also sought to add counts against the hospital for post-birth negligence in failing to detect and treat the baby's condition. The court granted the motion to amend the complaint. The issue presented was whether the statute of limitations had run on the informed consent claims so as to defeat the attempt to amend the complaint to allege such new causes of action. The court held that the two-year limitations period (Del. Code Ann. tit. 18, § 6856) was applicable to the informed consent claim and that the period began to run on the date of the amniocentesis. The court found that the informed consent claims related back to the date of the filing of the complaint and therefore were not time barred. The court held that the original complaint gave sufficient notice to the defendant that the claims arose from the amniocentesis. The court further found that the claim for punitive damages arising from the defendant's actual or constructive knowledge of the fetal injury prior to the performance of the tubal ligation was sufficient, if proved, to support the imposition of punitive damages.

* ## § 10.7 – Ultrasound: Uses

Page 170, add following first paragraph:

In *Shelton v. St. Anthony's Medical Center,* 781 S.W.2d 48 (Mo. 1989), the plaintiff went to the defendants for ultrasound tests on her developing child. The plaintiff sued the defendants for their failure to properly read and interpret the ultrasound pictures. They failed to determine that the child was developing without arms and with other severe defects. The trial court dismissed the complaint, and that dismissal was affirmed on appeal. The Missouri Supreme Court reversed and remanded the case. The court held that Mo. Ann. Stat. §§ 188.130.2 and 516.105 applied to the case. One statute bars claims based on allegations that "but for the negligence of the defendant the child would not have been born." That statute was applicable when the child was conceived prior to the effective date of the statute but born after the effective date. However, the mother, who could not bring a wrongful birth claim, could still pursue a claim for emotional distress arising out of the failure to inform. Such an emotional distress claim was not precluded by the statute, § 188.130.2, which provides: "No person shall maintain a cause of action or receive an award of damages based on the claim that but for the negligent conduct of another, a child would have been aborted."

* ## § 10.9 Fetal Heart Rate Monitoring

Page 178, add at the end of the section:

The plaintiffs brought suit arising out of the death of a fetus in utero. The plaintiff mother was under the care of the defendants and claimed that the defendant clinic failed promptly and properly to notify her obstetrician that fetal distress was occurring. The court granted the defendants' motion for summary judgment, holding that there was no evidence that any delay in alerting the physician to the loss of fetal heart tones was the cause of the fetus's death. There was evidence that the child was brain dead within a few minutes of the loss of heart tone, substantially before a cesarean section could be performed. *Switzer v. Newton Health Care Corp.,* 734 F. Supp. 954 (D. Kan. 1990).

In another case, the plaintiff parents alleged that a child was injured during his birth. The child allegedly was in fetal distress prior to the delivery, and this resulted in oxygen deprivation and brain damage. The plaintiffs claimed that the defendants failed to conduct adequate fetal heart monitoring, which could have prevented the injuries complained of. The court, in *Gillis v. United States*, 722 F. Supp. 713 (M.D. Fla. 1989), dismissed the case. The court recognized that the hospital had a duty to monitor the fetal heart rate. The mother had had an enema and was in the bathroom for a considerable period following her admission to the hospital. Upon admission, it was determined that the fetus was in stable condition. Subsequently, when the monitor was applied following the enema, the fetus was found to be experiencing late deceleration, and action was immediately taken. The question was whether the 50-minute delay in using the monitor after the initial examination constituted a breach of the duty of care. The court found that the standard of care required monitoring at least every 30 minutes. However, the bulk of the 50-minute period was taken up by the enema, during which time there could be no monitoring. The court found that there was no breach of duty; even if there was such a breach, it was not the cause of the oxygen deprivation which resulted in the injuries complained of.

§ 10.13 – Early Decelerations

Page 179, add at the end of the section:

Early decelerations usually are associated with benign fetal head compression (head compression stimulates the vagus nerve, which slows the fetal heart). However, there is some evidence that early decelerations may be associated with cord compression. Early decelerations that are severe and repetitive, especially in the company of meconium or other warning signs of fetal distress (e.g., tachycardia, late or variable decelerations), may induce early delivery. J. Pritchard & P. MacDonald, *Williams Obstetrics* 287 (15th ed. 1976).

§ 10.16 – Beat-to-Beat Variability

Page 184, add at the end of the section:

Diminished beat-to-beat variability is an ominous sign of fetal distress. Absent beat-to-beat variability (flat line instead of jagged appearance) is a red flag warning of impending fetal death. Internal fetal heart monitoring provides accurate recognition of beat-to-beat variability. External fetal heart monitoring does not allow accurate beat-to-beat fetal heart rate evaluation.

§ 10.17A Paper Speed in Electronic Fetal Heart Monitoring (New)

Many electronic fetal heart monitors currently in use in hospitals have the capability of recording fetal heart patterns and uterine contractions at either 1 cm/min or 3 cm/min. As early as 1975, the American College of Obstetricians and Gynecologists (ACOG) cautioned against the use of the slower paper speed for monitoring active labor. ACOG *Technical Bulletin No. 32* (June 1975) properly observed that pattern recognition is "difficult if not impossible" at the slow paper speed of 2 cm/min. and that, "where FHR abnormalities arise, the faster paper speeds will enhance FHR pattern recognition."

Practice Note. The author is presently involved in two cases in which the fetal heart monitor was set at the slower paper speed. In both cases, the plaintiff contends that the labor and delivery nurses were unable to recognize late and variable decelerations because of the compressing effect of the slow paper speed on these abnormal tracings. Also, in both cases, the manufacturer of the monitor has been joined as a defendant – the contention being that the manufacturer was negligent in equipping the machine with the 1 cm/min. speed switch and in not warning the operators of the equipment (nurses and physicians) that the slower paper speed should not be used to monitor active labors (especially not high-risk labors).

The only explanation for the 1 cm/min. feature is that, at the slower speed, less paper is used. This results in a cost savings of a few dollars and the added benefit of less cumbersome storage problems. However, when placed beside the cost of caring for a brain-damaged infant whose fetal distress was undetected because of the slow paper speed, there is no comparison, no justification, and no excuse for equipping monitors with the slow paper switch.

§ 10.17B Electronic Fetal Heart Monitor Tracings: Legal Issues (New)

The Nurses Association of the American College of Obstetricians and Gynecologists (NAACOG), in its *Technical Bulletin No. 7* (July 1980), made the following recommendation relative to the legal aspects of fetal heart monitor tracings and their storage:

> The fetal heart monitor tracings are a part of the patient's record and must be kept and maintained by the institution. The monitor tracings should include the patient's name, hospital number and the date and time of admission and delivery

in the case of intrapartum monitoring. The fetal monitor tracings are bulky and can take up space in the patient's medical record, making it cumbersome in medical record departments.

Each institution must determine its own system of storage for the monitor tracings *and assure their accessibility and availability.* The most acceptable solution to this problem is the microfilming of the entire tracing. Microfilming is expensive, however, and may be prohibitive in some institutions.

Emphasis added.

Practice Note. In connection with the fetal heart monitor, plaintiff's counsel should request production of (1) the fetal heart monitor strips; (2) the operating manual provided by the manufacturer for operations of the equipment; and (3) hospital protocol, rules, and instructions relating to indictions for use of fetal heart monitoring equipment. Counsel may also wish to consider a motion to allow inspection of the equipment in the event there is a concern about whether the machine was in proper working order at the time of the incident.

The sixth edition of *Standards for Obstetric-Gynecologic Services* (1985) has been released. There are several significant changes from previous additions of the ACOG standards. Perhaps the most interesting addition to the standards appears under the heading "Labor Surveillance": "Electronic fetal monitoring is highly sensitive but has low specificity; therefore, on the basis of fetal heart rate patterns alone, definitive cause and effect relationships between patterns and long-term outcome cannot be determined." This language bears a strong resemblance to the comments contained in the 1985 National Institutes of Health Study, *Prenatal and Perinatal Factors Associated with Brain Disorders* § 2.1 (NIH Publication No. 85-1149, U.S. Department of Health and Human Services, April 1985 relating to the accuracy of fetal heart monitoring as a diagnostic and prognostic modality.

§ 10.17C Role of the Nurse in Electronic Fetal Monitoring (New)

In 1979, the Committee on Obstetrics: Maternal and Fetal Medicine of The American College of Obstetricians and Gynecologists developed guidelines and recommendations regarding the appropriate use of electronic fetal heart monitoring in obstetrics. The guidelines supported the use of continuous electronic fetal heart monitoring in high-risk patients and low-risk patients who develop problems in the intrapartum period. In 1980, the Nurses Association of the American College of Obstetricians and Gynecologists (NAACOG) discussed the role of the nurse in electronic fetal heart monitoring in light of the committee's recommendations and guidelines, in its *Technical Bulletin No. 7* (July 1980). The purpose of the bulletin was "to present basic guidelines regarding the nurses' roles" in electronic fetal monitoring. The following is a list of the significant recommendations which appear in the bulletin.

1. Nurses who perform fetal monitoring "may be legally responsible for their actions and will be measured by their level of professional education; the established standards of care as defined by the professional nursing organization; . . . and in accordance with the Nurse Practice Act."

2. The nurse "is responsible for observing, assessing, evaluating, and intervening in accordance with the data received from the EFM."

3. The "ability to recognize and interpret fetal heart rate patterns and uterine activity is inherent in the nurses' role in EFM."

4. "During the electronic monitoring procedure, the nurse must continually observe and evaluate the tracing for ominous patterns."

5. "The charting of pertinent information on the monitor tracing is also the responsibility of the nurse."

6. "The fetal monitor tracings are a legal part of the patient's record and must be kept and monitored by the institution."

7. The obstetric nurse must possess "special training and instruction in preparing the patient, in attaching and operating the monitoring equipment, in pattern interpretation, and in making a nurse diagnosis based on the data received from the monitor tracing."

§ 10.18 Fetal Blood Sampling

Page 187, add at the end of the section:

Fetal scalp blood sampling has always been a controversial subject. Many obstetricians do not employ this technique; many hospitals do not provide the equipment or laboratory capabilities needed to conduct the test. Nonetheless, the ACOG has promoted the use of fetal scalp blood sampling and the benefits of this monitoring technique for many years. In 1977, ACOG *Technical Bulletin No. 4* (Jan. 1977) provided guidelines and indications for fetal scalp sampling, stating in unequivocal language that "if the indicators of fetal distress are suggestive of fetal compromise or if the fetal scalp pH ≤ 7.20 the infant should be delivered in the most expeditious manner."

CHAPTER 11

THE EVENTS OF LABOR AND DELIVERY

*

§ 11.10 — Pelvic Capacity

Page 204, add at the end of the section:

In *Stein v. Insurance Corp.*, 566 So. 2d 1114 (La. Ct. App. 1990), the plaintiff parents brought suit arising out of the allegedly negligent prenatal care and delivery of the child. The mother consulted with the defendant obstetricians and arranged for them to provide prenatal care and deliver the baby. A medical history was taken one year earlier, during the mother's first pregnancy, after which a normal child was born. For the second pregnancy, the defendant followed the normal examination procedure and ran a sonogram. At 37 weeks the defendant observed that the fetus's head was floating out of the pelvis, indicating that it had not dropped into the pelvic cavity. In an examination four weeks later, the defendant determined that the fetus was dropping into the pelvic cavity. At an examination one week later, the defendant believed that there was excess fluid but that the child was not an abnormally large baby. He planned to induce labor one week later. On that date, the mother checked into the hospital and pitocin was administered to induce labor. Four hours later, the pitocin was increased. The defendant examined the mother on several occasions and then performed an amniotomy. This permitted the child's head to drop into the pelvic cavity. The mother was given epidural anesthesia and was completely dilated. Nurses applied fundal pressure and the head started to emerge. The defendant attempted to use forceps but could not get a good grip. He performed an episiotomy and, after more fundal pressure and forceps, he removed the head up to the neck. At this point he determined that there was shoulder dystocia. Immediate delivery is required in such a situation, since the umbilical cord is totally compressed and the baby will suffer brain damage or death. The defendant tried several procedures and could not turn the infant. The nurse used superpubic pressure to dislodge the child. The baby weighed 11 pounds, 10 ounces. The child was born with a fractured right clavicle and fractured rib cage. She had right brachial plexus nerve damage that resulted in Erb's Palsy. The defendants were found not to have been negligent for failing to employ ultrasound to determine the size of the fetus. As the mother suffered from gestational diabetes, the failure to perform a 50-gram glucose loading test was also not a breach of the standard of care, and was not the cause of the injuries. This was supported by the evidence despite the fact that the fetus of a diabetic mother tends to have a greater risk of shoulder dystocia.

§ 11.15 Care of the Fetus and the Mother

Page 210, add after first paragraph:

The care of the mother and child is particularly critical at this time, as both are greatly at risk. In *Bubendey v. Winthrop University Hospital,* 151 A.D.2d 713, 543 N.Y.S.2d 146 (1989), the plaintiff mother sued the hospital arising out of her treatment during childbirth, seeking recovery for emotional distress. The appellate court affirmed dismissal of the suit because the plaintiff failed to allege that she sustained any independent physical injury attendant to the hospital's conduct relating to the birth. The only alleged injury was that she suffered extensively through the labor, which continued for many hours. She also claimed that the failure to admit her to the hospital resulted in alleged brain damage to the child, who died fours months later. The plaintiff mother claimed to have sustained "severe psychological trauma" as a result of the harm inflicted on her child. However, the court found that she could not recover for any distress normally attendant to birthing and extended labor in such a situation.

In *Ewing v. Aubert,* 532 So. 2d 876 (La. Ct. App. 1988), the surviving husband brought a wrongful death action for the death of his pregnant wife and the child's injuries. Judgment was entered on the jury verdict for the hospital. The appellate court affirmed the judgment, while finding that the verdict was supported by sufficient evidence that the defendant nurse was not negligent with regard to the rupture of the patient's uterus during labor. The defendant nurse specialist was found to be required to exercise a higher degree of care than other general nurses; thus, the plaintiff had to establish the standard for similar specialist nurses.

The nurse increased the dosage of the hormone pitocin to stimulate contractions. She failed to arrest labor and discontinue pitocin, where there was cephalopelvic disproportion, before the uterus ruptured. The evidence established that the increase of pitocin was not related to the rupture and that the nurse was not required to diagnose an arrest of labor; such a duty resided in the obstetrician. The obstetrician performed an emergency cesarean section, during which the mother died due to a massive amniotic fluid embolism. The child sustained severe anoxic brain damage prior to birth which rendered the child a spastic quadriplegic with cerebral palsy. Prior to this action against the nurse, the plaintiff settled with the obstetrician in the amount of the statutory limitation on damages.

* The plaintiff parents alleged that their child was injured during his birth. The child allegedly was in fetal distress prior to the delivery, and this resulted in oxygen deprivation and brain damage. The plaintiffs claimed that the defendants failed to conduct adequate fetal heart monitoring, which could have prevented the injuries complained of. The court, in *Gillis v. United States,* 722 F. Supp. 713 (M.D. Fla. 1989), dismissed the case. The court recognized that the hospital had a duty to monitor the fetal heart rate.

The mother had had an enema and was in the bathroom for a considerable period following her admission to the hospital. Upon admission, it was determined that the fetus was in stable condition. Subsequently, when the monitor was applied following the enema, the fetus was found to be experiencing late deceleration, and action was immediately taken. The question was whether the 50-minute delay in using the monitor after the initial examination constituted a breach of the duty of care. The court found that the standard of care required monitoring at least every 30 minutes. However, the bulk of the 50-minute period was taken up by the enema, during which time there could be no monitoring. The court found that there was no breach of duty; even if there was such a breach, it was not the cause of the oxygen deprivation which resulted in the injuries complained of.

* A plaintiff mother was injured in the course of delivery and sued a hospital and private diagnostic clinic for damages. Two months prior to the delivery, she consulted with the physician at the clinic and received assurances that, if in the course of the delivery she required epidural anesthesia, it would be administered by that particular physician or by an anesthesiologist who would insert the catheter. She was admitted to the hospital as a private patient of the clinic and its physicians. She was given an epidural anesthetic block to the epidural space of the spinal cord. The anesthesia was administered by a resident of the hospital. The first attempt to insert the catheter failed and punctured the layers covering the spinal cord, releasing spinal fluid. The second attempt struck a blood vessel. The third attempt was successful. Following the delivery, the plaintiff suffered various problems attributable to the puncture of the spinal cord covering and the loss of fluid. The trial court entered summary judgment for the defendants. That judgment was affirmed by the court, in *Labarre v. Duke University*, 99 N.C. App. 563, 393 S.E.2d 321 (1990). The plaintiff's breach of contract claim failed because there was no consideration supporting the promise that the physician or an anesthesiologist would administer the anesthetic. The tort claim of the plaintiff was also rejected, because she failed to allege that the resident who administered the anesthetic was negligent. Therefore, liability for those acts could not be imputed to the hospital.

*

§ 11.17 Delivery of the Fetus

Page 214, add before last paragraph:

The plaintiffs, child and parents, sued the obstetrician for injuries sustained by the child during delivery. The child sustained brachial plexus palsy. The defendant physician's expert witness admitted that the injuries were caused by the defendant's acts during the delivery. The physician attempted to turn the baby's head to rotate the shoulders after discovering shoulder dystocia. The issue was whether the application of pressure to the head constituted a breach of the duty of care. The appellate court upheld the trial court's judgment for the physician on the jury verdict, finding that the evidence supported the verdict. *Dunne v. Somoano,* 550 So. 2d 5 (Fla. Dist. Ct. App. 1989).

In *Armendarez v. Tarrant County Hospital District,* 781 S.W.2d 301 (Tex. Ct. App. 1989), the plaintiffs sued for injuries sustained by their son during delivery. They alleged that the hospital and the physicians were negligent in using vacuum extraction equipment and proceeding with a vaginal delivery, as opposed to performing a cesarean. The central issue was the application of governmental and official immunity. The trial court granted summary judgment for the defendants. The appellate court reversed, holding that there were questions of material fact precluding the grant of summary judgment. With respect to the issue of official immunity, the court held that physicians working at government hospitals are not immune to tort liability when their duties are the same as those performed by private physicians in private hospitals. However, there was a factual question as to whether the hospital residents were in a special position and were engaged in governmental functions such as might require the extension of immunity to them. With respect to the claims against the hospital district, the court held that Tex. Civ. Prac. & Rem. Code § 101.021 did not serve to extend immunity to claims arising from the negligent use of tangible property. This raised a factual issue as to whether the injuries were sustained due to the negligent use of the vacuum extractor or through other causes.

CHAPTER 12

OBSTETRICAL TRAUMA AND BIRTH INJURIES

§ 12.2 Cerebral Injuries

Page 220, add at the end of the section:

In *Henry v. St. Johns Hospital*, 159 Ill. App. 3d 725, 111 Ill. Dec. 503, 512 N.E.2d 1044 (1987), the child contracted cerebral palsy allegedly due to administration of a paracervical block during labor. The trial court entered a judgment in the amount of the $10 million jury verdict. The appellate court affirmed the judgment, holding that there was sufficient evidence to support a finding of negligence and causation. The drug manufacturer was also held liable. The court held that the manufacturer could sue the hospital and physician in contribution on theories of negligence, misuse of the product, and assumption of the risk. Expert testimony was properly introduced by the plaintiff to establish that use of the paracervical block in this case was a breach of the standard of care which proximately caused the child's injuries. The testimony established that the injuries were more likely than not caused by the breach.

The mother was given two blocks using the drug Marcaine. The first block was given by her physician, and the second by a resident without the authorization of her physician. Upon arriving at the hospital, her physician used a fetal heart monitor which showed a good fetal heart rate. The physician then attempted to induce labor. He inserted an internal fetal monitor and gave the block. He watched for 15 minutes and the fetal heart rate was still strong. One half hour later, the pain returned and the first-year resident administered the second block. After the second block, the child went into bradycardia lasting until the child was born. The physician was called back to the hospital and was told that bradycardia had developed. The child was in severe bradycardia for five minutes until the physician returned. The physician testified that it is not acceptable practice in the area to give the second block without the physician's authorization. Usually, such a second block should not be given within 90 minutes.

In *Willey v. Ketterer*, 869 F.2d 648 (1st Cir. 1989), applying New Hampshire law, suit was brought for damages suffered by a child born with cerebral palsy, claiming that the defendant hospital and obstetrician were negligent in delivery. The trial court entered judgment on the verdict for the defendant. The court of appeals reversed, ordering a new trial. The court held that the erroneous admission of evidence of febrile seizures suffered by the baby's sister, and the uncle's Down's Syndrome, constituted reversible error. Such evidence was not linked to cerebral palsy or used to show a genetic predisposition. Such a connection was promised by the defendant and the court admitted the evidence subject to the connection which was never made. The plaintiff moved to strike all references to the conditions at the close of all the evidence, as it was obvious that no link had been established. The defendant agreed, but the evidence had already been heard by the jury. There had been extensive discovery, and the defendant should have known that no connection could be demonstrated.

In *Ewing v. Aubert*, 532 So. 2d 876 (La. Ct. App. 1988), a surviving husband brought a wrongful death for the death of his pregnant wife and the child's injuries. Judgment was entered on the jury verdict for the hospital. The appellate court affirmed the judgment, while finding that the verdict was supported by sufficient evidence that the defendant nurse was not negligent with regard to the rupture of the patient's uterus during labor. The defendant nurse specialist was found to be required to exercise a higher degree of care than other general nurses; thus, the plaintiff had to establish the standard for similar specialist nurses.

The nurse increased the dosage of the hormone pitocin to stimulate contractions. She failed to arrest labor and discontinue pitocin, where there was cephalopelvic disproportion, before the uterus ruptured. The evidence established that the increase of pitocin was not related to the rupture and that the nurse was not required to diagnose an arrest of labor; such a duty resided in the obstetrician. The obstetrician performed an emergency cesarean section, during which the mother died due a massive amniotic fluid embolism. The child sustained severe anoxic brain damage prior to birth which rendered the child a spastic quadriplegic with cerebral palsy. Prior to this action against the nurse, the plaintiff settled with the obstetrician in the amount of the statutory limitation on damages.

Such injuries can be the result of a combination of prebirth negligence and negligence with regard to treatment in connection with the birth. In *Scott v. United States*, 884 F.2d 1280 (9th Cir. 1989), applying Alaska law, a child was injured prior to and during his birth at a military hospital. The district court entered judgment for the plaintiffs. The circuit court affirmed in part and reversed in part, holding that the trial court properly permitted recovery of damages arising from the effect of the child's spastic quadriplegia (cerebral palsy) on the parent-child relationship. The appellate court upheld the award of separate amounts for the child's past and future pain and suffering, as distinguished from an award for his past and future impairment.

The trial court was required, however, to recalculate the discount rate for the economic losses. Alaska law applied to determine the discount rate in this Federal Tort Claims Act case. The child was properly awarded $2 million for the injuries which rendered him incapable of any form of an independent life and required around-the-clock professional care. The trial jury awarded the child $8.75 million for future economic losses reduced to present value. The parents were awarded $350,000 for loss of the parent-child relationship. This case extensively discusses the damage perspective, but has no discussion of the underlying negligence on the part of the defendant which resulted in the injuries.

§ 12.3 Hypoxia

Page 221, add at the end of the section:

Clearly, hypoxia can cause a variety of severe injuries. In *Bradford v. McGee*, 534 So. 2d 1076 (Ala. 1988), the infant allegedly contracted cerebral palsy due to the negligence of the defendant physician and hospital. The jury returned a verdict for the plaintiff in the amount of $950,000. The trial court denied the defendant's motion for j.n.o.v. and granted the motion for a new trial. The Alabama Supreme Court affirmed and remanded, because of the possible prejudice of juror nonresponsiveness on voir dire with respect to material questions involving brain damage suffered by a relative in another personal injury case.

The applicable standard of care in such a case is established by reference to a national medical community. The plaintiff's expert testimony, which was extensively reported in this decision, introduced some evidence that the physician breached the applicable standard of care by failing to conduct fetal testing at 42 weeks. The plaintiff presented evidence that the physician's breach of the standard of conduct potentially caused the chronic hypoxia resulting in the cerebral palsy. The plaintiff's evidence must have selective application to one theory of causation, proving it to a probability. In this case, the plaintiff introduced sufficient evidence that hypoxia can cause cerebral palsy and that gestation periods greater than 42 weeks can deprive the fetus of essential oxygen. It was further contended that the child was negligently allowed to remain in the womb for a dangerously protracted period of time. The plaintiff failed to introduce sufficient evidence, however, to prove that the delay in performing a cesarean section cause the cerebral palsy.

§ 12.3A Iatrogenesis as a Cause of Cerebral Palsy: The Defense View (New)

There is no question that iatrogenesis is one cause of cerebral palsy. Failures in obstetrical care include traumatic forceps delivery, failure to recognize and treat fetal distress, failure to perform timely cesarean section, and failure to properly treat preeclampsia, to name but some. Such failures may

113

proximately cause brain damage and cerebral palsy. For example, the failure to recognize fetal distress may permit a state of hypoxia to progress to such an extent that brain cells are destroyed. Or, when the physician fails to timely extricate the fetus from a postmature uterine environment, the fetus may suffer permanent brain damage incident to uteroplacental insufficiency.

The known causes of cerebral palsy, then, include iatrogenesis, asphyxia, infection (i.e., TORCH), and metabolic and genetic factors. The most influential document advancing the defense viewpoint is, of course, the 1985 National Institutes of Health study, *Prenatal and Perinatal Factors Associated With Brain Disorders* (NIH Publication No. 85-1149, U.S. Department of Health and Human Services, April 1985). The study acknowledges iatrogenesis as a cause of cerebral palsy but posits that obstetric care, trauma, and birth complications account for a minority of cases of cerebral palsy.

In the last few years, the medical professional and defense bar have made a concerted effort in the literature and in the courtroom to prove that "almost nothing an obstetrician does or fails to do results in cerebral palsy." *See* K. Niswander, *Does Substandard Obstetric Care Cause Cerebral Palsy?*, Comtemporary OB/GYN 43 (October 1987). In his article, Dr. Kenneth R. Niswander reports the results of a study undertaken to relate the quality of obstetric care with poor outcome. His conclusion is that obstetrical malpractice is virtually never associated with cerebral palsy. Among conclusions reached by the author from various studies are the following:

1. Severe asphyxia rarely causes brain damage;
2. Determining the cause of cerebral palsy in an individual is nearly impossible;
3. Substandard obstetric care, especially failure to react to evidence of possible fetal asphyxia, is not causally related to cerebral palsy;
4. Obstetric intervention might not prevent cerebral palsy in cases of fetal asphyxia because:
   a. There has been no significant consistent change in the prevalence of cerebral palsy over many years;
   b. Most newborn asphyxia is not followed by cerebral palsy;
   c. Most cerebral palsy is not preceded by severe intrapartum asphyxia;
   d. The diagnosis of fetal asphyxia is imprecise;
   e. Fetal asphyxia may follow fetal brain damage.

The author suggests a three-part test that must be satisfied before a correlation between intrapartum asphyxia and cerebral palsy may be suggested. First, there must be documented severe newborn acidosis. Second, there must be evidence of systemic damage to at least two of the following systems: cardiovascular, gastrointestinal, hematologic, pulmonary, or renal. (The author contends that asphyxia severe enough to cause brain damage must also damage other organs.) Third, the newborn must have a stormy neurologic course (e.g., seizure activity).

§ 12.10 Hyperbilirubinemia

Page 226, add at the end of the section:

In *Rutledge v. Children's Mercy Hospital,* No. CV85-15580 (Mo. Cir. Ct., Jackson County July 12, 1985), *reported in* 29 ATLA L. Rep. 36 (Feb. 1986), a structured settlement with a present value in excess of $800,000 was reached for an infant whose hyperbilirubinemia was not properly treated. The plaintiff's mother presented at a hospital with premature membrane rupture at a gestational age of 35 weeks. Shortly after birth, with a weight of 2,200 grams, the infant developed respiratory distress and was transferred to the defendant hospital. On the second day of life, he was noted to be clinically jaundiced, and phototherapy was instituted. The next day his bilirubin level was 15.2, and two days later, it peaked at 19. Although the physicians decided to do an exchange transfusion, it was not performed for another 12 hours. During this time, the plaintiff began to experience "non-purposeful movements" and other symptoms reflecting bilirubin toxicity to the brain (kernicterus). At present, he suffers athetoid cerebral palsy. The suit alleged delay in instituting appropriate respiratory support resulting in deterioration of the plaintiff's condition and precipitating the development of kernicterus, failure to timely manage unconjugated hyperbilirubinemia and failure to supervise resident care and management of the plaintiff.

CHAPTER 13

PLACENTAL ABRUPTION

§ 13.1 Premature Separation of the Placenta

Page 228, add before last paragraph of section:

The plaintiffs sued a hospital for the death of their child two months after birth by cesarean section. They sued the physicians and the hospital. The trial court granted the defendants' motions for summary judgment. The appellate court reversed the summary judgment for the hospital. In *Albain v. Flower Hospital,* 50 Ohio St. 3d 251, 553 N.E.2d 1038 (1990), the Ohio Supreme Court reversed the appellate court judgment. The plaintiff mother was visiting friends when she started bleeding, and was rushed to the hospital. Because her obstetrician did not have staff privileges at that particular hospital, he agreed to have the on-call obstetrician handle the situation. The mother was examined and the on-staff obstetrician was called. The on-staff physician was seeing patients in her office and gave care orders. She told the nurse that she would be at the hospital at 5:30. She went home and was called there and told that she had been expected. She arrived at the hospital at 8:00. She consulted with the plaintiff's obstetrician and transferred the plaintiff to another hospital which had a neonatologist. At 9:30, the plaintiff was examined by her regular obstetrician and the staff obstetrician, who determined that there was a possible abruptio placentae. The baby was delivered by cesarean section two hours later. The infant had suffered from neonatal asphyxia and died two months later. The court held that the hospital could not be held liable under the plaintiff's claims of negligence for the granting of staff privileges. The granting of staff privileges does not impart the necessary level of control over a physician so as to impose liability in respondeat superior. The court also rejected the claim that the hospital had a nondelegable duty to assure that physicians with staff privileges performed in a nonnegligent manner. The court found that hospitals only have a duty to assure that those with staff privileges are competent, and even a competent physician can be negligent in any given case. The hospital did not violate any duty owned to the plaintiff by failing constantly to supervise the actions of those physicians with staff privileges. The court further rejected an attempt to impose liability on theories of agency by estoppel or ostensible agency.

§ 13.5 – Treatment

Page 232, add at the end of the section:

In a 1985 case, *Anguioni v. Glen Cove Community Hospital,* No. 1181/80 (N.Y. Sup. Ct., Nassau County, Mar. 1, 1985), *reported in* 28 ATLA L. Rep. 326 (Sept. 1985), the plaintiffs filed suit against an obstetrician and a hospital alleging negligent delay in responding to an emergency situation caused by abruptio placenta. The plaintiff mother was admitted to the defendant hospital in labor under the supervision of family practice residents. Thirty-five minutes after an external fetal monitor demonstrated late decelerations, without correction by oxygen administration or turning the patient on her side, an obstetrical resident contacted the attending physician who advised that they arrange for an emergency cesarean section. The anesthesiologist was not called for ten minutes. The membranes were ruptured and bloody amniotic fluid was returned. When the attending obstetrician arrived within one-half hour after he was called, the anesthesiologist had not yet arrived, and the wrong operating room had been set up. Twenty minutes later, the infant was delivered by cesarean section, suffering intrauterine hypoxia with meconium aspiration. He suffered neonatal seizures and was diagnosed as having spastic cerebral palsy. He requires complete custodial care. The plaintiff received $1.5 million in settlement.

§ 13.8 Placenta Previa – Diagnosis

Page 238, add at the end of the section:

Placenta previa raises serious risks to the infant and therefore requires timely and appropriate medical intervention. In *Kilker v. Mulry,* 437 N.W.2d 1 (Iowa Ct. App. 1988), a child sustained brain damage when the obstetrician ruptured the misplaced placenta during an investigative procedure. The trial court entered a verdict for the defendant. The appellate court affirmed the lower court, holding that there was a jury question as to negligence. The verdict had been entered on the claim that the defendant was not negligent in not earlier diagnosing the condition of placenta previa and that an earlier diagnosis would have prevented the exploratory procedure resulting in injury. Such a verdict was supported by the evidence. Shortly prior to birth, the mother was discovered to have placenta previa, that is, the placenta in front of the baby blocking the baby's egress into the birth canal. A cesarean section was then required. Prior to discovering the condition, the defendant used an amniotic hook, which ruptured the placenta and caused a massive hemorrhage. The loss of blood from the rupture could have resulted in the brain damage.

PLACENTAL ABRUPTION

In *Kavanaugh v. Nussbaum*, 71 N.Y.2d 535, 523 N.E.2d 284, 528 N.Y.S.2d 8 (1988), the trial court denied a motion to set aside a verdict on liability and entered judgment on some damage counts of the complaint. The appellate division modified the judgment and affirmed. The court of appeals affirmed and remitted the action, holding that the defendant obstetrician was not vicariously liable for the negligence of a physician who covered for him on the day prior to the birth. The evidence supported a finding of negligence and causation on the part of both the obstetrician and the emergency room physician. The plaintiff was awarded $1.5 million for pain and suffering and $740,000 for impaired earning capacity, which damages were apportioned between the defendants.

The child was born after only 31 weeks gestation, while in distress, and weighed only three pounds at birth. The 44-year-old mother went to the emergency room when she started bleeding. There was a question as to whether the child was injured due to placenta previa which should have been detected at the time. The next day, an internal examination of the mother was performed and, upon loss of the fetal heartbeat, a cesarean section was performed. The Apgar scores of the newborn were 1 at 1 minute, 5 at 5 minutes, and 4 at 10 minutes. The baby was transferred to another hospital with better neonatal facilities, where a tracheotomy was performed, but the child suffered permanent debilitating injuries.

CHAPTER 14

HYPERTENSIVE DISORDERS IN PREGNANCY

§ 14.4 – Eclampsia

Page 245, add after first paragraph:

Eclampsia poses serious risks to the mother. The results of improper treatment of the condition can result in the death of the mother in a variety of ways. In *Crumbley v. Wyant,* 188 Ga. App. 227, 372 S.E.2d 497 (1988), the patient died while bathing. A nursing assistant filled the bathtub and left the decedent, who was found 20 minutes later, unconscious, with her face in the water. She was resuscitated, but there was severe brain damage and she died shortly thereafter. The trial court entered judgment on the jury verdict for the defendant physician and hospital. The appellate court affirmed the lower court decision, and recognized that the codefendants had the right to cross-examine one another's witnesses on the issue of whether the plaintiff died from preeclampsia/eclampsia or from another cause. They could also cross-examine on the failure to diagnose the condition, the hospital's failure to report test results to the physician, and the claim that inadequate nursing care was provided. The court also recognized that there is a presumption that medical services are performed in a reasonably skillful manner.

§ 14.8 Signs and Symptoms

Page 249, add at the end of the section:

A baby was born at an Indian Health Service hospital. The plaintiffs claimed that the baby was injured due by the hospital's failure to treat the mother's hypertension and preeclampsia. It was alleged that these conditions resulted in oxygen deprivation to the fetus, thereby causing profound brain damage. The issue was raised as to the ability of the hospital to provide the mother and infant with proper care. The hospital was classified as a "level one" birth center; level one is the lowest level of care available and means that the hospital is equipped to handle only low-risk births. The protocols of the Indian Health Service require that, when it is determined that more intensive medical care is required, the patient should be taken to a hospital which can provide such care. This was the crux of the case. The court held that the plaintiff could recover only if she could establish that she had the warning signs of hypertension and preeclampsia and that the

119

hospital failed to recognize these signs and act pursuant to its protocols. Additionally, it would be necessary to establish that the violation of the protocols was the cause of the child's brain damage. The court detailed the facts of the pregnancy and the treatment plus the lack of facilities at the Indian Health Service hospital in question. The court held that the hospital was negligent in failing properly to monitor and treat the mother, and that that negligence was the cause of the injuries sustained by the child. The plaintiffs were awarded $2.5 million for the cost of caring for the child, $760,000 for lost earning capacity, and $160,000 for medical expenses already incurred. The court further awarded the grandmother the sum of $525,000 for the loss of consortium with her grandchild. The mother, on the other hand, was not entitled to any such award, since she had effectively abandoned the child, leaving it with the grandmother. *Anderson v. United States,* 731 F. Supp. 391 (D.N.D. 1990).

§ 14.9 Prevention and Treatment

Page 254, add at the end of the section:

The plaintiff sued the hospital and physicians arising out of alleged negligent management of her pregnancy, which resulted in a miscarriage. The plaintiff suffered from hypertension, which condition required special treatment and attention. The trial court dismissed the complaint as failing to state a claim. The appellate court, in *Coughling v. George Washington University Health Plan, Inc.,* 565 A.2d 67 (D.C. 1989), reversed. The court held that the plaintiff was entitled to be treated in a nonnegligent manner. The failure of the defendants to exercise the appropriate standard of care could support recovery without regard to whether there was a cause of action for the negligence that resulted in the injury to a viable fetus. The plaintiff's complaint alleged injuries that she actually sustained and not a wrongful death claim for loss of the fetus. The court further held that the plaintiff properly alleged a physical impact so as to support a claim for negligent infliction of emotional distress. The negligent treatment resulted in preeclampsia, which increased the plaintiff's risk of injury and destroyed her placenta. As a result of the negligence, she was required to submit to two painful procedures to remove the dead fetus from her uterus. Such allegations were sufficient to state a claim.

CHAPTER 17

TERATOGENIC AGENTS

§ 17.1 Introduction

Page 278, add at the end of the section:

Recently, the problem of the teratogenic effects of prescription drugs has spawned a spate of products liability actions. In *Brock v. Merrell Dow Pharmaceuticals,* 874 F.2d 307 (5th Cir. 1989), applying Texas law, a child was born with Poland's Syndrome (an absence of fingers or their shortening, with a corresponding decrease of the pectoralis muscle) following in utero exposure to Bendectin. The trial court entered judgment for the plaintiff. The appellate court reversed because of a lack of sufficient epidemiological proof to establish the essential element of causation. The appellate court held that the defendant was entitled to a j.n.o.v. The court recognized that there is no medical consensus that Bendectin is teratogenic, and found that the plaintiff failed to trace the etiology of the birth defect to the drug. The court looked to the manner in which causation was established in Agent Orange litigation and also to similar Bendectin cases such as *Richardson v. Richardson-Merrell, Inc.,* 857 F.2d 823 (D.C. Cir. 1988), which affirmed a j.n.o.v. granted for the defendant. The court did say, however, that while the lack of epidemiological proof was fatal to this case, that does not mean that such a lack will be fatal to all toxic tort cases.

Hull v. Merrell Dow Pharmaceuticals, 700 F. Supp. 28 (S.D. Fla. 1988), involved a birth defect allegedly caused by the mother's use of Bendectin during pregnancy. This case was removed from state to federal court. The defendant manufacturer then moved for summary judgment, which was granted. The court noted 30 human epidemiological studies finding that Bendectin is not teratogenic and held that, even if the drug could cause birth defects, its use seven weeks into the pregnancy did not cause the child's extensive leg and foot deformities. The manufacturer claimed that such ingestion was too late in the mother's pregnancy to cause the deformity complained of. The court cited *Lynch v. Merrill-National Laboratories,* 646 F. Supp. 856 (D. Mass. 1986), *aff'd,* 830 F.2d 1190 (1st Cir. 1987), which similarly granted summary judgment for the manufacturer in a case involving a similar limb defect.

Hagen v. Richardson-Merrell, Inc., 697 F. Supp. 334 (N.D. Ill. 1988), resulted from a birth defect to the child's hand allegedly due to exposure of Bendectin in utero. Bendectin was prescribed in June 1976 and was taken by the mother through the fourth month of the pregnancy. The defendant moved for summary judgment. The court held that there were material issues of fact as to the cause of the child's ectrodactyly, and therefore denied the motion. The defendant contended that the defect was genetic in nature and that it could not be held liable, as the drug is not a mutagen. The plaintiff contended that the drug is a teratogen which affected limb development. The court found that the plaintiff failed to establish fraud with regard to the manufacturer's labeling the drug safe and destroying fetal specimens, and held that punitive damages were not recoverable. The court determined that the failure of the manufacturer to use premarketing testing was not relevant to such a fraud claim. Falsifying test results was similarly irrelevant where the FDA investigated and concluded that variances in the testing were justifiable and further testing was conducted. The court further held that the claim for breach of warranty was time barred. The plaintiff had waited five years after the eight-year statute of repose was adopted before filing the strict liability claims. The eight-year statute was effective to bar such claims.

In *St. Amand v. Merrell Dow Pharmaceuticals,* 140 Misc. 2d 278, 530 N.Y.S.2d 428 (1988), the plaintiff child was born with Pierre-Robin Syndrome allegedly due to in utero exposure to the defendant's drugs. The mother also claimed that the obstetrician's management of the labor and delivery, coupled with the mother's taking of Bendectin, was the cause of the injuries. The manufacturer sought discovery of the mother's medical and employment records in order to discover other potential causes of the condition. The manufacturer was entitled to obtain the medical history of the mother, family history, and genetic factors to determine the etiology of the child's condition and whether such factors caused the syndrome, as opposed to exposure to the drug.

* In a Bendectin case, the plaintiff children, who were exposed to the drug in utero, sued the manufacturer of the drug on claims arising out of their birth defects (limb reductions). The court, in *Daubert v. Merrell Dow Pharmaceuticals, Inc.,* 727 F. Supp. 570 (S.D. Cal. 1989), granted the manufacturer's motion for summary judgment. The court held that the plaintiffs failed to provide any evidence of a causal connection between the injuries suffered and use of the drugs by their mothers. The plaintiffs had introduced expert testimony in support of their claims. The court rejected that testimony because the conclusions were based on in vitro, chemical, and animal studies. The court found that the testimony was insufficient, as experts in the field would have relied upon human epidemiological studies. The court also rejected the authority of an unpublished study which failed to conduct its own research but only reinterpreted prior studies. The court reviewed Federal Rule of Evidence 703 and found that the plaintiff's expert testimony failed to establish that the opinion was based on methodology usually relied upon by experts in the field. The court bolstered its decision by citing numerous other Bendectin cases, which also held that there was a lack of sufficient scientific proof of causation. For another case coming to the same result on similar issues, *see Cadarian v. Merrell Dow Pharmaceuticals, Inc.,* 745 F. Supp. 409 (E.D. Mich. 1989).

* In another Bendectin case, the child was born with one finger missing from each hand. The court, in *Wilson v. Merrell Dow Pharmaceuticals, Inc.,* 893 F.2d 1149 (10th Cir. 1990), applying Oklahoma law, affirmed the judgment on the jury verdict for the defendant drug company. The issue was whether the trial court should have given a missing-witness instruction when the manufacturer failed to call a geneticist to testify on causation. The appellate court held that the lower court properly exercised its discretion, as such testimony would have been cumulative. The trial court also properly permitted the use of sales charts which had graphs dealing with the frequency of birth defects in the general population as compared with sales of the drug, since this was a basis for the witness's expert opinion. Any defects in the charts were directed to the weight of such evidence and not its admissibility. The appellate court recognized the vast amount of scientific data which failed to establish a causal connection between use of the drug and the occurrence of birth defects.

* In *Bernhardt v. Richardson-Merrell, Inc.,* 892 F.2d 440 (5th Cir. 1990), applying Mississippi law, suit was brought for injuries sustained by a child as a result of in utero exposure to Bendectin taken by the mother during pregnancy. The child was born without fingers on one hand. In this case, the mother did not take the drug until the 54th or 55th day of her pregnancy. Medical evidence was introduced to the effect that fingers are found on the human fetus by the 44th day after conception. Therefore, fingers should have been present prior to the mother's use of the drug. Clearly, this destroyed the attempt to establish the required element of causation. The plaintiffs had submitted certified interrogatory answers, but such did not qualify as expert affidavits, which would have been required to counter the defendant's expert evidence. The answers to the interrogatories were, at best, only hearsay references to expert opinions. Therefore, this court affirmed the trial court's grant of summary judgment for the defendant.

* *Cosgrove v. Merrell Dow Pharmaceuticals, Inc.,* 117 Idaho 470, 788 P.2d 1293 (1989), is yet another Bendectin suit. In this case, strict liability and negligence claims were brought by the plaintiffs. The trial court entered judgment on the jury verdict, which was affirmed on appeal. The mother brought a claim against the manufacturer, but the manufacturer was properly granted summary judgment on that claim, as the suit was filed after the two-year statute of limitations (Idaho Code § 5-219) had run. The child was born without a portion of one arm and hand. The trial court gave the jury a list of special verdict questions. The first question on the list related to causation. The order of questions was not error even though most such lists start with issues of strict liability or negligence.

* In *Bealer v. Hoffman-La Roche, Inc.*, 729 F. Supp. 43 (E.D. La. 1990), the court granted the manufacturer's motion for summary judgment. The plaintiff had a therapeutic abortion after she learned she was pregnant, because she was taking the drug Accutane, which is associated with a high risk of birth defects. She sued the manufacturer on a claim that the drug was unreasonably unsafe. The court found that the warning was adequate, as a matter of law, where the manufacturer properly gave warnings and information to prescribing physicians. This court also cited other decisions upholding the sufficiency of the warning. The warning provided (729 F. Supp. at 45):

WARNING TO FEMALE PATIENTS

YOU MUST NOT TAKE ACCUTANE IF YOU ARE OR MAY BECOME PREGNANT DURING TREATMENT

Severe birth defects are known to occur in infants of women taking Accutane during pregnancy. The possibility that you may become pregnant must be ruled out by you and your doctor before you start Accutane therapy. Wait until the second or third day of your next normal menstrual period before beginning Accutane therapy. An effective form of contraception (birth control) should be discussed with your doctor. Contraception must be used for at least one month before beginning therapy and during therapy, and it must be continued for one month after Accutane treatment has stopped. Immediately stop taking Accutane if you become pregnant while you are taking the drug, and immediately contact your physician to discuss the desirability of continuing the pregnancy.

CHAPTER 18

OBSTETRICAL ANESTHESIA

§ 18.13 – Paracervical Block

Page 300, add at the end of the section:

In *Henry v. St. John Hospital,* 159 Ill. App. 3d 725, 111 Ill. Dec. 503, 512 N.E.2d 1044 (1987), the child contracted cerebral palsy allegedly due to administration of a paracervical block during labor. The trial court entered a judgment in the amount of the $10 million jury verdict. The appellate court affirmed the judgment, holding that there was sufficient evidence to support a finding of negligence and causation. The drug manufacturer was also held liable. The court held that the manufacturer could sue the hospital and physician in contribution on theories of negligence, misuse of the product, and assumption of the risk. Expert testimony was properly introduced by the plaintiff to establish that use of the paracervical block in this case was a breach of the standard of care which proximately caused the child's injuries. The testimony established that the injuries were more likely than not caused by the breach.

The mother was given two blocks using the drug Marcaine. The first block was given by her physician, and the second by a resident without the authorization of her physician. Upon arriving at the hospital, her physician used a fetal heart monitor which showed a good fetal heart rate. The physician then attempted to induce labor. He inserted an internal fetal monitor and gave the block, He watched for 15 minutes, during which time the fetal heart rate was still strong. One half hour later, the pain returned and the first-year resident administered the second block. After the second block, the child went into bradycardia lasting until the child was born. The physician was called back to the hospital and was told that bradycardia had developed. The child was in severe bradycardia for five minutes until the physician returned. The physician testified that it is not acceptable practice in the area to give the second block without the physician's authorization. Usually such a second block should not be given within 90 minutes.

Similarly, in *Ramon v. Farr,* 770 P.2d 131 (Utah 1989), the defendant physician injected the mother's cervix with anesthesia one hour before birth, during which the child sustained serious physical and mental defects. The question was presented as to whether the physician directly injected the child with the Marcaine. However, the plaintiffs did not introduce sufficient evidence to support the claim that an injection to the mother without injecting the child would have not affected the child. At birth the child seemed normal, but several hours later he showed symptoms of serious problems. The trial court entered judgment for the defendant. The appellate court held that, although the manufacturer's package insert does not per se establish the standard of care for physicians, such a use of the anesthetic was not recommended by the manufacturer, and the warning could be prima facie evidence of negligence. The package insert was evidence that should be considered by the jury. An issue was also raised as to the refusal of the court to give an offered instruction. Any error in refusing the instruction that parents are entitled to recovery if the physician fails to give information on a paracervical block procedure was harmless. The refused instruction read as follows:

> You are instructed that the manufacturers of Marcaine included a package insert which stated that "Until further clinical experience is gained, paracervical block with Marcaine is not recommended. Fetal bradycardia frequently follows paracervical block with some amide-type local anesthetics and may be associated with fetal acidosis," and that the *Physician's Desk Reference* contained an identical warning. The Defendants either knew or should have known of such warning. If you find that the Defendants nevertheless proceeded to use Marcaine as a paracervical block and that such use was a proximate cause of Plaintiffs' injuries, then, the fact that Defendants used Marcaine for a paracervical block contrary to written warning would be prima facie evidence of negligence by the Defendants. Prima facie means that such action by Defendants would not be conclusive, but that in the absence of other evidence which is convincing in repudiating the assumption, that such actions were reasonable and prudent, you should find in favor of the Plaintiffs and against one or both of the Defendants.

Other rejected instructions provided:

> In connection with the use of the drug Marcaine by the Defendants and your determination as to whether or not the Defendants were negligent by its use and/or whether or not the Defendant had a duty to inform [plaintiff] . . . of its use, you may take into consideration the fact that the manufacturer of Marcaine inserted a package insert with the drug used . . . warning that "Until further clinical experience is gained, paracervical block with Marcaine is not recommended. Fetal bradycardia frequently follows paracervical block with some amide-type local anesthetics and may be associated with fetal acidosis," and that the *Physician's Desk Reference* for 1980 contained exactly the same warning and that both Defendants were aware of such warning at the time Marcaine was used upon [plaintiff], but that neither Defendant informed [plaintiff] of such warning or told her that Marcaine would be used for a paracervical block.
>
> It is the settled general rule that in the absence of an emergency or unanticipated condition, a physician must first obtain the consent of the patient before treating or operating upon him or her.
>
> The relationship between a physician and his patient creates a duty in the physician to disclose to his patient any material information concerning the patient's physical condition and treatment. This duty to inform stems from the fiduciary nature of the relationship and the patient's right to determine what shall or shall not be done with his or her body. The scope of the duty is defined

by the materiality of the information in the decisional process of an ordinary individual. If a reasonable person in the position of the patient would consider the information important in choosing a course of treatment, then the information is material and disclosure is required. Once the duty to disclose certain information is established, then the physician's total breach of that duty presents to the jury the question of what damages were proximately caused by the breach of the duty.

Under Utah law, it shall be presumed that what the physician did to or for a patient was either expressly or impliedly authorized to be done. However, this is a rebuttable presumption and a patient may recover damages from a physician based upon the physician's failure to obtain the informed consent of the patient, upon showing [the elements of Utah Code Ann. § 78-14-5(1)].

*

§ 18.15 – Spinal Anesthesia

Page 302, add at the end of the section:

A plaintiff mother was injured in the course of delivery and sued the hospital and private diagnostic clinic for damages. Two months prior to the delivery, she consulted with her physician at the clinic and received assurances that, if in the course of the delivery she required epidural anesthesia, it would be administered by that particular physician or by an anesthesiologist who would insert the catheter. She was admitted to the hospital as a private patient of the clinic and its physicians. She was given an epidural anesthetic block to the epidural space of the spinal cord. The anesthesia was administered by a resident of the hospital. The first attempt to insert the catheter failed and punctured the layers covering the spinal cord, releasing spinal fluid. The second attempt struck a blood vessel. The third attempt was successful. Following the delivery, the plaintiff suffered various problems attributable to the puncture of the spinal cord covering and the loss of fluid. The trial court entered summary judgment for the defendants. That judgment was affirmed by the court in *Labarre v. Duke University*, 99 N.C. App. 563, 393 S.E.2d 321 (1990). The plaintiff's breach of contract claim failed because there was no consideration supporting the promise that the physician or an anesthesiologist would administer the anesthetic. The tort claim of the plaintiff was also rejected, because she failed to allege that the resident who administered the anesthetic was negligent. Therefore, liability for those acts could not be imputed to the hospital.

CHAPTER 19

INDUCTION OF LABOR

§ 19.1 Introduction

Page 305, add at the end of the section:

The artificial induction of labor may be a medical necessity under certain situations; it requires a timely and accurate diagnosis of the condition of both mother and child. In *Fabianke v. Weaver,* 527 So. 2d 1253 (Ala. 1988), the physician allegedly failed properly to determine the labor and delivery rate, which resulted in a premature birth and attendant injuries to the child. The child suffered respiratory distress due to its premature lungs, was intellectually deficient, and could have suffered a learning disability. The jury verdict awarded the husband $11,000 for medical expenses, the child $50,000 for pain and suffering, and nothing for the mother. The Alabama Supreme Court affirmed, on a finding that the testimony of a psychologist as to the potential connection between the respiratory distress and the child's condition was admissible. Also, a Philadelphia obstetrician-gynecologist was allowed to testify as an expert against the Alabama physician. The defendant physician admitted the premature birth, and a psychologist's testimony was therefore admissible where it was not used to prove the standard of care.

The claim sounded in the negligent induction of labor. The mother had been taking Norlestrin, a birth control pill, but suspected that she was pregnant. The defendant obstetrician determined that the baby was past due, according to his projected delivery date computed on the basis of conception prior to the mother's taking the drug. This was why he induced labor. It was below the standard of care to fail to determine whether the mother was pregnant prior to prescribing the pills.

§ 19.4 Chemical Induction

Page 307, add at the end of the section:

One case arising out of the use of pitocin was *Ewing v. Aubert,* 532 So. 2d 876 (La. Ct. App. 1988), wherein the surviving husband brought a wrongful death for the death of his pregnant wife and the child's injuries. Judgment was entered on the jury verdict for the hospital. The appellate court affirmed the judgment, while finding that the verdict was supported by sufficient evidence that the defendant nurse was not negligent with regard to the rupture of the patient's uterus during labor. The defendant nurse specialist was found to be required to exercise a higher degree of care than other general nurses; thus, the plaintiff had to establish the standard for similar specialist nurses. The nurse increased the dosage of the hormone pitocin to stimulate contractions. She failed to arrest labor and discontinue pitocin, where there was cephalopelvic disproportion, before the uterus ruptured. The evidence established that the increase of pitocin was not related to the rupture and that the nurse was not required to diagnose an arrest of labor; such a duty resided in the obstetrician. The obstetrician performed an emergency cesarean section, during which the mother died due to a massive amniotic fluid embolism. The child sustained severe anoxic brain damage prior to birth which rendered the child a spastic quadriplegic with cerebral palsy. Prior to this action against the nurse, the plaintiff settled with the obstetrician in the amount of the statutory limitation on damages.

§ 19.6 – Routes of Administration

Page 312, add at end of the section:

In a New York case, the plaintiff contended that an excessive dosage of Pitocin led to the decedent's uterine rupture and death.

In *Vialva v. City of New York*, 118 A.D.2d 701, 499 N.Y.S.2d 977 (1986), an action was filed on behalf of a woman who died of an amniotic fluid embolism as she was being prepared for cesarean section. Four days prior to her estimated due date, the decedent underwent a non-stress test which was questionably non-reactive.

Practice Note. A non-reactive (positive) non-stress test means that the fetal heart rate has not shown appropriate acceleration. A non-reactive test should alert the physician to the possibility of fetal distress and warrants the performance of an oxytocin challenge test. See § **6.14**.

The resident in charge of the plaintiff's case begin to administer Pitocin in order to induce or augment the patient's labor. At 5:00 p.m. the administration of Pitocin was begun with a dosage of four drops per minute to be increased two drops every ten minutes until the patient's labor pattern became acceptable. Pitocin was administered for a period of eight-and-a-half hours and was finally discontinued when the patient's contractions had reached a frequency of one per minute. At 4:00 a.m., some two-and-a-half hours after the discontinuation of Pitocin, the fetal heart rate dropped to bradycardic levels, and the decision was made to perform a cesarean section. However, as she was being prepped, the patient went into convulsions, began to hemorrhage, suffered a heart attack, and died. Autopsy revealed that the cause of death was an amniotic fluid embolism.

INDUCTION OF LABOR

Practice Note. Amniotic fluid embolism is a rare but lethal complication of late labor. The condition is caused when amniotic fluid from the amniotic sac enters the maternal bloodstream. The embolic occlusion of the pulmonary system causes respiratory distress and D.I.C. (disseminated intravascular coagulation). The mother and fetus usually succumb.

At trial, the plaintiff's experts testified that the decedent had died as a proximate result of the physician's negligent administration of Pitocin. Specifically, the plaintiff's obstetrical expert testified that the administration of Pitocin was contraindicated in the patient because the fetal head was not engaged in the patient's pelvis (i.e., the fetus was "floating") at the time the Pitocin infusion began. This, the experts testified, increased the risk of uterine rupture. The plaintiff's expert also testified that the patient had received an excessive amount of Pitocin over the eight-and-a-half-hour period, which caused titanic contractions, enhancing the likelihood of uterine rupture. The laceration or rupture of the patient's uterus, the experts said, allowed amniotic fluid to escape into the maternal circulation, causing the patient's death.

Practice Note. The plaintiff's expert testified also that the patient was not adequately monitored during the administration of Pitocin. In this regard, the medical records revealed that the decedent had not been checked between the hours of 12:30 a.m. and 1:30 a.m. The plaintiff's expert testified that the standard of care is to check a patient every 15 or 20 minutes during the time Pitocin is running.

It is interesting to note that the 1982 *ACOG Standards* state that the obstetrician must be in the labor area for the first 20 minutes after the administration of Pitocin is commenced. The 1985 standards drop this requirement but repeat the 1982 recommendation that the physician should be "readily accessible" to manage any complications that may arise during infusion. *ACOG Standards For Obstetric-Gynecologic Services* 35 (1985).

CHAPTER 20

FORCEPS

§ 20.14 Vacuum Extraction

Page 329, add to footnote 13:

In Stiles v. Sen, 152 A.D.2d 915, 544 N.Y.S.2d 259 (1989), the newborn died one half hour after birth. The surviving mother sued the physician and the hospital. The appellate court reversed the lower court grant of partial summary judgment for the defendants, as there were material questions of fact. There was a dispute as to whether the plaintiff had sustained a cervical or vaginal tear, arising out of the improper use of forceps, which would provide the physical injury necessary to support a claim for emotional distress arising out of the death of the infant. Such independent physical injury is required for a recovery of damages for emotional distress.

The plaintiff's obstetrician induced labor. He tried to deliver the baby with a vacuum extractor and failed. He then used forceps and the child was born alive with extensive trauma to scalp, skull, and brain. The mother was severely hemorrhaging and developed sinus tachardia. A cardiologist was consulted. The obstetrician had stated that the postpartum hemorrhage was not uncommon.

* In *Armendarez v. Tarrant County Hospital District,* 781 S.W.2d 301 (Tex. Ct. App. 1989), the plaintiffs sued for injuries sustained by their son during delivery. They alleged that the hospital and physicians were negligent in using vacuum extraction equipment and proceeding with a vaginal delivery, as opposed to performing a cesarean. The central issue was the application of governmental and official immunity. The trial court granted summary judgment for the defendants. The appellate court reversed, holding that there were questions of material fact precluding the grant of summary judgment. With respect to the issue of official immunity, the court held that physicians working at government hospitals are not immune to tort liability when their duties are the same as those performed by private physicians in private hospitals. However, there was a factual question as to whether the hospital residents were in a special position and were engaged in governmental functions such as might require the extension of immunity to them. With respect to the claims against the hospital district, the court held that Tex. Civ. Prac. & Rem. Code § 101.021 did not serve to extend immunity to claims arising from the negligent use of tangible property. This raised a factual issue as to whether the injuries were sustained due to the negligent use of the vacuum extractor or through other causes.

CHAPTER 21

BREECH PRESENTATION

*

§ 21.8 Management of Labor and Delivery

Page 342, add after last paragraph:

The plaintiffs, child and parents, sued an obstetrician for brachial plexus palsy injuries sustained by the child during delivery. The defendant physician's expert witness admitted that the injuries were caused by the defendant's acts during the delivery. The physician attempted to turn the baby's head to rotate the shoulders after discovering shoulder dystocia. The issue was whether the application of pressure to the head constituted a breach of the duty of care. The appellate court upheld the trial court's judgment for the physician on the jury verdict, finding that the evidence supported the verdict. *Dunne v. Somoano,* 550 So. 2d 5 (Fla. Dist. Ct. App. 1989).

In *Stein v. Insurance Corp.,* 566 So. 2d 1114 (La. Ct. App. 1990), the plaintiff parents brought suit arising out of the allegedly negligent prenatal care and delivery of the child. The mother consulted with the defendant obstetricians and arranged for them to provide prenatal care and deliver the baby. A medical history was taken one year earlier, during the mother's first pregnancy, after which a normal child was born. For the second pregnancy, the defendant followed the normal examination procedure and ran a sonogram. At 37 weeks the defendant observed that the fetus's head was floating out of the pelvis, indicating that it had not dropped into the pelvic cavity. In an examination four weeks later, the defendant determined that the fetus was dropping into the pelvic cavity. At an examination one week later, the defendant believed that there was excess fluid but that the child was not an abnormally large baby. He planned to induce labor one week later. On that date, the mother checked into the hospital and pitocin was administered to induce labor. Four hours later, the pitocin was increased. The defendant examined the mother on several occasions and then performed an amniotomy. This permitted the child's head to drop into the pelvic cavity. The mother was given epidural anesthesia and was completely dilated. Nurses applied fundal pressure and the head started to emerge. The defendant attempted to use forceps but could not get a good grip. He performed an episiotomy and, after more fundal pressure and forceps, he removed the head up to the neck. At this point he determined that there was shoulder dystocia. Immediate delivery is required in such a situation, because the umbilical cord is totally compressed and the baby will suffer brain damage or death. The defendant tried several procedures and could not turn the infant. The nurse used superpubic pressure to dislodge the child, who weighed 11 pounds, 10 ounces. The child was born with a fractured right clavicle and fractured rib cage, and had right brachial plexus nerve damage that resulted in Erb's Palsy. The defendants were found not to have been negligent for failing to employ ultrasound to determine the size of the fetus. The mother suffered from gestational diabetes, so the failure to perform a 50-gram glucose loading test was also not a breach of the standard of care, and was not the cause of the injuries. This was supported by the evidence despite the fact that the fetus of a diabetic mother tends to have a greater risk of shoulder dystocia.

§ 21.18 Cesarean Section Versus Vaginal Delivery

Page 350, add at the end of the section:

In *Juanita Doe v. Foundation Hospital,* No. 579593-0, (Alameda County, Cal. Sup. Ct. July 2, 1985), *reported in* 29 ATLA L. Rep. 35 (Feb. 1986), the plaintiff's mother alleged that her infant contracted a herpes infection during delivery as a result of the negligent failure of the obstetrician to perform a timely cesarean section.

One week prior to the infant's birth, the plaintiff's mother was admitted to the defendant hospital with a fever, vaginal discharge, and lip lesions. After the mother's membranes were ruptured, an internal monitor was placed on the infant. A cesarean section delivery was not performed until 20 hours after rupture. Subsequent to the birth, the plaintiff, who is now two and one-half years old, was diagnosed with herpes encephalitis, resulting in brain damage and quadriplegia. The plaintiff's suit alleged failure to test the mother for genital herpes during the hospitalization prior to the birth, failure to timely perform a cesarean section within four hours after rupture of the membranes to reduce the possibility of transmission of the genital herpes infection to the infant, negligence in placing an internal scalp monitor, which increased the likelihood that infection would travel into the brain, and failure to timely perform and receive a herpes culture report. The plaintiff received a structured settlement with a present value of $800,000.

In *Campbell v. Pitt County Memorial Hospital,* No. 86390558 (N.C. Ct. App. Feb. 17, 1987), Westlaw Allstates Database, the parents of Jennifer Campbell brought action against the hospital alleging negligence in connection with the vaginal delivery of their child, who was in a footling breech presentation. The evidence at trial indicated that the obstetrician and nursing staff knew the fetus was in the footling breech presentation at the time Mrs. Campbell was admitted to the hospital in labor. Nonetheless, the physician decided to proceed with a vaginal delivery. For several hours prior to delivery, the attending nurses observed signs of fetal distress. The attending nurse expressed her concern to the attending physician, but she did not contact her immediate supervisor when the doctor failed to address the fetal distress.

The umbilical cord was entangled around the baby's feet on delivery. Subsequently, Jennifer Campbell was diagnosed as suffering from cerebral palsy.

The jury entered a verdict on behalf of the plaintiffs, finding that the hospital was negligent in failing to make a reasonable effort to monitor and oversee the treatment of the laboring patient and her fetus by the attending physician. The trial court entered a judgment n.o.v., as to which the plaintiffs appealed.

The North Carolina Court of Appeals held that the defendant hospital, under the doctrine of corporate responsibility, owed a duty to make a reasonable effort to establish a mechanism for the prompt reporting of a situation which created a threat to the safety of a patient, that is, a situation of fetal distress. The court further held that the evidence supported the jury's determination that the hospital breached its duty to the Campbells and that as a direct and proximate result, Jennifer Campbell suffered hypoxia and resultant cerebral palsy. The court also held the evidence was sufficient to establish that the hospital breached its duty to ensure the parents' informed consent to the vaginal delivery of their footling breech baby had been obtained prior to delivery.

Practice Note. The North Carolina appeals court expressly recognized the doctrine of corporate responsibility, which involves the violation of a duty owed *directly* by the hospital to the patient, as a basis for liability apart and distinct from respondeat superior. The court, citing its earlier decision in *Bost v. Riley,* 44 N.C. App. 638, 262 S.E.2d 931 (1980), said:

> If a patient at a modern-day hospital has the reasonable expectation that the hospital will attempt to cure him, it seems axiomatic that the hospital have the duty assigned to make a reasonable effort to monitor and oversee the treatment which is prescribed and administered by a physician practicing at the facility.

The evidence established at trial that Mrs. Campbell had learned five weeks prior to delivery that her baby was in a breech presentation. Shortly after she was admitted to the hospital, the obstetrician confirmed the footling breech presentation by x-ray pelvimetry. He further confirmed the footling presentation by vaginal examination. The plaintiffs' experts properly testified at trial that the diagnosis of footling breech presentation clearly indicated that the fetus be delivered by cesarean section so as to avoid precisely what happened in this case – cord entanglement and resulting asphyxia.

The plaintiffs produced at trial a nurse expert, who testified that the physician had the primary responsibility of explaining the risks of the alternative methods of breech delivery (cesarean section and vaginal delivery) and that the nurses had the responsibility of making sure the patient fully understood the doctor's explanation of those risks. The nurse expert further testified that, in her opinion, had the physician and nurses fully explained the risks of vaginal delivery in a footling presentation, the parents would have opted for cesarean section. The court of appeals held that this testimony, as well as the testimony of the plaintiffs' physician experts, supported the jury's verdict that the hospital had failed to obtain the plaintiffs' informed consent.

CHAPTER 22

CESAREAN SECTION

§ 22.3 – Fetopelvic Disproportion

Page 357, add to footnote 3:

In Douzart v. Jones, 528 So. 2d 602 (La. Ct. App. 1988), the child was injured at birth. The parents appealed from a judgment for the physician. The appellate court affirmed, holding that there was insufficient evidence to hold the defendant physician liable for failing to anticipate that there was a probability of shoulder dystocia which might have required the performance of a cesarean section. Absent such evidence, the obstetrician could not be held liable for the child's mild Erb's palsy in his arm. The court rejected the locality rule for establishing the standard of care for the obstetrician specialist and applied a national standard. The plaintiffs, however, failed to prove the essential elements of the case, and the defendant's actions were found to be a reasonable exercise of his professional judgment.

The same mother's first child sustained shoulder dystocia, but the progress of the instant labor did not suggest the presence of the problem in this case. The chances of recurring dystocia are extremely rare. Shoulder dystocia occurs when one shoulder is trapped behind the mother's pelvis during delivery, after the exit of the infant's head. Such a situation often impairs the infant's breathing. In such a case, it is usually necessary to make a maximum incision on the back wall of the vagina to free the infant. The court also found that the defendant's failure to use a fetal heart monitor was not a breach of the standard of care, and, even if it was a breach, it did not have any causal connection to the injury in question.

In *Kavanaugh v. Nussbaum,* 71 N.Y.2d 535, 523 N.E.2d 284, 528 N.Y.S.2d 8 (1988), the trial court denied a motion to set aside a verdict on liability and entered judgment on some damage counts of the complaint. The appellate division modified the judgment and affirmed. The court of appeals affirmed and remitted the action, holding that the defendant obstetrician was not vicariously liable for the negligence of a physician who covered for him on the day prior to the birth. The evidence supported a finding of negligence and causation on the part of both the obstetrician and the emergency room physician. The plaintiff was awarded $1.5 million for pain and suffering, with $740,000 for impaired earning capacity, which damages were apportioned between the defendants.

The child was born after only 31 weeks gestation, while in distress, and weighed only three pounds at birth. The 44-year-old mother went to the emergency room when she started bleeding. There was a question as to whether the child was injured due to placenta previa which should have been detected at the time. The next day, an internal examination of the mother was performed and, upon loss of the fetal heartbeat, a cesarean section was performed. The Apgar scores of the newborn were 1 at 1 minute, 5 at 5 minutes, and 4 at 10 minutes. The baby was transferred to another hospital with better neonatal facilities, where a tracheotomy was performed, but the child suffered permanent debilitating injuries.

§ 22.8 – Fetal Distress

Page 361, add at the end of the section:

Fetal distress is one of the most prevalent causes of birth trauma. The case of *Reilly v. United States,* 665 F. Supp. 976 (D.R.I. 1987), was a Federal Tort Claims Act suit arising out of the negligence of the defendant naval obstetrician in the delivery of the child. The court held that liability could be imposed on the government for the failure of the obstetrician to meet the requisite standard of care, which breach resulted in the injuries. Rhode Island law was applied to determine the standard of care. The court ordered that amounts recovered for the child's lost earnings ($1.1 million) and for future medical and other care ($8.93 million) be placed in a reversionary trust. The court, however, refused to award noneconomic damages in addition to the child's pain and suffering ($1 million) without an answer from the Rhode Island Supreme Court on what noneconomic damages were available, that is, whether the parents could recover for their emotional distress, loss of consortium, and loss of the child's society. This case also contains an extensive discussion of various damage elements.

The evidence established that the defendant was negligent in the failure to perform a cesarean section even though the baby was clearly asphyxiated. There was negligence in failing to take measures to terminate the labor and in failing to use a heart monitor to track the progress of the fetus. The defendant was further negligent in using a vacuum suction technique on the baby's head while the baby was in such distress. At 3:35, the mother was admitted to the hospital. At 9:00, there was a deceleration of the fetal heart rate. The mother was not responsive to therapy, and labor was going on for an extended period. The baby was large and in the occiput position, all of which pointed to asphyxia. The defendant called for an operating room to perform a cesarean section, but then abandoned the idea. The defendant tried to have the mother push before the cervix was fully dilated. At 10:15, the defendant removed the fetal monitor: an absolute breach of the standard of care. Shortly thereafter, there was further dramatic deceleration.

Page 363, replace § 22.15 with the following §§ 22.15 through 22.15C:

§ 22.15 Anesthesia for Cesarean Section: Basic Considerations (New)

The frequency of cesarean sections has increased dramatically in recent years. From an incidence of 3 to 8 percent a decade ago, the present rate of cesarean sections is around 30 percent. G. Ostheimer, *Manual of Obstetric Anesthesia* 223 (1984). Indications for cesarean sections may be divided into elective and emergency indications.

Elective indications for cesarean sections include the following:

1. Dystocia, i.e. cephalopelvic disproportion
2. Fetal distress, e.g. uteroplacental insufficiency, preeclampsia
3. Breech presentation
4. Rh isoimmunization
5. Malpresentation.

Emergency cesarean section is indicated in a number of situations including the following:

1. Severe fetal distress
2. Prolapsed cord
3. Abruptio placenta
4. Failure to progress
5. Failed test of forceps
6. Placenta previa
7. Tetanic uterine contractions
8. Inability to endure labor.

Cesarean section imposes on the mother and the fetus an increased risk of morbidity and mortality in comparison to the risks inherent in a normal vaginal delivery. For the mother, the major stresses are to the heart and the respiratory system. For the fetus, the extent and severity of the stress imposed by cesarean section depend upon the maturity of the fetus, the type of duration of analgesia and anesthesia, and, of course, the quality of the anesthesia and obstetric care. J. Bonica, *Obstetric Analgesia and Anesthesia* 163 (2d ed. 1980).

Safe anesthesia for cesarean section requires skilled and experienced physicians and nurses, and proper equipment. The two basic approaches for cesarean section are *general* and *regional.* Both types of anesthesia are effective and safe, if performed by competent, technically skilled professionals. A recent article reports that 41 percent of pregnant women receive general anesthesia, 35 percent receive spinal anesthesia, and 21 percent receive epidural anesthesia. C. Gibbs, *Obstetrical Anesthesia: A National Survey*, Anesthesiology 65:298 (1986).

§ 22.15A General Anesthesia (New)

General anesthesia may be the preferred route of administration in the following situations, among others:

1. Hypovelemia
2. Hemorrhage
3. Severe, acute fetal distress
4. Regional anesthesia ineffective
5. Regional anesthesia contraindicated.

General anesthesia (*anesthesia* means loss of consciousness) is usually accomplished by the administration of intravenous thiopental (Pentothal). Thiopental is not used as the sole anesthetic agent. Rather, it is administered in a dose that puts the patient to sleep along with a muscle relaxant, succinylcholine. Cricoid pressure is maintained to prevent aspiration during this process and nitrous oxide plus oxygen is administered through a cuffed endotracheal tube. Some anesthesiologists also administer a low dose of halothane to insure a loss of consciousness. This balanced combination of drugs is designed to produce safe and effective anesthesia with minimal risks of maternal morbidity and mortality and newborn depression.

§ 22.15B – Advantages, Disadvantages, and Risks (New)

The use of general anesthesia for cesarean section has several advantages. General anesthesia is safe and reliable, when administered by highly skilled and experienced professionals. The patient is totally relaxed, unconscious, and unaware of the procedure; hence, the physician has an optimal situation for performing surgery. However, this condition of unconsciousness is also one of the disadvantages of general anesthesia, because the mother is unable to experience, watch, and participate in the birth of her child.

The major disadvantages of general anesthesia are much more serious, constituting risks to maternal and fetal well-being. These risks include maternal aspiration, esophogeal intubation, and narcotization of the newborn. See §§ **18.7, 18.8** and **18.9.** Causes of neonatal depression from general anesthesia include maternal hypoventilation, maternal hyperventilation, and reduced utero-placental perfusion. In addition, the effect of anesthetic drugs on the fetus may cause varying degrees of depression, depending upon such factors as the agent used and the induction-delivery time.

§ 22.15C Regional Anesthesia (New)

A number of drugs and methods are presently used to produce local or regional anesthesia for cesarean section. *Spinal anesthesia* refers to the introduction of a local agent into the subarachnoid space (subarachnoid block). Complications include maternal hypotension, total spinal blockade, and nausea, vomiting, and headache. Advantages of spinal anesthesia are substantial: There is low fetal exposure to the anesthetic agent; the patient is awake and able to experience her child's birth; there is no risk of aspiration; and the procedure is quick, simple, and very reliable.

Epidural anesthesia is frequently employed in cesarean section today. The injection of a local anesthetic into the epidural or peridural space effectively blocks the pain of uterine contractions and delivery. The use of epidural anesthesia for cesarean section carries obvious advantages: The patient is awake; there is no risk of aspiration; and it is quick, safe, and effective. There are certain disadvantages, however. These include the possibility of hypotension, central nervous stimulation (convulsion), inadvertent spinal anesthesia, and post-spinal headache.

CHAPTER 23

IMMEDIATE CARE OF THE NEWBORN

§ 23.1 Introduction

Page 368, add at the end of the section:

The plaintiffs sued the family physician and the hospital's high-risk team for negligence in the care of their newborn, which resulted in severe neurological deficits. The defendants claimed that the deficits were due to a pre-birth brain malformation and accompanying birth defects. The birth was difficult, and shortly thereafter the child showed the characteristics of hypotonia and other symptoms of perinatal asphyxia. The child was born with club feet and dysmorphic physical features, and also suffered from hypoglycemia. The trial court entered judgment on the jury verdict (10-2) for the defendants. The court of appeals, in *Richards v. Overlake Hospital Medical Center,* 59 Wash. App. 266, 796 P.2d 737 (1990), affirmed. The court held that the trial court committed harmless error in instructing the jury that the family physician was to be judged by the standard of a reasonably prudent family physician. The court properly rejected a plaintiffs' instruction seeking to base the standard of care on the expectations of society or of the patient. The court recognized that the jury found that the cause of the injuries was a prenatal event and not the care given after birth.

There was also an issue as to juror misconduct. One juror with a medical background reviewed the medical records which had been introduced into evidence and came to the conclusion that the defects were due to the mother's contracting influenza 20 weeks into the pregnancy. This opinion was shared with other jurors. The court upheld the trial court's finding that this was not juror misconduct requiring a new trial.

§ 23.3 Resuscitation

Page 370, add at the end of the section:

The American Academy of Pediatrics and the American College of Obstetricians and Gynecologists, in their 1983 publication, *Guidelines for Perinatal Care,* list a number of conditions which require the availability of skilled resuscitation at delivery. These conditions are:

141

1. Fetal distress, defined as (a) persistent late decelerations, (b) meconium staining, (c) cord prolapse, (d) scalp pH $\leq$ 7.25, and (e) severe variable decelerations with absent beat-to-beat variability
2. Cesarean section or mid-forceps delivery anticipated
3. Bleeding in the third trimester
4. Multiple births
5. Estimated birth weight $\leq$ 1500gf
6. Dysfunctional labor.

Once problems such as fetal distress are detected, it is necessary to assure proper respiration so as to prevent or mitigate further injuries. In *Bacon v. Mercy Hospital*, 243 Kan. 303, 756 P.2d 416 (1988), the parents and child sued the hospital, physicians, and pediatricians, claiming that they were negligent and that their negligence caused the child's cerebral palsy. The trial court entered summary judgment for the defendant. That judgment was affirmed, as no evidence was presented that the conduct of the defendants in the hours following the delivery caused the cerebral palsy. The court recognized the general tenet that negligence can never be presumed or inferred from a poor result; the plaintiff always has the burden of proof of negligence and causation. The etiology of the child's cerebral palsy required expert testimony. The plaintiff submitted affidavits after the motion for summary judgment was heard, but those affidavits were irrelevant bolstering of the materials previously supplied by the plaintiff, and should have been submitted in connection with the motion. Also, an insufficient connection was drawn between the medical texts to establish the plaintiff's claims or, at a minimum, to overcome the motion for summary judgment. The physicians testifying for the plaintiff were not experts on cerebral palsy. This severely undermined their testimony.

The mother had an uneventful pregnancy until 15 minutes prior to the delivery, when the fetal heart monitor registered a sudden severe brachycardia, then no discernable pattern. The umbilical cord was wrapped twice around the baby's neck, and the cord compression caused the autonomous nervous system to decelerate. The baby was delivered not breathing, cyanotic, and with a low heart rate. The physicians used a laryngoscope and endotracheal tube for resuscitation, and the baby was placed on a warming tray. There was a question as to whether a pediatrician should have been called in by the obstetrician at that point. There was severe bronchial and lung tissue resistance to the bagging and mouth-to-mouth resuscitation was used. It took between 30 and 45 minutes before the child recovered and turned pink.

§ 23.4 Evaluating the Newborn's Physical Status (Apgar Scores)

Page 371, add at the end of the section:

Practice Note. The Apgar score is "the traditional and most universal criteria for assessing the newborn's well-being in the delivery room." *Neonatology Pathophysiology And Management of The Newborn* 329 (G. Avery ed., 2d ed. 1981) [hereinafter *Neonatology Pathophysiology*]. The score is an indicator of the new-born's capacity to tolerate the stress of the labor process. A low Apgar score has traditionally been associated with hypoxia and asphyxia. A number of studies have demonstrated the correlation between a low 5-minute Apgar score and later neurologic damage and developmental handicap. *See, e.g.,* J. Drage, C. Kennedy, H. Berendes, et al: *The Apgar Score As An Index of Infant Morbidity,* Dev. Med. Child Neurol. 8:141a (1966). The incidence of cerebral palsy has been shown to increase with low late Apgar scores in infants with Apgars of 0 to 3 at 20 minutes. *Neonatology Pathophysiology* at 36. However, the Apgar score is not absolutely reliable as an indicator of late neurologic damage.

Some babies with fairly high Apgar scores may in fact be severely brain damaged. In one study, 55 percent of children with later cerebral palsy had Apgar scores of 7 to 10 at one minute, and 73 percent scored 7 to 10 at five minutes. K. Nelson & J. Ellenberg, *Apgar Scores as Predictors of Chronic Neurologic Disability,* 68 Pediatrics, 36-44 (No. 1, July 1981). In such instances, the reassuring Apgar score may have been influenced by fetal position changes or a late improvement in placental perfusion. By the same token, some babies with very low–even zero–Apgars may do well and display no late neurologic sequence. One study has found that even zero Apgars at birth may be compatible with "reasonable survival under efficient, prompt resuscitation." *Neonatology Pathophysiology* at 363, (citing H. Scott, *Outcome of Very Severe Birth Asphyxia,* Arch. Dis. Child. 52:620 (1977).

The controversy surrounding the accuracy and reliability of the Apgar scoring system as an indicator of asphyxia and a prognosticator of future neurologic sequalae, such as cerebral palsy, has increased in recent years with increasing medico-legal concerns in perinatal medical practice. One important aspect of this controversy has to do with the premise which states that "the one-minute Apgar score reflects the obstetrician's doing, where the five-minute score belongs to the pediatricians." M. Volk & M. Morgan, *Medical Malpractice: Handling Obstetric and Neonatal Cases* 698 (1986). As the authors of one medico-legal text observe:

> This arbitrary assignment of responsibility and the resulting attempts to draw distinct territorial boundaries have, in many cases, turned the delivery area into a war zone. The obstetrician is under intense pressure to produce a good product,

143

i.e., to deliver a baby with good Apgar scores. Additionally, if the infant does develop a neurologic problem at a later date, the presence of good Apgar scores may either ward off further investigations into the obstetricial care or may strenghten its defense . . . On the other side of the fence is the pediatrician or neonatologist who feels he or she is expected to successfully resuscitate any infant that he or she is handed. In his or her mind, there is one recurrent thought, imagining hearing the obstetricians telling the family, "I don't know what happened. The baby was fine when I handed him to the pediatricians."

Id.

The problem of inaccurate Apgar scoring does not appear resolvable in the present litigation-induced climate of paranoia. It would be helpful to have an independent "referee" to assign the Apgar score; this was the recommendation of the ACOG in the 1981 Precia II. Unfortunately, finding an impartial nurse or physician in the labor and delivery room or the nursery is not likely when the infant is born in a severely depressed condition with neurologic damage.

Thus, the plaintiff's attorney is left with the task of attacking the accuracy of the Apgar score (when the score is high, but the baby is born with brain damage) by impeaching the creditability of the scorer and by demonstrating contradictions in the labor record and/or the nursery records. For example, when the Apgar score is low, but the baby is severely distressed at birth, counsel may be able, through his expert's testimony, to raise the inference that this incongruity is the result of Apgar tampering.

The American Academy of Pediatrics, Committee on Fetus and Newborn, has published an important article entitled *Use and Abuse of the Apgar Score,* 78 Pediatrics, 1148-49 (Dec. 1986). In this article, the AAP makes the following pronouncement:

> [H]ypoxia leading to cerebral palsy can be presumed only when three criteria are met: (1) Apgar score is 0 to 3 at ten minutes (in the absence of other cause), (2) infant remains hypotonic for at least several hours and (3) infant has seizures . . . . To substantiate that hypoxia led to adverse neurologic outcome requires additional perinatal evidence such as Apgar scores of 0 to 3 at ten minutes, and early perinatal seizures, and prolonged hypotonia. One of these elements alone is insufficient evidence that prolonged or severe asphyxia has occurred.

This pronouncement by the AAP is certain to be an effective weapon in the defense of an obstetricial malpractice case. The class of cases of cerebral palsy which may be attributable to hypoxia has been narrowed considerably by the AAP.

The article is somewhat ambiguous, however. Although three criteria are established for the identification of hypoxia as the etiology of cerebral palsy (low Apgar, hypotonia, and seizure activity), the authors of the study refer to "additional perinatal evidence" which may substantiate hypoxia. Such additional evidence could include, for example, evidence of acidosis, fetal monitor tracings showing late decelerations, and the presence of thick meconium at the time of delivery.

Practice Note. In one case in which the author was involved, the parents of a brain-damaged baby had videotaped their child's delivery. The video tape record showing a floppy, unresponsive infant was a powerful evidentiary weapon in attacking the validity of a high Apgar score assigned by the pediatrician.

Comment. The following is an excerpt from an actual deposition of a labor and delivery nurse who was on duty when the plaintiff's fetus was demonstrating what one of plaintiff's experts would later refer to as the "death spiral" – periods of bradycardia followed by tachycardia. The infant in this case was born with a 0 Apgar and now suffers from athetoid cerebral palsy. At one point in the labor the nurse reinjected the epidural and concomitantly the fetal heart tones dropped to 48. Plaintiff's position was that the drop in FHTs and the subsequent periods of bradycardia and tachycardia were caused by umbilical cord compression. An intravascular injection was ruled out because the mother did not experience hypotension (if she did, it was not recorded). The hospital indicated in its Answers to Interrogatories that the fetal heart monitor tracings were "lost or destroyed."

Q. When you came on shift in the afternoon of October 30th, did Nurse Simpson make a shift report to you?

A. Yes.

Q. What did she tell you about Mrs. Nelson's progress in labor up to that point?

A. That she was progressing normally. Was 3 centimeters dilated and about 90% effaced, station was minus two. Fetal heart tones were in the 140-160 range.

Q. Did you read in the labor record that there had been meconium staining noted at the time she was admitted, at the time Dr. Carter ruptured Mrs. Nelson's membranes?

A. Yes.

Q. Did you place significance on this observation of meconium?

A. Well, just to watch the patient for any developing problem.

Q. Is meconium a sign of fetal distress?

A. Can be. Not necessarily, but can be.

Q. Is meconium a sign that there may be a problem with the oxygenation of the fetus?

A. Not necessarily. Can mean nothing at all. I've seen lots of babies who are born in meconium and do perfectly fine.

Q. But, meconium is noted in the literature as a red flag - a warning sign that the fetus may be in a compromised, or potentially compromised uterine environment.?

A. I suppose that is a possibility.

Q. Let's look at the record at 10:25 in the evening. Did you make the notation "FHT's dropped to 48 with epidural injection?"

A. Yes.

Q. First, let me ask you, did you make the epidural injection?

A. Reinjection.

Q. Right, excuse me, the reinjection. Was the doctor present when you made the reinjection?

A. No.

Q. What is the hospital's policy with respect to the nurse doing the reinjection?

A. I think it says that as long as the doctor is in the hospital, it is all right. I have always done this. It's Dr. Carter's policy to establish the epidural and to make the reinjections, but when he is with another patient or not available, then I or one of the other RN's who are trained to do it can do so.

Q. Before making the reinjection, did you do anything?

A. Aspirated the syringe to make sure we did not have an intravascular injection.

Q. Anything else at all?

A. Like what?

Q. I'm just asking the question. Did you take any other measures, make any other observations, at the time you made the reinjection?

A. No. That's all that is required. Reinject the measured amount of nesacaine, 3%, 7cc.

Q. All right, now in the records you wrote that upon the reinjection the FHT's dropped down to 48. Does this indicate an intravascular injection?

A. No.

Q. What is the basis of your opinion that this drop in FHT's did not signal an intravascular injection?

A. Because her blood pressure stayed normal. If it had gone into the vascular system directly, her blood pressure would have dropped and stayed down for some time. It did not drop.

Q. At least, you did not record a drop in the records.

A. It did not drop.

Q. It has been four years. Do you recall of your own memory, independent of the records, that her blood pressure did not drop?

A. Yes.

Q. We'll come back to that in a moment. Let me ask you now about what happened after the FHT's dropped to 48, in the next two and one-half hour period. First, is the record correct that the FHT's dropped at 10:25 and then, as the record says, "returned to normal" at 10:35?

A. Well, I'm sure they came back to normal right away, because we turned her and gave her oxygen and I am sure they came right back up to normal.

Q. The record indicates what happened. When an event occurs, you record it in the record?

A. Yes.

Q. And you recorded that the FHT's returned to normal at 10:35. This would indicate they were abnormal for a period of ten minutes?

A. You don't always record something the minute it happens.

Q. At 10:45, you wrote "FHT's going down to 100, slowly, then rising slowly." Did you record that note when it happened?

A. I assume so.

Q. Is your memory now fading?

A. I am sure that is recorded when it happened.

Q. All right. Now, that notation indicated bradycardia?

A. Yes.

Q. And it also indicates that there is a late deceleration?

A. Not necessarily late, but a deceleration, yes.

Q. If we had the monitor strips, we would see at 10:45 a late deceleration?

A. As I said, not necessarily late.

Q. Is a late deceleration one that begins after the onset of the contraction and then slowly recovers after the contraction is over?

A. Yes.

Q. Nurse Sweeney, you wrote at 11:00, FHT's stabilizing but going up, and the anesthesia record shows that at 11:00, the fetal heart tones went up to 160.?

A. Yes.

Q. Well, if the heart tones are going from 48 up to 160, how is that stabilizing?

A. By that it means the FHT's are going back to the baseline.

Q. What was the baseline?

A. Around 120-130, in that area.

Q. There are notations here showing 150, 148, 160. How do you get a baseline of 120-130?

A. That's an average.

Q. I see. What is the significance of the notation FHT's going up to 160? Is 160 tachycardia?

A. No.

Q. It isn't? How do you define tachycardia, Mrs. Sweeney?

A. Tachycardia is anything above 180. Up to 180 is normal.

Q. Where did you learn that?

A. From literature. Schooling. In-service.

Q. You learned from the literature that tachycardia begins at 180 in a fetus?

A. Yes.

Q. Is that what Dr. Carter instructed you in the in-services you've told us about?

A. Yes.

Q. And what Nurse Lowe, the nursing supervisor, told you was tachycardia?

A. Yes.

Q. So, if you saw on the fetal monitor these FHT's going up to 160, this would not be a cause of concern?

A. No.

Q. Certainly, then, you would not feel it important to notify the doctor?

A. Right.

Q. And at 11:20, you wrote "tachycardia continues". The anesthesia record now shows the FHT's are at 178, 180, and 186 around 11:20 to 11:30. Is it your testimony that tachycardia begins at 180?

A. Yes.

Q. So that when you saw the FHT's going up to 180, you now thought you had a problem, you had tachycardia?

A. I didn't think it was a problem.

Q. Is tachycardia significant in a laboring patient?

A. In the fetus?

Q. Yes.

A. No. Tachycardia in itself is not significant.

Q. Tachycardia in itself has no significance?

A. Right.

Q. Where did you learn that?

A. From everything I've been taught.

Q. That tachycardia has no clinical significance?

A. No significant clinical significance.

Q. Let me get this straight. Your testimony is that tachycardia, fetal tachycardia, has no significant clinical significance.?

A. That's what I've been taught.

Q. Does tachycardia take on any additional significance when you see, as in this case, that it was preceded by FHT's going down as low as 48, staying down for ten minutes, dropping down again to below 100?

A. The presence of decelerations does not make tachycardia significant. You can't add the decelerations to tachycardia and suddenly tachycardia takes on something different.

Q. All right. At 11:45 you make the notation, FHT's going down below 100 with contractions. That means you have a late deceleration?

A. Not necessarily late. Just a deceleration. An early deceleration.

Q. Well, since the hospital has told us in their answers to our interrogatories that the fetal heart strips for Mrs. Nelson's labor were lost or destroyed, you have nothing to show outside of these records which would support your opinion that these decelerations which are documented in the record were earlys, and not lates. Do you?

A. I remember them to be earlys. I am sure of that.

Q. All right. Now, at 12:15, you wrote in the records "large amount mec. staining." What is the significance of observing a large amount of meconium at this stage of labor, with the decelerations and tachycardia going on?

A. The significance is that meconium can be fetal distress.

Q. Does the tachycardia which you noted in the records take on added significance when it keeps company with meconium?

A. No.

Q. But, you've testified that meconium is a sign of fetal distress?

A. Yes.

Q. And large amount is an ominous sign?

A. Yes.

Q. Why did you not contact the doctor immediately upon observing the meconium?

A. I did contact him.

Q. Record shows you waited 20 minutes before notifying him. Do you see that?

A. I know I went and got him immediately.

Q. Sometimes, you wrote in the record exactly when things happened. Sometimes you didn't.

A. You can't always take time to write. You have to make the decision to act or to write, so I will take acting over sitting and writing in a case like this.

Q. Now, you didn't see fit to notify the doctor when you saw the FHT's going down at 10:45 and again at 11:00 and at 11:45. And, since you don't think tachycardia is important, you didn't notify him when you saw the heart tones rise up to 160 and on up to 180. Why do you suddenly think the doctor needs to know what is going on at 12:20 after waiting all this time?

A. Because when you have a lot of meconium, you know there is a problem, a potential problem, and the baby may need to be delivered. Up until that time, there was nothing going on with the FHT's or anything else.

Q. Just decelerations, accelerations, and late patterns?

A. There were several decelerations, several accelerations.

Q. Just so I can get this clear in my mind, is it your testimony that you did not believe that the decelerations and the tachycardia were indicating that fetal distress was going on, that this baby was suffering from hypoxia and asphyxia?

A. As I've already said, these are signs of a possible problem, that you watch what is going on, but in and of themselves, these kinds of fetal heart patterns are not fetal distress. But when I saw the meconium, then, yes, this is something the doctor has to be aware of right away.

Q. At any time during your shift, did the doctor come in and examine the patient?

A. Yes, the record is right there. At 11:00.

Q. That was the only time between the time you came on at 4:00, and the time you saw the doctor in the delivery room?

A. I'm sure he came into the labor room a number of times.

Q. It's not in the records. It's only in the records that he came in at 11:00.

A. Well, I know he did come in several times that are not in the records. I don't write down every single time the doctors come in and see the patient and look at the monitor.

Q. But you are supposed to write down every time he actually examines the patient?

A. Yes.

Q. And you wrote down every time he actually came in there and examined the patient? And that was once. Right?

A. That's all I wrote down.

Q. Did Dr. Carter ever tell you to get ready for a cesarean section?

A. No.

Q. Never mentioned it?

Q. I will represent to you, and this is a fact, that Dr. Carter has testified in this matter by way of deposition, and he has testified that he told you at 11:00 to be prepared for the possibility of a cesarean section. Is that testimony true?

A. If that's what he says.

Q. Well, is that or is that not the fact of what happened?

A. I don't remember him ever saying anything about a cesarean section. There was no reason for him to be talking about a cesarean section until right at the end, and then he went ahead right away and delivered the baby vaginally.

§ 23.5 External Cardiac Massage

Page 372, add at the end of the section:

In *Parker v. Southwest Louisiana Hospital Association,* 540 So. 2d 1270 (La. Ct. App. 1989), a child was severely brain damaged when one day old due to a cardiac arrest or apneic episode while the child was in the hospital nursery. The trial court entered a verdict for the defendant. The appellate court affirmed, while finding that the hospital complied with the requisite standard of care in observing a well baby at 10- to 15- minute intervals when the infant's condition did not require constant supervision. The court also found that the claimed failure of the staff properly to intubate the baby when they attempted resuscitation was not established by the evidence.

The complaint alleged a variety of failures to train and supervise the nursing staff. The complaint specifically alleged that the staff failed to call for a "Code Blue" immediately when the child was found to be in distress, and that the distress would have been discovered earlier had there been sufficient staff monitoring the children. The hospital had a separate nursery intensive care unit for children whose conditions required constant supervision, but this baby was normal and required no such extraordinary measures.

The case discussed the incidence of sudden infant death syndrome (SIDS), which is 2 in 1,000 babies from 3 weeks to 6 months old. This baby went into arrest within 24 hours of birth; SIDS incidence is approximately 1.5 per 100,000 at that age. Therefore, the occurrence of apnea is extremely rare in such a child. The court also recognized that a baby can turn blue within 60 to 90 seconds of when it stops breathing and that the amount of brain damage sustained by such a child is not indicative of the amount of time the baby was left unobserved.

§ 23.7 The Neonatal Examination

Page 376, add at the end of the section:

In *Montalbano v. North Shore University Hospital,* 154 A.D.2d 579, 546 N.Y.S.2d 408 (1989), the plaintiff parents sued the physician and hospital for malpractice arising out of the delivery of their child. The trial court's grant of summary judgment for the physician was reversed. The appellate court held that the physician's bare statements that he complied with the applicable standard of care, and that his actions were not the cause of the infant's injuries, were insufficient support for summary judgment in his favor. These statements were insufficient as a matter of law. The defendant physician also attempted to exculpate himself by claiming that he did not examine the child after the birth. This was also insufficient to support summary judgment, particularly since the parents alleged that the failure to examine constituted additional malpractice.

CHAPTER 29

ANALYSIS OF DAMAGES AND LOSS OF EARNING CAPACITY

§ 29.1 Summary of Costs for Recommended Health Care and Loss of Earning Capacities

Page 454, add at the end of the section:

In 1988, Florida enacted the Florida Birth Related Neurological Injury Compensation Plan, Fla. Stat. Ann. § 766.301 *et seq.* (West Supp. 1989). This statutory scheme provides special treatment for certain obstetrical injuries, in recognition of the tremendous cost increases in medical malpractice insurance of such practitioners vis-à-vis other physicians. The legislature recognized that the costs of birth-related neurological injuries are great. The statutory plan is the exclusive remedy for the child, parents, and other plaintiffs, and applies except where there is willful or wanton conduct. The statute of limitation is tolled by filing a claim with the compensation plan, but such must be filed within seven years of the birth. The claim is heard by a medical advisory panel. Upon finding that a neurological birth injury has occurred, the board shall make an award for medical and hospital expenses, including custodial care, but there can be no recovery for the benefits receivable for the government and certain insurance benefits. Additionally, there can be a periodic payment recovery to the parent which shall not exceed $100,000. Past expenses are to be paid immediately, and future expenses will be paid as they accrue. The plan is applicable to the patients of hospitals and participating physicians, who must notify their patients of their participation in the plan. The physicians participate in the plan through the payment of assessments.

§ 29.2 Periods of Health Care Costs and Loss of Earning Capacities

Page 455, add at the end of the section:

Clearly, in severe birth trauma cases, injuries can be horrific, resulting in the need for lifetime medical and other services. Accordingly, the future damages are large. In the case of *Scott v. United States*, 884 F.2d 1280 (9th

Cir. 1989), applying Alaska law, a child was injured prior to and during his birth at a military hospital. The district court entered judgment for the plaintiffs. The circuit court affirmed in part and reversed in part, holding that the trial court properly permitted recovery of damages arising from the effect of the child's spastic quadriplegia (cerebral palsy) on the parent-child relationship. The appellate court upheld the award of separate amounts for the child's past and future pain and suffering, as distinguished from an award for his past and future impairment.

The trial court was required, however, to recalculate the discount rate for the economic losses of income loss and medical expense. Alaska law applied to determine the discount rate in this case. The child was properly awarded $2 million for the injuries which rendered him incapable of any form of an independent life and which would require around-the-clock professional care. The trial jury awarded the child $8.75 million for future economic losses reduced to present value. The parents were awarded $350,000 for loss of the parent-child relationship. This case extensively discusses the damage perspective, but has no discussion of the underlying negligence on the part of the defendant which resulted in the injuries.

In *Reilly v. United States,* 665 F. Supp. 976 (D.R.I. 1987), a suit was brought arising out of the negligence of the defendant naval obstetrician in the delivery of a child. The court held that liability could be imposed on the government for the failure of the obstetrician to meet the requisite standard of care, which breach resulted in the injuries. Rhode Island law was applied to determine the standard of care. The court ordered that amounts recovered for the child's lost earnings ($1.1 million) and for future medical and other care ($8.93 million) be placed in a reversionary trust. The court, however, refused to award noneconomic damages in addition to the child's pain and suffering ($1 million) without an answer from the Rhode Island Supreme Court as to what noneconomic damages were available, that is, whether the parents could recover for emotional distress, loss of consortium, and loss of the child's society. This case also contains an extensive discussion of various damage elements.

The evidence established that the defendant was negligent in the failure to perform a cesarian section even though the baby was clearly asphyxiated. There was negligence in failing to take measures to terminate the labor and in failing to use a heart monitor to track the progress of the fetus. The defendant was further negligent in using a vacuum suction technique on the baby's head while the baby was in such distress. At 3:35, the mother was admitted to the hospital. At 9:00, there was a deceleration of the fetal heart rate. The mother was not responsive to therapy, and labor was going on for an extended period. The baby was large and in occiput position, all of which pointed to asphyxia. The defendant called for an operating room to perform a cesarean section, but then abandoned the idea. The defendant tried to have the mother push before the cervix was fully dilated. At 10:15, the defendant removed the fetal monitor, an absolute breach of the standard of care. Shortly thereafter, there was further dramatic deceleration.

§ 29.11   Other Professional Care

Page 463, add at the end of the section:

Educational and rehabilitation specialists may be required. In *Lininger v. Eisenbaum,* 764 P.2d 1202 (Colo. 1988), the suit involved claims for wrongful birth and wrongful life of a child who was born blind. The trial court dismissed the suit and the appellate court affirmed. The Supreme Court of Colorado affirmed in part and reversed in part, holding that the wrongful birth claim was viable, whereas the wrongful life claim was properly dismissed. The plaintiff parents claimed that if the defendant physicians had not been negligent in failing to determine that the first child's blindness was hereditary, the parents would not have had this second child. This stated a claim for recovery of extraordinary medical and educational expenses. The court overruled the decision in *Continental Casualty Co. v. Empire Casualty Co.,* 713 P.2d 384 (Colo. 1986), on the wrongful life claim. The court looked at the blindness as carrying the same type of monetary burden as would occur in any personal injury. There was an extensive review of these torts in other jurisdictions, but the court rejected the wrongful life claim, holding that the defendant's physicians did not owe a duty to the child.

In October 1981, the first child was born, and in March 1982 his vision problems were detected. A pediatric ophthalmologist, neuro-ophthalmologist, and another ophthalmologist each stated that the first child had congenital optic nerve hypoplasia. Therefore, the plaintiffs thought that the blindness might be genetic, but were assured by the defendants that it was not. The plaintiffs thought that another child could help the first child and sought further advice on the possibility that the second child would be born blind. The defendants again stated that the condition was not hereditary. In August 1983, the second child was born. Several months later, the child was diagnosed as being blind. It was then discovered that the blindness was due to Leber's congenital amaurosis, which is hereditary. The risk of the condition arising in the second child was one in four.

CHAPTER 33

CROSS EXAMINATION OF DEFENDANT PHYSICIAN AND EXPERT WITNESS

§ 33.10 Cross Examination of Defendant Obstetrician Regarding Traumatic Forceps Delivery, Cephalopelvic Disproportion, and Arrested Labor (New)

The following trial testimony was elicited on cross-examination of the defendant obstetrician. Plaintiff's attorney sought to establish that the defendant performed a high forceps delivery, a method of delivery which has been abolished from safe modern obstetric practice. Plaintiff's attorney also sought to establish that the delivery was complicated by an large (macrasomic) fetus and a cephalopelvic disproportion.

Q. Okay. Okay. Jewell Miller came into your office on February 14th of '85 as a part of her regular prenatal visits. Correct?

A. I assume it was a regular visit, yes. I think she had been in the week before.

Q. Sir?

A. I think she was on a week–may I look at this?

Q. Yes.

A. She was on weekly visits, and she was there on the 7th. So I would assume that the 14th was a regular visits.

Q. Okay. Do you recall any statements that were made between you and Jewell Miller on February 14th of '85?

A. No, I don't.

Q. Do you recall telling her that the baby had not dropped on that date?

A. I possibly could have.

Q. Because that's what your clinical findings indicated. Correct?

A. That's correct.

Q. And that you doubted that she would have the baby on the expected EDC date of 2/22/85?

A. I probably said that if she did, it would be a long labor, that she was not prepared, she was not ready, she was not engaged.

Q. Okay.

A. And that it would be a long labor for her to try to go natural.

Q. Do you recall her asking you whether or not she could go into labor with the baby not dropped?

A. I don't recall, but the answer I would give her would be yes, she could go into labor without the baby dropped.

Q. And did you indicate that if that happened that it would be a long labor that might result in a cesarean section?

A. I don't know if I said cesarean section, but I said it would be a long labor.

Q. But isn't that true?

A. There's always a chance.

Q. Okay. She in fact went into labor that same day. Correct?

A. Apparently so.

Q. Okay. And you wouldn't have expected that based on your examination that morning.

A. I've been doing this so long I don't expect anything any more. I just take it as it comes.

Q. But you didn't expect that, did you?

A. I wished she would not, because I did not think that her cervix was prepared.

Q. What does that indicate to you when the lady does go into labor and her cervix isn't prepared? What do you foresee as potential complications at that point?

A. Usually a long labor.

Q. Is that all?

A. Well, there's so many other factors involved that you just can't say.

Q. On 2/14 of '85 did you have any reason to believe that this was going to be an excessively sized baby? I'm talking about before she goes into the hospital.

A. As I stated earlier, I thought the baby was eight-and-a-half to nine pounds at that time.

Q. And that's based on fundal height?

A. From feeling the entire abdomen, yes.

Q. Well, an eight-and-a-half to nine-pound baby is still a pretty good size baby.

A. Still a nice baby, yes.

Q. What's a normal size baby?

A. I don't know what normal is.

Q. Well, what's the average size baby?

A. I don't know.

Q. Nobody's come up with any statistics on that?

A. I don't think.

Q. Okay. And at that point you felt like she had sufficient pelvic space to deliver this baby normally and naturally, on 2/14 of '85.

A. Yes, I did.

Q. Okay. You didn't believe there was any evidence that there might be cephalopelvic distribution at that time.

A. Disproportion?

Q. Disproportion, I'm sorry.

A. No, I did not.

Q. Doctor, is there any obstetrical procedure that you're not qualified to perform?

A. Could you rephrase the question?

Q. Well, there are a number of obstetrical procedures, are there not?

A. Yes, I would assume there are. Yes.

Q. Is there any of them that you're not qualified to perform?

A. Do you have one in mind that you can give me?

Q. No. I assume that you know what you can do and what you can't do.

A. I do not do vaccum extractions.

Q. Okay. So you don't feel qualified–

A. I was not trained to do vaccum extractions. I guess I could learn. I guess I could do them. It's not done here.

Q. Okay. Anything else you don't feel like you're qualified to perform?

A. The high forceps.

Q. By high forceps what do you mean?

A. When the baby's above the ischial spines.

Q. When you say the baby's above the ischial spines, what part of the baby are you talking about?

A. When the biparietal diameter is above the ischial spines, when you're in a minus station.

Q. When the biparietal diameter is above the ischial spines you consider that to be a high forceps delivery?

A. Yes, I do.

Q. And you don't feel qualified to do that?

A. Unless there was a dire emergency. I guess I could do it. I've never done it, so–I can't think of a reason to do it.

Practice Note. Here, the defendant obstetrician defines a high forceps delivery as one in which the "biparietal diameter is above the ischial spines, when you're in a minus station." This definition is not sufficiently precise to identify the proscribed high forceps operation.

Although it is generally said that engagement (sometimes called lightening) occurs when the parietal bones are at or below the ischial spines, mere engagement in this sense does not always justify classifying the forceps delivery a "mid" rather than a "high." Many obstetricians would not consider the level of the ischial spines, that is, 0 station, to be the dividing line between mid and high forceps procedures. One authority, Dr. Danforth, writes that forceps delivery should never be performed unless the fetal head is engaged in a station *below* +2, that is, deeply engaged. R. Benson, *Current Obstetric and Gynecologic Diagnosis and Treatment* 853 (2d ed. 1978). The point is that the higher the station at the time of delivery, the greater the risk of traumatic neurologic injury to the fetus.

Q. Okay. If the presenting part was at a plus one station, where would the biparietal diameter be? What station would it be at?

A. Below the ischial spines.

Q. Would it be?

A. Plus one.

Q. No, I said if the presenting part was at plus one–

A. Oh, I'm sorry.

Q. If the presenting part was at plus one, where would the biparietal diameter be?

A. Probably at zero.

Q. One centimeter above?

A. Probably somewhere in there.

Q. Okay. If the presenting part was at a plus one station would you consider that to be a high forceps delivery?

A. Probably a mid forceps.

Q. Why?

A. Well, I think the biparietal diameter would probably be at the ischial spines.

Q. That's assuming you didn't have any molding or caput?

A. Uh-huh.

Q. Did you have molding or caput in this delivery?

A. Yes, we did.

Q. You had quite a bit, did you not?

A. A moderate amount, yes.

Q. Do you know how many centimeters of molding or caput you had in this particular case?

A. No, sir.

Q. Did anybody ever make any measurements of that?

A. I don't know if they did or not, sir.

Q. Is that something normally done, making measurements of caput or molding after a delivery?

Practice Note. The reference to the molding of the fetal head and the caput succedaneum (edema over the presenting part, the head) in this baby is significant in at least two respects. First, the major issue under scrutiny in the defendant's testimony is whether he performed a high forceps delivery–which is strictly contraindicated in modern obstetrics–or a mid forceps delivery, which is not in favor among most obstetricians. If, as the defendant testified, the presenting part was at plus one station, and the presenting part had undergone swelling and molding, then the biparietal diameter was probably higher up than the ischial spines, that is, at the high forceps level. Second, the presence of severe molding is strong evidence of cephalopelvic disproportion and would indicate abandonment of an unsuccessful trial of forceps and performance of cesarean section.

A. I do not think so, sir, but I can't answer that.

Q. Okay. So then the two procedures that you've told me about that you don't feel qualified to perform would be high forceps delivery –

A. Yes.

Q. –and a vacuum extraction?

A. Yes.

Q. Any other obstetrical procedures that you can think of that you wouldn't be qualified to perform?

A. I would be uncomfortable doing a version and extraction. Although I haven't done them, I would be uncomfortable doing a version and extraction.

Q. What is that?

A. Where you turn the baby around.

Q. Okay. Is that different from rotation with forceps?

A. Yes, sir. It's turning the whole baby around.

Q. You feel comfortable and qualified in doing mid forceps deliveries?

A. Yes, sir.

Q. Okay. How may mid forceps deliveries had you done prior to February 15th of '85?

A. I don't know, sir.

Q. Had you done some?

A. Yes, sir.

Q. A number of them?

A. I've been doing them for over twenty years, yes sir.

Q. Well, I understand that, but, I mean, is that something that you commonly do?

A. I wouldn't say it was routine, but certainly, you know, eight to ten percent of the time.

Q. Okay. Mid forceps delivery means that the biparietal diameter is at or below zero?

A. Zero to plus one, yes, sir.

Q. If the biparietal diameter was at plus one, assuming a normal head without caput or molding, where would the presenting part be?

A. Probably plus two.

Q. Your calculations, then, are indicating that in a normal child the biparietal diameter is approximately one centimeter –

A. One to two centimeters.

Q. Okay.

A. We are talking about this much (indicating).

Q. When the baby – when the head is coming out of the vagina, is there a technical term for that, when the head is bulging the perineum? Is that what you call it?

A. Crowning is what I call it.

Q. Crowning? When you have crowning, at what station in the normal baby head would the biparietal diameter be at?

A. I guess plus three. I don't know.

Q. Okay. In February of '85 did you feel like you were qualified to deliver OP presentations?

A. Yes, sir.

Q. You felt qualified to do mid forceps deliveries?

A. Yes, sir.

Q. Did you feel qualified to handle situations involving cephalopelvic disproportion?

A. Yes, sir.

Q. Did you feel qualified to handle deliveries involving involving shoulder dystocia?

A. Yes, sir.

Q. And had you prior to February of '85 performed all of those specific situations, that is, shoulder dystocia, cephalopelvic disproportion, mid forceps deliveries, and OP presentations?

A. For about 22 years, yes, sir.

Q. Okay. Since February of '85 have you changed your techniques regarding any of these problems that we've discussed, shoulder dystocia, OP presentations, cephalopelvic disproportion?

A. Not that I can think of.

Q. Okay. In February – are you familiar with what we call the standard of care in obstetrics in Dallas, Texas back in February of '85?

A. I think so.

Q. Okay. And you were familiar with the standard of care regarding cephalopelvic disproportion?

A. Yes, sir.

Q. Forceps deliveries?

A. Yes, sir.

Q. And dystocia?

A. Yes, sir.

Q. Okay. You had Jewell Miller sign consent forms giving you the right to perform – do the labor and delivery on her?

A. The nurse had her sign. But, yes, it's with our routine orders.

Q. Other than that consent form, did you ever explain to Jewell Miller the risk involved in the labor and delivery of an infant?

A. I don't recall.

Q. You can't remember whether you did or whether you didn't?

A. (Witness shakes head).

Q. Is that something you would normally do with a patient?

A. What risk are you discussing?

Q. Well, the risk that the labor may not go according to the way it's supposed to and that you might have to do a cesarean section or there might be some type of cephalopelvic disproportion and that you might have to use forceps or the various complications that can arise in the normal course of a pregnancy or delivery?

A. Probably did not spell each one of them out, no.

Q. Okay. Do you recall any risk that you did inform her of?

A. That was two years ago, sir, and I don't recall specific conversations.

Q. Doctor, if we could now look at Mrs. Miller's labor records. Does it appear that she was admitted to E.R. with the notation dilated to plus one?

A. Yes.

Q. And 75 percent effacement?

A. Right.

Q. You had seen her earlier that morning and there was no effacement?

A. That's correct.

Q. Okay. What does that indicate to you, that between whatever time she came in to see you and the time she was admitted to the hospital she had become over 75 percent effaced?

A. That she was in early labor.

Q. Does that mean the baby's dropped now?

A. Not necessarily.

Q. It does signify that she is in labor, early labor.

A. I felt that it signified that she was in early labor.

Q. Okay.

A. You can dilate and efface and not be in labor, but the fact that she was having some kind of irregular contractions at the time and had changed her cervix from when I had seen her that day.

Q. Okay. It shows a minus two station—

A. Yes.

Q. And again, to you that meant that the biparietal diameter was at a minus two station—

A. Yes.

Q. —not the presenting part.

A. That's correct.

Q. Okay. It has the words soft and post, it looks like to me.

A. Means that instead of being firm like she had been in the office that day, it had softened up.

Q. Okay. The cervix, that is.

A. The cervix.

Q. Okay.

A. The cervix was posterior, which means it was back toward her rectum instead of just straight up.

Q. Do you consider the onset of labor to begin when the membranes rupture or when the contractions begin?

A. I consider it when there is progressive dilation and effacement of the cervix.

Q. Okay. Well, it says contraction since two thousand p.m., which would be 8:00 o'clock, or thirty minutes after her membranes ruptured. So when did you consider in her case her labor to have begun?

A. I can't answer that question.

Q. Why not?

A. Because I don't know when her cervix started to dilate and efface.

Q. Could it have dilated and effaced before her membranes ruptured?

A. Could have.

Q. So she could have been in labor for quite some time even at the time she was admitted to the hospital.

A. We don't have any evidence of that one way or the other.

Q. Okay. She's got clear after she says spontaneous rupture of each membrane, clear. Is that normal?

A. Yes.

Q. What is the converse to that? What, bloody or cloudy or what?

A. Uh-huh.

Q. That would indicate a problem?

A. Not necessarily, because they frequently have bloody show.

Q. Okay. And it also indicates that at the time she came in the emergency room, which was 9:03 p.m., that you were notified. Correct?

A. I guess so, yes. It says I was notified. I assume I was.

Q. Okay. Doctor, the first page again, back to the first page, you show that you did three operations? Number one was the mid forceps delivery.

A. Oh, I'm sorry.

Q. Number two, a midline episiotomy, and number three, a repair of a third degree extension.

A. Yes, sir.

Q. Let's take those one at a time. Again, I asked you this before, but I forgot what your testimony was. What do you consider a mid forceps delivery?

A. When the biparietal diameter is at zero plus one.

Q. Okay. If you have an OP presentation – someone has told me that if it's an OP presentation it's always a mid forceps delivery. You can never have an OP presentation without mid forceps. Do you disagree with that or agree?

A. I disagree with that.

Q. Okay. Why?

A. Because I've delivered OPs without forceps. Without mid forceps, excuse me.

Q. Is there a difference in the forcep itself as to whether it's a mid forcep or a low forcep?

A. Not necessarily.

Q. Or does that basically depend on where the child's biparietal diameter's at when you classify it as a mid versus a low forceps?

A. You can use the same forceps.

Q. Okay. What station was the child's head at when you did the forceps delivery?

A. I thought it was plus one.

Q. Meaning the biparietal diameter was at plus one, not the presenting part.

A. That's correct.

Q. If the presenting part was a plus one, where would the biparietal diameter be?

A. Probably at zero.

Q. Zero or perhaps minus one.

A. That's conjecture. I would say probably zero.

Q. Okay. But it could be one to two centimeters above the presenting part.

A. Could be.

Q. Okay. You've got that you did a midline episiotomy. Is that the same thing as a median epistiotomy?

A. No, it's not.

Q. Okay. Could you explain the difference?

A. A median is off to the side, and a midline is down the middle.

Q. What's a medio-lateral episiotomy?

A. That's what I'm saying. I must have misunderstood your question, then.

Q. Okay. In other words, the episiotomy that you did was directly from the vagina down toward the anus?

A. Yes, sir.

Q. Why did you do a midline episiotomy rather than a medio-lateral episiotomy?

A. I've always done midline episiotomies.

Q. Regardless of the circumstances?

A. Yes, sir.

Q. Apparently the episiotomy that you did wasn't big enough. Would you agree with that?

A. Yes, sir, we made it larger.

Q. Okay. You made it larger or when the head came out it lacerated?

A. I made it larger and then the head extended it some.

Q. Okay. Well, let me ask you this. You originally made an episiotomy that was how long?

A. Down to the rectal sphincter.

Q. Okay. When did you extend that?

A. When–I don't recall the exact moment that we did it.

Q. Well, was it right at the end of delivery?

A. No.

Q. When was it?

A. It was a little bit before the end of the delivery.

Q. And you extended it how far?

A. Probably that far. I went in and cut the muscle through and then extended it up to the rectum a little bit.

Q. Into the anal sphincter?

A. Yes.

Q. Okay. When the child's head was delivered it even extended it more.

A. A little but more, yes, sir.

Q. Indicating what?

A. It was posterior and couldn't flex up.

Q. Indicating that the head was larger than you thought it was going to be?

A. No.

Q. It didn't.

A. No.

Q. The fact that your episiotomy tore when the child's head came through doesn't indicate to you that the head was larger than you expected?

A. No.

Q. Was the head larger than you expected?

A. I don't think so.

Q. Was the child larger than you expected?

A. A little larger than I expected.

Q. What was the circumference of the child's head after delivery?

A. I don't recall, sir.

Q. Do you have any notes reflecting that?

A. No, sir I don't.

Q. Have you researched the hospital chart to see if they have any notes?

A. No, sir, I did not.

Q. Did you make any notations as to what the actual size of the biparietal –

A. No, I didn't.

Q. –diameter of the child was after deliver.

A. No, I didn't.

Q. Would that be significant to you in any way?

A. No, sir, it wouldn't.

Q. You have a third degree extension, and I notice in other places in the records, such as the recovery room form, the summary of recovery and delivery, they have that it was a fourth degree extension.

A. Some places that you train when you go into the rectum it's a fourth degree. Where I trained it's an extension of a third degree.

Q. That's the worst type of extension you can have.

A. I don't know if it's the worst, but it certainly is–with a midline episiotomy it happens.

Q. It was a large baby. Larger than what you had counted on and estimated?

A. Yes. It was a big baby.

Q. And I believe you've already testified, and tell me if I'm correct, that based on the fact that it was a nine-pound four-and-one-quarter-ounce baby that would have indicated that your fundal height measurements were low?

A. I don't think I said that.

Q. Okay. Well, were they not low?

A. I told you that I thought the baby weighed somewhere in the neighborhood of eight-and-a-half to nine pounds.

Q. Okay. Do you have any reason as to why the fundal height measurements that you made did not correspond to the weight of the baby?

A. It is very difficult to say inside the uterus what the baby is going to weigh.

Q. Okay. If you had known that the baby was going to be this big before you did the delivery of the child, would you have done it any differently? I'm asking you if you knew this before.

A. No. I thought Ms. Miller's pelvis was adequate, and I thought she had progressed adequately.

Q. Okay. Do you still think her pelvis was adequate?

A. It's always easy to look back and say.

Q. Well, I'm not trying to say it's not, but I'm just asking you do you still think her pelvis –

A. If I had to do it over again, I would do it the same way, yes.

Q. You would?

A. Knowing what I know now, you mean?

Q. Yes.

A. Of course not.

Q. Knowing what you know, what would you have done?

A. I probably would have operated on it at 12:00 o'clock the night before.

Q. You would have done a C section?

A. Probably.

Q. You state that the baby had evidence of severe shoulder dystocia; is that correct?

A. Yes, sir.

Q. Okay. You make that sound like a condition. Is it a condition, shoulder dystocia?

A. It's a very rare occurring thing.

Q. Okay. Dystocia means difficult delivery; isn't that correct?

A. Difficulty, yes.

Q. Okay. What you're trying to say there is you had difficulty delivering the baby because of difficulty in delivering the shoulder.

A. Yes, sir.

Q. One shoulder or both shoulders?

A. One shoulder.

Q. One?

A. Yes, sir.

Q. The right or the left?

A. I think it was the left, but I don't remember, sir.

Q. Okay. You don't mention anything in your discharge summary about head dystocia. Don't you agree with me that there was a lot of head dystocia in this delivery?

A. I wouldn't necessarily call it head dystocia, but –

Q. What would you call it?

A. I don't know what I would call it.

Q. Well, tell me what else was the problem besides shoulder dystocia.

A. That was the major problem.

Q. You can't have shoulder dystocia until the head's delivered; is that correct?

A. That's correct.

Q. Because the shoulder's going to hang up on the rim of the pelvis.

A. That's correct.

Q. And it can't hang up on the head of the pelvis until the medicine is delivered.

A. It will hang on the symphysis, excuse me.

Q. Okay. But only after the head is delivered.

A. That's correct.

Q. But weren't you having a lot of problems before the head was ever delivered?

A. Well, as we got, as I told you, the forehead out, then it was very difficult, yes.

Q. Okay. The forehead, but you didn't get the entire head out.

A. That's correct.

Q. And you can't have shoulder dystocia until you get the entire head out.

A. That's right.

Q. So you had a lot of problems just getting the head out. Would you agree with that?

A. Yes, sir.

Q. And would you agree with me that that's called head dystocia or cephalic dystocia?

A. I don't know what I would call it.

Q. Well, the reason I say that, in reading the – and you may not even have this chart, but there was also a chart on the baby.

A. Yes, sir.

Q. Have you read that chart?

A. No, sir.

Q. Dr. Nale, the pediatrician, says delivery was under epidural anesthesia with mid forceps delivery under occiput posterior presentation. Delivery was difficult with head and shoulder dystocia. My question, I guess, again is would you agree that –

A. We had difficulty with the head, yes.

Q. Would you agree with me that you had more difficulty with the head than you really had with the shoulder?

A. No, sir.

Q. Would you agree with me that it was not until you used the third set of forceps that you ever delivered the head?

A. I used two sets of forceps.

Q. You didn't use three sets of forceps?

A. No, sir.

Q. Okay.

A. There were three sets of forceps out.

Q. Okay.

A. The routine ones I normally use.

Q. Okay.

A. Because the child was molding, I wanted to use another pair. I brought the baby down and changed forceps and attempted to rotate it with the Kielland forceps.

Q. Okay.

A. And the head would not rotate easily, so my thinking was that we were committed to delivering the baby.

Q. Okay. We will back up to that in just a minute.

A. Yes.

Q. Was there also evidence of cephalic-pelvic disproportion in her delivery?

A. I did not think so.

Q. Okay. What would be indications of that, Doctor?

A. Failure to progress.

Q. Wasn't there a failure to progress in this case?

A. I did not think so.

Q. What do you consider a normal progression rate?

A. I think every one of them is different.

Q. Doctor, if you assume, as Williams assumes, that station refers to the presenting part, and you do your forceps operation when the station is minus two, that's a high forceps delivery?

A. If that's what you assume.

Q. Because the biparietal diameter would be way up at minus four or higher.

A. Yes.

Q. But, you say that station refers to biparietal diameter so, a minus two station means the biparietal diameter is two centimeters above the ischial spines.

A. Yes, sir.

Q. According to the Williams Obstetrics classification that means that the presenting part—

A. Yes, sir.

Q. —is two centimeters above the ischial spines, correct, according to what you read a while ago?

A. Yes.

Q. And again, it's your statement that the people over there at Garland use your classification rather than the presenting part?

A. Yes.

Q. Okay. Do you know for a fact that that's the way they do things?

A. I don't know anything for a fact, sir.

Q. Okay. Well, she stayed at minus two station that entire two-and-a-half hours. She didn't descend at all. Would you agree with that?

A. I would agree with that.

Q. You stated a while ago that she had a good course of descent, but that doesn't seem to show that she's descending any at all.

A. I didn't think she was in active labor.

Q. And again, it gets me back to what do you mean by active labor.

A. Progressively dilating.

Q. Okay.

A. And effacement.

Q. Okay. Well, she had effaced over 75 percent. We know that. That's progressive, isn't it?

A. She could have done that without going into labor.

Q. Okay. Generally, I hate to keep using these words normally and generally, but isn't it true that in the first pregnancy, a woman with her first delivery, that she's engaged at the time labor begins?

A. More frequently than not.

Q. All right. What does it indicate to you when that hasn't occurred?

A. It can indicate that she's not in good labor.

Q. Okay. Do you agree with the statement that in the primigravida at a minus two station or above at term in labor runs a known probability of over 50 percent section rate due to abnormal presentation and cephalic pelvic disproportion?

A. I don't know what the percentage would be, but I would think it would be higher than if she were engaged.

Q. So that's a clue to you already, since she comes in at a minus two, even if you take your calculations as being correct, that there's at least a probability that you're going to have an abnormal presentation and that you're going to have cephalopelvic disproportion.

A. That's always—there's always a chance of that, yes.

Q. All right. I know there's a chance of it. There's a chance of anything. My question to you was isn't it probable based on the fact that when she came into labor she was at a minus two station?

A. I would say that it was more likely—

CROSS EXAMINATION

Q. Than not?

A. No. Than if she were engaged.

Q. Okay. Did you consider that when they told you she was at a minus two station in labor?

A. You always take everything into consideration. But I also took into consideration that she was not having regular contractions.

Q. In the first stage of labor what is considered normal for frequency and duration of contractions?

A. The entire first stage?

Q. Does it change over the first stage?

A. I think it does.

Q. Okay. Well, give me a summary of what you feel like is normal good steady contractions as far as frequency and duration's concerned.

A. Two to three minutes lasting 30 to 45 seconds, something like that, 45 seconds.

Q. Two to three minutes in frequency?

A. Yes, sir.

Q. And 45 seconds?

A. Thirty to 45 seconds.

Q. What about in the second stage of labor? Does that change?

A. The contractions may get a little more intense.

Q. Does frequency stay the same?

A. Frequency stays about the same.

Q. Two to three minutes?

A. Yes.

Q. They may become more intense, maybe up to a minute?

A. Maybe, yes sir.

Q. Okay. Well, if you will look under contractions, under frequency and duration, starting about five minutes till 12 o'clock, doesn't it show that she is having a frequency of two to three every two to three minutes and an intensity of 60 seconds?

A. I'm sorry, where are you?

Q. First page, labor notes, down at 2355.

A. Yeah.

Q. According to the standards that you just gave me, that is even better than good contractions as far as frequency and duration are concerned. Wouldn't you agree?

A. I wasn't there to evaluate them, so I don't know.

Q. Well, based on what's written in the records, Doctor. I realize that you weren't there. It says that she's having a frequency of two to three – every two to three minutes and that they are lasting 60 seconds. You just got through telling me that if you had them every two to three minutes and they lasted from 30 to 45 seconds you felt like that was good.

Based on that record, then, would you agree that she at least at that point is starting to have –

A. Contractions.

Q. – contractions?

A. Yes, sir.

Q. But she continues not to descend. Would you agree with that?

A. Well, at 1 o'clock there's nothing, except it says now they are five minutes apart, lasting 30 seconds, and then it's irregular contractions at 1 o'clock.

Q. Well, she stays at a minus two station from the time she came to the hospital, which was – the emergency room was 9 o'clock p.m., and stays at a minus two station, according to these records, until 7:30 the next morning, or close to 11½ hours, where she didn't descend at all. That wasn't significant to you?

A. Well, when I came – excuse me. When I came out at 4 o'clock I did not think she was having good labor pains. I examined her. I felt them. I thought they were irregular and not really of any significant pattern or of good quality.

Q. Well, let's look at page three of the labor record. You've been at minus two ever since she's been in the hospital and now it's 6:20 a.m., 11 hours labor, and she's still at minus two. And the record shows rapid dilation with the Oxytocin you ordered and basically, complete dilation and only moving two centimeters. That's a terribly slow descent, wouldn't you agree?

A. Yes, sir.

Q. A lousy labor course. It should be descending at about one centimeter per hour?

A. About one centimeter an hour, yes, sir, be happy with that, first baby.

Q. What rate of descent do you like to see per hour?

A. You obviously like them at plus three the whole time.

Q. Sure. But you don't get that.

A. No.

Q. What do you like to see as far as rate of descent per hour?

A. Well, they usually will stay about where they are, zero minus one, until they complete.

Q. Okay. So you don't have any descent without complete dilation?

A. You can have people at plus one, yes. I mean, that's what you – that's obviously ideal, plus two.

Q. Okay. After you have complete dilation what do you like to see as far as the rate of descent? I'm not talking about the station. I'm talking about how quick you get the descent per hour.

A. Well, I would like for them to do it in 10 or 15 minutes, but, unfortunately, very few will do that. I think up to an hour and a half, two hours.

Q. An hour and a half to two hours to be where?

A. To be at plus one, plus two.

Q. Well, when you're at plus one, you're still pretty high up there, aren't you?

A. Yes.

Q. Even if you look at the way you calculate it, which is if the biparietal diameter's at plus one, you're still pretty high up there.

A. Well, it's below the spine. I wouldn't say it was high up there.

Q. And if you use the method that's used in Williams Obstetrics, which is the presenting part being at plus one, that means that the biparietal diameter is just at zero or perhaps above. Correct?

A. Probably at zero.

Q. Okay. So, Doctor, your statement, then, is that—where did you have engagement in this lady? At what time did you have engagement? When was the patient engaged?

A. I consider engagement when the baby is in the inlet.

Q. Right. Well, when was that?

A. I thought she was in the inlet the entire time.

Q. So you felt like the lady was engaged when she came to the hospital.

A. Yes.

Q. Okay. Because, again, you're stating that it's the biparietal—

A. Yes, sir.

Q. —diameter that you judge stations by.

A. Yes, sir.

Q. All right, now looking ahead to the delivery notes, the notes indicate you first applied forceps at plus one. You felt the head, and you have previously testified that there was molding and you could feel the caput. Didn't that tell you the biparietal diameter might be a whole lot higher than plus one?

A. No, sir, because I could feel the ears this time. Of course, she was under anesthesia.

Q. Okay. You could feel the ears?

A. Yes, sir.

Q. Where were the ears at?

A. (Indicating).

Q. Were they at plus one?

A. Yes, sir.

Q. But would you agree that she did have a lot of molding—

A. Yes, sir, she had molding.

Q. —and caput at that time?

A. She had molding and caput, yes, sir. As I said, the presenting part to me was at plus two.

Q. Okay. What were your findings in the delivery room when you made your exam?

A. They were essentially the same.

Q. That she was at a plus one station, complete effacement, complete dilation?

A. Yes, sir.

Q. That there was a large amount of caput and swelling?

A. There was caput. I wouldn't say there was a large amount, but certainly caput.

Q. Was there a large amount of molding?

A. There was molding present.

Q. Okay. Then what did you do, Doctor?

A. I felt that we were not going to get any further lower.

Q. Why?

A. I felt the baby was occiput posterior, and felt that we were not getting the kind of pushing we were getting. I mean, she just couldn't push the baby for the epidural.

Q. In other words, you attribute the failure of the baby to descend because of the mother's weakness in contractions?

A. No, sir. I didn't say that.

Q. Well, tell me why you didn't –

A. I didn't think she was able to push because of the epidural.

Q. So the epidural shouldn't have been given?

A. I didn't say that.

Q. Well, why was the epidural given?

A. To try to relieve her pain.

Q. But –

A. Relax her.

Q. But you were giving her a lot of pain medication for that, weren't you?

A. That's the other thing. I don't like to keep giving pain medication, because it goes through the placenta.

Q. So you gave her the epidural, but you stated that it was the epidural that kept her from doing enough pushing to expel the baby, in your opinion.

A. In my opinion, she was not able to push hard enough, that's correct.

Q. Okay. But at the last time that we at least have her contractions monitored she was having real good contractions.

A. Yes, sir.

Q. So what makes you say that?

A. I didn't say the contractions. I said the pushing. I'm sorry.

Q. She wasn't pushing hard enough.

A. That's right, sir.

Q. Okay. So you decided to do a forceps delivery.

A. Yes, sir.

Q. Okay. It says in this note here prepared for delivery, pushing with contractions, forceps applied by Dr. Johnson. What kind of forceps?

A. Okay. I was going to use the Simpson forceps, but because she had molding I didn't put them on. I changed and asked them for the McLean forceps.

173

CROSS EXAMINATION

Q. Is it your testimony under oath that you didn't put the Simpson forceps on?

A. I do not recall putting the Simpson forceps on. I put my hand in there, put them in there. I didn't like the way it felt, and I took them out. But I never applied the forceps.

Q. So you put them in, and you didn't like the way they felt?

A. Yes, sir.

Q. And then you took them out.

A. Yes, sir.

Q. Now, you realize that Mr. and Mrs. Miller are watching everything that you do.

A. Yes, sir, I do.

Q. Because she's got a mirror up there where she can see.

A. Yes.

Q. And he's standing there behind you, and he's watching what you're doing.

A. Yes, sir.

Q. And your testimony is that you didn't pull with the first set of forceps?

A. I don't recall pulling with the first set of forceps. But this has been two years ago, so –

Q. Okay. So you just tried them on for fit, and they didn't fit, and you took them out.

A. I didn't like the way they felt.

Q. Why didn't you like the way they felt?

A. They just didn't feel like they were fitting like the way I wanted them to fit.

Q. Okay. Then you changed forceps. Right?

A. Yes, sir.

Q. To the Tucker-McLean forceps?

A. Yes, sir.

Q. What kind of forceps are the Tucker-McLean forceps?

A. They are a forcep that is better if the head's somewhat molded.

Q. They are better than Simpson forceps –

A. I think so.

Q. – if you've got a molded head?

A. Yes, sir.

Q. Are these rotating forceps or pulling forceps or both?

A. They can be used either way.

Q. Okay. Were you going to attempt to deliver the baby OP, or were you going to attempt –

A. I was going to attempt to rotate the baby.

Q. Okay. You were going to attempt to rotate to OA and deliver.

A. Yes, sir.

Q. You realize you had a choice there.

A. Yes, sir.

Q. You could have delivered OP.

A. OP, yes, sir.

Q. So did you try to rotate?

A. Yes, sir.

Q. Okay. With the Tucker-McLean forceps.

A. I tried, but the Tucker-McLeans are not, I don't think, as good as the Kiellands.

Q. For rotating.

A. Yes, sir.

Q. Okay. You tried to rotate with the Tucker-McLean, though. Correct?

A. Did not try. I gave it (indicating) to see if it would turn, and it would not turn.

Q. But you said you gave it a—you mean you gave it a rotating rather than a pulling turn.

A. I gave it a rotating turn, yes. I'm sorry.

Q. Did you give it a pulling turn?

A. Yes, sir, I did.

Q. Did you pull before you rotated, or did you rotate and then pull?

A. I pulled and then tried to rotate.

Q. So you tried to deliver OP, then, by pulling.

A. Wanted to see how it would come down, and it came down some. Then I tried to rotate it, and it wouldn't rotate.

Q. You did get descent when you tried pulling?

A. That's right.

Q. How much descent?

A. The top of the head was at the introitus.

Q. Was the head bulging the perineum?

A. It was right to the perineum. It was not bulging.

Q. Could you see the baby's head?

A. Yes, sir. Yes, sir.

Q. How much of the head, just the very—

A. That much (indicating).

Q. A little bit? Just the crown?

A. More than the crown. That much a least (indicating).

Q. What you were seeing was the caput, though.

A. Yes, sir.

Q. Okay. Did you feel like when you had the Tucker-McLean forceps on that you had good traction?

A. Yes, I did.

Q. Did it slip on you any?

A. No, sir.

Q. Okay. You gave it a trial of forceps, then, with the Tucker-McLean?

A. And pulled it down, yes, sir.

Q. Okay. But you didn't get it out.

A. No, sir.

Q. Okay. Why didn't you do a C-section at that point?

A. Because I don't think that I could have gotten the baby back up. I think the baby was down so far I could not push it back up or pull it back up or grab it back up.

Practice Note. The record clearly illustrates that a cephalopelvic disproportion existed. There was a clearly documented failure of descent. The defendant should have recognized the cephalopelvic disproportion early on and prepared for a cesarean section. A so called "trial of forceps" contemplates the situation in which the physician is aware of a troublesome cephalopelvic relationship but considers the likelihood of a safe vaginal delivery to be strong enough that a trial of forceps is warranted. However, when any difficulty is encountered, the trial *must* be abandoned and cesarean section performed. The defendant OB in this case should have abandoned his forceps and commenced preparation for a stat cesarean section.

Q. In other words, it is your testimony that you don't think you can do a C section when the baby's head is at the, say, plus three station?

A. I think it would have been very, very chancy, yes.

Q. So when you used the Tucker-McLean forceps you pulled, giving me the impression that you were trying to deliver OP.

A. If it would have come easily OP, I was going to try to deliver it OP, yes.

Q. So you were going to try to deliver it OP first.

A. Yes.

Q. And then since you were unsuccessful—

A. It came down, but it still—I was not satisfied.

Q. So it came down, but what?

A. The head came down, okay, but did not come out.

Q. Okay. Did you try to get it out?

A. No.

Q. Why not?

A. It was still—there was that much from coming out (indicating).

Q. Were you pulling pretty hard on it?

A. I would say moderately, yes.

Q. How long did you pull on the baby's head?

A. I never looked at the clock.

Q. Well, it shows, the chart shows, that once you started putting forceps on at about, oh, say 1 o'clock, the baby was delivered at 1320, so you were in there about 20 minutes using forceps. Would you agree with that?

A. Not the whole time, no sir.

Q. What were you doing the rest of the time?

A. Well, as I told you, we put the first set of forceps on, was not happy with them.

Q. Okay.

A. Took them off.

Q. You could figure that out pretty quick, couldn't you ?

A. That's why I didn't use them. I just felt uncomfortable with it, so that's why I changed. So I had to get out another pair of forceps.

Q. Okay. You don't know how long you used the Tucker-McLean forceps?

A. No, sir. It was not long. I just don't – you know, I don't look at the clock. It seems like forever.

Q. So you got her down to a plus three station with that second set of forceps.

A. What I would consider a plus three, plus two, plus three.

Q. And the reason you didn't – and the reason you didn't go for a C section at that point was because you felt like now you had pulled it down too much and it was too late to do a C section?

A. Yes, sir.

Q. So you try – well, according to you, your second set of forceps, the Kierllands –

A. Keillands.

Q. Keillands?

A. Yes, sir.

Q. They are rotating forceps.

A. Yes, sir.

Q. You had already tried to rotate with the Tucker-McLean?

A. Yes, sir.

Q. And that didn't work. Correct?

A. That's correct.

Q. So then you tried to rotate – did you try to pull with the Kielland forceps, or did you simply try to rotate?

A. I tried to rotate with the Kiellands, and again the baby did not want to rotate.

Q. Okay. So then what did you do?

A. I delivered it posteriorly.

Q. By pulling with the Kiellands?

A. Yes, sir.

Q. Tell me about how you delivered it. What happened? You're having all these problems. You can't rotate it. You can't – well, you've tried pulling with the Tucker-McLeans, but you've gotten to a point that it won't go any further?

A. Well, I just didn't want to keep pulling with the Tucker-McLeans. I'm sure I could have pulled on. I just felt I could change forceps and do better by rotating the baby.

177

Q. Were you panicking at this point?

A. I was not happy. I wouldn't say I panicked, no.

Q. Did you feel like you were causing trauma to the child's head as you were delivering the child?

A. No, I didn't.

Q. You didn't?

A. That's why I changed forceps.

Q. I'm talking about when you used the Kielland forceps and you tried to rotate and it wouldn't rotate.

A. I didn't try to rotate it that hard.

Q. Okay. Well, but then you tried to pull again.

A. Pulled it.

Q. My question is did you use a lot of force with the Kielland forceps when you were pulling?

A. Probably had to use more than I would normally use, yes.

Q. Did you feel like you were causing trauma to the baby's head when you were using the Kielland forceps and finally delivered the child?

A. I did not, no.

Q. Tell me about what happened with the Kielland forceps when you pulled, when you finally got the child to come out. What happened?

A. Well, after we got this much delivered, then pulled the baby on out and tried to turn the baby's head. And the shoulders came up under the symphysis, and I couldn't deliver the shoulders at all.

Q. So what we've been talking about up to this point was the problems you were having just getting the head out. Right?

A. Yes, sir.

Q. And then once you got the head out the baby's head would not turn?

A. Well, it turned to the side.

Q. Is that normal or abnormal?

A. That's normal.

Q. Okay. But the shoulder hung up.

A. Yes, sir.

Q. Okay. It's not unusual for you to have shoulder dystocia when you have head dystocia. Wouldn't you agree, Doctor?

A. Not necessarily.

Q. It's not unusual for you to have shoulder dystocia when you have an OP presentation.

A. Not necessarily.

Q. Okay. What does that mean?

A. Well, you can have shoulder dystocia with an anterior delivery that you've had no problem with.

Q. Is it more common to have shoulder dystocia with an OP presentation?

A. I don't think so.

Q. Is it more common to have shoulder dystocia when you have head dystocia?

A. I don't know.

Q. So you didn't get the head out until you used the Kielland forceps?

A. That's correct.

Q. How long did it take you after you got the head out before you could deliver the shoulders?

A. I didn't look at the clock. It seemed forever.

Q. The reason I ask you that, Doctor, is there's nothing in the labor notes about shoulder dystocia or difficulty delivering the shoulder. But this did happen? Is that correct?

A. That's when I had Harry and them pushing so hard.

Q. Well, let's back up here. You've got them pushing all the way back up to when you were applying the first set of forceps. That's before you got the head out. Correct?

A. The most of the pressure given by whoever was giving it, and I don't know who was giving it, was to get the shoulders out. And I don't recall whether it was Harry or Dale or who.

Q. Okay. But you will agree with me that you didn't have the head out – you didn't get the head out with the Simpson forceps because you didn't even use –

A. I didn't really even pull on those, no, sir.

Q. You didn't get the head out with the Tucker-McLean forceps. Correct?

A. Got it down to about a plus two, plus three.

Q. But you didn't get the head out.

A. No, sir, I did not.

Q. And it took you – the Kierllands?

A. Kiellands.

Q. Kiellands, excuse me, forceps for you to get the head out itself.

A. Yes, sir.

Q. And that was after you used more pressure than you would normally use.

A. Yes, sir.

Q. And then once you got the head out you started having the problems with the shoulder.

A. Yes, sir.

Q. Did you break the clavicle of the shoulder?

A. I could have. I do not know.

Q. You could have? I mean intentionally.

A. I did not intentionally. I'm sorry.

Q. Okay.

A. And I did not hear it, and it did not appear to be fractured.

Q. How did you get the shoulder out?

A. How did I get the shoulder out?

179

Q. I may have asked you that, but tell me again.

A. Posterior pressure to the baby's head to pull it down trying to get it out from under there and then took my other hand – my hand, excuse me, and rotated it over the baby's shoulder and pulled it down.

Q. Have you ever had as hard a delivery as this one?

A. It would certainly rank with one of the hardest, yes.

Q. Let me describe something for you, Doctor, that my clients have told me that they observed when you were trying to deliver this baby, and you tell me if you agree or disagree.

A. Yes.

Q. That when you were trying to pull the baby's head out with the forceps that they could see the very slight bit of the baby's scalp, but once you let go of the forceps it would suck back in. Does that sound right to you?

A. It probably moved up a little, yes. I wouldn't say it sucked back in.

Q. Well, the head would disappear?

A. I wouldn't say disappeared, no.

Q. Okay. So you would disagree with that statement.

A. Yes. It may have gone up a little.

Q. Does that indicate that something's hanging up in there? What was keeping you from getting the child out?

A. I don't know.

Q. Do you think it was because the head was so large?

A. I don't know.

Q. You don't have an opinion one way or the other?

A. No, sir.

Q. It couldn't have been shoulder dystocia because you hadn't delivered the head yet.

A. That's right.

Q. Do you think she had a contracted pelvic outlet?

A. That's a possibility.

Q. That's the one measurement that you never made, isn't it, Doctor?

A. That is a very rough measurement.

Q. You did make a measurement?

A. I said that is a very rough measurement.

Q. But, you didn't make any measurement.

A. No, I did not measure that.

Q. Okay. Do you still believe that there was no cephalopelvic disproportion regarding this pregnancy or this delivery?

A. Yes, I do.

Q. You do believe that there was?

A. No, I'm sorry.

Q. You don't believe that there was?

A. I don't believe there was, no. I believe she had an adequate pelvis.

Q. Would you agree with me that you gave it more than just a trial of forceps?

A. No.

Q. You wouldn't agree with me?

A. No.

Q. Do you know what we mean by a trial of forceps?

A. Yes, I do.

Q. What do we mean?

A. When you attempt to deliver vaginally and can't get the forceps on or can't deliver.

Q. You can't get the forceps on?

A. On.

Q. Well, doesn't trial of forceps mean that if you're going to use forceps, you put them on and you gently and firmly give it pulls, but if it doesn't work, then you abandon them? Isn't that the trial of forceps?

A. I–

Q. Never heard of that word?

A. I've heard the word, yes.

Q. But you don't really know what it means.

A. Yes.

Q. You do or you don't?

A. I do.

Q. Well, am I wrong, or am I right?

A. You're using the word gently, and I don't know what the word gently means.

Q. Well, you were saying something about trial of forceps meant that you couldn't get the forceps on.

A. That would be one definition, that you can't get the forceps on at all.

Q. What's the other definition?

A. That you're not able to bring the baby down.

Q. Okay. And isn't that the case–

A. I felt the baby was coming down, in my judgment.

Q. Doctor, would you agree that this was a high application of forceps?

A. No.

Q. Why?

A. Because I felt the baby was at a plus one.

Q. Okay. And the presenting part was when the baby was at plus one?

A. When the biparietal diameter was at plus one, I would say plus two, plus three.

Q. Okay. Did you feel like there was two centimeters of caput or molding?

A. I don't recall.

Q. It says in the labor notes on the fourth page–right before you delivered the baby it says fetal heart tone regulated?

A. Should have been regular.

Q. Regular?

A. Regular.

Q. So there were no signs of fetal distress during the entire delivery, that you're aware of?

A. I always tell them to list between each contraction.

Q. And you don't have any listed?

A. I'm sorry?

Q. And you don't have any listed.

A. No.

Q. So that means there weren't any.

A. Well, I mean, at 3:10 they took one. I'm sorry, at 1310. Excuse me. Not after 1310.

Q. Excuse me. Explain to me what you're saying.

A. Well, I may have misunderstood your question.

Q. I said were there any signs of fetal distress in this delivery.

A. No.

Q. Okay. When did Dr. Rubane come into the delivery room?

A. A few minutes after we delivered the baby.

Q. The baby was already delivered.

A. Yes, sir.

Q. Did you call him in, or did somebody else?

A. I had the nurse call.

Q. Dale?

A. I don't recall.

Q. You're sure he wasn't in there during the delivery?

A. I don't think so.

Q. Okay. Do you know why he was called in?

A. Because we had an Apgar 3 baby.

Q. Okay. And what kind of doctor is Dr. Rubane?

A. He's a pediatrician.

Q. After the delivery of the child did you notice that there was severe molding and caput?

A. I would say there was caput. I wouldn't say it was severe.

Q. You wouldn't say it was severe?

A. I really don't recall.

Q. Okay. Did you feel like the head was oversized?

A. No.

Q. You didn't?

A. No.

Q. Was there noticeable trauma on the head? Did you observe—

A. No.

Q. —evidence of trauma?

A. No, I did not.

Q. What did the child look like, if you can recall?

A. I don't recall.

Q. You didn't observe it?

A. Well, obviously I worked with it until the pediatrician got there.

Q. I know, but you didn't observe any abnormalities with the child?

A. And we were really trying to get the baby to get good breaths and pink up. No, I did not.

Q. Okay. Why was the child given 45 seconds of oxygen?

A. That's very common, to give them oxygen after delivery, especially with an Apgar 3. You want to be sure they are well oxygenated.

Q. Okay. When did you do the episiotomy?

A. When I pulled down with the Tucker-McLean forceps.

Q. After you –

A. After I was pulling, yes.

Q. After you were pulling with the Tucker-McLean?

A. Yes.

Q. So you did the episiotomy after the forceps were inserted?

A. Yes, sir.

Q. And after you were pulling.

A. Yes, sir, when the perineum was –

Q. Bulged?

A. Yes, sir.

Q. Were there any conversations that you can recall today between you or anybody in the delivery room concerning what had happened?

A. No, sir.

Q. Did anyone during or after delivery question your technique of delivery?

A. No, sir.

Q. Did anyone during or after delivery tell you that you should have done a cesarean section earlier?

A. No, sir.

Q. I think I've already asked you this. Did you feel everyone in the delivery room did what they were supposed to do?

A. Yes, sir.

Q. Would you agree that the age of the difficult forceps delivery's in the past?

A. No, sir.

Q. I just want to make sure I'm correct on this forceps sequence. You tried to deliver OP. That didn't work with the Tucker-McLean forceps. Then you tried to rotate with the Tucker-McLean forceps, but you could not get any rotation.

Then you abandoned the Tucker-McLean forceps, used the Kielland forceps, tried to rotate with the Kielland forceps, but could not get any rotation, and then pulled with the Kielland forceps and delivered the head.

A. Yes, sir.

Q. Is that the correct sequence of events?

A. Yes, sir.

Q. Okay. Would you also substantiate and agree that the head never showed through the introitus?

A. Introitus, yes, sir.

Q. Until you used the forceps?

A. Yes, sir, I would agree to that.

Q. And that the head never bulged the perineum until you used the forceps.

A. Yes, sir.

Practice Note. The baby was born with an Apgar score of 3 at five minutes. Subsequently, the baby was diagnosed as suffering from severe brain damage incident to a traumatic forceps delivery.

§ 33.11 Formal Settlement Presentation in Brachial Plexus-Erb's Palsy Case (New)

The materials in this section are modeled after a written settlement presentation prepared by the author for submission to the agents and attorneys of the defendant obstetrician and defendant hospital. The materials were presented in a leather notebook. Each page was enclosed in a plastic sheet protector; each section was neatly organized and divided. Family photographs were mounted on blue paper and captions were placed underneath photographs of the injured child and her parents. The written materials were distributed to opposing counsel and the insurance carrier after the author had presented a video brochure in his offices. A large settlement was obtained following the presentation of the video and written brochure.

NORMAN HERRELL *ET AL.* SETTLEMENT BROCHURE

TABLE OF CONTENTS

CROSS EXAMINATION

I. SUMMARY OF FACTS

In 1981, plaintiff Sandra Herrell, mother of Jana Herrell, was admitted to Mercy Hospital in labor. She was one week past her E.D.C. (estimated date of confinement). This was Sandra's first pregnancy. She was attended by her obstetrician, Dr. Weber, and his partner, Dr. Frank. Sandra was started on IV Pitocin and, according to the labor and delivery notes, progressed to a vacuum-extracted delivery of an 8-pound, 12-ounce female, over midline episiotomy with a third degree extension and cervical laceration. Dr. Frank delivered the child and he noted in the discharge summary that there was "shoulder dystocia with resultant brachial plexus injury and fracture of the infant's right clavicle."

The Labor Progress Chart (see Section IIIA) depicts an abnormal labor curve. Specifically, Sandra Herrell's labor was characterized by an arrested descent. In other words, Sandra's fetus was too large to safely and expeditously navigate the birth canal. Despite clinical signs that the baby was large, and in the face of an abnormal labor curve, Dr. Frank failed to perform an indicated cesarean section, as a result of which Sandra's first-born (Emily) suffered the same injury sustained by our client, four-year-old Jana Herrell, Emily's younger sister.

In 1984, Sandra Herrell returned to Dr. Weber for management of her second pregnancy. Dr. Weber was well aware of the difficult labor and shoulder dystocia which had complicated Sandra's 1981 delivery. Dr. Weber possessed all of the office and hospital records from the 1981 delivery. Dr. Weber assumed care of Sandra of September 7, 1985. On that date, an ultrasound was performed for the first and only time, despite Sandra's previous history of protracted labor and shoulder dystocia. Dr. Weber did not order x-ray pelvimetry. There is no indication he made any effort to clinically assess the fetal size. No evaluation of the patient for gestational diabetes was ever ordered by Dr. Weber. Again, it is significant that Dr. Weber did not perform serial ultrasounds to determine the growth character-istics and eventual size of the fetus.

Sandra was admitted to the hospital on April 27, 1984 for induction of labor. She was noted to be 2 cm dilated, 50 percent effaced and at minus 2 station. *Sandra never progressed beyond minus 1.* Sandra's abnormal labor was a tragic medical history that was repeating itself. Dr. Weber attempted a vaginal delivery and, just as had happened in 1981, a shoulder dystocia developed. The result was a brachial plexus injury, Erb's palsy, and a permanent disfiguring, disabling injury to Jana's right arm and shoulder.

Unfortunately, unlike her older sister, Jana did not recover from her brachial plexus injury. She has been diagnosed as having a combined Erb's-Klumpke's palsy. She will always have a short arm. Her emotional health has been permanently impaired. Her capacity to enjoy life and to earn an income have been impaired. Her parents, Sandra and Norman Herrell, have suffered the torment and mental anguish only parents of crippled children can understand.

Dr. Weber's negligence in this case amounts to a heedless and reckless disregard of the rights, safety, and welfare of Jana Herrell and her parents. Dr. Hale will testify that the failure of Dr. Weber to learn from the history of the 1981 disaster, and to keep the highest index of concern and suspicion in Sandra's 1984 pregnancy amounts to gross negligence.

Dr. Hale will tell the jury that Mercy Hospital must share the responsibility for Dr. Weber's gross and reckless management of Sandra's labor and delivery. This corporate responsibility arises from the very fact that Dr. Weber was allowed to practice high-risk obstetrics at the hospital. The hospital knew, or should have known, that Dr. Weber had flunked his boards on one occasion, literally "ducked out" of a second scheduled board examination and, on a third occasion simply failed to show for a scheduled examination. The hospital knew, or should have known, that the ACOG examiners who flunked Dr. Weber criticized his total lack of understanding of the management of abnormal labor and the indication for cesarean section.

Mercy Hospital's corporate irresponsibility in failing to revoke or restrict Dr. Weber's obstetrical privileges imposes liability on the hospital for gross negligence. See *Birchfield v. Texarkana Memorial Hospital,* 747 S.W.2d 361 (Tex. 1987). Thus, Mercy Hospital and Dr. Weber face astronomical damages when the jury returns its verdict finding gross negligence in the care and management of Sandra and Jana Herrell.

II. FAMILY PROFILE

Practice Note. Under this section the author presented color photographs depicting Jana Herrell's injured arm. We also included photographs of Jana's mother, father, and older sister. The photographs were mounted on dark blue construction paper; quotes from the medical records and interviews with the plaintiff's experts and parents were typed under the photographs as explanatory captions.

III. MEDICAL HISTORY

Practice Note. This portion of the brochure contains the labor and delivery records and other pertinent information concerning both the 1981 and 1984 labor and delivery of the Herrell children. We also included the reports of the subsequent treating neurologist, Dr. Jones, and the subsequent treating pediatric orthopedic surgeon, Dr. Goodwin.

NEURO DIAGNOSTIC CLINIC, P.C.
105 Armstrong Road
Toledo, Ohio 79800
(555) 398-8000

HERRELL, JANA LEIGH   EMG NCV # 452   April 2, 1986
DOB 04/27/84   Toledo Rehab Center
                                                            Dr. Jones

HISTORY: Brachial birth injury on left. Somewhat improved over time. (Sister with
            Erb's palsy, recovered by 6 months.)

NERVE CONDUCTION STUDIES

Sensory Nerve Action Potentials   *Latency (msec) Amplitude (uV)*
Left Median to Index Finger   No response elicited
Left Ulnar to Little Finger   No response elicited

Motor Nerve Conduction Velocity/Distal Latency (msec)/Velocity (msec)
Left Median to Abductor Pollicis Brevis 2.20 32.2 (Normal for age)
Left Ulnar to Abjuctor Digiti Quinti (?)0.24 19.8 (slow for age)

ELECTROMYOGRAPHY

Muscles Tested: Left biceps, triceps, brachiordialis, abductor pollicis brevis, first
dorsal interosseous, extensor digitorum communis.

Left cervical paraspinals.

Findings:

(1) Silence at rest, normal motor unit potentials, compete recruitment
patterns in left biceps, triceps, brachioradialis, left cervical paraspinals.

(2) Silence at rest normal motor unit potentials, giant motor unit potentials
and incomplete recruitment patterns in extensor digitorum ommunis.

(3) Complex high frequency discharges, fibrillations and positive sharp
waves at rest, normal motor unit potentials and incomplete recruitment patterns
in left abjector pollicis brevis.

(4) Normal insertional activity, fibrillations and positive sharp waves at rest,
normal motor unit potentials and complete recruitment patterns in left first
dorsal interosseous.

IMPRESSION: Abnormal study.

Absent sensory nerve action potentials and slow ulnar nerve conduction velocity are consistent with lesion of brachial plexus (distal to dorsal root ganglion). Absence of denervatoin potentials in paraspinals is not diagnostic but helps confirm this.

Denervation potentials in hand muscles is consistent with lower plexus involvement and ongoing dysfunction of nerve but not total destruction.

Giant motor unit potentials are consistent with healing (reinnervation) in damaged nerves.

_____

Joseph Jones, M.D./yl

CROSS EXAMINATION

Orthopedics Associates
Robert Goodwin, M.D.
401 Pasadena Circle
Toledo, Ohio 79800

HERRELL, JANA LEIGH

May 23, 1984: She is a month old. I saw her when she was a neonate and because of a tough delivery, she had a mixed Erb's-Klumpke's palsy of the left upper extremity. She was starting to show some very fine spontaneous movement before discharge from the hospital, but since I've seen her (which was about a month ago) she is beginning to get a little activity of her left deltoid. With gravity eliminated she can very minimally abduct the left shoulder. She has some atrophy of the supra and infraspinati muscles around the shoulder blade, and this makes her left shoulder blade wing a little bit and also shows a little bit more prominence of the spine of the scapula. She still lacks wrist extension, holding her hand in palmar flexion and has some intrinsic wasting of the left hand. And as a result of the intrinsic wasting, she cannot fully extend the fingers. Thusly, she has not only auxiliary nerve involvement, but radial nerve involvement. This would imply that the major injury was probably to the posterior quarter of the brachial plexus.

I would like to see Jana in one month in order to identify more muscular activity and also in order to document what muscles have started to show some return. RAG:kf

June 22, 1984: She is now 3 months old and has a mixed Erb's Klumpke's Palsy, but there has been some return of more structural motion in her left upper extremity than before. She is now flexing her fingers more fully, she can extend the fingers, but she still does *not* have wrist extension against gravity. She is now pronating and supinating the forearm against gravity very well. She still does not have biceps flexion and biceps activity of the elbow, but she can extend against resistance. She can abduct the shoulder a little bit, but not much. She is getting more sensibility in the arm and seems to be more responsive to pin-prick stimulus. I would like to see her in six weeks. RAG:kf

August 15, 1984: Jana is now 3-½ months old. She was born with a combination of an Erb's-Klumke's palsy.

Today, on examination, by comparison to 2 months ago, she is now showing me some active muscle tone in the radial wrist extensors, although she still has a wristdrop. Sometimes during the examination, I can detect a little active extension of the wrist against gravity. Her grasp is greater, so that the profundi and sublimi seem to be working fairly nicely. She can oppose the thumb, so that the opponens is working. She can now abduct and forward elevate her shoulder. The scapula on the left side is not as prominent as it was, and so I think she is developing some muscle tone of the supra and infrasppinati. She definitely has muscle tone in the deltoid and she is generating good muscle tone in the triceps. There's still no biceps activity as seen by the absence of elbow flexion. She is working her brachial radialis and the supinators and pronators are also working. Therefore, I see some magnitude of improvement since the last time I saw her.

192

Also, the little lump from the torticolis is diminishing and her neck moves from side-to-side with equal ease indicating that the tightness of the sternocleidomastoid on the right is less significant. The patient is to see me in three months. RAG:kf

November 13, 1984:   Jana Leigh is here today four months after her last visit and now I'm recording that she does have some active wrist extension. She has active digital extension. The wrist drop is not so prominent. I feel muscular activity in the biceps and I really do think that she is starting to be able to flex the elbow. She still cannot abduct the shoulder fully. She has a little prominence of the left scapula and this is the lateral border of the scapula due to some imbalance of the musculature around the scapula. The parents were reassured. And since Jana is just 6 months old, I do feel that there will be more time for improvement. RAG:kf

March 26, 1985:   Patient NOT Seen. LETTER TO DR. JONES. RAG:kf

October 8, 1985:   Jana Leigh is seen today for a six-month checkup. She has Erb's-Klumpke's palsy. The hand is being used more and more. She has lack of full extension of the long finger. She has a little clawing of the little finger or fifth finger, and she has slight adduction contracture of the thumb of her left hand. Her wrist extension is good. She does not have good triceps function, for when she falls, the elbow buckles. She can flex the elbow well but she cannot extend it. She walks with the elbow postured in slight flexion. She has no abduction of the shoulder.

She is improving and she continues to improve.

I will try to research the possibility of exploration of the brachial plexus to see what we can do.

As far as I can tell, the fifth nerve root is out and perhaps the seventh or eighth nerve root is out or weak. This may be a cervical avulsion rather than a brachial plexus injury.

April 16, 1986:   The Herrells were here today. I am not recommending surgery for the brachial plexus just yet. The EMG study was done showing giant motor unit potentials consistent with healing or reinnervation of damaged nerves. This was done by Dr. Jones. I'll discuss the case with Dr. Jones. RAG:kf

IV. LIABILITY

Practice Note. Under this section, we provided ACOG (American College of Obstetrics and Gynecology) documents chronicling Dr. Weber's unsuccessful history before the American Board of Obstetrics and Gynecology. We were able to obtain Dr. Weber's board history through requests for production served on counsel for the defendant hospital. That board history contained the following documents:

A. Dr. Bud Weber's Board History

1. ACOG Oral Examination Report of Board Action on 02/07/80. This two-page report is marked in bold black letters "FAIL," making it a perfect trial exhibit, as well as potent material for the written brochure. On the critique page, the board examiners wrote of Dr. Weber (among other criticisms), "Dr. Weber's criteria for cesarean section for failure to progress: 'I can just tell when they weren't making progress.' . . . very limited ability to interpret FHR [fetal heart monitor strips]."

Of course, in Jana Herrell's case, it was precisely this total lack of understanding of the criteria for cesarean section for failure to progress that led to Jana's brachial plexus injury.

ACOG Oral Examination Report of Board Action on 12/12/85. The 1985 report states: "[Dr. Weber] after reporting to the examiner's room, decided that he was not prepared to take the examination. After a conversation with Dr. Cavett he decided to leave without being examined."

This exhibit is obviously an insurance defense lawyer's nightmare – particularly the hospital's lawyer. Corporate responsibility requires, at a minimum, that the hospital restrict or place under supervision an obstetrician who is so unqualified to take his boards that he ducks out after taking the time and expense to travel to the examination site.

Note: This document is relevant on the issues of the hospital's knowledge of Dr. Weber's lack of knowledge and experience, although it is not relevant on the issues of Dr. Weber's negligence on the date in question.

ACOG Report of Board Action from 1981. This report says simply, although eloquently, "No Show."

Report of Obstetrical Expert, Vicki Hale, M.D. Dr. Hale, our obstetrical expert, appeared in the videotape presentation. We excerpted portions of Dr. Hale's interview in the written brochure. Dr. Hale discusses the negligence and liability of both Dr. Weber and the hospital.

B. Vicki Hale, M.D.

IN THE DISTRICT COURT OF TOLEDO COUNTY, OHIO
171ST JUDICIAL DISTRICT

NORMAN HERRELL and SANDRA HERRELL, Individually and as Next Friends of JANA HERRELL, a Minor,	* * * * *	
vs.	* *	No. 87-3440
BUD WEBER, M.D., BUD WEBER, M.D., P.A., and MERCY HOSPITAL.	* * *	

EXCERPTS FROM INTERVIEW WITH DR. VICKI HALE, EXPERT WITNESS

Date Taken: August 30, 1988

Interviewed by: Scott M. Lewis

SCOTT M. LEWIS: Doctor, let's turn our attention now to 1984. And Mrs. Herrell once again come under Dr. Weber's care; is that correct?

DR. VICKI HALE: Yes.

MR. LEWIS: Is he charged with the knowledge of what went on in the first pregnancy?

DR. HALE: Yes.

MR. LEWIS: Is he required, based upon this serious injury that occurred in 1981 to the child, is he required to keep that in mind and to act appropriately to prevent that from happening a second time around?

DR. HALE: Every minute he's dealing with it.

MR. LEWIS: And would a reasonably prudent physician have been on guard and kept a high index of suspicion for a macrosomic infant the second time around?

DR. HALE: That's an understatement. I think most reasonably prudent clinicians would be literally terrified of this happening again because you have to remember that this is one of the most terrifying things that can occur to the physician who is delivering the patient and only the head comes out.

MR. LEWIS: Let's look, Doctor, at Trial Exhibit No. 7 which is the labor progress chart from the 1984 delivery of Jana Herrell. Looking at that chart, is there anything that you can tell us in terms of the labor curve whether it's a normal or an abnormal curve?

CROSS EXAMINATION

DR. HALE: Well, this is not a normal curve. Here the patient is minus two when she comes in and she never gets past minus one. Ever. These curves never cross, not on this paper.

MR. LEWIS: For Dr. Weber not to have understood what was going on with this labor, for him not to have intervened to prevent this disaster, which you said was obviously coming. Is that an act of negligence?

DR. HALE: I think that that is a uniform word that's used, and so I would use it because it is a definable entity, but I don't think it's adequate. I just don't comprehend what was done here. I don't know anybody else who would do this sort of thing. Put a patient on the table as I say at minus one with a history that we've all discussed, et cetera, et cetera, and try to attempt a delivery.

MR. LEWIS: Is that an example of gross negligence in your experience and background?

DR. HALE: I think it's incompetent to – you know, that's where I would start.

MR. LEWIS: Do you place any responsibility on Paris hospital for what happened to Jana Herrell, in view of what you said about Dr. Weber's conduct of this labor?

DR. HALE: Obviously, this can't be his first act of incompetence. Such acts don't exist in a vacuum unless a physician for some reason is acutely, physically, mentally, and emotionally not himself on one particular occasion, then such patients as we see here are isolated. And, indeed, I know having been on a previous case of Dr. Weber's and seeing his testimony as taken in deposition regarding that case that Dr. Weber was involved in a number of cases and indeed the hospital had to have known that he was involved in a number of cases. And one would presume that prudence would dictate that they would have investigated in some way, shape or form something about those cases. I would have to also believe that unless the nurses were grossly negligent, they would have informed the chief of service that some negligent forms of behavior were occurring in a chronic manner on the delivery end.

MR. LEWIS: Doctor, we have discussed one of these exhibits which we will introduce at trial. This is a blowup of the oral examination results from Dr. Weber's attempt to pass the boards back in 1980. As you see, the result of that is F-A-I-L. Doctor, I want to ask you to look at page two of this board examination result and ask you to look at number one under weaknesses prescribed to Dr. Weber by the examiners. Will you read that for us, please?

DR. HALE: It says, "Number 1. Patient management. Criterion for cesarean section or failure to progress." This is something that they have discussed with him. His answer to that was simply, "I can just tell when they aren't making progress." That apparently was his answer to a question which they wanted described in detail.

MR. LEWIS: Doctor, as I understand in reading this document, the board examiners are criticizing Dr. Weber back in 1980 for not being able to understand how to deal with a failure to progress. Would that be correct?

DR. HALE: That's correct.

MR. LEWIS: And is that, in fact, exactly what happened in 1981 with the Herrell child and in 1984 with Jana Herrell?

DR. HALE: That's also correct.

MR. LEWIS: All right. So the weaknesses that they found in Dr. Weber went on to manifest themselves in his care of Mrs. Herrell and her children in this case?

DR. HALE: Unquestionably.

MR. LEWIS: Now, Doctor, if we could place ourselves in the position of the hospital and you on the medical staff of Mercy Hospital in 1984, would this information which is contained in the board documents of 1980, would this information be of interest to you in judging Dr. Weber's competence to be a member of the staff and to deliver babies?

DR. HALE: Unquestionably.

MR. LEWIS: And what would your judgment be if you were on the hospital credentials committee or the administration if you knew this information?

DR. HALE: I would either say that the gentleman couldn't practice at my hospital, or if he were allowed to practice, he would have to be under strict supervision.

MR. LEWIS: Do you feel, based upon your experience and training and specifically your experience on the medical staff of the hospital, that the hospital has some duty to investigate and discover information in a physician's board history?

DR. HALE: They certainly failed. They should, I think, have looked into it more closely to understand why. If they chose not to look into it to understand why, then they should have certainly not allowed him to practice either at all or by himself.

MR. LEWIS: If Mercy Hospital had in 1980 availed themselves with this information, which we obtained, and had acted upon it by terminating Dr. Weber's privileges or circumscribing them appropriately, do you believe based upon a reasonable medical probability that Jana Herrell would be a normal, healthy, and unimpaired child today?

DR. HALE: Without a doubt.

MR. LEWIS: Doctor, this is a blowup of the oral examination form from the American Board when Dr. Weber appeared in 1981 and apparently "no showed." Does that have any significance in terms of the present case?

DR. HALE: I believe that it does. Physicians who are preparing for the oral examinations, particularly a physician who has failed his first oral examination, I would have to believe would spend months preparing. In addition to this as you know they have to prepare their case records again to be sent in which takes a very long time, and I would have to believe that Dr. Weber would have spent a great deal of time to prepare and to be ready the second time. It has great professional significance and only an incredible catastrophe or an act of God would have kept the average practitioner from not showing, I believe, for a second oral examination. For Dr. Weber not to have shown for any reason other than the two that I've indicated, would have to indicate that for whatever reason he didn't consider this important enough or he simply felt too incompletely prepared and perhaps some fear of failure, had second thoughts and then didn't come.

MR. LEWIS: Let's look at a copy from the American Board of Obstetrics and Gynecology oral examination in December of 1985. What does that note indicate?

DR. HALE: Well, they say the third time is the charm. Dr. Weber apparently came in for the examination. He reported to the examiner. And when faced with his examiners, simply turned and left, saying suddenly that he just wasn't prepared. The doctor who apparently – it looks like a bow – Dr. Joseph Bowman here apparently conferred with one of his other physicians and decided to let him leave without being examined. This I think was an act of kindness because they truly could have simply considered him a failure. It was – not being prepared is exactly what they would have found on the oral examination. They just simply couldn't have handled it and he slipped away. This, however, simply is unfortunately what you would expect as an outcome from examining the case we've just examined, knowing that here is another case that I've had a chance to look at and beside that knowing from his depositions that there had been other cases and his attitudes that he takes. This is simply a proof in writing of what is evident of the small knowledge I have of him and obviously should have been evident to everybody he worked with including and obviously the hospital.

MR. LEWIS: Doctor, let's assume contrary to the actual fact in this case that Mercy had acted reasonably and had obtained Dr. Weber's board history beginning back in 1980 and knew that he had failed the examination in 1980 and knew about his other experiences before the board. Do you have any opinions to whether or not based upon that board history Mercy should have allowed Dr. Weber to practice obstetrics?

DR. HALE: I think based upon the board history of the failure in 1980, the specific comments made about the failure which we have already outlined, his subsequent decision not to show up for his next scheduled examination and then his abject withdrawal from his final examinations and that there was indeed no reason for him even to take it.

MR. LEWIS: Doctor, can you summarize your opinions with respect to the conduct of Dr. Weber and Mercy Hospital in this case?

DR. HALE: As far as Dr. Weber, he clearly had a responsibility to his patient. He did not in any way, shape or form that I can find meet any of his responsibilities. He showed to me no gram of real professional competence. There was a tiny glimmer when he decided to at least admit her one day previous to her EDC, but he had laid no ground work for that whatsoever really as far as what he ever intended to do because it turned out he never really had a plan. And finally by his lack of planning, his lack of being observant during her labor that she did not descend properly, then bring her in for forceful delivery from her minus one station with a very large baby clearly resulted in the direct damages to the child which will haunt that child and family for the rest of its life. As far as the hospital, I believe it has a duty to every patient that enters that hospital to have screened its physicians so that a patient can feel that if Dr. Weber practices in this hospital, the hospital must find him competent, it has reason to believe he is competent. It's a big institution, it's a big building. The patient sees this edifice and is impressed and thinks that there is some cerebration behind it, that it is not just a physical piece of architecture. It lives, it breathes and cares for the patients that go in. And the hospital indeed did have that duty. I don't believe that the hospital performed that duty and I think that we've adequately deleted that and we have without any doubt come to the conclusion that the lack of performance of that duty directly affected the outcome of this case, there would be no case if the duty had been followed and that duty in the case of the hospital could simply have been said if Dr. Weber was even allowed to practice there to say you must have someone look over your shoulder, someone to come in, check make sure everything is okay and that they agree with you. This case occurred in the middle of the day. The entire staff was available, everybody, so you can't say it was in the middle of the night. There really aren't any excuses.

MR. LEWIS: Doctor, is this a case on the part of Dr. Weber as well as Mercy Hospital, is this a case of simple negligence or is this a case of conscious indifference?

DR. HALE: I would say that it is a case of negligence compounded by a lack of ability on the part of the physician. And I think what appears to be indifference on his part, a lack of thoughtfulness, no thought if one can defined indifference as not bothering to think. The hospital—I just don't know why they did what they did and why they let it go as they have and had. It certainly could be interpreted as a thoughtful indifference because they had to have known. They just simply had to have known.

MR. LEWIS: If Dr. Weber and the people at Mercy had fulfilled their responsibility to our client, would in all medical probability Jana Herrell be a normal healthy and physically unimpaired child today?

DR. HALE: There's absolutely no question in my mind that this patient in other hands and in another hospital would have had a fine result and she would be a happy child today in a happy family and this is just an incredible travesty of what medicine is supposed to be.

C. Medical Literature

Practice Note. Under part C of the Liability section, the author provided excerpts from J. Pritchard, P. MacDonald & N. Gant, *Williams Obstetrics,* (1985) and other treatises.

D. JCAH Requirements

Practice Note. Under part D of the Liability section, we provided the insurance carrier with Standard I of the JCAH Accreditation Manual for Hospitals. Standard I imposes upon the hospital the responsibility to insure that only those physicians ". . . offering evidence that their training and/or experience, current competence, professional ethics . . . are adequate to assure the medical staff and governing body that any patient treated by them will receive optimal achievable quality of care . . ." are allowed to serve on staff. *JCAH Accreditation Manual for Hospitals* 197 (1984).

Practice Note. Clearly, while board certification is only a benchmark as a basis for privilege delineation (*JCAH Accreditation Manual for Hospitals* 198 (1984), repeated failure to achieve board certification should be a red flag to the hospital administration and credentials committee. When a physician, such as Dr. Weber, has failed to achieve certification, then successful clinical experience must be demonstrated and reflected in the privilege file. *Id.* In Dr. Weber's case, the hospital knew or should have known of Dr. Weber's clinical incompetence and his history of litigation, as well as his board failures.

V. DAMAGES

Practice Note. Under the Damages section, we included a summary of damages, with case citations supporting our claims for all items of damages. Also included under this section was a document titled "An Evaluation of Economic Damages," prepared by plaintiff's economic consultant and expert, Dr. Dillman. His summary of economic damages is excerpted in the materials that follow.

Portions of the videotape interview with Jana's subsequent treating orthopedic surgeon, Dr. Goodwin, were excerpted under the damages portion of the written brochure for the purpose of demonstrating the expert testimony plaintiffs would introduce at trial on the issue of Jana's serious and permanent physical and emotional injuries. Dr. Goodwin also comments on the mental anguish suffered by the parents as a result of having to observe and deal with Jana's palsy, her deformity, and her own emotional injuries.

CROSS EXAMINATION

A. Damages Summary

The following figures are based on present value and represent the minimum probable jury verdict on special issues which will be submitted at trial.

Impairment of future earning capacity for Jana Herrell (minimum)	$ 200,000
Impairment of household service	196,590
Past medical expense	17,678
Future medical expenses (minimum)	18,000
Future medical commodities (minimum)	5,000
Past, present and future pain and suffering for Jana Herrell	150,000
Past, present and future mental anguish for Jana Herrell	250,000
Permanent disfigurement of Jane Herrell	250,000
Past, present and future mental anguish for Norman and Sandra Herrell	200,000
Exemplary damages against Dr. Weber	200,000
Exemplary damages against Mercy Hospital	200,000
Total (potential jury verdict)	$1,687,268
Settlement demand to Bud Weber, M.D., and Mercy Hospital	$1,000,000

Impairment of Future Earning Capacity for Jana Herrell. In Texas it is clearly established that the measure of damages, where the injured person is a child, is the loss of earning capacity, and not actual wages lost. *Greyhound Lines, Inc. v. Craig,* 430 S.W.2d 573 (Tex. Civ. App. 1968).

Dr. Dillman will testify that Jana has suffered a substantial impairment of her future earning capacity. He will testify that the present value of her future earning capacity is $1,840,040.

Impairment of Household Services. Loss of household services for a housewife is firmly established as an element of recovery in a personal injury suit. *Hicks Maintenance v. Vanlandingham,* 444 S.W.2d 663 (Tex. Civ. App. 1969). The following areas of endeavor are to be considered by the jury in awarding damages for impaired household services:

Chauffeur
Cook
Dietitian
Dishwasher
Food buyer

Gardener
Housekeeper
Laundress
Maintenance worker
Child care
Practical nurse
Seamstress

Dr. Dillman and Dr. Goodwin will testify that a functionally one-armed person such as Jana Herrell will be unable to perform most of those duties enumerated above and will have extreme difficulty in performing the others.

Past Medical Expenses. Jana Herrell's medical expenses, for which her parents Norman and Sandra are responsible, total approximately $20,000. Copies of all medical expenses incurred to date will be provided counsel.

Future Medical Expenses. Dr. Dillman has provided us with a report indicating that the present value of future medical services over Jana's lifetime would be $126,270. Dr. Dillman has evaluated the costs of future medical commodities to be approximately $42,478.

Plaintiffs' submit that the costs of Jana's future medical expenses, including surgery, therapy, and other modalities of treatment, would have a minimum reasonable value of $25,000.

Physical Pain and Suffering of Jana Herrell. Physical pain and suffering is a distinct element of recovery for mental anguish based upon physical pain or injury. *Leyndecker v. Harlow,* 189 S.W.2d, 706 (Tex. Civ. App. 1945).

Mental Anguish of Jana Herrell. Mental anguish is a proper element of damages in a personal injury suit. It is more than a mere disappointment, anger, resentment or embarrassment . . . It includes a mental sensation of pain, resulting from such painful emotions as grief, severe disappointment, indignation, wounded pride, shame, despair and/or public humiliation.

Permanent Disfigurement of Jana Herrell. When, as a result of the defendants' wrongful acts the plaintiff has suffered unsightly changes in her physical appearance, she may recover damages for disfigurement as an element separate and distinct from damages for pain and suffering or mental anguish. *Houston Transit Co. v. Felder* 208 S.W.2d 880 (Tex. 1948).

Mental Anguish of Norman and Sandra Herrell. A person other than the victim of a tort may receive damages for past, present and future mental anguish as a bystander who witnesses the injury of a close relative. *Jannette v. Deprez,* 701 S.W.2d 56 (Tex. Ct. App. 1985).

CROSS EXAMINATION

B. Report of Robert Goodwin, M.D.

Practice Note. The following excerpts from our videotape brochure were placed in the Damages section of our written brochure for the purpose of previewing the trial testimony of Jana's subsequent treating orthopedic surgeon. Dr. Goodwin's testimony addresses Jana's physical injuries as well as the emotional components of her deformity. Note, also, that plaintiff's expert addresses the parents' injuries.

SCOTT M. LEWIS: I would like to ask you a few questions about the videotape.

DR. ROBERT GOODWIN: Yes.

MR. LEWIS: You saw that Jana was unable to abduct her arm. Is this the same condition that she's had all along?

DR. GOODWIN: Yes, sir. And for qualification of abduct, that means elevate the arm.

MR. LEWIS: In all probability, will she always have that trouble with her arm?

DR. GOODWIN: Yes, sir. Something more important I think than hair care is dressing, Jana cannot lift her arm to put it through a sleeve of a blouse, a sundress, or any other form of a coat. And so she's always going to have to learn to slip her arm through the sleeve and then with her right arm pull it up over, get into it with her right arm and then bring it in front of her.

There's another thing that I noticed that has been brought out in the physical findings that I have exhibited in my notes is that she can't flex the elbow this way because of weakness of the biceps muscle. So any activity that requires bringing something from down below her waist level up in front of her even though no abduction is necessary, but bringing something from the table and bringing it up to here is going to be impaired.

MR. LEWIS: Okay. And she has a shortness of the left arm. Can you explain that?

DR. GOODWIN: All palsied extremities grow at a different rate than the normal extremities; therefore, bone length is compromised as well as muscular circumference compromised. This just simply reflects that nerve function also dominates growth function, too; and if nerve function is impaired, then there will be a growth function impairment also. This will extend until she is skeletal mature, age 15 or 16, then the growth problem will not be a matter to be dealt with.

I can't give you an estimate of how short she will ultimately be but in my experience with other Erb's palsied afflicted children there can be as much as three inches of shortening of the limb by the time of skeletal maturity.

MR. LEWIS: And skeletal maturity arrives at about age 15 or 16. Is that correct?

DR. GOODWIN: For women.

MR. LEWIS: For women. So she's always going to have a short arm and it may in fact be shorter than it is now in comparison to the right arm?

DR. GOODWIN: That's possible.

MR. LEWIS: Now, we saw that Jana had difficulty, in fact, couldn't pick up a ball and couldn't pick up other articles. Is that something that will ever get any better in your opinion?

DR. GOODWIN: No. She'll learn to compensate more and more with use of the right upper extremity, but the limited use of the left upper extremity has reached its maximum improvement.

MR. LEWIS: Doctor, in your experience with patients who have Erb's palsy, Klumpke's palsy, is there an emotional component that goes with these children?

DR. GOODWIN: Yes, sir.

MR. LEWIS: Can you tell us what that is, sir?

DR. GOODWIN: Well, as Jana gets along in years, particularly preteen and teen years, her difference from other children will be a factor. It will be not only noticeable to Jana but to other children. The preteen years are particularly cruel years. The teen years are more understanding years. In fact, in the teen years any individual, high school or junior high, who has a disability or an affliction and perseveres is usually well-respected by their peers. But the preteen years and the elementary grades can be particularly cruel ones and can have an emotional impact. There will be an impact upon her emotional stability as well as the family stability and that has already shown that it has had an impact upon the family emotions dealing with this problem.

MR. LEWIS: In what way, sir.?

DR. GOODWIN: I think that the mother and father for a long time if I might say and be–I don't want to encroach upon their emotions but if I might say they may have had some very difficult times dealing with the fact that I tried to be kind and yet explicit that Jana had a problem that I didn't feel would completely resolve after about 12 months or 18 months. That was difficult for them to deal with and to accept and there was a lot of denial at first. I think now as time passes they are dealing with that. The denial is being less of a factor and acceptance is becoming more positive for them.

TABLE OF CASES

CASES

Case	*Book §*
Brock v. Merrell Dow Pharmaceuticals, 874 F.2d 307 (5th Cir. 1989)	§§ 8.5, 17.1
Bubendey v. Winthrop Univ. Hosp., 151 A.D.2d 713, 543 N.Y.S.2d 146 (1989)	§§ 6.7, 11.15
Bulala v. Boyd, 239 Va. 218, 389 S.E.2d 670 (1990)	§§ 3.3, 4.18, 6.8, 7.11
Burke v. Rivo, 406 Mass. 764, 551 N.E.2d 1 (1990)	§§ 6.2, 8.2, 8.7
Butler v. Rolling Hill Hosp., 382 Pa. Super. 317, 555 A.2d 205 (1989)	§ 8.7
Buzniak v. County of Westchester, 156 A.D.2d 631, 549 N.Y.S.2d 130 (1989)	§ 6.7
Byrd v. Wesley Medical Center, 237 Kan. 215, 699 P.2d 459 (1985)	§§ 6.5, 8.7
Cadarian v. Merrell Dow Pharmaceuticals, Inc., 745 F. Supp. 409 (E.D. Mich. 1989)	§§ 5.1, 8.5, 17.1
Campbell v. Pitt County Memorial Hosp., No. 86390558 (N.C. Ct. App. Feb. 17, 1987)	§ 21.18
Carson v. Muru, 424 F.2d 825 (N.H. 1980)	§ 6.14
Castrigano v. E.R. Squibb & Sons, 546 A.2d 775 (R.I. 1988)	§ 8.5
Coleman v. Atlanta Obstetrics & Gynecology Group, P.A., 194 Ga. App. 508, 390 S.E.2d 856 (1990)	§§ 2.7, 4.4
Continental Casualty Co. v. Empire Casualty Co., 713 P.2d 384 (Colo. 1986)	§§ 8.7, 29.11
Corley v. Commonwealth Edison Co., 703 F. Supp. 748 (N.D. Ill. 1989)	§ 9.8
Cosgrove v. Merrell Dow Pharmaceuticals, Inc., 117 Idaho 470, 788 P.2d 1293 (1989)	§§ 7.2, 8.5, 17.1
Coughling v. George Wash. Univ. Health Plan, Inc., 565 A.2d 67 (D.C. 1989)	§§ 9.6, 14.9
Cowe v. Forum Group, 541 N.E.2d 962 (Ind. Ct. App. 1989)	§ 8.9
Crumbley v. Wyant, 188 Ga. App. 227, 372 S.E.2d 497 (1988)	§ 14.4
C.S. v. Nielson, 767 P.2d 504 (Utah 1988)	§§ 6.2, 8.7
Dalley v. Utah Valley Regional Medical Center, 791 P.2d 193 (Utah 1990)	§§ 3.3, 4.17
D'Angelis v. Zakuto, 383 Pa. Super. 65, 556 A.2d 431 (1989)	§ 4.9
Daubert v. Merrell Dow Pharmaceuticals, Inc., 727 F. Supp. 570 (S.D. Cal. 1989)	§§ 5.1, 8.5, 17.1
Denham v. Burlington N. R.R., 699 F. Supp. 1253 (N.D. Ill. 1988)	§ 6.6
Denny v. United States, 1971 F.2d 365 (5th Cir. 1948), *cert. denied*, 337 U.S. 919 (1949)	§ 2.10
Dohn v. Lovell, 187 Ga. App. 523, 370 S.E.2d 789 (1988)	§ 8.2
Douzart v. Jones, 528 So. 2d 602 (La. Ct. App. 1988)	§§ 4.5, 22.3
Dunne v. Somoano, 550 So. 2d 5 (Fla. Dist. Ct. App. 1989)	§§ 5.1, 11.17, 21.8
Enright v. Eli Lilly & Co., 141 Misc. 2d 194, 533 N.Y.S.2d 224 (Sup. Ct. 1988)	§§ 6.7, 8.5

CASES

INDEX

INDEX

ISBN 0-471-54059-5